U.S. COAST GUARD
FAMILY HEALTH CARE GUIDE

The Office of Health and Safety provides you with this family medical guide to help you evaluate and understand many common medical conditions. By becoming familiar with the information in this book, you can reduce the anxiety and uncertainty that often surround illness and injury. We hope this guide becomes a valuable home resource for you and your family.

You can use the guide to:
* Identify and treat minor conditions that do not require professional medical attention;
* Identify important signs and symptoms requiring prompt or immediate professional medical attention;
* Help you treat medical emergencies until professional help arrives.

* *

For health benefits information, including advice on obtaining health care from Coast Guard, Department of Defense, or civilian professionals, call your local Health Benefits Advisor (HBA). The telephone number is available from your local Coast Guard unit.

MY LOCAL HBA NUMBER IS:

_____

If you cannot reach your local HBA, if you require additional information, or if you have other concerns, call the Coast Guard's nationwide Health Benefits Hot Line at 1-800-9-HBA-HBA.

* *

This *AMA Guide to Your Family's Symptoms* and the HBA program are part of the Coast Guard's commitment to continually improve your access to quality health care. We want to increase the availability of accurate medical information so you and your family can make better health care decisions. Your continued good health, safety, and well-being are the Commandant's top priority.

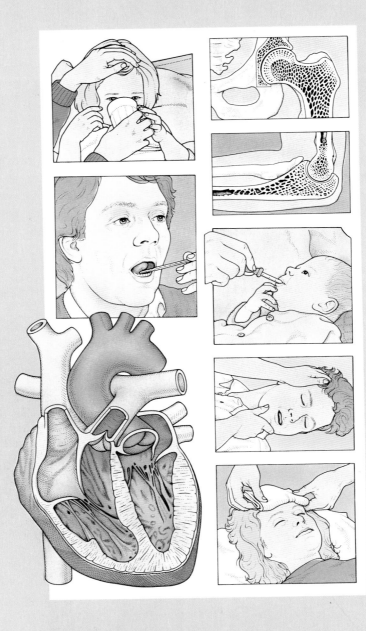

THE AMERICAN MEDICAL ASSOCIATION

GUIDE TO YOUR FAMILY'S SYMPTOMS

(formerly titled *The AMA Home Medical Adviser*)

Medical Editors Charles B. Clayman, MD
Raymond H. Curry, MD

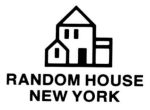

**RANDOM HOUSE
NEW YORK**

The American Medical Association Guide to Your Family's Symptoms was conceived, written, and designed by Dorling Kindersley Limited, in association with the American Medical Association.

American Medical Association

Executive Vice President	James S. Todd, MD
Vice President, Corporate and Consumer Affairs	Steven V. Seekins
Publisher, Consumer Books Division	Heidi Hough

Editorial Staff

Medical Editors	Charles B. Clayman, MD Raymond H. Curry, MD
Managing Editor	Dorothea Guthrie
Senior Editor	Lori A. Burnette
Editor	Robin Fitzpatrick Husayko

Consultants

Byron J. Bailey, MD
Bruce M. Berkson, MD
Frederick C. Blodi, MD
Philip D. Darney, MD
Richard N. Foltz, MD
Norman Fost, MD
Richard Goldberg, MD
Ian D. Hay, MD, PhD
Nicholas C. Hightower, Jr., MD
Linda Hughey Holt, MD

Jeffrey R. M. Kunz, MD
Burton J. Kushner, MD
Dennis Maki, MD
Harriet S. Meyer, MD
Ronald M. Meyer, MD
Brian O'Leary, MD
Sylvia Peterson
Domeena C. Renshaw, MD
Carlotta M. Rinke, MD
Joseph H. Skom, MD

Philip D. Shenefelt, MD
Alfred Soffer, MD
Thomas N. Thies, DDS
Howard Traisman, MD
David T. Uehling, MD
Maurice W. Van Allen, MD
William J. Weigel, MD
Jody W. Zylke, MD
American Dental Association

Dorling Kindersley Editorial Staff

Medical Editor: Dr. A. J. Smith; *Medical Consultants:* Dr. H. B. Valman, Dr. T. J. L. Richards, Dr. S. M. M. Kinder; *Project Editor:* Cathy Meeus; *Art Editor:* Dinah Lone; *Editorial Director:* Amy Carroll

Library of Congress Cataloging-in-Publication Data

The American Medical Association guide to your family's symptoms / American Medical Association. — 1st updated pbk. ed.
p.   cm.
Rev. ed. of: The American Medical Association home medical adviser.
1st American ed. © 1988.
Includes index.
ISBN 0-679-74128-3 (tr. pap.)
1. Medicine, Popular.
2. Symptomatology—Popular works.
I. American Medical Association.
II. American Medical Association
home medical adviser.
RC81.A5434   1992   91-51014
Manufactured in the United States of America
2 4 6 8 9 7 5 3
First Updated Paperback Edition

Preface

For most people, most of the time, that miraculous machine we call the human body functions with remarkable reliability. It does, however, require maintenance and occasional repair.

When symptoms appear—when your body sends out signals that something is wrong—the trouble may be only a minor illness. It may be a cold or some other self-limiting ailment from which you will recover with or without medical intervention.

But minor symptoms, sometimes even a headache or a cough, can also be the first warning of a more serious problem. The symptom charts in this book are designed to help you interpret body signals more accurately, allowing you to distinguish between what may be a minor problem and what may require professional medical attention. These charts will also help you decide how long you, as a concerned but sensible person, should wait before seeking medical help.

This book is not intended to teach you medical diagnosis; no book can do that. Only your doctor can definitively diagnose and treat most illnesses. But this book can give you a more informed understanding of your symptoms and provide medically approved answers to everyday questions. In addition, this volume includes illustrated sections on first aid and emergency treatment.

The self-help symptom charts in this book were developed under medical supervision, tested on patients, and reviewed by American medical authorities. We are pleased to add *The AMA Guide to Your Family's Symptoms* to the American Medical Association's Home Health Library.

James S. Todd, MD
Executive Vice President
American Medical Association

Contents

The human body

The symptom charts

Useful information

1 Children's charts
page 49

2 General medical: men and women
page 145

3 Special problems: men
page 233

4 Special problems: women
page 249

How to use this book

The American Medical Association Guide to Your Family's Symptoms has been designed as a ready reference to enable the reader not only to understand how his or her body works, but to determine whether something has gone wrong and what to do about it. Information is divided among three major sections—The human body, The symptom charts, and Useful information.

The human body

The first section of the book looks at the human body, beginning with conception and fetal growth and a child's developing systems and skills, on through to the adult body, both male and female. In addition to infant growth, the developmental milestones—intellectual, physical, social, and emotional—experienced by all children are presented in pictures and charts.

Each of the adult body's major systems—such as the circulatory, respiratory, or reproductive system—is illustrated to show how it works. Special symptoms boxes point out a few of the things that could go wrong and list the charts that deal with those problems. Here, too, you will find a discussion of what happens in pregnancy and how to safeguard your own and your family's health, including advice on fitness, diet, exercise, and avoiding bad health habits.

The symptom charts

At the core of the book are 147 charts that concentrate on the most common symptoms experienced by men, women, and children. Each chart deals with a specific symptom and then explores some of the possible diagnoses. Finding the probable cause is simply a matter of answering YES or NO to questions. You will then be advised on what to do next—for instance, consult your doctor without delay. All you need to know about these charts is found on page 38—How to use the charts.

For convenience, children's symptoms are confined to 53 special children's charts. Because symptoms may have different causes at different ages, they are divided among Babies under one, Children: All ages, and Adolescents.

Charts for men and women are also broken down into different sections. Sixty charts cover general medical problems of men and women; 10 charts cover special problems of men; and 24 charts concern special problems of women (including problems of pregnancy and childbirth).

There are three ways to find the chart you need—whether it's from the children's, general medical, or special problems sections. Pain-site maps, system-by-system chartfinders, and chart indexes are individually presented for men, women, and children. Refer to pages 40–48.

Useful information

The third section contains information that will help you deal with illness or injury at home and record useful personal medical data. Essential first aid, home health care, and a medications guide are illustrated, as are growth and height and weight charts, and a complete set of family medical records. Finally, there is room to list emergency telephone numbers so they'll always be at hand.

The human body

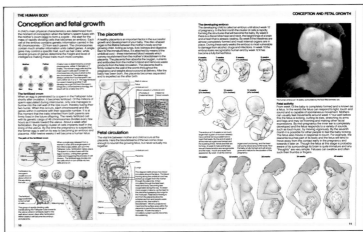

The symptom charts

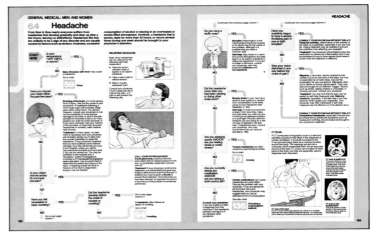

Useful information

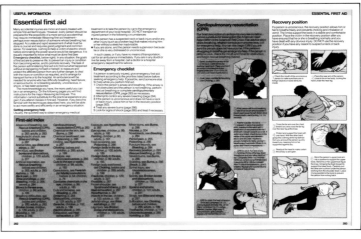

The human body

Conception and fetal growth

A child's main physical characteristics are determined from the moment of conception when the man's sperm fertilizes the woman's ovum (egg) to form a zygote – the start for the mass of rapidly dividing cells that becomes an embryo. Each cell of the embryo contains genetic information carried in the 46 chromosomes – 23 from each partner. The chromosomes contain much smaller information units called genes. A single gene may control a specific trait, such as hair color, while several groups of genes determine height and potential level of intelligence.

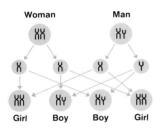

Woman **Man**

Girl **Boy** **Boy** **Girl**

A baby's sex is determined by a single chromosome, either X (female) or Y (male). The woman's egg cells and the man's sperm cells each contain 23 chromosomes, one of which is the sex chromosome. The mature egg always carries the X but the sperm can carry either an X or a Y. The egg fertilized by a sperm bearing another X will develop into a girl (XX), but if the sperm brings the Y chromosome to the egg, the result will be a boy (XY).

The fertilized ovum

When an egg is penetrated by a sperm in the fallopian tube shortly after ovulation, it becomes fertilized. Of the millions of sperm ejaculated during intercourse, only one has managed to burrow into the cell wall of the ripe ovum, thereby fusing the nuclei of the egg and sperm. When this occurs, the 23 chromosomes contained in the egg combine with the 23 chromosomes contained in the sperm. It is at this moment that the traits inherited from both parents are firmly fixed in the future offspring. The newly fertilized cell with its genetic cargo of 46 chromosomes divides every few hours as it travels toward the uterus. About a week after fertilization, the growing cluster of cells implants itself in the lining of the uterus.

The path of the fertilized ovum

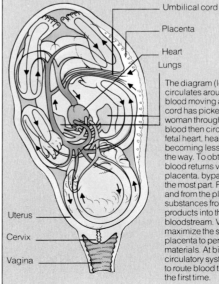

Fallopian tubes
Ovaries
Uterus
Vagina
Cervix

When a single egg released from a woman's ovary and a single sperm of the millions ejaculated join in the fallopian tube, fertilization takes place. The sperm's nucleus fuses with the egg's nucleus, uniting their genetic matter and triggering the process of cell division. The fertilized egg divides into two cells, each of which in turn divides into two cells, and so on.

Fertilization by one sperm usually occurs about a third of the way along the tube.

The fertilized egg subdivides to form a cluster of cells.

Maturing egg

This group of rapidly dividing cells travels along the fallopian tube toward the uterus, where it embeds itself in the wall about 7 days after fertilization. Within weeks it will become the embryo and placenta.

The placenta

The placenta is an important factor in the successful growth and development of your baby. This disc-shaped organ is the lifeline between the woman's body and her growing child. The placenta is connected to the fetus by the umbilical cord, which is composed of three intertwined blood vessels. The placenta serves as lungs, kidneys, and digestive tract for the fetus, absorbing the oxygen, nutrients, and antibodies from the woman's blood and removing waste products from the fetal circulation. The placenta is firmly rooted to the wall of the uterus throughout pregnancy and weighs about a pound at delivery. After the baby has been born, the placenta becomes separated and is expelled as the afterbirth.

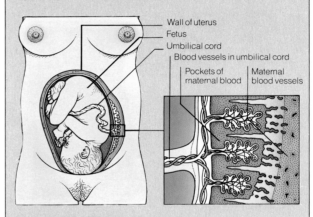

Wall of uterus
Fetus
Umbilical cord
Blood vessels in umbilical cord
Pockets of maternal blood
Maternal blood vessels

Fetal circulation

The vital link between the woman and the fetus occurs at the placenta. Here the bloodstreams of the two come close enough to nourish the growing fetus, but never actually mix together.

Umbilical cord
Placenta
Heart
Lungs
Uterus
Cervix
Vagina

The diagram (left) shows how blood circulates around the fetus. The blood moving along the umbilical cord has picked up oxygen from the woman through the placenta. The blood then circulates through the fetal heart, head, and body, becoming less oxygenated along the way. To obtain more oxygen, the blood returns via the heart to the placenta, bypassing the lungs for the most part. Fetal blood flowing to and from the placenta absorbs substances from and expels waste products into the woman's bloodstream. Villi (tiny projections) maximize the surface area within the placenta to permit the exchange of materials. At birth, the baby's circulatory system abruptly changes to route blood through the lungs for the first time.

From embryo to fetus

The developing fertilized egg is called an embryo until about the 12th week of pregnancy. In the first month the cluster of cells grows rapidly. By week 6 there is a discernible head and neck, the beginnings of a brain, and a heart that is beating. By week 8 most of the internal organs have formed. During these early weeks the embryo is most vulnerable to damage from alcohol and other drugs and from infections. In week 10 the embryo looks human and by the end of week 12, when all major organs are functioning, it is a fully formed fetus.

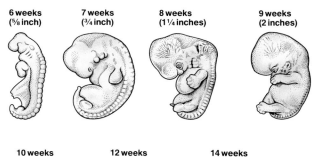

6 weeks
(⅝ inch)

7 weeks
(¾ inch)

8 weeks
(1¼ inches)

9 weeks
(2 inches)

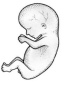

10 weeks
(2½ inches)

12 weeks
(3½ inches)

14 weeks
(4⅘ inches)

The embryo at 5 to 6 weeks is not much larger than a grain of rice but has a central nervous system and a heart that beats. By the end of week 8 all the internal organs are formed and the budding limbs, hands, and feet are forming. At week 9 male and female sexual characteristics are recognizable and the nose, mouth, and eyes have appeared. By the end of week 12 all the internal organs are functioning, and the heart can pump blood around the body.

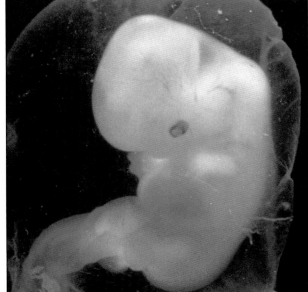

The human embryo at 7 to 8 weeks, surrounded by the fluid-filled amniotic sac.

Fetal activity

From the end of week 12 the fetus is completely formed. In the uterus the fetus can respond to light, touch, and sound and is capable of spontaneous movement. Pregnant women can usually feel movements around week 17, but well before this time the fetus is kicking, curling its toes, stretching its arms and legs, and may be smiling and making other facial expressions. By mid-pregnancy the inner ear is completely developed and the fetus responds to a variety of sounds, such as loud music, by moving vigorously. By the seventh month it is possible for other people to feel the fetus kicking. The fetus also moves in response to touch. For example, if the placenta touches part of its body, the fetus tends to move away from this contact early in the pregnancy and toward it in the later stages of pregnancy.

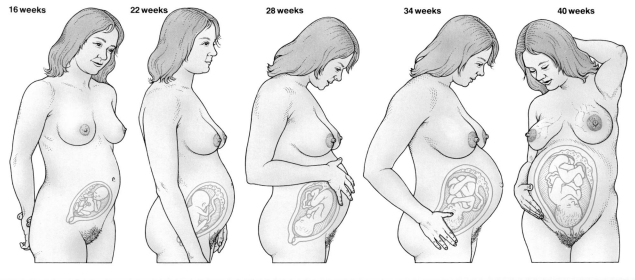

16 weeks　　**22 weeks**　　**28 weeks**　　**34 weeks**　　**40 weeks**

The newborn baby

At birth the placenta stops supplying the baby with oxygen and food and stops taking away waste products. A baby is born with certain instincts and reflexes that help him or her survive the first few days of life. For example, during breast-feeding, a baby will reflexively attach to the mother's nipple and suck, and a baby's bladder empties automatically. A small or premature baby may require special treatment at birth because some of the body's systems, particularly the respiratory system, may be immature. A premature baby may have difficulty breathing, feeding, and maintaining his or her body temperature. In an incubator the baby can be carefully monitored and protected from infection until the baby's body systems become more fully developed.

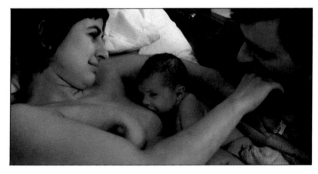

The appearance of the newborn

The newborn baby, with its oddly proportioned body and blotchy skin, may look very different from the perfect little bundle his or her parents had imagined.

The head
The head of the newborn baby may seem far too large and heavy for his or her tiny body. At birth the head is a quarter the size of the trunk, by 2 years it is a fifth, and in the 18th year only an eighth. A newborn rarely has a perfectly round head. Pressure on the head and the movement of the bones in the skull to protect the brain during birth commonly lead to temporary changes in the shape of the head.

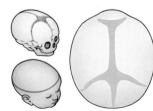

The fontanelles
At birth, the skull bones are made up of areas of cartilage with soft areas between them. The larger of these soft spots—which are areas of thick membrane—are known as the fontanelles. A baby has two main fontanelles, one at the front and one at the back of the head. During birth the areas of cartilage interlock, protecting the brain from damage.

The eyes
Red, puffy eyes are common among newborns because of the tremendous pressure exerted on the head during birth. This swelling diminishes within a few days. Many babies appear to be squinting because of the folds of skin at the inner corners of the eyes. These are normal and usually become less noticeable a week after birth. If your baby is still squinting after 1 month, consult your pediatrician.

The mouth
Blisters may appear on the newborn's upper lip or in the mouth at any time while the baby is nursing. These are harmless and will eventually disappear. The tongue of the new baby grows from the tip during the first year, so that it appears to be more firmly anchored than an adult's tongue. By the first birthday the tongue is fully mobile.

The skin
The newborn's skin is rarely perfect. Red or blue patches, jaundice, and small white spots are common. A baby who has been undernourished in the uterus or a baby of an exceptionally long pregnancy is likely to have wrinkled skin. The skin usually clears up by the end of the first month.
Vernix: At birth the baby is covered with a white, greasy substance called the vernix. This is a natural protection against minor skin infections and is washed off the baby after birth.
Lanugo hair: At birth parts of the baby's body are often covered with hair, called lanugo hair. This may be a soft fuzz on the head or a very coarse layer over the shoulders and down the back. The lanugo hair is normal and usually rubs off after 1 to 2 weeks.

Other skin conditions occur in some newborn babies and not in others.
Peeling skin: Some babies are born with a dry, peeling skin on the palms or soles of the feet. This is not eczema and disappears in a few days.
Cradle cap: Some babies have patches of thick, yellow scales over their scalps. Daily shampooing and treatment with petroleum jelly, baby oil, or mild ointment containing salicylic acid (a softening agent) will remove cradle cap.
Variable skin tone: The newborn's hands and/or feet may appear bluish and at times the upper half of the baby's body may be paler than the lower half. This is due to immaturity of the circulation and goes away as the baby's circulatory system matures.
Blue patches: Sometimes called "mongolian spots," these look like bruises, but in fact are patches of pigment beneath the skin. They are harmless, but usually permanent, and are more common in babies with dark skin tones.
Birthmarks: Most red marks on the baby's skin are caused by pressure exerted during birth and will fade away naturally. Sometimes small red streaks on the eyelids, forehead, and nape of the neck are caused by enlarged blood vessels near the surface of the skin. These red marks also will fade. Ask your doctor about any large or unusual birthmark.
Skin eruptions: Some babies develop a rash that is red and blotchy with small white spots. The condition usually lasts only a few days and disappears without treatment.
Spots: New babies get all sorts of spots, most of which form because the newborn's skin and pores do not yet function efficiently. Red spots with yellow centers and white spots across the nose should never be squeezed. They will disappear after a few days.

Sexual characteristics
A slight swelling of the breasts in babies of both sexes is completely normal. Swelling may occur in the first few days after birth and is caused by the flood of hormones from the mother, which may affect the baby as well. The baby's breasts may even have a tiny amount of milk in them, which should be left alone because of the risk of infection. The swelling will go down in a few days. The genitals of both boys and girls at birth are larger in proportion to the rest of their bodies than at any other stage in their development. The presence of maternal hormones may cause a little extra swelling in the first days after birth and the vulva or scrotum may also look red or inflamed. The swelling and inflammation subside as soon as the baby's body rids itself of excess hormones from the mother.

The umbilical cord

The umbilical cord, which has served as the fetus's lifeline throughout its time in the uterus, is painlessly cut after the placenta has been delivered. The cord is first tied and then cut, leaving 3 or 4 inches of stump attached to the baby. The stump shrivels and drops away within 10 days or so. Sometimes the baby develops a small bulge near the navel, called an umbilical hernia. Though it may protrude more when the baby cries, it is not a cause for concern and usually disappears within the first 4 years of life.

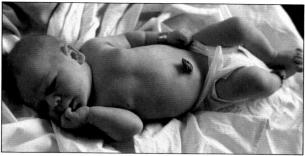

Tests on the newborn

The following tests are performed on the newborn in order to detect any defects. The chances of curing defects are much greater if problems are detected at birth.

- Backbone—checked for a swelling or ulcer, which may indicate spina bifida
- Navel—checked for a swelling typical of an umbilical hernia
- Face and mouth—checked for cleft lip and palate
- Face and hands—checked for features of Down's syndrome: upward slanting eyes, puffy eyelids, and abnormal palm creases
- Anus—checked for imperforate (closed) anus
- Feet—checked for clubfoot
- Hips—checked for dislocation of the hip
- Eyes—checked for discharge and physical defects

Blood tests on the newborn

Tests for phenylketonuria (a metabolic disease) and thyroid hormone deficiency—both preventable causes of mental retardation—are usually done within 1 week of birth. The phenylketonuria test may be repeated at 1 month. Additional blood tests may be performed to check the level of the chemical bilirubin in the body if the baby is jaundiced, or to check for any familial biochemical disorder.

Reflexes and movements

Every newborn comes into the world with an instinctive set of reflexes intended to protect and sustain life. A baby whose breathing is blocked will struggle to clear his or her nose and mouth. Voluntary movements become obvious at about 3 months.

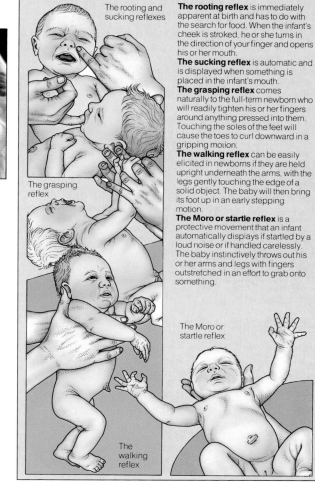

The rooting and sucking reflexes

The grasping reflex

The walking reflex

The Moro or startle reflex

The rooting reflex is immediately apparent at birth and has to do with the search for food. When the infant's cheek is stroked, he or she turns in the direction of your finger and opens his or her mouth.

The sucking reflex is automatic and is displayed when something is placed in the infant's mouth.

The grasping reflex comes naturally to the full-term newborn who will readily tighten his or her fingers around anything pressed into them. Touching the soles of the feet will cause the toes to curl downward in a gripping motion.

The walking reflex can be easily elicited in newborns if they are held upright underneath the arms, with the legs gently touching the edge of a solid object. The baby will then bring its foot up in an early stepping motion.

The Moro or startle reflex is a protective movement that an infant automatically displays if startled by a loud noise or if handled carelessly. The baby instinctively throws out his or her arms and legs with fingers outstretched in an effort to grab onto something.

The Apgar score

At birth, five simple tests are carried out to assess the general well-being (particularly the breathing) of a newborn baby. A score between 0 and 2 is given for each of the following physical signs and the total is known as the Apgar score. A score of 4 or less indicates severe breathing difficulties (asphyxia). Most babies score between 7 and 10. The test is performed once and repeated after 5 minutes, by which time the score has usually improved.

What is tested	Points given		
	2	1	0
Color	Pink all over (white babies) or pink lips and palms (nonwhite babies)	Blue extremities	Blue all over
Breathing	Regular	Irregular	Absent
Heart rate	More than 100 beats a minute	Less than 100 beats a minute	Absent
Movement	Active	Some movement	Little or no movement
Reflex response	Cries	Whimpers	Absent

The growing child

At the moment of conception, one complete cell is formed; this cell contains the genetic information—passed on or inherited from each parent—that determines not only the sex of the new child, but also many of his or her specific characteristics. Different genes define physical traits, such as height, build, and skin type, and the rate at which a child develops. Therefore, a child whose parents were relatively late in walking, speaking, or reaching puberty is likely to follow a similar pattern of development. Physiological traits are also genetically determined—a child may inherit a susceptibility to certain diseases. The effects of inherited physiological traits, however, can be modified. For example, if a child has a susceptibility to ear infections, prompt treatment each time the symptoms occur should ensure against any permanent damage. Poor or healthy teeth are inherited; parents can safeguard the teeth of the young child by having him or her brush with a toothpaste containing fluoride. (See *Toothache,* chart 36.)

A growing body requires both nutrients and exercise. A child who eats a well-balanced diet (see *Eating a healthy diet,* page 34, and *The components of a healthy diet,* page 119), and regularly plays or participates in sports (see *Getting enough exercise,* page 34) will usually develop normally and establish a basis for long-term good health.

Emotional development

From birth a child has individual needs that, in infancy, reflect themselves in the baby's feeding and sleeping patterns. The infant is entirely dependent on the parents for all his or her physical and emotional needs. Gradually this dependence lessens as children become more able to do things for themselves and begin to make friends. The environment in which a child grows plays a vital part in this development. A child is usually able to adjust to changing needs and demands (for example, at school) with relative ease if the home environment is loving and secure.

As a child develops certain skills (see *Milestones,* page 17), his or her personality begins to be revealed. For example, between the 1st and 3rd years, children are often hard to handle as they practice and build on newly found skills (see *The terrible twos,* page 88).

Some children are constantly physically and emotionally restless, and are known as hyperactive—a type of behavior that is at one end of the spectrum of "normal" development. Such children demand a great deal of patience and understanding and, occasionally, help from outside the family (see *Hyperactivity,* page 89).

During nursery and school years every child's environment expands beyond the family as the child begins to form new relationships, independent from those formed at home. The time of greatest emotional and social development is during adolescence. The physical development of puberty, which marks the transition from childhood to adulthood, is accompanied by increased hormonal activity that affects all adolescents' feelings about themselves. For the teenager, adolescence is usually a time of experimentation. (See also *Adolescent behavior problems,* chart 51.)

Changing proportions and features

There are two growth spurts in the development of a child, one during the first year of life, and the other during puberty. From the first year, the rate of growth gradually declines to reach its lowest point immediately before puberty begins.

At birth, a baby's head is about ¼ of his or her body length and as wide as the shoulders. The legs account for ⅜ of the body length. Gradually these proportions change, so that by adulthood the head is about ⅛ and the legs ½ of the total body length.

Until puberty begins, the male and female are, on average, of similar height and build. During puberty, however, differences in stature between the male and female become significant. On average, the male grows taller; the male's height increases by 11 inches (28 cm) and the female's by 8 inches (20 cm). Change begins in the legs and progresses to the trunk, where most of the growth occurs. Muscle bulk increases—particularly in the male, whose chest, shoulders, and arms become noticeably broader. In both sexes the forehead becomes more prominent and the jaw and chin lengthen. During adolescence the diameter of the head grows and the skull thickens by 15 percent. In the adolescent female, the pelvis broadens; layers of fat form on the hips; and the breasts develop, usually as the first sign of puberty. (See also *Delayed puberty,* chart 50, and *The reproductive system,* page 21.)

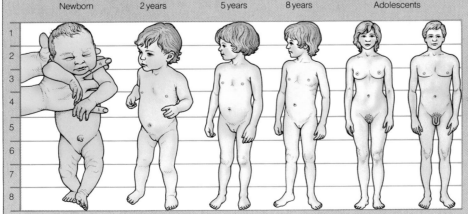

Newborn 2 years 5 years 8 years Adolescents

During the first 18 years of life the body is constantly growing and changing. In this time it undergoes radical change—in total body length, weight, proportion, and shape. The features of the face gradually become more defined. At birth the weight of a baby equals around 5 percent of its young adult weight. In the first year alone, a baby's weight triples. By the end of the second year, the baby will weigh about four times its birth weight. By the age of 10, 50 percent of the young adult weight has been reached. Between infancy and adolescence the legs change from ⅜ of the total body length to ½, and the head from ¼ to ⅛.

Developing skills

From the moment an infant enters the world, his or her life is a constant process of development and maturation. Within 3 months, the instinctive reflexes present at birth have given way to voluntary responses, and the process of thinking, learning, and developing skills is well on its way. No two babies are ever the same and, although the pattern of development is constant, the rate of progress varies greatly from one child to another. Your child may crawl and walk months later than your friend's. Your baby will eventually sit, stand, crawl, and walk at his or her own pace. Every passing week brings new accomplishments in muscle coordination and manipulative ability.

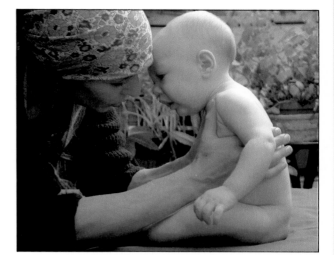

Physical skills

Hand and eye coordination

Learning to put what the eyes see together with what the hands do is called "hand-eye coordination." During the first 8 weeks of life the infant looks at things without touching them and touches things without looking at them. As soon as an object passes out of the baby's limited visual range, it is as though it never existed. Until the baby discovers its hands, he or she only passively gazes at a toy. First the baby must be able to see the object clearly and want what he or she sees. Then it's a matter of knowing where his or her hand is in space and being able to gauge the distance between the two. Next comes the tricky maneuvering of hand and arm that enables the baby to actually grab hold of the object.

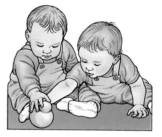

Most babies enjoy being propped up in a sitting position so that they can look around and be a part of things. You can help your baby practice sitting up by supporting the tummy and shoulders as you talk to him or her, so that he or she raises the head to look up at you. In this way the muscles of the neck and shoulders are gradually strengthened. By the time the baby is 8 or 9 months old, he or she will be able to sit up, look over a shoulder, and reach forward without losing balance.

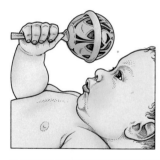

From about the second or third month, the baby begins to link seeing with doing. Now, when a rattle is seen the baby tries to keep it in view and do something with it. At first he or she can only swipe at it, but later the hand opens wide, and grasping fingers curl tightly around the toy. When the rattle moves, it makes a noise, drawing the baby's attention from the sight of the toy back to the motion of his or her hands. In this way the coordination between hand and eye is further reinforced and the baby gains a sense of his or her control over objects.

Sitting

Most babies gradually are able to sit up without support by about 8 or 9 months. It is only at this time that the baby has gained sufficient strength in the neck, shoulders, and trunk to enable him or her to sit up without toppling over. Until he or she can hold the head and torso steady, you can help your child to develop the necessary strength by introducing him or her to games using the muscles needed for grasping, pulling, and pushing.

Crawling

Crawling demands from babies a good deal of strength, balance, and complicated maneuvering. Before babies can get going, they must develop enough muscular control to hold their heads up and support their body weight on the forearms while lying on their tummies. Then they must get into position by tucking their knees up under them, raising their bottoms into the air, and summoning enough balance to finally shove off. It is no easy task and most babies do not accomplish it until they are 8 or 9 months old.

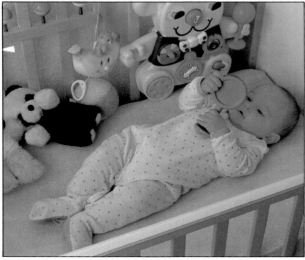

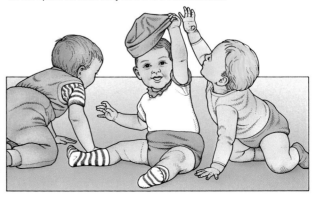

At about 9 or 10 months a child will begin trying to stand on his or her own. Because back, leg, and foot muscles will still be a bit wobbly, it helps a child to have something to pull up with and to hang on to. If this is a piece of furniture, make sure it is solid and won't tip over.

When a baby is ready to start walking, his or her willingness to do so may exceed his or her balance. Push toys require supervision. Infant walkers do not lead to earlier walking and, because of their speed, can be dangerous; falls down stairs while an infant is in a walker are common. Do not use walkers, which cause many injuries, and always supervise your child. Eventually, crawling and tottering will give way to sure steps.

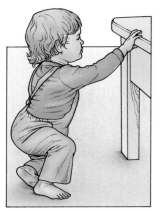

Safety tips
A child's newly developed mobility means that he or she is far more vulnerable to accidents than ever before. His or her agility will most certainly exceed his or her ability to sense danger; parents must take sensible precautions. (See *Preventing accidents,* page 34.)

The sitting baby
Most babies, from as early as 6 weeks, like to be propped up so that they can look around. A bouncing seat is ideal, but the baby must be securely fastened and the seat placed on a nonskid surface. If you prop your baby up in an adult chair or on the floor, make sure he or she is surrounded by plenty of pillows so that he or she does not tip over. Choose sturdy infant furniture and strollers that the baby cannot pull over as he or she tries to stand.

The crawling baby
A crawling baby must be carefully watched. Make sure the area is clean, smooth surfaced, and free of loose wires, sharp edges, or unstable furnishings and open hearths. Trailing tablecloths, low-hanging plants, breakables, and the dog's water bowl should be removed. Always have safety gates across stairways. Lock any door that you don't want the baby to go through. Never leave a crawling baby unsupervised.

The walking baby
Toddlers who can walk can reach and climb, so don't leave windows open. Banisters should be too narrow to squeeze through and stairways should be fenced off. Swinging or sliding doors should be locked and locks must be out of reach. Possible hiding places, like cabinets, trunks, and old kitchen appliances (such as refrigerators), must be securely fastened.

Turn all the handles of pots and pans away from the front of the stove or install a guard around it. Never leave anything that is boiling or hot unattended and make sure that all sharp kitchen utensils are out of reach.

Glass doors should have clearly visible stickers on them and yard gates should be firmly shut. Lock away all medicines. Never leave small objects lying around that your child can put into his or her nose or ears and never leave your child unsupervised.

Walking
All babies are born with a walking reflex, but real walking comes much later, with the baby taking his or her first unsupported steps anytime between 9 and 18 months of age. At first the child walks clinging to the furniture or to you, then he or she begins to negotiate the space between supports. Later, the baby begins to toddle, managing a few paces in open space between one support and the next. The day that the baby walks without support, with legs and elbows stretched wide apart for balance, is one of great excitement and pride for everyone.

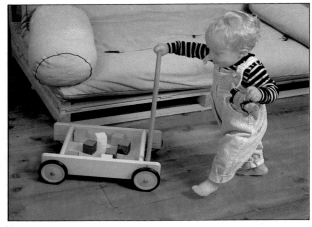

Standing
As early as 5 or 6 months, babies love to be held in a supported standing position. By 7 months they may be hopping from one foot to another, and at 9 months some can place one foot in front of the other while supported. Imagine a child's excitement when he or she discovers how to stand on his or her own two feet. It is not until the baby is 10 or 11 months old that he or she gains enough control over the lower leg muscles to stand up. By then he or she will stand with the whole of his or her body weight on the feet. Once a child has pulled himself or herself into a standing position, the child may take another week or so to learn how to sit back down again.

Milestones

The ages below are *average* times by which children achieve certain skills. Each child develops individually and may progress earlier or later.

6 weeks
- Smile

10 weeks
- Roll over from a sideways position on to the back

4–6 months
- Raise head and shoulders from a face down position
- Sit up with some support

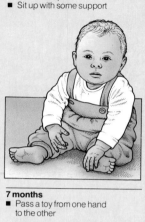

7 months
- Pass a toy from one hand to the other

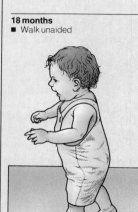

8 months
- Try to feed himself or herself with a spoon
- Sit up unsupported

9 months
- Rise to a sitting position

12 months
- Understand simple commands
- Stand unsupported for a few seconds

18 months
- Walk unaided

2½–3 years
- Stay dry during the day

3 years
- Talk in simple sentences
- Stay dry during some nights

4 years
- Get dressed and undressed (with a little help)

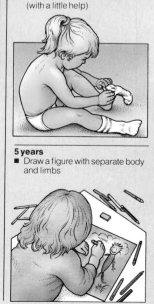

5 years
- Draw a figure with separate body and limbs

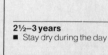

Social behavior

Playing

Play is a child's work and toys are the tools of the trade. As much as they need food, warmth, and love, children need play to enlarge their understanding of the world around them. Playthings are the stimuli that spur a child to explore his or her universe intelligently, and, while it is important to provide a child with a variety of materials and activities, it is just as essential to provide the space in which to enjoy them. While children's play is their work, work can be their play, and you will find that from about 12 to 18 months children like to imitate housework.

Sharing

Toddlers move gradually from independent play to cooperative play at around 3 years. Sharing is hard to learn and, although toddlers will not always play together in complete harmony, they will begin to learn tolerance and cooperation.

Discipline

Sensitive parents use discipline in a positive way, to teach rather than to punish. The parent must define clearly for the child what is or is not acceptable behavior, trying to intervene before problems arise, telling the child what to do as much as what not to do. Throughout the exhausting work of parenting, it can help to remember that your young child loves you, admires you, and identifies with you. Set limits, but show love and have fun too.

Fears and separation

As your baby becomes more physically capable, he or she begins to learn that he or she is an individual separate from you. Then, and again later, infants become wary of strangers and will cling to the parent. Phases of stranger anxiety are a part of normal development. Other fears come and go. By age 2 most children will have shown at least one fear of some sort. Even an imaginary monster is real to the child, and parents should be patient and sympathetic, reassuring the child that he or she will be protected. From age 2 to 3, the child learns to separate easily from the parent. Children need to learn on their own that what or who goes away will come back. This is a milestone to pass.

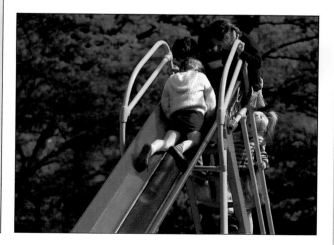

Your child's body

The skeleton

The skeleton is the body's framework, a rigid structure consisting of more than 200 bones that act as levers for the muscles to pull against to perform movement. The skeleton is a rigid structure that gives support and protection to the body by surrounding and enclosing the vital organs contained within the head, chest, and abdomen. At birth the skeleton consists mostly of cartilage, which is a soft, fibrous, and elastic tissue that works along with bone to build the mature skeleton.

Structure of the bone

Within the hard structural part of the bone, the cells are arranged in thousands of cylinders that help distribute the forces acting on the bones. The marrow, the fatty center of the bone, produces most of the body's white blood cells and all of its red blood cells. In a young child, all bone contains blood cell–producing marrow (the marrow is active only in some bones in an adult). Bone is made of minerals–calcium and phosphate– that give strength and rigidity.

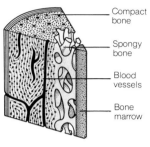

- Compact bone
- Spongy bone
- Blood vessels
- Bone marrow

How bones develop

During childhood, bone forms within the cartilage at specific stages of development until, during adolescence, the skeleton matures to its adult state.

Bone is an active, living, but hard tissue that grows, develops, and renews itself. Old bone cells are constantly reabsorbed and new ones formed. During childhood the skeleton undergoes a process of constant remodeling and strengthening. Growth of the long bones takes place mainly in one region–the epiphysis, or the growing end of the bone. Injury to this region can impair growth. Exercise and adequate supplies of vitamins (particularly vitamin D) and minerals (particularly calcium) and protein in the diet encourage the growth of healthy bones. (See also *Getting enough exercise,* page 34, and *The components of a healthy diet,* page 119.)

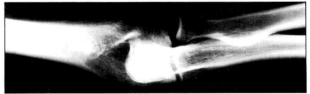

Adult's elbow joint

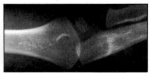

Child's elbow joint

These X-ray films show what happens to bones as they are forming. The actual shape of each bone is present at birth. The bones in the child's arm are made up of areas of cartilage (not visible on the X-ray) and bone (visible as solid areas). As a child develops, the cartilage is converted to bone. By early adulthood this conversion is complete.

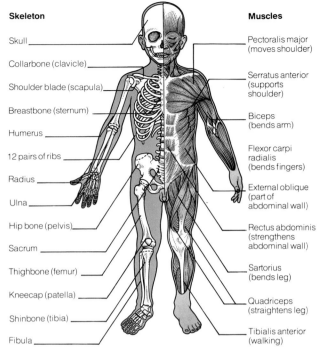

Skeleton

- Skull
- Collarbone (clavicle)
- Shoulder blade (scapula)
- Breastbone (sternum)
- Humerus
- 12 pairs of ribs
- Radius
- Ulna
- Hip bone (pelvis)
- Sacrum
- Thighbone (femur)
- Kneecap (patella)
- Shinbone (tibia)
- Fibula

Muscles

- Pectoralis major (moves shoulder)
- Serratus anterior (supports shoulder)
- Biceps (bends arm)
- Flexor carpi radialis (bends fingers)
- External oblique (part of abdominal wall)
- Rectus abdominis (strengthens abdominal wall)
- Sartorius (bends leg)
- Quadriceps (straightens leg)
- Tibialis anterior (walking)

Muscles

All movement of the body and its internal organs is carried out by the muscles. These are made up of thousands of individual fibers that contract to produce movement. There are two types of muscle: the voluntary muscles, which carry out body movements, and the involuntary (smooth) muscles, which are responsible for movement within the body (such as the rhythmic propulsion of food through the digestive tract). Muscles thrive on work; exercise improves the circulation of blood in the muscles, increases their bulk, and improves their chemical efficiency (see *Getting enough exercise,* page 34). A baby is born with certain instinctive reactions known as reflex movements. Gradually, these change as the central nervous system and the muscles develop, allowing the young child to steadily increase control over the body. (See *Brain and nervous system,* opposite page.)

How muscles grow

While still in the uterus, a baby moves vigorously and continues to do so at birth. However, the muscles are not yet fully developed and they require a nutritious diet, exercise, and hormones to mature properly. After puberty, the male hormones promote greater size and strength in boys' muscles. Exercise is imperative for proper muscle growth; without it muscle will actually shrink. Children who are physically active have stronger, better-coordinated muscles than children who are inactive.

Symptoms

Common problems include fracture of the bones, dislocation of joints, and muscle strains. Most injuries sustained are minor. A child who lies still or refuses to move an injured limb has probably sustained a serious injury, while a child who can still use an injured arm or hand during play is unlikely to have done much damage.

Occasionally the spine tends to curve sideways, and this condition, known as scoliosis, needs early recognition for satisfactory treatment.

See also the following diagnostic charts: **45** Painful arm or leg **46** Painful joints **47** Foot problems

Symptoms

Muscles that are underused or overused are more susceptible to damage. When a muscle is underused, it actually shrinks and becomes flabby. Inactivity further promotes muscle-wasting and weakness. Damage to muscles from overuse normally produces pain, stiffness, and sometimes

inflammation and swelling. Muscles may occasionally become weak or painful as a result of viral infection.

See also the following diagnostic charts: **14** Fever in children **26** Rash with fever **45** Painful arm or leg **46** Painful joints **47** Foot problems.

The heart and circulation

The heart is the center of the body's circulatory system. It is a muscle made up of two pumps. Each pump is divided into two compartments linked by valves. The main pumping compartments are the right and left ventricles. Blood, which carries nutrients and oxygen to all parts of the body and takes away waste products, is pumped throughout the body by the heart, first to the lungs, where oxygen is added and carbon dioxide is eliminated. The blood then goes back to the heart, passes through the left atrium, down into the left ventricle, and on to the brain and all body organs, via the aorta. Arteries carry blood away from the heart, and veins return the blood to it. When the blood returns to the heart it enters the right atrium, passing through the tricuspid valve to the right ventricle, which pumps it on to the lungs for fresh oxygen. In the fetus, two temporary paths that close shortly after birth allow the blood to bypass the nonfunctioning lungs. (See also *Heart and circulation,* page 24 and *Fetal circulation,* page 10.)

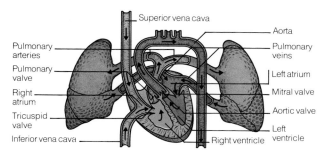

Symptoms

If a baby has congenital heart disease, it is generally discovered during routine tests done at birth. Rapid breathing and difficulty eating in an infant and poor physical development in a child are occasionally symptoms of a heart disorder. Serious heart disorders in children are rare, but congenital heart disease accounts for almost half the major physical defects present at birth.

The respiratory system

Respiration is more than just breathing – it encompasses the entire process by which oxygen reaches your child's body cells and is used by them to produce energy. It also includes the elimination of carbon dioxide and water, the waste products of the process. The respiratory system consists of the lungs and the tubes (bronchi) through which the air passes on its way to and from the lungs. Air breathed in through the nose and mouth passes down the trachea (windpipe) and enters the lungs through the bronchi and smaller bronchioles. The lungs themselves are spongelike organs made up of millions of air sacs called alveoli. It is through these tiny sacs that oxygen passes into the bloodstream and carbon dioxide passes out to be exhaled. Throughout this process the diaphragm – a sheet of muscle between the chest and abdomen – is rhythmically contracting and relaxing, allowing the rib cage and lungs to expand and pull in air, and then to contract and exhale the air.

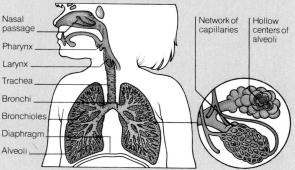

Nasal passage
Pharynx
Larynx
Trachea
Bronchi
Bronchioles
Diaphragm
Alveoli

Network of capillaries | Hollow centers of alveoli

Symptoms

The most common breathing problems in childhood are caused by infections and asthma. Young children are particularly susceptible to viruses until they have developed immunity to the common ones; after this they catch fewer colds. Sore throat, runny nose, coughing, and raised temperature often accompany a cold. Fast, noisy, and difficult breathing are symptoms of breathing disorders. An asthmatic child has attacks in which the small airways in the lungs become narrow and so make breathing difficult. Asthma attacks tend to become less frequent as the child grows.

See also the following diagnostic charts: **3** Fever in babies **9** Feeling sick **14** Fever in children **18** Headache **31** Runny or stuffed-up nose **32** Sore throat **33** Coughing **34** Fast breathing **35** Noisy breathing

The brain and nervous system

A child's ability to develop both physical and mental skills is largely determined by the gradual development of the nervous system (see diagrams below). This is made up of the brain and spinal cord (central nervous system) and a network of nerves (peripheral nervous system). The nervous system controls both conscious activities and unconscious body functions, such as digestion (see *Brain and nervous system,* page 26).

Development of the nervous system

The nervous system is made up of billions of nerve cells, which detect information from inside and outside a child's body. At birth, the connections between the nerve cells are immature. In addition, the brain, which receives messages from and transmits information to the nerves, is only partially developed. The nervous system matures gradually, enabling a young child to control internal organs (such as the bladder) and to develop a wide range of skills, including walking and speaking (see *Milestones,* page 17).

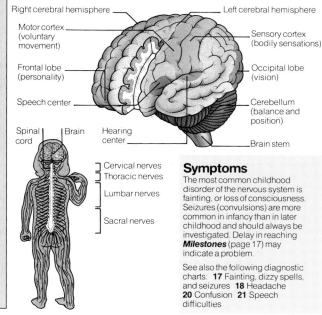

Right cerebral hemisphere
Motor cortex (voluntary movement)
Frontal lobe (personality)
Speech center
Spinal cord | Brain
Hearing center

Left cerebral hemisphere
Sensory cortex (bodily sensations)
Occipital lobe (vision)
Cerebellum (balance and position)
Brain stem

Cervical nerves
Thoracic nerves
Lumbar nerves
Sacral nerves

Symptoms

The most common childhood disorder of the nervous system is fainting, or loss of consciousness. Seizures (convulsions) are more common in infancy than in later childhood and should always be investigated. Delay in reaching **Milestones** (page 17) may indicate a problem.

See also the following diagnostic charts: **17** Fainting, dizzy spells, and seizures **18** Headache **20** Confusion **21** Speech difficulties

The senses

Each of the five senses is in working order from the moment a child is born. Newborn babies are thought to have a sense of smell because they do have a sense of taste and the two are inextricably linked. A newborn is able to see from the moment of birth but can only discriminate brightness and movement. Babies are able to sense sound vibrations in the uterus and can hear at birth. Babies also react to touch in the uterus, moving first away from and then toward the placenta. At birth, babies respond with pleasure to gentle, warm pressure on their backs and stomachs.

Hearing
The ear, as described on page 103, is important both as a means of communication and as the body's center of balance.

Sight
The instruments of sight are the eyes, which begin in the embryo as two fledgling "buds" from the brain. The eyeball is a complex structure consisting of three layers. The sclera is visible as the white of the eye; the choroid layer is rich in blood vessels that supply the sensitive inner lining of the eyeball; and the retina contains the light-sensitive nerve cells that pick up images and transmit the information through the optic nerve to the brain. It is in the brain that these images are decoded to allow vision.

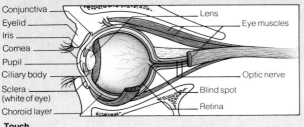

Conjunctiva
Eyelid
Iris
Cornea
Pupil
Ciliary body
Sclera (white of eye)
Choroid layer
Lens
Eye muscles
Optic nerve
Blind spot
Retina

Touch
It is known that the fetus in the uterus reacts to touch because it moves away from the surrounding placenta early in the pregnancy but toward it later on. At birth, the newborn reacts instinctively to touch by gripping any object placed in his or her hand and likewise will respond with sucking reflexes to a gentle stroking on the cheek. Most babies react with pleasure to warmth, softness, and gentle pressure, and physical contact is an essential need from the moment of birth on. By the time a child is 1 year old, his or her sense of touch is developed well enough to know a cuddly toy just by the feel of it.

Taste
The child's taste buds identify different tastes in the same manner as the adult's. Particular tastes are detected at specific areas on the tongue: bitterness at the back, sourness at the sides, saltiness at the front, and sweetness on the tip. Bitter, acid, or sour tastes cause a baby to grimace, turn away, or cry. Babies can also distinguish between different levels of sweetness and will suck longer and harder at a bottle of sweetened water than plain or only slightly sweetened water. By the toddler stage a child easily knows chocolate cookies from vanilla.

Smell
The sensitive hairlike endings of the olfactory nerves project into the nasal passage. They detect odors in the air and pass the information to the olfactory bulbs, which are linked directly to the brain. One of the first associations a baby makes is with his or her mother's smell, recognizing and responding to it as a source of comfort, pleasure, and food.

Olfactory nerve
Nasal cavity

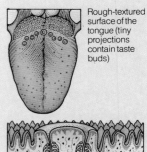

Rough-textured surface of the tongue (tiny projections contain taste buds)

Symptoms
The main symptom of disorder in any of the senses is partial or total loss of sensitivity. There may be pain or other symptoms affecting the sensory organ concerned. The most common ear problem is infection. Symptoms include earache, itching, fever, and discharge from the ear. If your baby fails to respond to sounds, you should suspect hearing loss. Common childhood eye problems are infections and irritations that cause pain, itchiness, redness, and discharge. A neglected squint may eventually lead to impaired vision.

See also the following diagnostic charts: **27** Eye problems **28** Disturbed or impaired vision **29** Painful or irritated ear **30** Deafness **31** Runny or stuffed-up nose **32** Sore throat

The digestive system

The system of organs responsible for carrying out the digestive process is known as the digestive tract. This tract extends from the mouth to the anus. Food is broken down so that the minerals, vitamins, carbohydrates, fats, and proteins it contains can be absorbed into the body.

Symptoms
Gastroenteritis (infection of the digestive tract) is the most common digestive disorder of childhood. Symptoms include vomiting, diarrhea, and abdominal pain. Vomiting and diarrhea can cause dangerous loss of fluid. If this fluid is not replaced, a child may become seriously dehydrated.

See also the following diagnostic charts: **7** Vomiting in babies **8** Diarrhea in babies **37** Vomiting in children **38** Abdominal pain **39** Loss of appetite **40** Diarrhea in children **41** Constipation **42** Abnormal-looking bowel movements **43** Urinary problems

Mouth
Digestion begins in the mouth when, as food is chewed, enzymes in the saliva break down certain carbohydrates. The tongue and the muscles of the pharynx then propel the mixture of food and saliva (called a bolus) into the esophagus and down into the stomach.

Stomach
Food may spend from 30 minutes to an hour or two in the stomach, where it is churned and partially digested by acid and enzymes until it is a semiliquid substance (called chyme). After passing into the duodenum, the chyme is broken down further by digestive juices from the liver and pancreas.

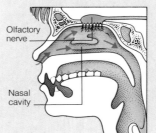

Esophagus
Pancreas

Salivary glands

Duodenum
The duodenum is the first part of the small intestine, into which the partially digested food (chyme) from the stomach passes for further breakdown.

Small intestine
The final stage of digestion is completed in the small intestine, where the nutrients are split into chemical units small enough to pass through the wall of the intestine into the network of blood vessels and lymphatics, which carry the nutrients to the liver.

Large intestine (colon)
Undigested material passes in semi-liquid form from the small intestine into the large intestine, where most of the water content is reabsorbed into the bloodstream. The semisolid waste that remains moves down into the rectum, where it is stored until it is expelled from the body through the anus. The addition of fiber to the diet may increase the efficiency with which the large intestine can properly eliminate waste products.

Rectum

The lymphatic system

The lymphatic system consists of the lymph glands or nodes, found mainly in the neck, armpits, and groin, and the small vessels that connect these glands, called the lymphatics. The lymph nodes contain white blood cells that defend the body against infection. When infection occurs, the lymph nodes may swell and become tender. Lymphocytes (white blood cells) are released from the glands into the bloodstream. The spleen is also part of the lymphatic system, but it has other functions, including control of the circulation of red blood cells.

Symptoms
Glands that swell during an infection are actually lymph nodes. Swollen, tender glands behind the ear are a sign of ear infection, those below the ear and jaw may indicate tonsillitis, and those in the back of the neck may mean German measles (rubella).

See also the following diagnostic charts: **9** Feeling sick **15** Swollen glands **26** Rash with fever **29** Painful or irritated ear **32** Sore throat **33** Coughing

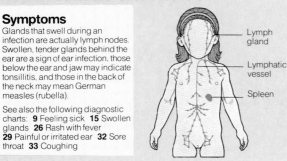

Lymph gland

Lymphatic vessel

Spleen

The endocrine system

The endocrine glands manufacture hormones and distribute them to all parts of the body via the bloodstream. These hormones regulate the body's internal chemistry; its responses to hunger, stress, infection, and disease; and its preparation for physical activity.

Pituitary gland
The pituitary gland is a peanut-sized organ located beneath the brain. The most important role of the pituitary, often called the "master gland," is to stimulate and coordinate the functions of the other endocrine glands, which produce their own hormones. It also manufactures growth hormones, which regulate growth during childhood.

Thyroid gland
The thyroid gland is located at the front of the throat, just below the Adam's apple. It produces the hormones that control the conversion of food into energy and the rate at which the body needs energy to continue to function.

Parathyroid glands
The parathyroids produce a hormone that controls the level of calcium and phosphorus—essential for healthy bones and efficient functioning of nerves and muscles.

Adrenal glands
The adrenal glands lie above the kidneys and produce hormones that help regulate the amounts of sugar, salt, and water in the body, as well as the shape and distribution of body hair. These glands also produce epinephrine, which increases blood flow to the muscles, heart, and lungs during excitement or stress.

Pancreas
The pancreas lies at the back of the abdomen, behind the stomach. It makes enzymes that pass into the duodenum (the upper part of the small intestine), where they help to digest food. The pancreas also produces the hormones insulin and glucagon, which play an integral part in regulating the sugar level in the blood.

Ovaries (female) and testicles (male)
The ovaries in the adolescent female and the testicles in the adolescent male produce the hormones responsible for the onset of puberty. In the female the ovaries are also responsible for the production of the ova (eggs); in the male the testicles produce sperm. The hormones secreted by these glands determine the development of male and female sexual characteristics.

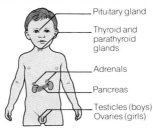

Pituitary gland

Thyroid and parathyroid glands

Adrenals

Pancreas

Testicles (boys) Ovaries (girls)

Symptoms
Disorders can occur when the level of a hormone changes. Symptoms of diabetes mellitus, a deficiency in the level of insulin in the body, include thirst and abnormally frequent urination. Delay in the onset of puberty may be the result of a hormonal disorder. Consult your doctor.

See also the following diagnostic charts: **10** Slow growth **40** Diarrhea in children **43** Urinary problems **50** Delayed puberty **51** Adolescent behavior problems

The urinary system

A baby's reflexes automatically expel urine from the bladder. A child learns control of bladder and bowels when he or she is physiologically and mentally ready to do so (see *Toilet training,* page 127). Also, a child urinates more frequently than an adult because children have smaller bladders (see *The structure of the urinary tract,* page 125).

Symptoms
Infection in the urethra or bladder, causing pain when your child passes urine, is the most common disorder of the urinary system. Pain or a change in the number of times your child passes urine in a day, or a change in its color, may indicate an underlying disorder.

See also the following diagnostic charts: **8** Diarrhea in babies **40** Diarrhea in children **41** Constipation **42** Abnormal-looking bowel movements **43** Urinary problems **44** Toilet-training problems

The reproductive system

Boys
In the male fetus, the organs of reproduction (the testicles) lie in the abdomen and descend into the scrotum shortly before birth. The male's reproductive system usually matures between the ages of 11 and 17, with the enlargement of the penis and the ability to ejaculate sperm.

The male reproductive system consists of the external genitalia—two testicles within the scrotum, and the penis—and a series of internal organs: the prostate gland, two seminal vesicles, and two tubes known as the vas deferens. Sperm are continually manufactured in each testicle and pass into the epididymis, where they mature for 2 to 3 weeks. They then pass into the vas deferens for storage before ejaculation.

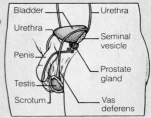

Bladder

Urethra

Urethra

Seminal vesicle

Penis

Prostate gland

Testis

Scrotum

Vas deferens

Girls
The ovaries in a baby girl contain all the ova (eggs) that will ever be produced in her life. At puberty, usually between 11 and 14 years, production of the female sex hormones begins, which stimulates the beginning of menstruation.

The female genital system includes the vagina, the ovaries, the uterus, and the fallopian tubes. The uterus begins to enlarge at puberty. The ovaries produce the female hormones and provide storage for the eggs. Eggs pass from the ovaries through the fallopian tubes to the uterus. The vagina is the birth canal.

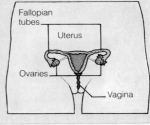

Fallopian tubes

Uterus

Ovaries

Vagina

Symptoms
Boys: Symptoms of a genital disorder include pain, swelling, and inflammation and should always receive medical attention. Problems include internal damage as a result of external injury to the groin and infection of the urinary tract. Less commonly, the foreskin of the penis may be too tight.

Girls: The most common genital problem experienced by young girls is inflammation and irritation of the external genital area. Pain when urinating and abnormal frequency in urinating are common symptoms of a genital disorder. Delay in the onset of puberty only rarely indicates a serious underlying problem, but should be investigated in both girls and boys.

See also the following diagnostic charts: **43** Urinary problems **48** Genital problems in boys **49** Genital problems in girls **50** Delayed puberty

Your body

The skeleton

The skeleton gives form, support, and protection to the body. It consists of more than 200 bones, supplemented by pieces of cartilage. Cartilage is a tough, elastic material, which forms an important complement to bone, especially where a combination of strength and flexibility is required. The bones, especially the long bones of the limbs, act as levers operated by the muscles, allowing movement. Some bones serve to protect the organs they enclose and some contain the bone marrow, where red blood cells are formed. The bones are living material with cells that are constantly replacing old bone with new bone cells. To maintain healthy bones, you need adequate amounts of protein, calcium, and vitamins—particularly vitamin D—in your diet.

Joints

The separate bones of the skeleton are interconnected by joints. There are several types of joints. Fixed (suture) joints hold the bones firmly together, allowing no movement, as in the skull. Partly movable (cartilaginous) joints allow some flexibility, as in the bones of the spine. Freely movable (synovial) joints provide great flexibility in several planes of movement, as in the shoulder.

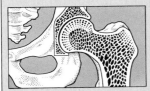

Ball-and-socket joints
Ball-and-socket joints, such as those in the hip and shoulder, permit maximum range of movement. In the hip, the top of the thighbone is nearly spherical and slots into a semi-circular socket in the pelvic bone. The ball-and-socket joints allow movement in virtually every direction.

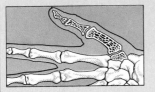

Saddle joints
Saddle joints allow both side-to-side and back-and-forth motion. There is a saddle joint in the thumb, without which it would be extremely difficult to grasp either large or small objects.

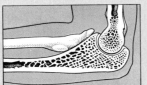

Hinge joints
Hinge joints, which are found in the fingers, toes, elbows, and knees, allow movement in one direction only. The two bones that meet at the hinge are held together by tough fibrous ligaments and the ends of the bones are cushioned in lubricating fluid.

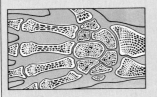

Gliding joints
Gliding joints in the carpal bones of the wrists slide in motion similar to the saddle joints, side-to-side and back-and-forth, but the movement is more restricted. With age, the movement of the joints can become less smooth and increasingly difficult.

Symptoms
Symptoms of joint problems include pain, swelling, and stiffness. Osteoarthritis, a degeneration of the joints, commonly affects the neck, hands, hips, and knees. Rheumatoid arthritis attacks the connective tissue around the joints, causing inflammation and disability.

See also the following diagnostic charts: **108** Painful or stiff neck **112** Painful or swollen joints **113** Painful knee

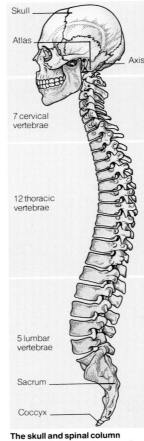

The skull and spinal column
At the base of the skull is an opening through which the spinal cord connects with the brain. The cord itself runs through the spinal column, which is made up of 24 separate, and some fused, vertebrae. The vertebrae form a protective casing for the spinal cord.

Skull
Atlas
Axis
7 cervical vertebrae
12 thoracic vertebrae
5 lumbar vertebrae
Sacrum
Coccyx

Symptoms

The most common problems affecting the skeleton of people of all ages include fractures of the bones as a result of injury and damage to the joints and ligaments as a result of injury or degeneration. Bone infections and tumors are rare. Symptoms of disorders of the skeleton include pain, swelling, and inflammation (redness and heat) around the affected part.

See also the following diagnostic charts: **107** Back pain **108** Painful or stiff neck **109** Painful arm **110** Painful leg **111** Foot problems **112** Painful or swollen joints **113** Painful knee

The structure of bone
The structure of bone combines strength with lightness and a degree of flexibility. Bone itself is made up of protein hardened with mineral salts, principally calcium and phosphorus. The outer (compact) bone contains blood and lymph vessels and the inner (spongy) bone has a honeycomb structure for lightness. In the center of the long bones is a cylindrical cavity filled with bone marrow. The marrow inside the bones is a fatty material containing blood-forming tissues that produce the red and white blood cells.

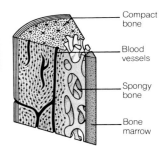

Compact bone
Blood vessels
Spongy bone
Bone marrow

Muscles

Movement of the body and its internal organs is carried out by the muscles—soft tissue arranged in fibers that can contract and relax to produce movement. There are two distinct types of muscle: the voluntary muscles, which control body movement, and the involuntary muscles, which are responsible for movement within the body—for example, those responsible for the rhythmical contraction of the digestive tract that propels food along its length.

Muscles thrive on work and normally remain in good condition if used regularly. Exercise increases the size of muscles and improves the circulation of blood to them, thereby increasing their capacity for strenuous activity. Conversely, inactivity leads to muscle-wasting and weakness.

Involuntary muscles
Involuntary muscles are not under conscious control. They do not contract or relax in response to your decision to make a movement. Instead, they work automatically. Both types of involuntary muscles—smooth and cardiac—are in continuous use, maintaining such functions as respiration, digestion, circulation, and contraction of the heart.

Heart
Intestines

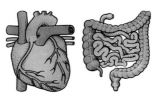

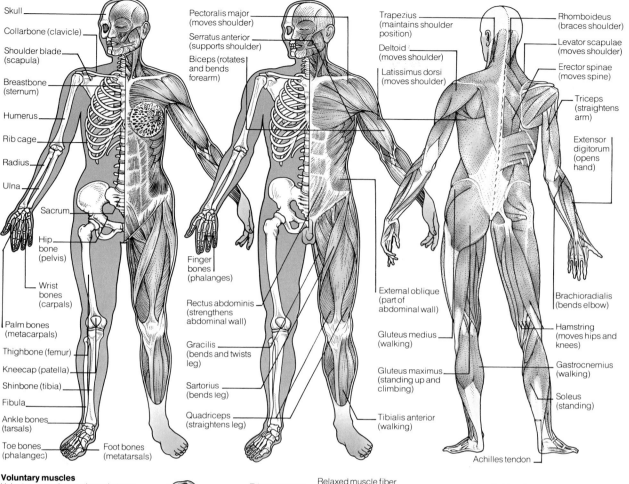

Skull
Collarbone (clavicle)
Shoulder blade (scapula)
Breastbone (sternum)
Humerus
Rib cage
Radius
Ulna
Sacrum
Hip bone (pelvis)
Wrist bones (carpals)
Palm bones (metacarpals)
Thighbone (femur)
Kneecap (patella)
Shinbone (tibia)
Fibula
Ankle bones (tarsals)
Toe bones (phalanges)
Foot bones (metatarsals)

Pectoralis major (moves shoulder)
Serratus anterior (supports shoulder)
Biceps (rotates and bends forearm)
Finger bones (phalanges)
Rectus abdominis (strengthens abdominal wall)
Gracilis (bends and twists leg)
Sartorius (bends leg)
Quadriceps (straightens leg)

Trapezius (maintains shoulder position)
Deltoid (moves shoulder)
Latissimus dorsi (moves shoulder)
External oblique (part of abdominal wall)
Gluteus medius (walking)
Gluteus maximus (standing up and climbing)
Tibialis anterior (walking)

Rhomboideus (braces shoulder)
Levator scapulae (moves shoulder)
Erector spinae (moves spine)
Triceps (straightens arm)
Extensor digitorum (opens hand)
Brachioradialis (bends elbow)
Hamstring (moves hips and knees)
Gastrocnemius (walking)
Soleus (standing)
Achilles tendon

Voluntary muscles

Voluntary muscles are those that can be consciously controlled. Only the skeletal muscles—those that connect bones or cartilage—are voluntary in motion.

Skeletal muscles are attached to bone, either directly or through tendons, and can bend and straighten joints in response to specific stimuli

The upper arm

Biceps muscle
Brachialis muscle
Triceps muscle
Humerus

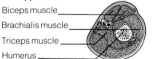

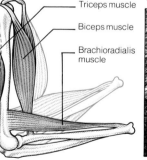

Triceps muscle
Biceps muscle
Brachioradialis muscle

Relaxed muscle fiber

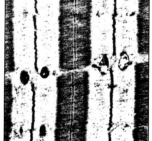

Contracted muscle fiber

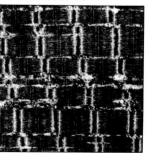

Muscle biopsies

A muscle biopsy is a microscopic examination of a small sample of muscle tissue for signs of disease. The photographs shown here are of very thin slices of healthy muscle, magnified 8,000 times. Each fiber is made up of fibrils bound together by a membrane. Each fibril contains two different proteins that are arranged in parallel filaments, creating the wide, dark stripes (myosin molecules) and the light stripes (actin molecules) seen in the photographs at left. In a relaxed muscle (left), the stripes overlap only slightly. In a contracted muscle (lower left), the fibers slide over each other, shortening the length of muscle.

How muscles work

Our muscles have been called the body's engine. They account for almost half the body weight and convert chemical energy into force that is exerted on the tendons and, through them, to the bones and joints. Most muscles usually work in groups, where the contraction of one muscle is accompanied by the relaxation of another. During contraction, a muscle shortens in length by as much as 40 percent to bring closer together its points of attachment on two different bones. Most voluntary muscles are fixed to two or more adjacent bones, often by means of a fibrous tendon. When a muscle contracts, the bones to which it is attached move.

Symptoms

Damage to muscles from injury normally produces pain, stiffness, and sometimes inflammation and swelling. Muscles may also become weak or painful as a result of viral infection.

See also the following diagnostic charts: **107** Back pain
108 Painful or stiff neck
109 Painful arm **110** Painful leg
112 Painful or swollen joints
113 Painful knee

The heart and circulation

The heart is a muscular pump with four chambers into which the major blood vessels enter, carrying blood to and from the rest of the body. As the chambers rhythmically expand and contract, valves between the chambers ensure that blood flows in the correct direction.

Blood transports oxygen and nutrients (see *Blood analysis,* page 146) to all parts of the body and carries away waste products. It circulates via the arteries, which carry oxygenated blood, and the veins, which return "used" blood to the heart.

Good blood circulation is essential for the health of every organ in the body. Good circulation in turn depends partly on the efficient functioning of the heart muscle and partly on the ease of blood flow through the arteries.

The good health of the circulatory system depends on the blood vessels remaining free from any obstruction, such as fatty deposits or blood clots. It is also important that the pressure of the circulating blood does not exceed certain levels. High blood pressure (hypertension) may damage the blood vessels or increase the risk of blockage of the blood vessels. For advice on reducing the risks of diseases of the heart and circulation, see *Coronary heart disease,* page 221.

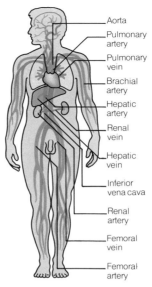

- Aorta
- Pulmonary artery
- Pulmonary vein
- Brachial artery
- Hepatic artery
- Renal vein
- Hepatic vein
- Inferior vena cava
- Renal artery
- Femoral vein
- Femoral artery

The circulatory system
The circulatory system carries blood to and from every part of the body. The center of the system is the heart. Arteries carry blood away from the heart; veins return blood to the heart.

Arteries and veins
The walls of arteries are four layers thick, providing strength for the high-pressure flow of blood forced through the arteries. Arteries and their various branches (arterioles) are surrounded by muscle, which allows them to dilate or contract to regulate blood flow. Veins have less elastic, less muscular walls. Valves in the veins stop blood from flowing in the wrong direction.

Heart chambers
The heart is divided into two by a septum. Each side has two chambers—an atrium and a ventricle—linked by a one-way valve. The left atrium and ventricle control oxygenated blood, and those on the right control de-oxygenated ("used") blood. The septum prevents the two types of blood from mixing.

Symptoms
The symptoms of impaired circulation depend on the organs or region affected. Heart disease may cause chest pain, palpitations, or breathlessness; poor circulation to the brain may cause fainting, dizziness, or confusion; circulation problems in the limbs may cause pain or swelling.

See also the following diagnostic charts: **63** Faintness and fainting **65** Dizziness **66** Numbness or tingling **69** Forgetfulness and confusion **90** Difficulty breathing **105** Palpitations **106** Chest pain **109** Painful arm **110** Painful leg

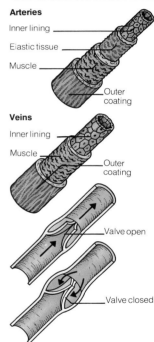

Arteries
- Inner lining
- Elastic tissue
- Muscle
- Outer coating

Veins
- Inner lining
- Muscle
- Outer coating
- Valve open
- Valve closed

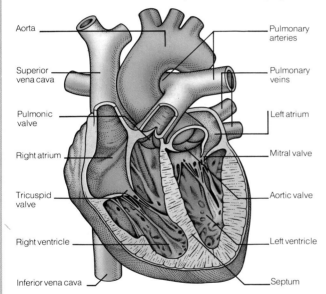

- Aorta
- Superior vena cava
- Pulmonic valve
- Right atrium
- Tricuspid valve
- Right ventricle
- Inferior vena cava
- Pulmonary arteries
- Pulmonary veins
- Left atrium
- Mitral valve
- Aortic valve
- Left ventricle
- Septum

Blood circulation through the heart and lungs

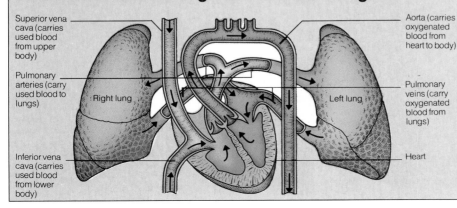

- Superior vena cava (carries used blood from upper body)
- Pulmonary arteries (carry used blood to lungs)
- Right lung
- Inferior vena cava (carries used blood from lower body)
- Aorta (carries oxygenated blood from heart to body)
- Pulmonary veins (carry oxygenated blood from lungs)
- Left lung
- Heart

De-oxygenated ("used") blood is carried back to the heart via the superior and inferior branches of the vena cava, which enters the right atrium. The blood then passes into the right ventricle and is pumped along the pulmonary arteries to the lungs. As blood passes through the network of small blood vessels surrounding the lungs, it absorbs oxygen from the breathed-in air and discharges waste carbon dioxide to be breathed out. The newly oxygenated blood then returns to the heart via the pulmonary veins, enters the left atrium, and then passes into the left ventricle. The oxygenated blood is then pumped through the aorta to all parts of the body.

The respiratory system

Respiration is more than just breathing—it encompasses the entire process by which oxygen reaches your body's cells and is used by them to produce energy. It also includes the elimination of carbon dioxide and water, the waste products of the process. Respiration involves the rib cage, diaphragm (the internal sheet of muscle between the chest and abdomen), and the respiratory tract. The respiratory tract includes the lungs and the tubes (bronchi and bronchioles) through which air passes on its way to and from the lungs. Air is breathed in through the nose and mouth and passes down the trachea (windpipe) and through a branching tree of tubes —the bronchi and bronchioles—to the alveoli, the air sacs in the lungs. The respiratory system can be damaged by repeated exposure to tobacco smoke or pollutants, or by infections. People who smoke and/or live in areas of severe air pollution are more likely to have chronic bronchitis, an inflammation of the mucous membranes that line the bronchi.

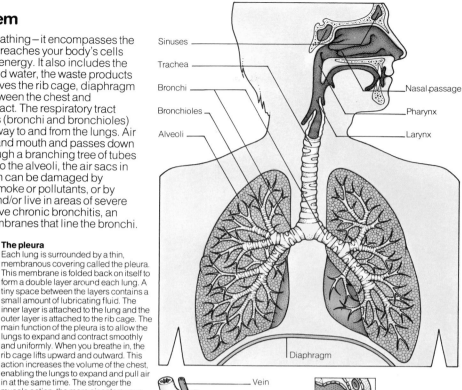

Sinuses
Trachea
Bronchi
Bronchioles
Alveoli
Nasal passage
Pharynx
Larynx
Diaphragm

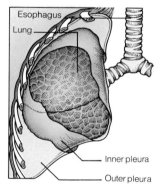

Esophagus
Lung
Inner pleura
Outer pleura

The pleura
Each lung is surrounded by a thin, membranous covering called the pleura. This membrane is folded back on itself to form a double layer around each lung. A tiny space between the layers contains a small amount of lubricating fluid. The inner layer is attached to the lung and the outer layer is attached to the rib cage. The main function of the pleura is to allow the lungs to expand and contract smoothly and uniformly. When you breathe in, the rib cage lifts upward and outward. This action increases the volume of the chest, enabling the lungs to expand and pull air in at the same time. The stronger the muscle action, the more air enters your lungs.

How you breathe

Air you breathe in through your nose is warmed and moistened by small blood vessels very close to the nasal cavity before the air passes into the lungs. In addition, tiny hairs that line the nose filter the air of foreign particles that might get into the lungs. When you breathe in, the diaphragm, which is dome-shaped when relaxed, is pulled flat. At the same time, muscles between your ribs contract and pull the rib cage up and out. These movements enlarge the volume of your chest, enabling the lungs to expand and pull in air. When you breathe out, the chest muscles and diaphragm relax, causing the rib cage to sink and the lungs to contract and squeeze out the air.

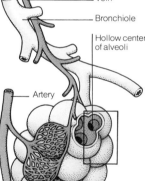

Vein
Bronchiole
Hollow center of alveoli
Artery
Network of capillaries

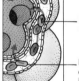

Flow of oxygen into red blood cells
Flow of carbon dioxide from red blood cells

How oxygen enters the blood
The lungs are spongelike organs made up of millions of tiny air sacs called alveoli. The thin linings of these sacs contain minute blood vessels, and here the vital exchange of oxygen and carbon dioxide takes place. The alveoli bring the blood into close contact with the inhaled air, allowing oxygen to pass into the bloodstream and carbon dioxide to pass out for exhalation.

Bronchoscopy
This view of the inside of the lungs (below right) shows the trachea dividing into the two main tubes, or bronchi, which lead into the lungs.

Symptoms

The most common respiratory disorders are caused by infection, and lead to bronchitis (inflammation of the lining of the tract) or pneumonia (inflammation of the lung tissues themselves). Infection may cause chest pain or soreness in the throat, and/or result in the production of excessive amounts of mucus. Coughing is a common symptom of respiratory disorders. If the breathing mechanism is severely damaged, there may be shortness of breath.

See also the following diagnostic charts: **85** Runny nose **86** Sore throat **87** Hoarseness or loss of voice **88** Wheezing **89** Coughing **90** Difficulty breathing **106** Chest pain

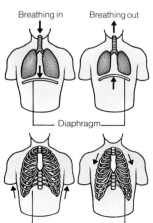

Breathing in
Breathing out
Diaphragm
Rib cage

Bronchogram of the lungs
A small amount of liquid visible on X-rays outlines the pattern of the bronchi and bronchioles.

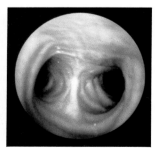

The brain and nervous system

The brain and nervous system together provide the control mechanism for conscious activities, such as thought and movement, and for unconscious body functions, such as breathing and digestion. Nerves also provide the means by which we register sensations, such as pain and temperature. The brain and nervous system require a constant supply of oxygenated blood. Disruption of the blood flow to any part of the system is one of the most common causes of malfunction of the brain and nervous system.

Brain cells are permanently damaged if their blood supply stops for more than 5 minutes. Ruptured or blocked blood vessels in the brain can have serious consequences, including permanent disability.

Injury, infection, degeneration, tumors, and diseases of unknown cause may also affect the brain and nervous system. Certain disorders may arise out of abnormal electrical activity or chemical imbalances in the brain.

The brain

The human brain lies protected inside the bones of the skull. It consists of millions of nerve cells (neurons) and nerve pathways capable of an infinite variety of intercommunications upon which individual intelligence and creativity depend. The brain is by far the most complex organ in the body and many aspects of its structure and function are not yet fully understood. Certain parts of the brain control different bodily functions. The two cerebral hemispheres—the cerebellum and the brain stem—constitute nearly 90 percent of brain tissue and control conscious thought and movement, as well as interpretation of sensory stimuli. The cerebellum regulates subconscious activities, such as coordination of movement and balance. The brain stem connects the rest of the brain to the spinal cord and contains nerve centers that govern the automatic functions, such as respiration, that sustain life.

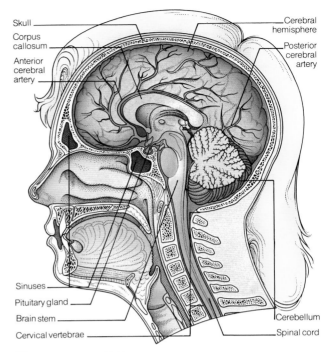

Skull — Corpus callosum — Anterior cerebral artery — Cerebral hemisphere — Posterior cerebral artery — Sinuses — Pituitary gland — Brain stem — Cervical vertebrae — Cerebellum — Spinal cord

The nervous system

The brain and spinal cord together make up the central nervous system, with the spinal cord serving as the link between the brain and the rest of the body. Motor pathways that carry stimuli from the brain to various organs of the body descend through the spinal cord, while sensory pathways from the skin and other sensory organs ascend through the spinal cord, carrying messages to the brain. A network of peripheral nerves links the central nervous system to other parts of the body and directs the conscious control of muscles and the unconscious control of organ function.

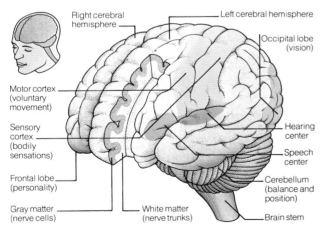

Right cerebral hemisphere — Left cerebral hemisphere — Occipital lobe (vision) — Motor cortex (voluntary movement) — Sensory cortex (bodily sensations) — Hearing center — Speech center — Frontal lobe (personality) — Cerebellum (balance and position) — Gray matter (nerve cells) — White matter (nerve trunks) — Brain stem

The spinal cord

The spinal cord is made up of numerous bundles of nerve fibers carrying messages to and from the brain. Connected to it and running throughout is the peripheral nervous system, which controls voluntary and involuntary actions. There are 12 pairs of such nerves radiating from the brain and 31 pairs from the spinal cord.

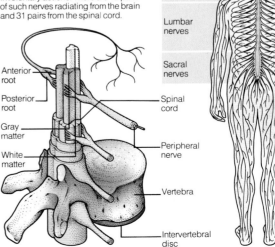

Anterior root — Posterior root — Gray matter — White matter — Brain — Spinal cord — Cervical nerves — Thoracic nerves — Lumbar nerves — Sacral nerves — Spinal cord — Peripheral nerve — Vertebra — Intervertebral disc

Symptoms

The symptoms of brain and nervous system disorders depend on the part of the system affected and may include pain, loss of sensation, and weakness. Brain disorders may cause a variety of psychological symptoms as well as physical symptoms, such as headache, drowsiness, confusion, or hallucination.

See also the following diagnostic charts: **63** Faintness and fainting **64** Headache **65** Dizziness **66** Numbness or tingling **67** Twitching and trembling **68** Pain in the face **69** Forgetfulness and confusion **70** Difficulty speaking **72** Depression **107** Back pain

The senses

The senses are the means by which we monitor our environment. Five separate systems receive different types of stimuli: the eyes; the ears (sound and balance); the nose; the tongue; and the sensory nerves in the skin (touch), which allow us to feel pain and changes in temperature.

The eyes

The instruments of sight are the eyes, which begin in the embryo as two "buds" from the brain. It is in the brain that nerve impulses from images recorded by the eyes are decoded to allow vision. The eye has six separate muscles that swivel it to look at objects in different directions. Normal vision depends on the refractive, or light-bending, power of the lens and cornea. Light rays entering the eye focus on the retina, forming the image the brain interprets.

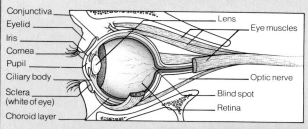

Conjunctiva
Eyelid
Iris
Cornea
Pupil
Ciliary body
Sclera (white of eye)
Choroid layer
Lens
Eye muscles
Optic nerve
Blind spot
Retina

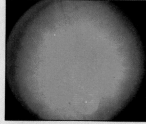

Ophthalmoscopic view of the retina
Vision results from the stimulation of nerve cells in the retina, signaling patterns of light intensity and color that are decoded by the brain. In the photograph at right, the pale disc is the optic disc, where all the nerves come together and leave the eye on the way to the brain. The retinal blood vessels can be seen radiating from the disc.

The ears

The ears, involved not only with hearing but with posture and balance, consist of an outer, middle, and inner part. The outer ear includes the visible, external flap of skin and cartilage, and the auditory canal. The canal is protected by hairs and sweat glands that secrete wax to trap foreign particles. The middle ear, behind the eardrum, contains the three smallest bones in the body—the hammer, anvil, and stirrup—which link the eardrum to the inner ear. The inner ear contains the cochlea (the organ of hearing) and the organs of balance. Vibrations from the eardrum are converted to nerve impulses that the brain perceives as sound.

The pinna (earflap) not only protects the ear but acts as a directional range finder, channeling sound toward the eardrum.

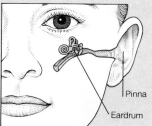

Pinna
Eardrum

Symptoms

The main symptom of any disorder of the senses is partial or total loss of sensation. There may also be pain or other symptoms affecting the sensory organ concerned.

See also the following diagnostic charts: **65** Dizziness
66 Numbness or tingling
80 Painful or irritated eye
81 Disturbed or impaired vision
82 Earache   **83** Noises in the ear
84 Deafness

Smell

Odors are detected by the olfactory nerves. These hairlike organs project into the top of the nasal cavity and absorb and analyze molecules from the inhaled air. The sense of smell may be damaged by smoking or temporarily impaired by colds or allergies. Permanent loss of smell may occur following nerve damage, sometimes as a result of a skull fracture, or may be caused by a disorder affecting the part of the brain that interprets smell sensations.

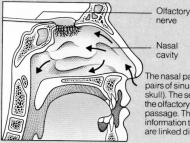

Olfactory nerve
Nasal cavity

The nasal passage is linked to several pairs of sinuses (air-filled cavities in the skull). The sensitive hairlike endings of the olfactory nerves project into the nasal passage. They detect odors and pass the information to the olfactory bulbs, which are linked directly to the brain.

Taste

The main taste organs are the taste buds, which are located in hairlike papillae that project from the upper surface of the tongue. They can distinguish four basic tastes: sweet, sour, salt, and bitter. Specific areas on the tongue detect particular tastes. The sense of taste is associated with the sense of smell, which helps us to differentiate a greater range of flavors. Loss of the sense of smell is the most common cause of an impaired sense of taste, but certain drugs and, occasionally, a deficiency in zinc or vitamin A may have the same effect.

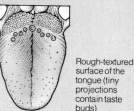

Rough-textured surface of the tongue (tiny projections contain taste buds)

The tongue
The taste buds for each taste are located on a specific area of the tongue. Bitterness is at the back, sourness at the sides, saltiness at the front, and sweetness at the tip.

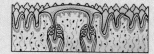

Touch

The sense of touch, which includes all skin sensations, is conveyed through nerves from receptors that lie under the surface of the skin. A different type of receptor is responsible for monitoring each of the main sensations. The number of receptors varies from one part of the body to another. The fingertips and the area around the mouth have a large number of receptors, whereas the skin of the middle back has very few. The sense of touch may be impaired by damage to the skin's nerve endings following an injury, by any disease that damages nerve fibers, or by a condition affecting the brain and/or nervous system.

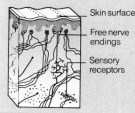

Skin surface
Free nerve endings
Sensory receptors

The sensation of touch is associated with a specific type of receptor embedded at various levels within the skin. Free nerve endings respond to gentle pressure and moderate heat and cold. Enclosed nerve endings register pressure and others respond to vibration and stretch. Thermal receptors respond to sensations of heat and cold, signaling the hypothalamus in the brain to adjust body temperature.

The digestive system

The system of organs responsible for carrying out the digestive process is known as the digestive tract. This tract, which extends from the mouth to the anus, breaks down food so that minerals, vitamins, carbohydrates, fats, and proteins can be absorbed into the body.

The mouth
Digestion begins in the mouth when, as food is chewed, enzymes in the saliva break down certain carbohydrates. The tongue and the muscles of the pharynx propel the mixture of food and saliva, known as the bolus, into the esophagus and down into the stomach.

The digestive organs

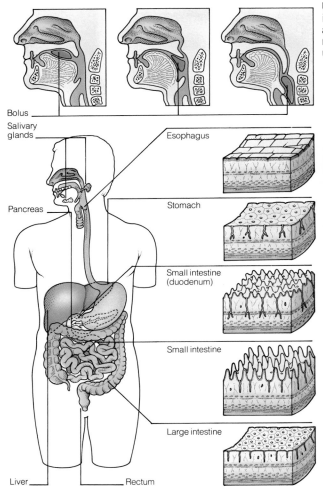

Bolus
Salivary glands
Esophagus
Pancreas
Stomach
Small intestine (duodenum)
Small intestine
Large intestine
Liver
Rectum

The stomach and duodenum
Food spends from 30 minutes to an hour or two in the stomach, being churned and partially digested by acid and enzymes, until it becomes a semiliquid substance (called chyme), which then passes into the duodenum, the upper part of the small intestine. Here the chyme is broken down further by digestive juices from the liver and pancreas.

The small intestine
The final stage of digestion is completed by enzymes farther along in the small intestine, where nutrients are split into chemical units small enough to pass through the wall of the intestine into the network of blood vessels and lymphatics.

The large intestine
Undigested food in liquid form flows from the small intestine into the large intestine, where most of the water content is absorbed back into the body. The semisolid waste that remains moves down into the rectum, where it is briefly stored until it is released through the anus as feces.

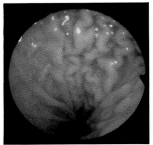

Endoscopic view of stomach
This photograph shows the lining of part of the stomach adjacent to the duodenum. Its circular muscles are partially contracted. See *Endoscopy*, page 201.

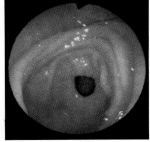

Endoscopic view of duodenum
This photograph shows characteristic circular folds of membrane that make up the surface of the duodenum.

The liver

The liver is the single largest internal organ in the body. It is dark reddish-brown and fills the upper right-hand part of the abdomen behind the lower ribs. The nutrients extracted from food by the digestive system are carried through the portal vein to the liver. The liver plays a vital role in regulating the composition of the blood and other essential chemical reactions in the body. Its functions include the production and storage of proteins, the storage of sugar and fats, the neutralization of substances toxic to the body, the breakdown of drugs, the manufacture of bile (a fluid that passes into the duodenum, where it helps to break down fatty food), and the manufacture and storage of red blood cell components.

Symptoms
The digestive system reacts quickly against irritants such as contaminated food, which may cause vomiting and/or diarrhea.

See also the following diagnostic charts: **56** Loss of weight

94 Vomiting **95** Recurrent vomiting **96** Abdominal pain **97** Recurrent abdominal pain **98** Swollen abdomen **99** Excess gas **100** Diarrhea **101** Constipation **102** Abnormal-looking bowel movements

Symptoms
Symptoms of a deteriorating liver may include loss of appetite, anemia, nausea, vomiting, and weight loss. There may be abdominal discomfort and indigestion. With extensive liver destruction, the legs and abdomen may fill with fluid and jaundice may

appear. The patient may become disoriented and confused.

See also the following diagnostic charts: **54** Feeling under the weather **55** Tiredness **56** Loss of weight **69** Forgetfulness and confusion **95** Recurrent vomiting **97** Recurrent abdominal pain

The lymphatic system

This system consists of the lymph nodes or glands (found mainly in the neck, armpits, and groin) and the small vessels, called the lymphatics, that connect the nodes. The lymph nodes contain lymphocytes, a type of white blood cell that defends the body against infection. The lymph nodes and the spleen act as barriers to the spread of infection by trapping any infection-carrying microbes that travel along the lymphatic vessels, preventing them from reaching vital organs. If you have an infection, the lymph nodes near the surface of the skin often become visibly swollen and sometimes painful.

The spleen

The spleen is, in effect, a large lymph gland involved in iron metabolism, blood cell storage, and the manufacture and destruction of blood cells. When red blood cells become old or defective, the spleen helps the liver filter them out of the bloodstream. The spleen also produces cells that help to destroy foreign bacteria.

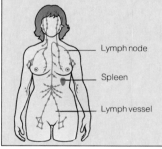

Lymph node

Spleen

Lymph vessel

Symptoms

In the majority of cases, swollen glands indicate that the lymphatic system is working normally – protecting your body against infection. In some cases, however, they may indicate a more serious underlying disorder.

See also the following diagnostic chart: **62** Lumps and swellings

The endocrine system

Endocrine glands manufacture hormones and distribute them to all parts of the body via the bloodstream. These hormones help to regulate the body's internal chemistry; its responses to hunger, stress, infection, and disease; and its preparation for physical activity. The hypothalamus (located in the brain) drives the pituitary gland to stimulate the other endocrine glands, thereby indirectly controlling many of the endocrine organs.

Hormone-producing glands

Pituitary gland

Thyroid and parathyroid glands

Adrenal glands

Pancreas

Ovaries

Testicles

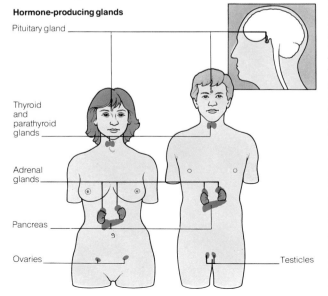

The pituitary gland

The pituitary gland is a peanut-sized organ situated just beneath the brain. The pituitary, often called the "master gland," stimulates and coordinates the functions of the other endocrine glands – the thyroid, the adrenals, and the ovaries or the testicles – so that they produce their own hormones. It also manufactures growth hormone and hormones to control the volume of urine, the contraction of the uterus during labor, and skin pigmentation.

The thyroid gland

This gland is located at the front of the throat, just below the Adam's apple. It is responsible for producing the hormones that control the body's metabolism (the conversion of food into energy) and it is the hormone that is involved in the metabolism of bone.

The parathyroid glands

These glands are situated behind the thyroid. The hormone they produce controls the levels of calcium and phosphorus, which are essential for healthy bones and for the efficient functioning of nerves and muscles.

The adrenal glands

The adrenal glands lie directly above the kidneys. Each adrenal consists of two parts – the cortex and the medulla – that have separate functions. The adrenal cortex produces steroid hormones, which help to regulate the amounts of sugar, salt, and water in the body, and influences the shape and distribution of body hair. The adrenal medulla produces epinephrine and norepinephrine, the hormones that increase the flow of blood to the muscles, heart, and lungs so that they are prepared to deal with excitement or stress.

The pancreas

The pancreas lies at the back of the abdomen, behind the stomach. It makes enzymes that pass down into the duodenum, the upper part of the small intestine, where they help to digest food. The pancreas also produces the hormones insulin and glucagon, which play an important part in regulating the glucose level in the blood. Glucose is the main source of energy for all the body's cells, and insulin stimulates the cells to absorb it in sufficient amounts.

The ovaries

Ovaries are endocrine glands that produce sex hormones (estrogen and progesterone) and ova (eggs). A woman is born with all the ova she will have – about 1 million ova at birth, decreasing to 40,000 at puberty. The ovaries are bean-shaped and about ½ inch long.

The testicles

The testicles are located in the pouch of skin known as the scrotum. The hormone they produce, testosterone, is responsible for the onset of puberty and the development of such characteristics as a deep voice and the male body shape and pattern of hair growth. It also influences developing sperm cells.

Symptoms

Disorders usually occur when the level of a particular hormone increases or decreases, upsetting the body's chemistry. Any disorder and the symptoms involved depend on which hormone is affected. For instance, if production of the hormone insulin is disrupted, the most common endocrine gland disorder, diabetes mellitus, may result. Changes in hormonal levels are also responsible for the physical changes in your body during puberty.

See also the following diagnostic charts: **55** Tiredness **56** Loss of weight **57** Overweight **60** Excessive sweating

The urinary system

The urinary system is responsible for filtering the blood and expelling the resulting waste fluid from the body. The organs of the urinary system consist of two kidneys, two ureters, the bladder, and the urethra (the tube through which urine passes out of the body). The male urethra is about 10 inches (25 cm) long and provides an outlet for semen as well as urine. In the female, the urethra is much shorter, about 1 inch (2.5 cm) long and lies just in front of the reproductive organs. Because of its close proximity to the anus and vagina, a woman's urinary tract is much more susceptible to infection.

How the urinary tract works

The kidneys are responsible for filtering waste substances from the blood. The filtered liquid passes into the central section of the kidney, where certain chemicals are reabsorbed to maintain the levels of acids, salts, and water in the body. The liquid that remains is urine. Urine passes down the ureters into the bladder, which is kept closed by a ring of muscles (called the urinary sphincter), and is then released periodically from the body through the urethra.

The urinary tract

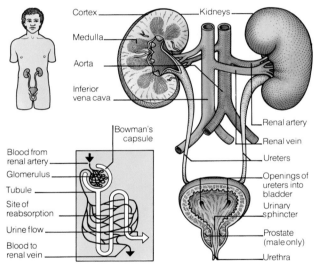

How the kidneys filter blood

Each kidney consists of millions of filtering units that are supplied with blood from the renal artery, via a cluster of minute blood vessels called glomeruli. Each cluster is surrounded by a cup-shaped organ called a Bowman's capsule, which is joined to the tubule. This is the point where the filtration takes place—filtered material is condensed to make a small amount of urine, which then passes through the tubules and down to the bladder.

Symptoms

Disorders of the urinary system are fairly common, caused in most cases by infection in or near the bladder. Infections usually enter the body via the urethra. Difficulty passing urine or any increase in the volume of urine passed may be a symptom of a more serious underlying disorder such as an obstruction. Pain when you urinate or discharge from the urethra may be caused by a sexually transmitted disease (for men, see page 238; for women, see page 262).

See also the following diagnostic charts: **104** General urinary problems **117** Painful urination **132** Painful urination

The male reproductive system

The male reproductive system is responsible for the manufacture and delivery of sperm. The organs of the reproductive system become fully developed at puberty (between the ages of 12 and 15). These organs are partly external (the scrotum containing the testicles, and the penis) and partly internal (the prostate and the organs that collect and store sperm).

Male urogenital organs

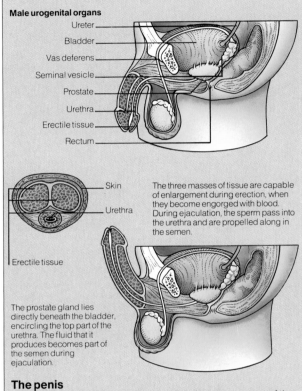

The three masses of tissue are capable of enlargement during erection, when they become engorged with blood. During ejaculation, the sperm pass into the urethra and are propelled along in the semen.

The prostate gland lies directly beneath the bladder, encircling the top part of the urethra. The fluid that it produces becomes part of the semen during ejaculation.

The penis

The penis is the organ through which the greater part of the urethra passes. Erection of the penis is usually caused by physical stimulation or sexual desire. The soft, spongy tissue becomes filled with blood, making the penis lengthen and stiffen. Also, partial erection may occur during sleep.

The testicles

The testicles, also known as the testes, produce the male hormone testosterone, and, with the help of this hormone, form sperm (see *Sperm production*, page 247). Testosterone is also responsible for the development of male genitals, for the growth of male facial and body hair, and for the deepening of the male voice.

Symptoms

Most disorders of the reproductive system affect the external organs. If you notice discharge from the urethra, this is likely to be caused by a sexually transmitted disease (page 238). Blood in the semen is usually the result of vigorous sexual activity, though in some cases it may be the result of a serious disorder, such as tuberculosis. Any swelling, with or without pain, or any change in the appearance of your testicles or penis is a sign of an underlying disorder.

See also the following diagnostic charts: **115** Painful or swollen testicles **116** Painful penis.

Breasts

The breasts, or mammary glands, produce milk to nourish a baby, and are also secondary sex characteristics. The layer of skin over the breast is smoother than elsewhere on the body. The skin of the nipple and its surrounding area (called the areola) is particularly thin and contains sweat glands and sebaceous (oil) glands. The nipple is cylindrical or conical in shape and responds to sexual arousal by becoming erect. Each of a woman's breasts consists of 15 to 20 groups of milk-producing glands embedded in fatty tissue. Milk ducts run from the gland through the core of the nipple, and open at the tip. During pregnancy, the release of specific hormones from the placenta and the pituitary gland causes the breasts to enlarge and produce milk.

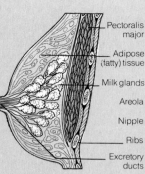
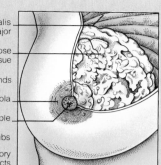

- Pectoralis major
- Adipose (fatty) tissue
- Milk glands
- Areola
- Nipple
- Ribs
- Excretory ducts

The breasts are supported by muscles, ligaments, and fatty tissue. The milk-producing glands are grouped into lobes, which radiate out from the nipple. In a girl of 10 or 11 years, the nipple begins to protrude while the areola around it swells outward. Glandular tissue and fat beneath increase rapidly and the areola flattens over the breast as it takes on a circular shape.

Breast development

The size and shape of a woman's breasts vary from one woman to another and at different times of life when female hormones are especially active, as during the menstrual cycle, pregnancy, and lactation. A fetus begins to develop breasts at about 5 months, and at birth there is a nipple with primitive milk ducts already present. The rush of hormones surging through the woman just before delivery sometimes affects the fetus as well, and the baby is born with slightly enlarged breasts that may even secrete milk in the first few days after birth. This discharge and the swelling quickly subside. As a young girl approaches adolescence, her body begins to develop the female shape and the breasts show the first signs of sexual development. The largest part of the breast is made up of glandular tissue supported in fat. The breast has no surrounding wall and merges with the fat underneath the skin. The breasts contain no muscle and exercise does not directly affect their size or shape.

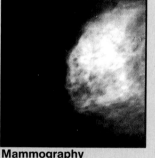

Mammography

Mammography, an X-ray procedure, produces a picture of the internal structures of the breast. Lumps and variations in consistency and increased density of breast tissue may be an indication of cancerous conditions. Every woman should have a mammogram done once between ages 35 and 40, every 1 to 2 years between 40 and 50, and annually after 50.

Symptoms

Lumps or swelling in the breasts should be examined by your doctor. Most growths are benign cysts or tumors. A malignant lump may or may not be painful and the skin over it may be dimpled or creased. Sometimes there is a dark discharge from the nipple.

See also the following diagnostic charts: **124** Breast problems **146** Breast-feeding problems

The female reproductive system

The organs of the female reproductive system include the two ovaries, each connected to the uterus by a fallopian tube, and the vagina, the passage that leads from the uterus to the external genitalia. Every month, one of the ovaries releases an egg into the fallopian tube. If the egg is fertilized, it embeds itself in the lining of the uterus. If the egg is not fertilized, it is shed, along with the lining of the uterus, during menstruation.

The external organs

The genitals consist of the mons pubis, the area of tissue and skin covered by pubic hair; the labia majora, two large lips of skin encircling the vaginal opening; the labia minora, two small lips of skin surrounding the clitoris inside the labia majora; and the clitoris, which is analogous to the male penis and is the most sensitive part of the genitalia, increasing in size and becoming erect during sexual arousal. This group of structures is known as the vulva.

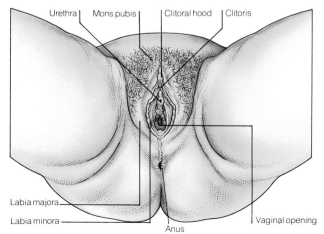

- Urethra
- Mons pubis
- Clitoral hood
- Clitoris
- Labia majora
- Labia minora
- Anus
- Vaginal opening

The internal organs

The internal reproductive organs in a woman—two ovaries and fallopian tubes, the uterus, cervix, and vagina—are surrounded by the bones of the pelvis. The uterus lies in the center of the pelvis, with the bladder in front and the rectum behind, and is supported in a double fold of elastic ligament.

The vagina, which is about 3 inches long, is the muscular passage between the uterus and the external genitals. The vagina allows blood to be shed during menstruation, allows entry of the penis during intercourse, and, during childbirth, provides a passage for the baby.

The cervix is a narrow, thick-walled structure, located in the lower front part of the uterus and leading to the top of the vagina. The inner part of the cervix is the opening between the uterus and the vagina.

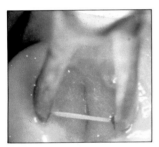

The opening of the cervix into the vagina is called the os. During a pelvic examination, the doctor checks the cervix and vaginal walls for any abnormalities. A sample from the cervix, called a Pap smear, is taken and sent to a laboratory where it is examined for signs of cancer or conditions that might lead to cancer. This procedure should be done every 1 to 3 years, or as your doctor recommends.

The uterus is a hollow, pear-shaped organ located at the front of the lower abdomen, behind the bladder. It is composed of powerful muscles, the strongest in the human body, which can accommodate a fully formed fetus, push it down the birth canal, and then return to original size within 6 weeks. The walls of the uterus are made of solid, smooth muscle lined with endometrium, the tissue that forms the site for implantation of the fertilized egg. If the egg is not fertilized, the thickened lining of the endometrium is shed during menstruation.

The fallopian tube is the site where the sperm meets the mature ovum (egg) shortly after ovulation. The tube is about 4 inches long and is funnel-shaped, ending in a fringe of fingerlike projections. The inner lining of the tube is covered by cells that help transport the ripe egg from the ovaries, along the tube, and into the uterus.

The ovaries are endocrine glands in the lower abdomen. They produce eggs and secrete the hormones estrogen and progesterone, which determine female characteristics and the pattern of menstruation. At birth, the ovaries contain all the ova a woman will ever have. Each ovary contains tens of thousands of eggs. During a woman's fertile years, one ovum ripens and is released into the fallopian tube each month; this is the process of ovulation. Fertilization of the egg released by the ovary is the beginning of pregnancy.

Cross section of an ovary

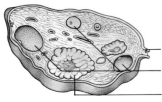

The egg ripens within a follicle inside the ovary. Halfway through the menstrual cycle the follicle ruptures, expelling the mature egg into the fallopian tube.

Ripening follicles

Corpus luteum

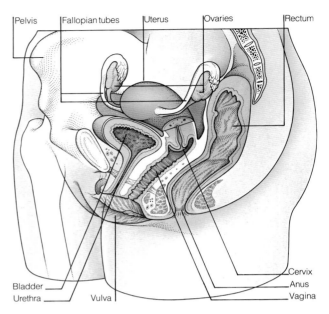

Pelvis | Fallopian tubes | Uterus | Ovaries | Rectum

Cervix
Anus
Vagina

Bladder
Urethra
Vulva

The menstrual cycle

The onset of the menstrual cycle (called the menarche) usually occurs in a girl between the ages of 11 and 14 years. The menstrual periods may be irregular for the first year or two as the process of ovulation becomes established. The entire cycle usually lasts about 28 days, but varies among women. Each stage in the menstrual cycle is regulated by a combination of hormones and chemicals produced in the hypothalamus of the brain, the pituitary gland, and the ovaries. During the days before ovulation, the hormones act to thicken the lining of the uterus, which becomes engorged with blood. If a fertilized egg reaches the uterus, the lining will be ready for implantation. If the egg is not fertilized, the thickened lining is not required and is shed about 14 days after the start of ovulation. After the age of about 45, periods become irregular and eventually cease altogether.

The month-long process of egg-ripening, egg release (ovulation), and shedding of the lining of the uterus is called the menstrual cycle.

During the few days prior to ovulation, the lining of the uterus is thickening and becoming engorged with blood. This prepares the uterus for implantation of a fertilized egg.

Each month one of the two ovaries releases an egg. The egg travels down the fallopian tube to the uterus. This part of the cycle takes 5 days.

A woman is fertile and can become pregnant anytime within a day or two before or after ovulation occurs.

Symptoms

The most common problems of the reproductive system are difficulties with menstrual periods, most often premenstrual tension and pain, irregular and heavy bleeding, or a change in the pattern of menstruation. Any change in the color or consistency of vaginal discharge is often a symptom of an infection in the vagina, uterus, or fallopian tubes. Problems can occur after menopause if the vaginal walls become dry and sore.

See also the following diagnostic charts: **125** Absent periods **126** Heavy periods **127** Painful periods **128** Irregular vaginal bleeding **129** Abnormal vaginal discharge **130** Genital irritation **134** Painful intercourse **137** Failure to conceive

Pregnancy

Pregnancy and childbirth involve unique changes in the physical and emotional chemistry of a woman. An understanding of how and why these changes occur and which symptoms are normal or abnormal can help ease concerns about what is happening to the body. If a woman is generally healthy, she should have little difficulty during pregnancy, although most women have some symptoms (such as nausea). If you think you might be pregnant, see your doctor for confirmation and arrange to have regular prenatal (before birth) checkups.

Your changing body
Several changes take place in the body during pregnancy. The most obvious is the absence of menstrual periods. Early in pregnancy nausea or vomiting ("morning sickness") may occur.

The breasts usually become enlarged, and a tingling sensation may be noticed in the nipples. The skin around the nipples may darken and the small lubricating glands in this area may become more prominent, creating small bumps.

The uterus is normally about the size and shape of a pear. In early pregnancy, as the uterus begins to grow, it presses on the bladder, causing a pregnant woman to feel the need to pass urine more frequently than usual. For the first 3 months of pregnancy, the size of the uterus does not change very much, but the enlargement becomes more noticeable in the fourth month. By the end of the fifth month, when the fetus is about 8 inches long, the increase in size becomes more rapid. By the end of the pregnancy, the total weight of the uterus, fetus, and amniotic fluid is about 16 pounds.

The skin also changes during pregnancy. The skin around the nipples and the upper part of the cheeks and forehead may darken. Some women have a dark line extending from the navel down to the pubic hair. This coloring should fade, but may not disappear altogether after delivery. Stretch marks may appear on the stomach, breasts, buttocks, and thighs, but these marks usually fade in time.

The teeth are affected by the high levels of progesterone produced during pregnancy, which cause the gums to become spongy and soft, inviting infection. Meticulous oral hygiene is essential during these months.

The joints become more pliant in pregnancy because the ligaments that bind them soften in response to hormonal action. This means that joints are more likely to stretch and ache, especially in the lower back and pelvis. Exercise, good posture, and well-fitting supportive shoes can relieve much of the discomfort.

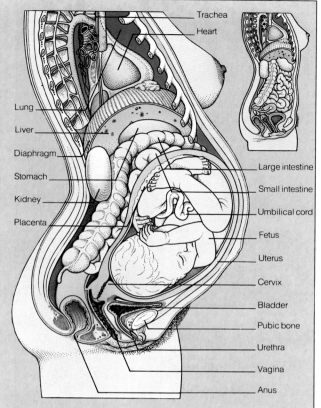

Trachea
Heart
Lung
Liver
Diaphragm
Stomach
Kidney
Placenta
Large intestine
Small intestine
Umbilical cord
Fetus
Uterus
Cervix
Bladder
Pubic bone
Urethra
Vagina
Anus

The vital functions
During pregnancy the heart must work harder to circulate blood through the uterus and placenta. The circulation to the breasts, kidneys, skin, and even gums also increases. During pregnancy the volume of blood increases by about 2½ pints and by the end of the second trimester the heart is working 40 percent harder to circulate the extra fluids around the body.

The lungs must also work harder during pregnancy to keep the increased volume of blood supplied with oxygen. Pressure on the lungs by the enlarging uterus may cause feelings of breathlessness, which is aggravated by the physical effort of carrying around the extra weight of the fetus and amniotic fluid. Breathing exercises may bring relief.

In early pregnancy the enlarging uterus may irritate the bladder, which may need emptying more often. In later pregnancy the pressure of the growing baby on the bladder also causes increased frequency of urination.

After childbirth
Hormonal effects on the muscles, which were essential for childbirth, may cause a new mother to tire easily. For this reason, it is essential to get sufficient rest in the days and weeks following the birth. It is quite common to feel depressed around the third or fourth day after childbirth when milk "comes in." This is a result of the action of hormones that stimulate the breasts to produce milk, which can cause emotional fluctuations as well. If depression worsens or lasts for more than 2 weeks, consult your doctor. (See also *Depression after childbirth*, chart 147.)

Symptoms
During pregnancy, sudden high levels of hormones may cause nausea and vomiting, as well as backaches as a result of softening of the ligaments that support the back. If a pregnant woman develops an unexplained rash with fever, German measles (rubella) is a possibility. Because the virus may damage the developing fetus, consult your doctor immediately (see Rash with fever, chart 79).

See also the following diagnostic charts: **55** Tiredness **138** Nausea and vomiting in pregnancy **139** Skin changes in pregnancy **140** Back pain in pregnancy **141** Heartburn in pregnancy **142** Vaginal bleeding in pregnancy **143** Shortness of breath in pregnancy **144** Ankle-swelling in pregnancy **145** Am I in labor? **146** Breast-feeding problems **147** Depression after childbirth

Keeping your child healthy

As a parent, you can help your child avoid many illnesses and health problems by providing a basic framework of good health care. This framework should consist of a well-balanced diet, plenty of exercise, reasonable safety precautions, and regular medical checkups. You can't always prevent your child from getting sick, but, if you follow the advice on this page, you'll provide your child with a foundation for good health that should help him or her recover from any illness. With your guidance and encouragement, your child can establish a pattern of healthy living for the rest of his or her life.

Eating a healthy diet
A child who eats a well-balanced diet that contains sufficient quantities of essential nutrients (see *The components of a healthy diet,* page 119) is likely to grow and develop at the expected rate and will be less susceptible to, and more likely to recover from, many of the minor illnesses of childhood. Children who establish good eating habits often continue them as adults.

Your main concern should be to provide your child with all the nutrients his or her body needs for healthy growth and day-to-day functioning. You can start by breast-feeding (see *Breast- and bottle-feeding,* page 61). As your child grows older, provide a balanced diet of a variety of nutritious foods, including poultry, fish, meat, beans and legumes, dairy products, whole-grain products (including breads and cereals), and fresh fruit and vegetables. Keep processed foods to a minimum and limit your child's consumption of sugary foods, which can lead to obesity and tooth decay, and foods high in salt and fat, which can contribute to illness later in life. Children under age 2 have different nutritional requirements from older children (for example, they require more fat and cholesterol in the foods they eat); your doctor can help you choose the right foods for your child's stage of development.

Children are notorious for their peculiar eating habits; a child may eat nothing but peanut butter sandwiches one day, nibble on nothing but fruit the next, and wolf down a perfectly balanced meal the third day. If you offer a highly nutritious selection of foods each day and don't force them on your child, the chances are good that, over the course of a week, he or she will get all the nutrition needed to grow and develop.

A good breakfast might be whole-grain cereal with milk (high in fiber and vitamins); a glass of orange juice (high in vitamins); whole-grain toast with margarine, jam, or fruit spread (high in fiber and carbohydrate; moderate in protein); and eggs (high in protein). A typical lunch might be a peanut butter sandwich on whole-grain bread (high in fiber; moderate in carbohydrate and protein); a vegetable (high in fiber and vitamins); low-sugar, low-fat oatmeal cookies (high in carbohydrate and fiber); and milk (high in protein and vitamins). A typical dinner might consist of a baked potato with grated low-fat cheese (high in protein and carbohydrate; medium in fiber and vitamins); fish (high in protein); vegetables (high in fiber and vitamins); fresh fruit (high in fiber and vitamins); and milk (high in protein and vitamins).

Getting enough exercise
Exercise is essential for children. It helps them develop strong muscles and a healthy heart and lungs. Encourage your child to exercise. Give your baby a safe environment (see box below) so he or she can play freely on the floor. Take your toddler on frequent playground outings and walks; don't confine him or her to the stroller. Many children develop sedentary life-styles from watching television all day; encourage your older children to spend more time outdoors in active play. Organized sports are fine, but any activity that gets your child up and running is a good choice. What's most important is to find activities your child enjoys. Better yet, make exercise something the whole family can enjoy.

Preventive medical care
Every child should be taken to visit the doctor for regular checkups. These visits will give you the opportunity to discuss your child's progress and any matters of concern, and will ensure that minor problems are noticed before they become more serious.

The most important element in preventive medical care for your child is immunization against a range of infectious diseases (see *Immunization,* page 97). Immunization must be part of your child's regular health care program. Your doctor can advise you on an appropriate immunization schedule.

Preventing accidents

Accidents are a common cause of injury and death in children and account for a high proportion of visits to the emergency room. You can prevent many accidents by taking steps to ensure that your child's environment is safe. The following checklist offers some basic precautions.

- Take a course in child safety and infant cardiopulmonary resuscitation (CPR). Your local Red Cross can supply information.
- Keep all medicines, dangerous chemicals, and sharp objects out of reach.
- Post the numbers of your doctor, fire department, and the nearest poison control center. Keep a bottle of syrup of ipecac (which induces vomiting) on hand, but do not use it without first consulting the poison control center. Be aware that even common house plants such as philodendrons and poinsettias can be poisonous if swallowed; keep such plants out of reach.
- Crawl around the floor to get an infant's-eye view of your home; remove any small objects your child could swallow accidentally, pad all sharp corners, and secure any wobbly bookshelves or tables. Secure the cords of any blinds so that they don't dangle.
- Put nonskid stickers on the bottom of the tub.
- Turn all pot handles in on the stove and use the back burners. Teach your child the meaning of "hot."
- Put childproof plastic covers on all exposed electric sockets. Make sure no electrical cords dangle from appliances.
- Install safety latches on drawers, doors, and toilet lids.
- Throw away plastic bags or store them in a safe place to prevent suffocation. Lock or remove the doors from unused major appliances such as refrigerators.
- Put safety gates at the bottom and top of stairs.
- Place stickers on any clear glass at your child's eye level to make the glass easily visible.
- Place your child in an approved car seat *every time* you ride in the car.
- Teach your child safety rules for crossing the street.
- Make sure your child wears a safety helmet when riding a bicycle. Check his or her bicycle to make sure that brakes, tires, and lights are in good condition. Helmets, kneepads, and wrist guards should be mandatory when your child is skating or skateboarding.
- Teach your child to swim.
- Teach your child fire safety rules.

Safeguarding your health

Your health and susceptibility to disease are determined partly by your life-style and partly by inherited factors. Whether or not you come from a long-lived, healthy family, reducing the risk factors in your life—by improving your diet, reducing your alcohol intake, giving up smoking, and getting more exercise—can help keep you physically fit and prevent disease. You can improve your physical well-being at any age by adopting a healthier life-style according to the guidelines described below.

Exercise

To be physically fit, a person must exercise regularly. Exercise helps the body in three ways: it maintains mobility and body strength and conditions the heart and lungs. Physical activity makes you breathe more deeply to get oxygen into your lungs, and your heart beats faster to pump blood to the muscles. There are many health benefits from exercise (see *Fitness and exercise,* page 36); the more activities you undertake that involve a high degree of physical exertion, the greater the benefit. Exercise will also help you lose weight, if combined with a sensible diet (see *How to lose weight,* page 151). It will boost the number of calories you burn and tone up muscles. Exercise also helps regulate your appetite.

Weight

Being overweight (see the weight chart on pages 302 and 303) is dangerous for your health. It increases the risk of serious disorders, such as diabetes and high blood pressure and related conditions (such as heart disease and stroke), and exacerbates the symptoms of many other disorders. Most people can achieve and maintain an ideal weight if they follow a sensible weight loss diet (see *How to lose weight,* page 151). It is far easier to prevent yourself from becoming overweight by eating a healthy, balanced diet and exercising; adjusting the quality and quantity of what you eat can prevent weight gain. (See *Age and increasing weight,* page 150.)

Smoking and alcohol

If you smoke, quit. Smoking is the main cause of many serious illnesses (see *The dangers of smoking,* page 196), including lung cancer and diseases of the heart and circulation. If you smoke regularly, you are probably reducing your life expectancy by about 5 minutes with each cigarette you smoke. By giving up smoking, your chances of having tobacco-related diseases lessen with each successive year. Smoking often accompanies the use of alcohol, a drug that can damage your health. You may be putting your health at serious risk if you regularly drink excessive amounts of alcohol (see *The effects of alcohol,* page 146) even if drinking never becomes an addiction. For example, you may risk obesity, high blood pressure, and cirrhosis (damage to the liver). Even moderate amounts of alcohol can adversely affect your health. The action of alcohol on the body and mind depends on the concentration of alcohol in the blood, and so varies from person to person. Men tend to feel the effects of the same amount of alcohol slightly later than women, in part because women have less of the stomach enzymes that break down alcohol. Factors such as the type of alcoholic beverage you drink and the speed at which you drink also affect the action of alcohol.

Diet

Diet plays a fundamental part in determining general health. In order to function efficiently, your body needs adequate amounts of each of the various nutrients included in the table below. It is important that you avoid eating too many processed foods, which are not high in nutrients but are high in calories. An excessive amount of refined carbohydrates in the form of white flour foodstuffs and simple sugars has been linked with obesity and a variety of diseases related to obesity. Eating too much fat has been related to heart and arterial disease. People whose diets are extremely high in fats and sugars may have elevated levels of blood cholesterol and triglyceride, the two blood fats that have been linked with obstructed blood flow and hardening of the arteries that lead to the heart.

Proteins	Carbohydrates
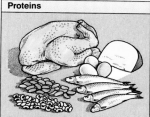	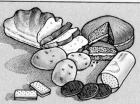
Proteins are needed for growth, repair, and replacement of body tissues. Proteins are found in legumes (such as beans, lentils, or peas) and cereals, as well as in meat, fish, and dairy products. **Diet advice:** Try to avoid eating too much beef, lamb, and pork, which have higher fat contents. Instead, eat skinless poultry, fish, and vegetable protein sources such as legumes, nuts, and grains.	Carbohydrates are a major source of energy, but eaten in excess they are stored in the body as fat. They are available as natural sugars and starches present in cereals, grains, and root vegetables. **Diet advice:** Eat unrefined products such as whole-grain bread and brown rice, which also contain fiber and other nutrients, and green and yellow vegetables and potatoes. Avoid eating white bread and refined cereals, which have few nutrients.

Fats	Fiber
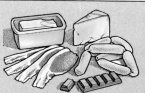	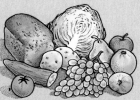
Fats are a concentrated source of energy that provide more calories than any other food. Saturated fats are found mainly in animal products, dairy products, and eggs. Monounsaturated fats are most commonly found in poultry, margarine, and olive oil. Polyunsaturated fats are found in fish, corn oil, and safflower oil. **Diet advice:** Intake of saturated fats should be kept to a minimum.	Fiber is the indigestible residue of plant products that passes through the digestive system. **Diet advice:** While fiber contains no energy value or nutrients, it is important for regular bowel movements, because it adds bulk to the stools.

Minerals	Vitamins
Minerals and certain salts are needed in minimal quantities. These include iron, potassium, calcium, and sodium, which is found in salt. **Diet advice:** Too much salt in the diet may be harmful for some people.	Vitamins are complex chemical compounds needed in small quantities by the body to regulate metabolism and to help with the conversion of carbohydrates and fats into energy. **Diet advice:** Vitamins may be destroyed by lengthy cooking, so eat steamed or raw vegetables and fruit regularly.

Fitness and exercise

Regular exercise benefits your health. You will sleep better, wake more refreshed, feel more alert, and be able to concentrate much longer. Exercising regularly will help you control your weight (see *Exercise and weight loss,* page 149) and help you build up your stamina—your staying power and endurance—which will in turn improve your physical and mental capacity for everyday activities. Research has shown that regular strenuous physical activity can help prevent and alleviate minor depression. There is evidence that regular weight-bearing exercise, such as walking briskly, can help delay the process of bone thinning (osteoporosis), a disorder common in postmenopausal women.

The benefits of exercise
Regular exercise has also been shown to help prevent coronary artery disease.

Heart, lungs, and arteries: Regular, vigorous activity will increase the strength and resiliency of the heart and lungs, helping them to become more efficient and less prone to disease. Exercise may also decrease blood pressure, thereby reducing the risk of hardening of the arteries. Research has linked vigorous activity with an increase in high-density cholesterol in the blood, which interferes with fat deposition in the arteries.

Joints: Regular exercise will maintain the strength and flexibility of your joints. Underuse contributes to stiffening and weakness of the ligaments that support and protect the joints. Your muscles will also become weak and flabby with lack of use.

Muscles: Exercise increases muscle tone, thereby conditioning the entire body. Exercise of a muscle or muscle group leads to increase in the size, strength, and number of muscle cells and the strength of their attachment to bones.

Your exercise routine

Three 20-minute sessions a week at regular intervals will put you on the road to fitness and well-being. Choose a moderate level of activity; you should never exert yourself to the point where you feel dizzy or faint. It is important to find an activity that you enjoy, or you may lack the motivation to continue your exercise routine over a period of time.

Sensible precautions
If you are thinking of starting a new sport or other form of exercise training, and if you are not accustomed to regular exercise, remember the following points:

- Do not be overambitious at first in the goals you set for yourself; it is safer to try to increase your level of fitness gradually.
- Make sure that your clothing and equipment are suitable.
- Always do some warm-up exercises (see right) before each session, to reduce the likelihood of sprains and strains.
- If any exercise or movement becomes painful, stop at once. Pain is a sign of damage.

Warning

Consult your doctor before starting any exercise activity for the first time if you are in any of the following categories:

- If you are over 60 years of age, or if you are over 40 and have not exercised regularly since reaching adulthood.
- If you are a heavy smoker (i.e., you smoke more than 20 cigarettes a day).
- If you are overweight (see the weight chart on pages 302 and 303).
- If you are under a doctor's care for a long-term health problem, such as high blood pressure, heart disease, diabetes, or kidney disease.
- If you are pregnant.

Warm-up exercises

You can reduce the risk of pulled muscles and torn ligaments by doing some gentle exercises to stretch and loosen the muscles and ligaments before you begin your exercise routine. Repeat the exercises described here for about 15 minutes before each exercise session, and for 5 minutes afterward.

(1) Head and neck
Slowly roll your head in a full circle, bending your neck backward at the back of the circle and flexing it forward at the front. Try to relax the muscles in your forehead as well as the shoulder muscles while gently rotating your head.

(2) Shoulders and chest
Extend both arms in front of you. Lift them above your head, placing the palms together. Keeping your arms straight, lower them toward your sides, holding them at shoulder height.

(3) Backs of the legs
Stand with your feet wide apart and hands on hips. Lean forward, bending at the hips and keeping your back straight. Lower your arms toward the floor in front.

(4) Trunk
Stand with your feet about shoulder-width apart and your arms by your sides. Bend sideways from the waist toward the right, allowing your right hand to slide down the leg to below the knee. Straighten up and do a similar bend to the left.

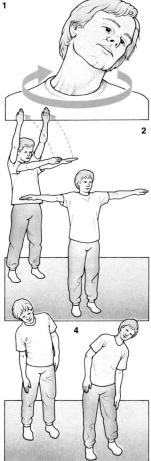
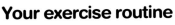
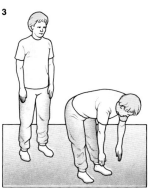

AIDS

The AIDS epidemic has spread rapidly throughout the world over the last decade, causing serious illness and death. The challenge of stemming the epidemic has become more complex, as more means of transmission have been discovered. Currently, there is no cure for AIDS.

What is AIDS?

AIDS is acquired immune deficiency syndrome, a serious condition in which the body's immune system is impaired and cannot protect the individual from a variety of severe infections.

AIDS is caused by the human immunodeficiency virus (HIV). A person who has HIV in his or her bloodstream is considered to be infected. Not everyone who is infected with HIV has AIDS, and it is not known what percentage of people with HIV will develop AIDS. However, it is thought that eventually, all or almost all of those infected will develop AIDS.

How does a person get HIV?

HIV is usually sexually transmitted. Most of the cases of HIV in this country were acquired through sexual contact (vaginal intercourse, anal intercourse, and, possibly, oral sex) with someone who was infected with HIV. The second major means of HIV transmission is the sharing of contaminated needles by intravenous drug users. One to 2 percent of the total number of reported cases have occurred in each of the following groups: blood transfusion recipients, hemophiliacs (who acquired the disease from contaminated infusions of clotting factor, a protein derived from blood), and babies born to women who were infected at the time of childbirth. Since 1985, the nation's blood supply has been screened for HIV. The chance of getting HIV today from a blood transfusion or an infusion of clotting factor is extremely small.

How common is AIDS?

As of June 1991, there were 179,694 reported cases of AIDS in the US; more than 114,300 people with AIDS had died. Current estimates are that at least 1 million Americans are HIV-infected. In the US, about 57 percent of people with AIDS are homosexual or bisexual men. More than 10 percent of all people with reported cases of AIDS are women. The number of cases of AIDS acquired from heterosexual contact has increased in the US.

The History of AIDS

AIDS probably began in Africa and was introduced in the US around 1959. In 1981, the Centers for Disease Control (CDC) in Atlanta, Georgia was alerted to reports of cases of a rare lung infection in previously healthy homosexual men in Los Angeles and then in New York.

A little later, cases of a rare tumor, Kaposi's sarcoma, were also reported in young homosexual men. Soon it appeared that there was a rapidly increasing epidemic of conditions associated with depression of the immune system. These conditions were observed not only in homosexuals but also in intravenous drug users and hemophiliacs, suggesting that transmission was related to blood as well as to sexual activity. An infective cause seemed likely and in 1983 French and American workers identified the virus responsible. In 1986 the virus was renamed HIV.

What are the symptoms of HIV infection?

Initial symptoms of HIV infection may include sore throat, fever, or lymph node swelling – similar to symptoms of mononucleosis. Later stages may involve persistent fever, weight loss, and diarrhea; neurologic changes such as dementia or nerve problems; infections that cause fever, severe pneumonia, and general sickness; and cancers of the lymphatic system, or a cancer of the skin and internal organs called Kaposi's sarcoma.

Could I be HIV-infected?

Currently, there is a two-part screening test for antibodies to HIV. However, a person can be infected for an unknown length of time – from 2 weeks to 6 months or more – before the body makes antibodies to the virus that can be detected by a test. People who think they may be infected with HIV should consult their doctors for testing and evaluation. Public health clinics and centers for people with AIDS also offer confidential testing.

How can I avoid getting AIDS?

Abstinence from sex and monogamy (having a long-term sexual relationship with one and only one person who is having sex only with you) are the most effective ways to avoid getting HIV. A person who has never had sex with an infected individual, has never used intravenous illicit drugs, and has never received a blood transfusion or hemophilia clotting factor therapy is extremely unlikely to get AIDS. People currently at high risk of HIV infection are homosexual men, heterosexuals who are having sexual intercourse with an infected person, intravenous drug users, and children born to infected women.

Safe sex is an important means of preventing the spread of HIV infection. Men must use condoms correctly so that HIV is less likely to be passed to or acquired from their partners. HIV can be transmitted during anal and vaginal sexual intercourse, and possibly also during oral sex. A man should put on a condom as soon as he gets an erection. After intercourse, he must withdraw his penis right away, holding the condom at the base so that no semen is spilled. A condom should never be reused.

Can my child get HIV from a classmate?

No child has ever contracted HIV infection from an infected classmate, and there is no medical reason for an HIV-infected child to stay out of school. HIV is acquired only from mixing of body fluids, as occurs during intimate sexual contact. Studies of families in which one person has HIV show that no family members have ever become infected from eating the same food, kissing, or sharing utensils with the person with HIV.

Can I get AIDS from my doctor?

Exceptional cases have been reported in which a patient appears to have acquired HIV from an infected doctor or dentist. These cases are being investigated. However, because HIV transmission requires intimate contact, and because health care workers take precautions such as washing their hands carefully and wearing gloves and masks, HIV transmission from a doctor, dentist, nurse, or other health care worker is extremely unlikely.

Is there a treatment for AIDS?

Reported cases of AIDS so far have all been fatal. However, effective treatment is available to delay the onset of AIDS, to treat AIDS-related infections, and to prolong the lives of people with AIDS. Experimental drugs are available to treat patients at all stages of infection. Vaccines to prevent AIDS are under study.

How to use the charts

The 147 charts in this book have been compiled to help you find probable reasons for your symptoms. Each chart shows in detail a single symptom—for instance, vomiting, headache, or a rash—and explores the possible causes by means of a logical series of questions, each answerable by a simple YES or NO. Your responses will lead you to a clearly worded end point, which suggests what may be wrong and offers advice on whether your disorder requires professional attention. To see how the charts work, examine the sample chart below and study the explanatory notes. Make sure you understand the meanings of the systematized action codes that indicate the relative urgency of the need to consult a doctor (see *What the instructions mean,* opposite page).

Note that every chart is numbered and has a title defining or describing the key symptom. An introductory paragraph provides further description and explanation of the purpose of the chart. Read this paragraph carefully to make sure you have chosen the most appropriate pathway toward an analysis of your problem; then proceed as indicated in the chart itself. Always begin with the first question and follow through to the end point that fits your special situation. In many cases, extensive boxed information accompanying the chart will enhance your understanding of specific diagnoses as well as likely treatment for underlying disorders. Always read through such information (except, of course, in emergencies, when swift action is essential).

It is important to consult the *correct* chart at the *correct* time. For instructions on how to recognize and define your symptom and how to choose the precise chart you need, turn to page 40.

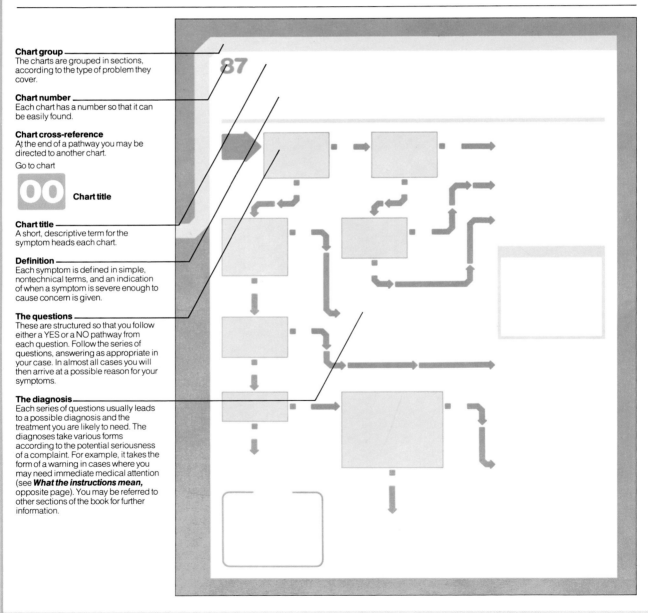

Chart group
The charts are grouped in sections, according to the type of problem they cover.

Chart number
Each chart has a number so that it can be easily found.

Chart cross-reference
At the end of a pathway you may be directed to another chart.

Go to chart

00 **Chart title**

Chart title
A short, descriptive term for the symptom heads each chart.

Definition
Each symptom is defined in simple, nontechnical terms, and an indication of when a symptom is severe enough to cause concern is given.

The questions
These are structured so that you follow either a YES or a NO pathway from each question. Follow the series of questions, answering as appropriate in your case. In almost all cases you will then arrive at a possible reason for your symptoms.

The diagnosis
Each series of questions usually leads to a possible diagnosis and the treatment you are likely to need. The diagnoses take various forms according to the potential seriousness of a complaint. For example, it takes the form of a warning in cases where you may need immediate medical attention (see *What the instructions mean,* opposite page). You may be referred to other sections of the book for further information.

WARNING: Though self-treatment is recommended for many minor disorders, remember that the charts provide only likely diagnoses. If you have any doubt about the diagnosis or treatment of any symptom, always consult your doctor.

What the instructions mean

EMERGENCY
GET MEDICAL HELP NOW!

The condition may threaten life or lead to permanent disability if not given immediate medical attention. Get medical help by the fastest means possible, usually by calling the local emergency response system (often 911). Depending on the level of care available in your area, it may be faster to take the person to the hospital yourself.

CALL YOUR DOCTOR NOW!

There is a possibility of a serious condition that may warrant immediate treatment and perhaps hospital admission. Seek medical advice immediately – day or night – usually by telephoning your doctor, who will then decide on further action. If you are unable to make contact with your doctor within an hour or so, emergency action (left) may be justified.

CONSULT YOUR DOCTOR WITHOUT DELAY!

The condition is serious and needs urgent medical assessment, but a few hours' delay in seeking treatment is not critical. Seek your doctor's advice within 24 hours.

Consult your doctor

A condition for which medical treatment is advisable, but for which reasonable delay is unlikely to lead to problems. Seek medical advice as soon as practical.

Discuss with your doctor

The condition is not urgent and the need for specific treatment is unlikely. However, your doctor's advice may be helpful. Seek medical advice as soon as practical.

Boxed information

On most charts there are boxes containing important additional information to expand on either a diagnosis or a form of treatment. See the information and self-help boxes below.

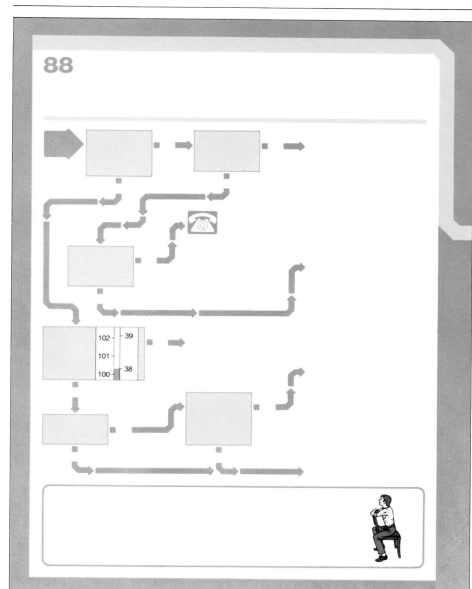

WARNING

Symptoms that indicate an immediate danger to life are highlighted in these boxes. Where appropriate, steps that can be taken while waiting for medical help to arrive are explained.

FIRST AID

Where symptoms may require either simple first-aid or lifesaving measures, you will find boxed information on what action you should take.

INFORMATION

These boxes expand on the possible diagnoses and likely forms of treatment for specific symptoms. For example, several of the boxes contain an explanation of a particular medical procedure. Where applicable, self-help treatment is included.

SELF-HELP

Where self-help measures may be effective in dealing with a symptom, advice is given on ways in which you may alleviate the problem.

How to find the chart you need

There are three ways of finding the appropriate chart for your symptom. You can use the *Pain-site map,* the *System-by-system* chartfinder, or the *Chart index,* depending on the nature of the symptom and where it is located. Whichever method you choose to find the correct chart, you will be given the title of the appropriate charts and its number.

1 Pain-site map

If you or a child is in pain, the quickest way to find the correct chart is by reference to the pain-site map for children (below), men (page 43), or women (page 46).

2 System-by-system chartfinder

If you know the body system affected but are unsure how to define the symptom, consult the system-by-system chartfinder for children (opposite page), men (page 44), or women (page 47).

3 Chart index

When you have no difficulty naming the symptom, consult the chart index for children (page 42), men (page 45), or women (page 48). If you or someone else has more than one symptom at the same time, concentrate on the symptom that causes the most distress.

1 Children's pain-site map

Consult this section to find the correct diagnostic chart for your child's symptom if he or she is suffering from pain in any part of the body. The illustrations below indicate possible areas of pain and are keyed in to the titles and numbers of the charts that deal with pain in that part of the body.

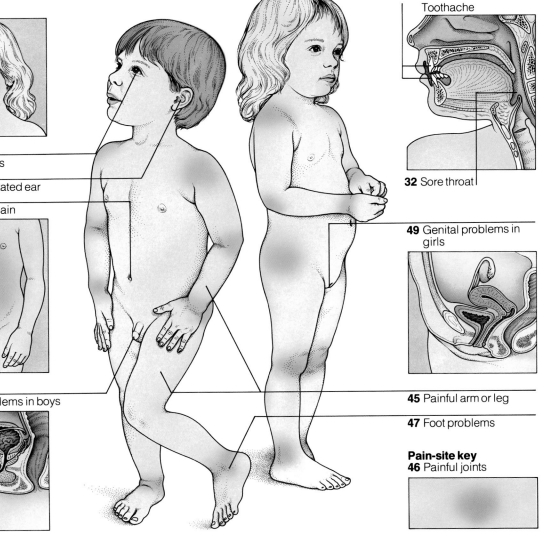

18 Headache

27 Eye problems

29 Painful or irritated ear

38 Abdominal pain

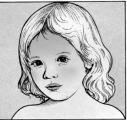

48 Genital problems in boys

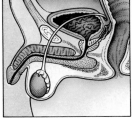

Toothache

32 Sore throat

49 Genital problems in girls

45 Painful arm or leg

47 Foot problems

Pain-site key
46 Painful joints

2 Children's system-by-system chartfinder

Consult this section if you know what part of the body or which body system your child's symptom originates in. A list of the charts that deal with each of the main body systems is given under each main heading. Select the chart that most closely seems to fit your child's symptom.

General symptoms

Babies under one
1 Slow weight gain
2 Waking at night
3 Fever in babies
5 Excessive crying
6 Feeding problems

Children: all ages
9 Feeling sick
10 Slow growth
11 Excessive weight gain
12 Sleeping problems
13 Drowsiness
14 Fever in children
15 Swollen glands

Adolescents
50 Delayed puberty
53 Adolescent weight
   problems

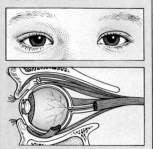

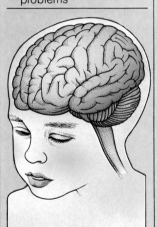

Head, brain, and psychological symptoms

Children: all ages
13 Drowsiness
17 Fainting, dizzy spells, and seizures
18 Headache
19 Clumsiness
20 Confusion
21 Speech difficulties
22 Behavior problems
23 School difficulties

Adolescents
51 Adolescent behavior problems
53 Adolescent weight problems

Eye and sight symptoms

27 Eye problems
28 Disturbed or impaired vision

Ear and hearing symptoms

29 Painful or irritated ear
30 Deafness

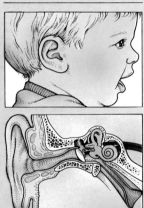

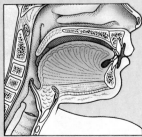

Mouth, tongue, and throat symptoms

32 Sore throat
36 Toothache

Skin, hair, and nail symptoms

Babies under one
4 Skin problems in babies

Children: all ages
16 Itching
25 Spots and rashes
26 Rash with fever

Adolescents
52 Adolescent skin problems

Muscle, bone, and joint symptoms

45 Painful arm or leg
46 Painful joints
47 Foot problems

Respiratory symptoms

31 Runny or stuffed-up nose
32 Sore throat
33 Coughing
34 Fast breathing
35 Noisy breathing

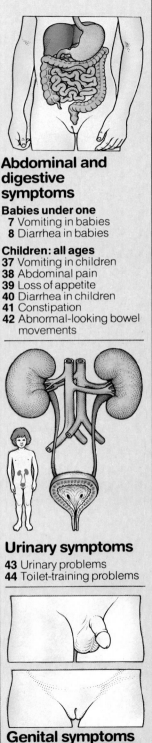

Abdominal and digestive symptoms

Babies under one
7 Vomiting in babies
8 Diarrhea in babies

Children: all ages
37 Vomiting in children
38 Abdominal pain
39 Loss of appetite
40 Diarrhea in children
41 Constipation
42 Abnormal-looking bowel movements

Urinary symptoms

43 Urinary problems
44 Toilet-training problems

Genital symptoms

48 Genital problems in boys
49 Genital problems in girls

3 Children's chart index

Consult this index if you think that you know the correct name for the symptom. The chart titles and their numbers are listed alphabetically, together with possible alternative names for symptoms (for example, *Raised temperature* for *Fever,* or *Swellings* for *Swollen glands*). In this section you will also find the titles of information boxes dealing with symptoms that do not have a separate chart.

A

Abdominal pain **38**
Abnormal-looking bowel movements **42**
Abnormal-looking urine **43**
Acne **52**
Adolescent behavior problems **51**
Adolescent skin problems **52**
Adolescent weight problems **53**
Aggressiveness **22**
Appetite, loss of, all ages **39**; adolescents **53**
Arm, painful **45**

B

Balance, loss of **17**
Behavior problems, all ages **22, 23**; adolescents **51**
Blackheads **52**
Blocked nose **31**
Blood in the bowel movements **42**
Boils **25**
Breathing, fast **34**; noisy **35**

C

Clumsiness **19**
Confusion **20**
Constipation **41**
Convulsions **17**
Coughing **33**
Crying, excessive **5**

D

Deafness **30**
Delayed puberty **50**
Destructiveness **22**
Diarrhea, babies **8**; all ages **40**
Disobedience **22**
Disturbed vision **28**
Dizzy spells **17**
Drooping eyelid **27**
Drowsiness **13**

E

Ear, painful or irritated **29**
Excessive crying **5**
Excessive weight gain, all ages **11**; adolescents **53**
Eye problems **27, 28**

F

Fainting **17**
Fast breathing **34**
Feces, abnormal-looking **42**
Feeding problems **6**
Feeling sick **9**
Fever, babies **3**; all ages **14**
Fever, rash with **26**
Feverish convulsions, babies **3**; all ages **14**
Foot problems **47**

G

Gas, babies **5**; all ages **38**
Genital problems, boys **48**; girls **49**
Glands, swollen **15**
Growth, slow **10**

H

Hair problems **24**
Headache **18**
Hearing difficulties **30**
High temperature, babies **3**; all ages **14**

I

Impaired vision **28**
Irritated ear **29**
Itching **16**

J

Joints, painful **46**

L

Late-rising in the morning **13**
Loss of appetite, all ages **39**; adolescents **53**
Loss of consciousness **17**
Leg, painful **45**
Lumps **15**

N

Nail problems **24**
Noisy breathing **35**
Nose, runny or blocked **31**

O

Overweight, all ages **11**; adolescents **53**

P

Painful arm **45**
Painful ear **29**
Painful joints **46**
Painful leg **45**
Puberty, delayed **50**

R

Raised temperature, babies **3**; all ages **14**
Rashes **25, 26**
Rash with fever **26**
Regurgitation **7**
Run down, feeling **9, 13**
Runny nose **31**

S

Scalp problems **24**
School difficulties **23**
Seizures **17**
Seizures, feverish, babies **3**; all ages **14**
Sight, disturbed or impaired **28**
Skin problems, babies **4**; adolescents **52**

L

Sleeping late **13**
Sleeping problems, babies **2**; all ages **12**
Slow growth **10**
Slow weight gain, babies **1**; adolescents **53**
Sore throat **32**
Speech difficulties **21**
Spots **25**
Squint **27, 28**
Stomachache **38**
Swellings **15**
Swollen glands **15**

T

Temperature, high, babies **3**; all ages **14**
Throat, sore **32**
Tiredness **13**
Toilet-training problems **44**
Toothache **36**

U

Urinary problems **43, 44**

V

Violence **22**
Vision, disturbed or impaired **28**
Vomiting, babies **7**; all ages **37**

W

Waking at night, babies **2**; all ages **12**
Warts **25**
Weight gain, excessive, all ages **11**; adolescents **53**
Weight loss, babies **1**; adolescents **53**
Weight gain, slow **1**
Withdrawal **22**

1 Men's pain-site map

Pain in any form, whether mild or severe, is the body's way of telling you that something is wrong. Pain may be referred (originating in one part of the body and felt in another) or localized at the site of an injury. In any case, pain that persists should never be ignored or masked through the indiscriminate use of pain-killing drugs. Consult this section to find the correct chart for your symptom if you have pain in any part of your body. The illustrations below indicate possible areas of pain and are keyed to the titles and numbers of the charts that deal with pain in that part of the body.

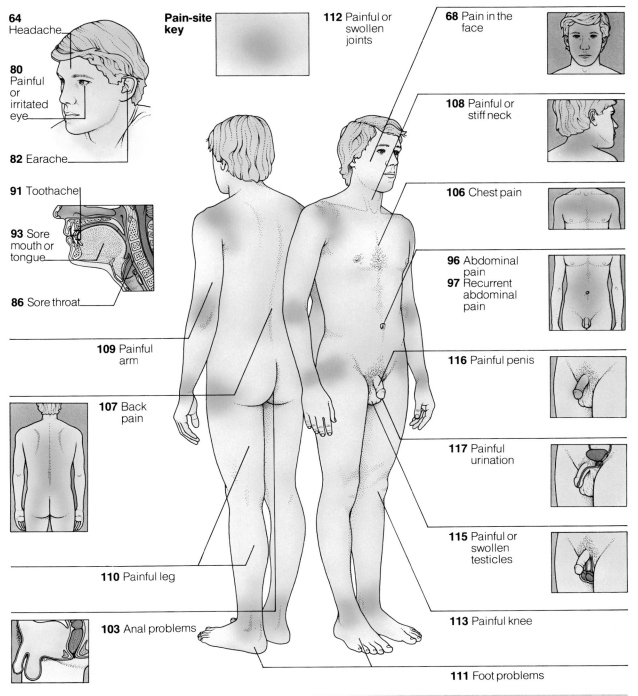

64 Headache

80 Painful or irritated eye

82 Earache

91 Toothache

93 Sore mouth or tongue

86 Sore throat

109 Painful arm

107 Back pain

110 Painful leg

103 Anal problems

Pain-site key

112 Painful or swollen joints

106 Chest pain

96 Abdominal pain
97 Recurrent abdominal pain

116 Painful penis

117 Painful urination

115 Painful or swollen testicles

113 Painful knee

111 Foot problems

68 Pain in the face

108 Painful or stiff neck

2 Men's system-by-system chartfinder

Consult this section if you know what part of the body or which body system your symptom originates in. A list of the charts that deal with each of the main body systems is given under each main heading. Select the chart that most closely seems to fit your symptom.

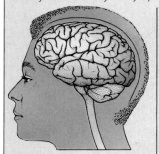

Head, brain, and psychological symptoms

63 Faintness and fainting
64 Headache
65 Dizziness
66 Numbness or tingling
67 Twitching and trembling
68 Pain in the face
69 Forgetfulness and confusion
70 Difficulty speaking
71 Disturbing thoughts and feelings
72 Depression
73 Anxiety

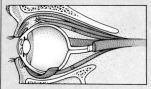

Eye and sight symptoms

80 Painful or irritated eye
81 Disturbed or impaired vision

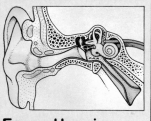

Ear and hearing symptoms

82 Earache
83 Noises in the ear
84 Deafness

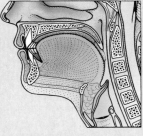

Mouth, tongue, and throat symptoms

86 Sore throat
91 Toothache
92 Difficulty swallowing
93 Sore mouth or tongue

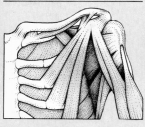

Muscle, bone, and joint symptoms

107 Back pain
108 Painful or stiff neck
109 Painful arm
110 Painful leg
111 Foot problems
112 Painful or swollen joints
113 Painful knee

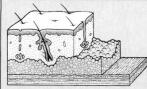

Skin, hair, and nail symptoms

60 Excessive sweating
61 Itching
62 Lumps and swellings
74 Hair and scalp problems
75 Nail problems
76 General skin problems
77 Spots and rashes
78 Raised spots or lumps
79 Rash with fever
114 Baldness

General symptoms

54 Feeling under the weather
55 Tiredness
56 Loss of weight
57 Overweight
58 Difficulty sleeping
59 Fever

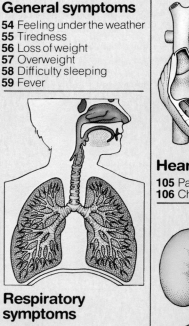

Respiratory symptoms

85 Runny nose
86 Sore throat
87 Hoarseness or loss of voice
88 Wheezing
89 Coughing
90 Difficulty breathing
106 Chest pain

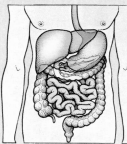

Abdominal and digestive symptoms

94 Vomiting
95 Recurrent vomiting
96 Abdominal pain
97 Recurrent abdominal pain
98 Swollen abdomen
99 Excess gas
100 Diarrhea
101 Constipation
102 Abnormal-looking bowel movements
103 Anal problems

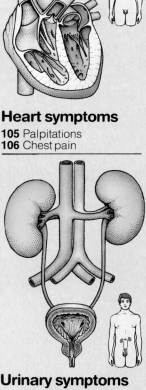

Heart symptoms

105 Palpitations
106 Chest pain

Urinary symptoms

104 General urinary problems
117 Painful urination

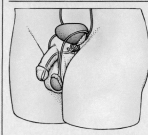

Genital symptoms

115 Painful or swollen testicles
116 Painful penis

Sexual symptoms

118 Erection difficulties
119 Premature ejaculation
120 Delayed ejaculation
121 Low sex drive
122 Fertility problems
123 Contraception

3 Men's chart index

Consult this index if you think that you know the correct name for your symptom. The chart titles and their numbers are listed alphabetically, together with possible alternative names for symptoms (for example, *Raised temperature* for *Fever*). In this section you will also find the titles of information boxes dealing with symptoms that do not have a separate chart.

A

Abdomen, swollen **98**
Abdominal pain **96;** recurrent **97**
Abnormal-looking bowel movements **102**
Abnormal-looking urine **117**
Abnormal thoughts **71**
Anal problems **103**
Anxiety **73**
Arm, painful **109**

B

Back pain **107**
Bad breath **93**
Baldness **114**
Blood, coughing up **89**
Blood in bowel movements **102**
Blood in semen **116**
Blood in vomit **94, 95**
Body odor **60**
Bowel, irritable **97**
Bowel movements, abnormal-looking **102;** blood in **102;** hard **101;** soft **100**
Breathlessness, **90**
Bruising **77**

C

Chest pain **106**
Confusion **69**
Constipation **101**
Contraception **123**
Coughing **89**
Coughing up blood **89**

D

Deafness **84**
Delayed ejaculation **120**
Depression **72**
Diarrhea **100**
Difficulty breathing **90**
Difficulty sleeping **58**
Difficulty speaking **70**
Difficulty swallowing **92**
Disturbed vision **81**
Disturbing thoughts and feelings **71**
Dizziness **65**
Drowsiness **55**

E

Ear, noises in the **83**
Earache **82**
Ejaculation, delayed **120;** premature **119**
Elbow, painful **109**
Erection difficulties **118**
Excess gas **98, 99**
Excess weight **57**
Excessive sweating **60**
Eye, painful or irritated **80**
Eye problems **80, 81**
Eyestrain **80**

F

Face, pain in the **68**
Fainting **63**
Faintness **63**
Feces, abnormal-looking **102;** blood in **102;** hard **101;** soft **100**
Feeling under the weather **54**
Feelings, disturbing **71**
Fertility problems **122**
Fever **59**
Fever, rash with **79**
Foot problems **111**
Forgetfulness **69**

G

Gas, excess **99**
General skin problems **76**
General urinary problems **104**

H

Hair problems **74, 114**
Headache **64**
Heart flutterings **105**
High temperature **59**
Hoarseness **87**

I

Impaired memory **69**
Impaired vision **81**
Irritable bowel **97**
Irritated eye **80**
Itching **61**

J

Joints, painful or swollen **112**

K

Knee, painful **113**

L

Leg, painful **110**
Loss of voice **87**
Loss of weight **56**
Low sex drive **121**
Lumps **62, 78**

M

Memory, impaired **69**
Mouth, sore **93**
Mumps and sterility **122**

N

Nail problems **75**
Nausea **94**
Neck, painful or stiff **108**
Noises in the ear **83**
Nose, runny **85**
Nosebleeds **85**
Numbness **66**

O

Overweight **57**

P

Painful arm **109**
Painful elbow **109**
Painful eye **80**
Painful joints **112**
Painful knee **113**
Painful leg **110**
Painful neck **108**
Painful penis **116**
Painful shoulder **109**
Painful testicles **115**
Painful urination **117**
Pain in the face **68**
Palpitations **105**
Panic attacks **73**
Penis, painful **116**
Premature ejaculation **119**

R

Raised lumps on the skin **78**
Raised spots on the skin **78**
Raised temperature **59**
Rash with fever **79**
Rashes **76, 77, 78**
Recurrent abdominal pain **97**
Recurrent vomiting **95**
Run down, feeling **54, 55**
Runny nose **85**

S

Scalp problems **74**
Sex drive, low **121**
Shoulder, painful **109**
Sickness **94, 95**
Skin problems, general **76**
Sleeping, difficulty **58**
Sore mouth **93**
Sore throat **86**
Sore tongue **93**
Speaking, difficulty **70**
Spots **76, 77, 78**
Stiff neck **108**
Stomach ache **96, 97**
Stress **73**
Swallowing, difficulty **92**
Sweating, excessive **60**
Swellings **62, 78, 115**
Swollen abdomen **98**
Swollen joints **112**
Swollen testicles **115**

T

Temperature, high **59**
Tension **73**
Testicles, painful or swollen **115**
Thoughts, disturbing **71**
Throat, sore **86**
Tingling **66**
Tiredness **55**
Tongue, sore **93**
Toothache **91**
Trembling **67**
Twitching **67**

U

Urinary problems **104**
Urination, painful **117**
Urine, abnormal-looking **117**

V

Varicose veins **110**
Vision, disturbed or impaired **81**
Voice, loss of **87**
Vomiting **94, 95;** recurrent **95**

W

Weight, excess **57;** loss of **56**
Wheezing **88**
Worrying **73**

1 Women's pain-site map

Pain in any form, whether mild or severe, is the body's way of telling you that something is wrong. Pain may be referred (originating in one part of the body and felt in another) or localized at the site of an injury. In any case, pain that persists should never be ignored or masked through the indiscriminate use of pain-killing drugs. Consult this section to find the correct chart for your symptom if you have pain in any part of your body. The illustrations below indicate possible areas of pain and are keyed to the titles and numbers of the charts that deal with pain in that part of the body.

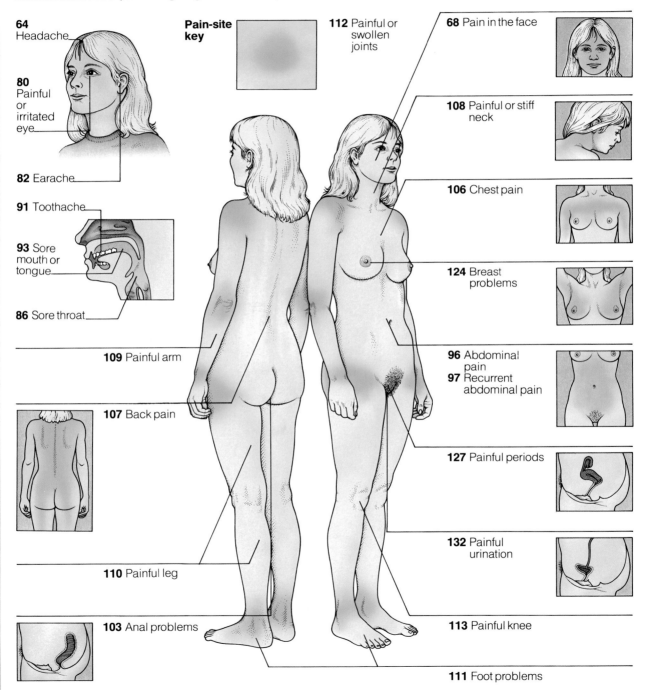

64 Headache

80 Painful or irritated eye

82 Earache

91 Toothache

93 Sore mouth or tongue

86 Sore throat

109 Painful arm

107 Back pain

110 Painful leg

103 Anal problems

Pain-site key

112 Painful or swollen joints

68 Pain in the face

108 Painful or stiff neck

106 Chest pain

124 Breast problems

96 Abdominal pain
97 Recurrent abdominal pain

127 Painful periods

132 Painful urination

113 Painful knee

111 Foot problems

2 Women's system-by-system chartfinder

Consult this section if you know what part of the body or which body system your symptom originates in. A list of the charts that deal with each of the main body systems is given under each main heading.

General symptoms

54 Feeling under the weather
55 Tiredness
56 Loss of weight
57 Overweight
58 Difficulty sleeping
59 Fever

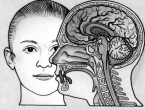

Head, brain, and psychological symptoms

63 Faintness and fainting
64 Headache
65 Dizziness
66 Numbness or tingling
67 Twitching and trembling
68 Pain in the face
69 Forgetfulness and confusion
70 Difficulty speaking
71 Disturbing thoughts and feelings
72 Depression
73 Anxiety
147 Depression after childbirth

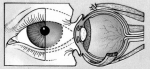

Eye and sight symptoms

80 Painful or irritated eye
81 Disturbed or impaired vision

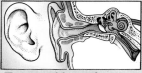

Ear and hearing symptoms

82 Earache
83 Noises in the ear
84 Deafness

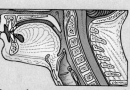

Mouth, tongue, and throat symptoms

86 Sore throat
91 Toothache
92 Difficulty swallowing
93 Sore mouth or tongue

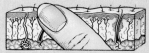

Skin, hair, and nail symptoms

60 Excessive sweating
61 Itching
62 Lumps and swellings
74 Hair and scalp problems
75 Nail problems
76 General skin problems
77 Spots and rashes
78 Raised spots or lumps on the skin
79 Rash with fever
139 Skin changes in pregnancy

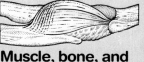

Muscle, bone, and joint symptoms

107 Back pain
108 Painful or stiff neck
109 Painful arm
110 Painful leg
111 Foot problems
112 Painful or swollen joints
113 Painful knee
144 Ankle-swelling in pregnancy

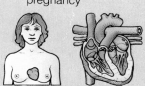

Heart symptoms

105 Palpitations
106 Chest pain

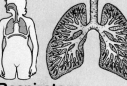

Respiratory symptoms

85 Runny nose
86 Sore throat
87 Hoarseness or loss of voice
88 Wheezing
89 Coughing
90 Difficulty breathing
106 Chest pain

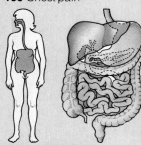

Abdominal and digestive symptoms

94 Vomiting
95 Recurrent vomiting
96 Abdominal pain
97 Recurrent abdominal pain
98 Swollen abdomen
99 Excess gas
100 Diarrhea
101 Constipation
102 Abnormal-looking bowel movements
103 Anal problems
138 Nausea and vomiting in pregnancy
141 Heartburn in pregnancy

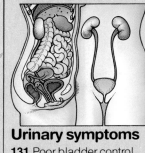

Urinary symptoms

131 Poor bladder control
132 Painful urination
133 Abnormally frequent urination

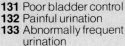

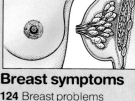

Breast symptoms

124 Breast problems
146 Breast-feeding problems

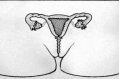

Gynecological symptoms

125 Absent periods
126 Heavy periods
127 Painful periods
128 Irregular vaginal bleeding
129 Abnormal vaginal discharge
130 Genital irritation

Sexual symptoms

134 Painful intercourse
135 Loss of interest in sex
136 Choosing a contraceptive method
137 Failure to conceive

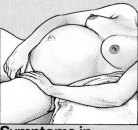

Symptoms in pregnancy

138 Nausea and vomiting in pregnancy
139 Skin changes in pregnancy
140 Back pain in pregnancy
141 Heartburn in pregnancy
142 Vaginal bleeding in pregnancy
143 Shortness of breath in pregnancy
144 Ankle-swelling in pregnancy
145 Am I in labor?
146 Breast-feeding problems
147 Depression after childbirth

Women's chart index

Consult this index if you think that you know the correct name for your symptom. The chart titles and their numbers are listed alphabetically, together with possible alternative names for symptoms (for example, *Raised temperature* for *Fever*). In this section you will also find the titles of information boxes within the charts.

1 Children's charts

Babies under one

All ages,

Adolescents,

1 Slow weight gain

It is important to keep a regular check on your baby's weight gain because failure to put on weight can be a sign of problems. Your baby is likely to be weighed whenever you visit your pediatrician, where any problems are likely to be noticed and dealt with. It is also a good idea for you to keep your own chart of your baby's progress so you can reassure yourself that your baby is developing normally. Using the growth charts below, compare your baby's weight gain and increase in head circumference as measured by your pediatrician with the average for babies of similar birth weight. Do not worry if your baby's progress does not exactly follow the curve shown; there can be many normal variations to this pattern (see Growth patterns in infancy, below). Only if you can find no normal explanation for your baby's failure to gain weight at the expected rate should you consult the diagnostic pathways on the facing page. Use the growth charts on pp. 298-299 to record your baby's length and weight.

For children over 1 year, see chart 10, Slow growth

GROWTH PATTERNS IN INFANCY

The growth charts on pp.298-299 allow you to record your baby's growth and to compare his or her progress with the standard weight gain for small, average and large babies. Most babies follow these standard curves, but there are many possible variations, most of which are quite normal. The charts on this page show some common examples of how your baby's growth may differ from the usual pattern. Remember that length, weight and head circumference are interrelated. When your pediatrician assesses the size of your baby, he or she is looking at the relationship among them. Above all, don't worry if your child appears to be growing slowly; consult your pediatrician.

Short mother and tall father
A short mother is likely to have a smaller-than-average baby. But, if the father is tall and the baby is ultimately going to take after him, the baby's growth chart is likely to show a rapid increase in both weight and head circumference in the first few months of life.

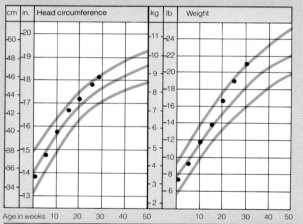

Tall mother and short father
A tall mother is likely to have a larger-than-average baby. However, if the father is short and the baby is going to take after him, the baby is likely to gain weight and increase his or her head circumference at a slower rate than normal for the first few months.

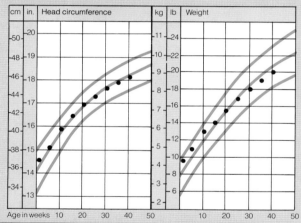

Gaining too little weight
This chart shows a baby who is gaining too little weight. The head is growing normally for an average-sized baby, but the weight gain curve is flattening out and approaching that for a small baby. In this case you should consult the diagnostic chart opposite.

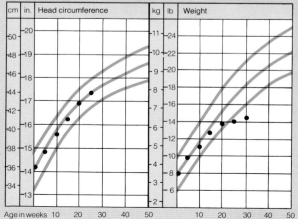

Gaining too much weight
This chart shows a baby who was of average weight at birth, but whose weight has consistently risen at a faster rate than his or her head circumference, so that the weight curve now relates to that of a larger-than-average baby (see chart 11, *Excessive weight gain*).

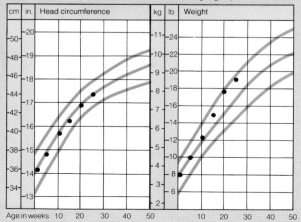

START HERE

Does your baby seem sick – for example, is he or she slow at feeding, lethargic or irritable?

YES →

An underlying illness may be causing your baby's slow weight gain. Consult your physician.

NO

Is your baby entirely breast-fed?

YES →

Do you offer to feed your baby whenever he or she cries?

YES →

Insufficient milk supply may mean that your baby is not getting enough nourishment. However, if your baby is over 3 months, he or she may be ready to start eating solid food. Discuss the problem with your physician or nurse, who may recommend adding bottles or advise you on weaning.

NO

Undernourishment may be the cause of slow weight gain.

Self-help: Crying is your baby's way of letting you know he or she is hungry. Imposing a strict feeding routine may prevent your baby from receiving the necessary amount of milk, and may also lead to a reduction in your milk supply (see *Breast- and bottle-feeding*, p. 61). So always offer to feed your baby whenever he or she cries, even if the baby sometimes refuses to feed. If your baby does not start to gain weight normally within 2 weeks, consult your physician.

NO

Is your baby entirely bottle-fed?

YES →

Do you offer to feed your baby whenever he or she cries?

YES →

Might you be adding too much water or too little liquid concentrate or milk powder when mixing the formula?

YES →

NO

Undernourishment may be the cause of slow weight gain.

Self-help: Crying is your baby's way of letting you know he or she is hungry. Imposing a strict feeding routine may prevent your baby from receiving the necessary amount of milk. So always offer to feed your baby whenever he or she cries, even if the baby sometimes refuses to feed. If your baby does not start to gain weight normally within 2 weeks, consult your physician.

NO

Does your baby always finish every drop of the formula?

YES →

NO

Overdilution of the formula may mean that your baby is not receiving adequate nourishment.

Self-help: Always follow the instructions on the container exactly when mixing your baby's formula. If you think your baby is thirsty, offer cooled, boiled water separately. If your baby does not start to gain weight normally within 2 weeks, consult your physician.

Consult your physician if you are unable to make a diagnosis from this chart.

Increasing appetite may mean that your baby needs more food than you are offering, even if you are giving the correct amount for your baby's age.

Self-help: Always offer more formula than you think necessary and let your baby feed until satisfied. If your baby is over 3 months, he or she may be ready to start eating solid food. If your baby does not start to gain weight normally within 2 weeks, or if you need advice on weaning, consult your physician.

WEIGHT LOSS IN THE NEWBORN

Most babies lose about 5 oz (150 g) in weight during the first week of life. This is perfectly normal and is not a sign that your breast-milk supply is inadequate or that your baby is underfed. Most babies start to put on weight again on the fifth day and have regained their birth weight by the time they are 10 days old. Thereafter weight gain should continue at a steady rate.

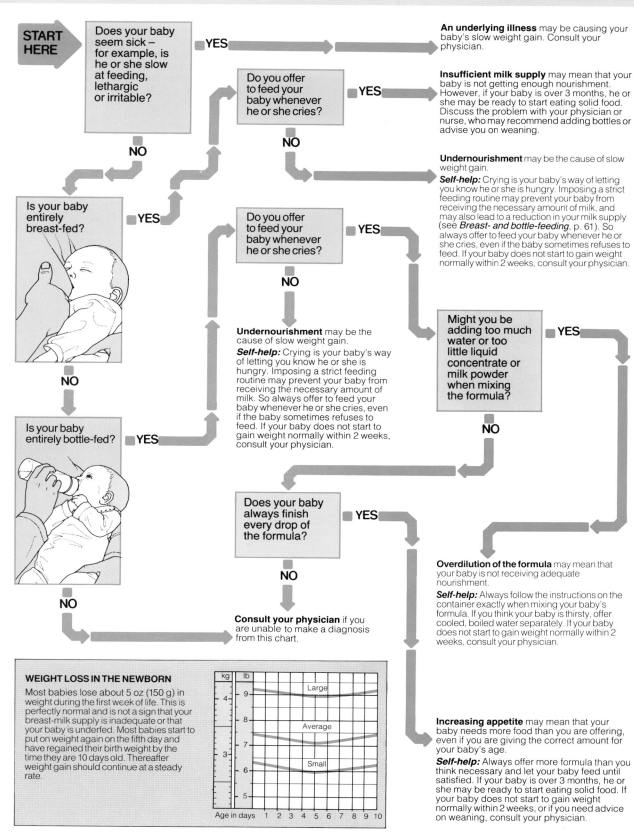

Large

Average

Small

Age in days 1 2 3 4 5 6 7 8 9 10

2 Waking at night

Most babies wake at regular intervals through the day and night for feedings during the first few months. Consult this chart only if you think your baby is waking more frequently than is normal for his or her age, if you **have difficulty settling your baby at night or if your baby who has previously slept well starts to wake during the night. Diaper rash can sometimes cause a baby to wake at night; see p. 57.**

For children over 1 year, see chart 12, Sleeping problems

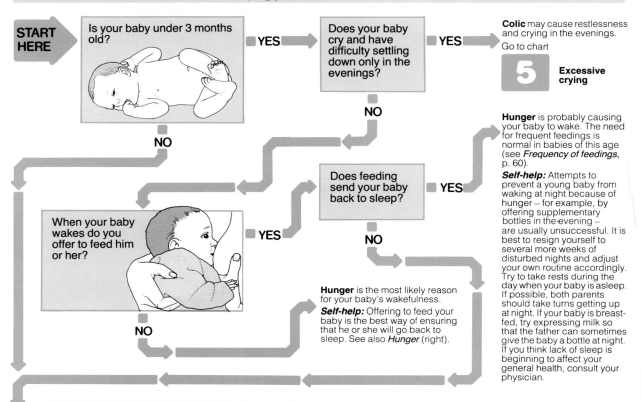

START HERE

Is your baby under 3 months old?

Does your baby cry and have difficulty settling down only in the evenings?

YES → YES →

Colic may cause restlessness and crying in the evenings.

Go to chart

5 **Excessive crying**

NO

NO

Does feeding send your baby back to sleep?

YES

When your baby wakes do you offer to feed him or her?

YES

NO

NO

Hunger is the most likely reason for your baby's wakefulness.
Self-help: Offering to feed your baby is the best way of ensuring that he or she will go back to sleep. See also *Hunger* (right).

Hunger is probably causing your baby to wake. The need for frequent feedings is normal in babies of this age (see *Frequency of feedings*, p. 60).

Self-help: Attempts to prevent a young baby from waking at night because of hunger – for example, by offering supplementary bottles in the evening – are usually unsuccessful. It is best to resign yourself to several more weeks of disturbed nights and adjust your own routine accordingly. Try to take rests during the day when your baby is asleep. If possible, both parents should take turns getting up at night. If your baby is breast-fed, try expressing milk so that the father can sometimes give the baby a bottle at night. If you think lack of sleep is beginning to affect your general health, consult your physician.

HELPING YOUR BABY SLEEP

Young babies (under 4 months)
In the first few months of life a baby will sleep when fed and comfortable; the most you can do to help your baby sleep is to ensure that these basic needs of food, warmth and comfort are provided. Concentrate on adjusting your own routine so that you sleep when your baby does to prevent yourself from becoming overtired by disturbed nights. The following suggestions may help you to cope more easily:

- Try to take rests during the day when your baby is asleep.
- Take turns with your partner getting up at night when your baby cries.
- If your baby is breast-fed, express some milk so that your partner can sometimes give the baby a bottle at night.
- Move your baby into a separate room as soon as you feel ready, preferably before the age of 6 months.

Older babies (4 to 12 months)
Most babies who are past the stage of needing frequent night feedings benefit from a regular bedtime routine. A baby who has learned to go to bed without fuss during the first year is less likely to have problems later on. In general, it is best to be firm and predictable, but this should

not prevent you from making the bedtime ritual affectionate and fun. Your baby needs to be reassured that going to bed is not a form of punishment. Some suggestions for increasing the chances of problem-free bedtimes are listed below:

- Always carry out the preparations for bed in the same order – for example, supper, bath, quiet playtime, a breast- or bottle-feeding, and then into the crib for the night.
- Avoid too much excitement in the hour or so before bed.
- Make your baby's room as inviting as possible with plenty to look at on the walls and favorite toys in the crib.
- Provide a night-light if your baby seems to be frightened of the dark.
- Do not be too ready to go to your baby if he or she whimpers in the night. He or she may simply be making noises while asleep, and going into the room may wake your baby unnecessarily.
- If your baby cries in the night, do whatever is necessary to settle him or her (giving a drink or changing a diaper) as quickly and quietly as possible. Do not let your baby persuade you to play, otherwise he or she may learn that waking at night can be fun.

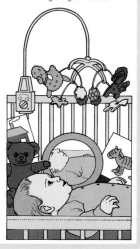

Help your baby not to feel lonely or bored in the crib by providing plenty of interesting things to look at.

Go to next page

Continued from previous page

Has your baby previously slept well at night?

YES →

Does your baby seem sick in any way – for example, is his or her temperature 100°F (38°C) or above?

YES →

A physical illness can easily disrupt a baby's sleep. Depending on your baby's additional symptoms, go to the appropriate chart elsewhere in this book.

When your baby woke, was he or she crying and difficult to console?

YES →

NO

NO

NO

Does your baby sleep in the same room as you?

YES →

Sharing the same room can result in unnecessarily disturbed nights for you and your baby. This may be because you make sounds that disturb your baby or – and this is more likely – the closeness of your baby may make you overaware of his or her movements during sleep. This may cause you to think that your baby is waking when he or she is only whimpering in his or her sleep. Many babies are restless sleepers and, if left alone (unless actually crying), will continue to sleep.

Self-help: If possible, move your baby into his or her own room. You are less likely to be disturbed by anything less than a true cry.

Earache, possibly as a result of an infection of the middle ear, is a common cause of waking at night and distress in a baby who has previously slept well.

Go to chart

29 **Painful or irritated ear**

NO

Is the room where your baby sleeps cold AND do you usually find your baby's covers have been kicked off during the night?

YES →

Cold may be waking your baby.

Self-help: A baby who moves a great deal while asleep and kicks off the bedclothes can be kept warm at night by a sleeping sack or a warm sleeper suit.

NO

Has there been any domestic crisis or possible cause for anxiety in recent weeks – for example, a move to a new house or a recent absence of the mother or father?

YES →

Anxiety is a possible cause for disrupted sleep even in a young baby. Even comparatively small changes in domestic routine can upset some babies.

Self-help: It may take several days to reassure your baby that there is no cause for anxiety. During this time try to ensure that there are no further changes of routine. When your baby wakes at night, offer a drink and a hug, but make sure that your baby understands that he or she will be put back in the crib. Otherwise, there is a danger that your baby will get into the habit of waking and expecting to play. See also *Helping your baby sleep* (opposite).

The need for the comfort and reassurance of your presence is the most common explanation for waking at night when a baby is past the stage of needing night feedings.

Self-help: From an early age, make every effort to stick to a set routine for putting your baby to bed. Your baby should be taught to understand that you will not allow him or her to get up again until morning. If your baby wakes at night, offer a drink but try to avoid picking him or her up. Do not stay with your baby any longer than is necessary to reassure him or her of your presence and to reassure yourself that all is well. If your baby cries when you leave the room, resist going back in. Crying for a few minutes will do your baby no harm and he or she will soon go back to sleep.

NO

SLEEPING PATTERNS

No two babies have the same sleeping pattern or the same sleep requirements, so do not make the mistake of thinking that your baby is abnormal if he or she sleeps less than a friend's baby of the same age. The typical sleeping patterns described here are given simply as examples, and your own baby's routine will almost certainly be different. However, the gradual transition from spending most of the day and night asleep to spending nearly the whole day awake and nearly the whole night asleep is likely to apply to most babies.

Newborn
A newborn baby spends most of the time asleep, waking for feedings about every 3 hours. After the first few months, most babies will sleep longer at night, perhaps only waking once. Wakeful periods in the day will probably become more prolonged.

6 months
By the time a baby is 6 months old, he or she is likely to sleep most of the night, but may wake briefly for a feeding in the early hours of the morning. He or she will be awake for most of the day, but will probably need a nap in the morning and in the afternoon.

1 year
A 1-year-old baby usually sleeps throughout the night without waking (between 10 and 12 hours on average). At this age, a baby will probably need only one major nap during the day.

☐ Awake
☐ Asleep

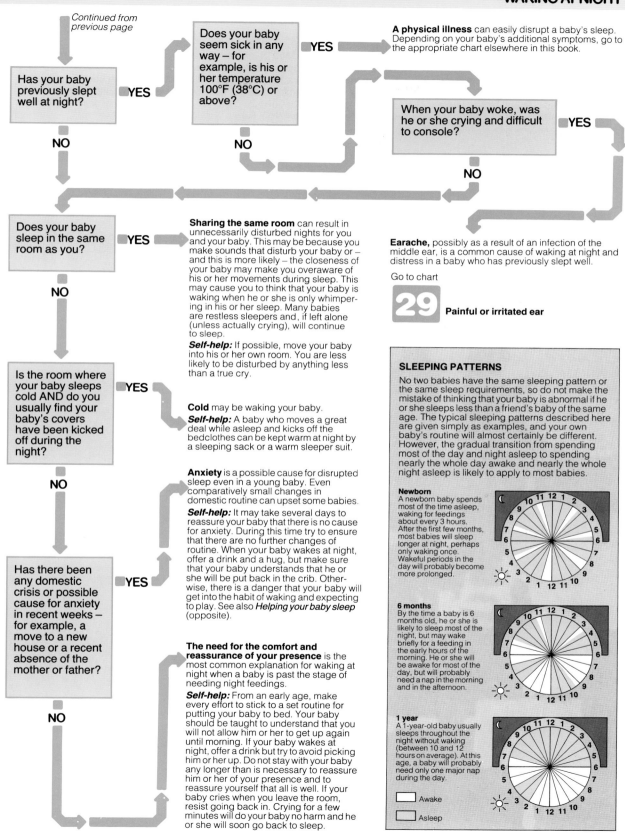

3 Fever in babies

A fever or above-normal body temperature is usually caused by infection. (Viral and bacterial infections are discussed on p. 66.) You may suspect that your baby has a fever if the forehead feels hot, if your baby is sweating more than usual, or if he or she seems sick. Taking your baby's temperature using a clinical thermometer as de-scribed in the box opposite will enable you to confirm your suspicions. Normal temperature may vary from 97° to 99°F (36° to 37.5°C). Minor fluctuations within this range are never a cause for concern if your baby seems otherwise well. Consult this chart if your baby's temperature rises above this level.

For children over 1 year, see chart 14, Fever in children

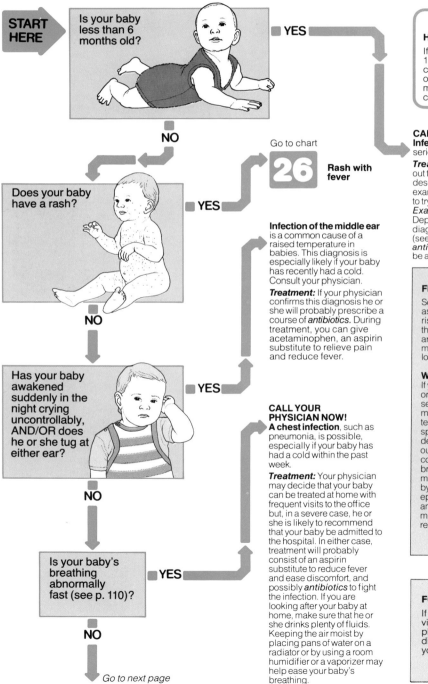

START HERE

Is your baby less than 6 months old?

YES

NO

Does your baby have a rash?

YES

Go to chart

26

Rash with fever

NO

Has your baby awakened suddenly in the night crying uncontrollably, AND/OR does he or she tug at either ear?

YES

NO

Is your baby's breathing abnormally fast (see p. 110)?

YES

NO

Go to next page

Infection of the middle ear is a common cause of a raised temperature in babies. This diagnosis is especially likely if your baby has recently had a cold. Consult your physician.

Treatment: If your physician confirms this diagnosis he or she will probably prescribe a course of *antibiotics*. During treatment, you can give acetaminophen, an aspirin substitute to relieve pain and reduce fever.

CALL YOUR PHYSICIAN NOW!
A chest infection, such as pneumonia, is possible, especially if your baby has had a cold within the past week.

Treatment: Your physician may decide that your baby can be treated at home with frequent visits to the office but, in a severe case, he or she is likely to recommend that your baby be admitted to the hospital. In either case, treatment will probably consist of an aspirin substitute to reduce fever and ease discomfort, and possibly *antibiotics* to fight the infection. If you are looking after your baby at home, make sure that he or she drinks plenty of fluids. Keeping the air moist by placing pans of water on a radiator or by using a room humidifier or a vaporizer may help ease your baby's breathing.

WARNING

HIGH FEVER

If your baby's temperature rises above 102°F (39°C), whatever the suspected cause, you should call your physician at once. This is because high temperatures may be caused by a serious infection and can lead to convulsions in some babies.

CALL YOUR PHYSICIAN NOW!
Infections at this age are unusual but may be serious.

Treatment: Until you see your physician, carry out temperature-reducing measures as described on p. 288. Your physician will examine your baby and, perhaps, order tests to try to make an exact diagnosis (see *Examination by the physician,* p. 67). Depending on whether your physician diagnoses a viral or bacterial infection (see p. 66), he or she may prescribe *antibiotics.* Admission to the hospital may be advised.

FEVERISH CONVULSIONS

Some babies have convulsions (also known as febrile seizures) when their temperatures rise too quickly. During such a convulsion, the arms and legs will shake uncontrollably and the baby may turn blue in the face. This may last for several minutes or sometimes longer.

What to do
If your baby has a feverish convulsion, lay him or her stomach down on a flat surface, and seek medical help at once. While waiting for medical help, attempt to reduce your baby's temperature by removing the clothing and sponging him or her with tepid water as described on p. 288. If your child vomits, clean out his or her mouth with your finger. The convulsion will not damage your baby's brain, and it will usually stop by itself in a few minutes. If your child has a convulsion caused by fever, it *does not mean* that your child has epilepsy. Some children, however, do have an underlying problem, and your physician may want to do more tests after your child recovers.

FOREIGN TRAVEL

If your baby develops a fever soon after a visit to a hot climate, be sure to tell your physician. Your baby may have caught a disease that is rare in this country, one that your physician might not otherwise suspect.

Continued from previous page

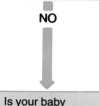

Does your baby have a clear discharge from the nose AND/OR has he or she been coughing?

YES

Measles is a possibility if your baby has been in contact with the disease within the past week or so. The appearance of a rash within the next few days will confirm the diagnosis. (See *Comparison of childhood infectious diseases,* p.97.) Otherwise, a generalized viral infection is likely. Consult your physician.

Treatment: For both types of illness, your physician is likely to recommend that you take steps to reduce your baby's temperature (see p.288) while the infection runs its course for the next week or so. Call your physician at once if your baby becomes drowsy or unresponsive, or if he or she refuses to drink.

NO

Is your baby unusually drowsy or irritable?

YES

CALL YOUR PHYSICIAN NOW!
Meningitis (inflammation of the membranes surrounding the nervous system, caused by viral or bacterial infection) may be the cause, especially if your baby has also vomited.

Treatment: Your baby will probably be admitted to the hospital where he or she will be given a *lumbar puncture* (p. 74) to make an exact diagnosis. Your child will be given fluids and possibly *antibiotics* (if the infection is bacterial) intravenously.

NO

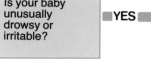

Has your baby had diarrhea AND/OR been vomiting?

YES

CONSULT YOUR PHYSICIAN WITHOUT DELAY!
Gastroenteritis (infection of the digestive tract) is the most likely cause of such symptoms.

Treatment: If the diagnosis is confirmed, your physician is likely to recommend that you follow the guidelines for treating gastroenteritis described in the box on p. 63. However, if your baby's symptoms are severe, or if there are signs of dehydration (see *Persistent vomiting,* p. 62), your physician may advise admission to the hospital, where fluids can be given intravenously.

NO

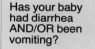

Has your baby been refusing solid food?

YES

A throat or mouth infection is the most likely explanation for the problem.

Self-help: Follow the advice on treating a sore throat on p. 107. Do not force your baby to eat if pain makes swallowing difficult, but make sure he or she drinks at least 1 ½ pints of fluid a day. Consult your physician if your baby is no better in 48 hours or develops any of the danger signs in the box on p. 106.

NO

Is your baby very warmly dressed AND/OR is he or she in warm surroundings?

YES

Overheating, caused by too much clothing or by excessively warm surroundings, can cause a baby's temperature to rise.

Self-help: In general, babies do not need to wear much more clothing than an adult in similar conditions and will be comfortable in a room temperature of 60° to 68°F (15° to 20°C). A baby crib should never be placed next to a radiator. If your baby has become overheated, removing any excess clothing and moving the baby to a slightly cooler (though not cold) place will soon reduce any fever. If your baby's temperature is not down to normal within an hour, consult your physician.

NO

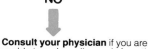

Consult your physician if you are unable to make a diagnosis from this chart.

HOW TO TAKE A BABY'S TEMPERATURE

The best way to take your baby's temperature is rectally. This is an accurate method and will not hurt your baby.

1 Use a rectal thermometer which has a short, round tip. When you buy it, the package must specify rectal.

2 Shake the thermometer with firm downward flicks of the wrist so that the mercury runs down into the bulb and reads well below the "normal" mark.

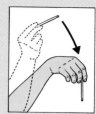

3 Place the baby over your knees holding the thermometer lightly between the index and middle finger. Dip the thermometer in petroleum jelly and insert slowly, without forcing, in the rectum. Hold in place for 3 minutes.

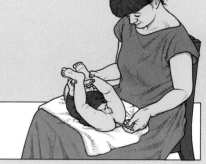

4 Remove the thermometer and look at it, turning until you get a clear reading. Using this method, you can consider your baby feverish if his or her temperature is 100°F (38°C) or above.

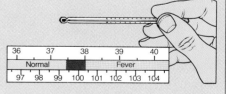

36	37	38	39	40
Normal			Fever	
97 98	99 100	101	102 103	104

4 Skin problems in babies

The skin of newborn babies is sensitive and can easily become inflamed as a result of minor irritations such as prolonged contact with urine or stools, overheating or rubbing against rough fabrics. Such rashes are usually no cause for concern, although you should deal with the cause. Rashes and other skin abnormalities that occur for no apparent reason, or that persist, should always be brought to your physician's attention. Medical advice should be sought promptly if your baby has a rash and seems sick.

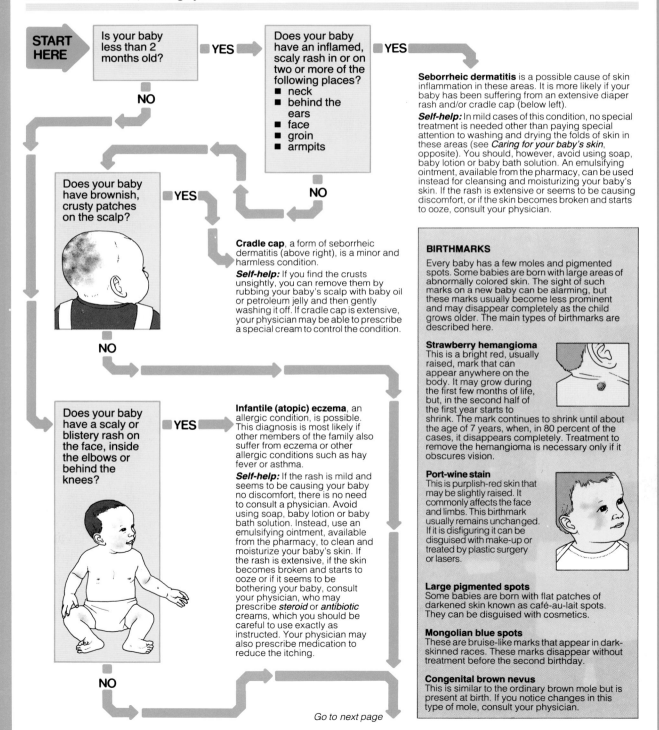

START HERE

Is your baby less than 2 months old?

YES → Does your baby have an inflamed, scaly rash in or on two or more of the following places?
- neck
- behind the ears
- face
- groin
- armpits

YES →

Seborrheic dermatitis is a possible cause of skin inflammation in these areas. It is more likely if your baby has been suffering from an extensive diaper rash and/or cradle cap (below left).

Self-help: In mild cases of this condition, no special treatment is needed other than paying special attention to washing and drying the folds of skin in these areas (see *Caring for your baby's skin*, opposite). You should, however, avoid using soap, baby lotion or baby bath solution. An emulsifying ointment, available from the pharmacy, can be used instead for cleansing and moisturizing your baby's skin. If the rash is extensive or seems to be causing discomfort, or if the skin becomes broken and starts to ooze, consult your physician.

NO ↓

Does your baby have brownish, crusty patches on the scalp?

YES ↓ **NO**

Cradle cap, a form of seborrheic dermatitis (above right), is a minor and harmless condition.

Self-help: If you find the crusts unsightly, you can remove them by rubbing your baby's scalp with baby oil or petroleum jelly and then gently washing it off. If cradle cap is extensive, your physician may be able to prescribe a special cream to control the condition.

NO ↓

Does your baby have a scaly or blistery rash on the face, inside the elbows or behind the knees?

YES →

Infantile (atopic) eczema, an allergic condition, is possible. This diagnosis is most likely if other members of the family also suffer from eczema or other allergic conditions such as hay fever or asthma.

Self-help: If the rash is mild and seems to be causing your baby no discomfort, there is no need to consult a physician. Avoid using soap, baby lotion or baby bath solution. Instead, use an emulsifying ointment, available from the pharmacy, to clean and moisturize your baby's skin. If the rash is extensive, if the skin becomes broken and starts to ooze or if it seems to be bothering your baby, consult your physician, who may prescribe *steroid* or *antibiotic* creams, which you should be careful to use exactly as instructed. Your physician may also prescribe medication to reduce the itching.

NO ↓

BIRTHMARKS

Every baby has a few moles and pigmented spots. Some babies are born with large areas of abnormally colored skin. The sight of such marks on a new baby can be alarming, but these marks usually become less prominent and may disappear completely as the child grows older. The main types of birthmarks are described here.

Strawberry hemangioma
This is a bright red, usually raised, mark that can appear anywhere on the body. It may grow during the first few months of life, but, in the second half of the first year starts to shrink. The mark continues to shrink until about the age of 7 years, when, in 80 percent of the cases, it disappears completely. Treatment to remove the hemangioma is necessary only if it obscures vision.

Port-wine stain
This is purplish-red skin that may be slightly raised. It commonly affects the face and limbs. This birthmark usually remains unchanged. If it is disfiguring it can be disguised with make-up or treated by plastic surgery or lasers.

Large pigmented spots
Some babies are born with flat patches of darkened skin known as café-au-lait spots. They can be disguised with cosmetics.

Mongolian blue spots
These are bruise-like marks that appear in dark-skinned races. These marks disappear without treatment before the second birthday.

Congenital brown nevus
This is similar to the ordinary brown mole but is present at birth. If you notice changes in this type of mole, consult your physician.

Go to next page

Continued from previous page

Does your baby have an area of inflamed skin or spots confined to or spreading from the diaper area?

YES →

Is the rash mainly around the anus?

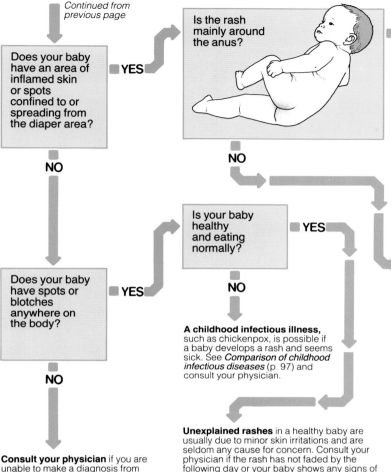

YES

Irritants that occur naturally in your baby's bowel movements may inflame the skin around the anus, causing diaper rash. This is most likely to occur with diarrhea, which makes the bowel movements more alkaline.

Self-help: Change the diaper as soon as it becomes soiled. Wash your baby well and apply a protective cream (see also *Caring for your baby's skin*, below). Consult your physician if diaper rash persists for more than 10 days. If your baby is passing unusually watery or frequent bowel movements, he or she may have an infection.

Go to chart

8

Diarrhea in babies

NO

NO

Is your baby healthy and eating normally?

YES

Generalized diaper rash is usually due to prolonged contact with wet diapers. Substances in the urine react with chemicals in the bowel movements to produce ammonia, which is irritating to a baby's skin. This type of diaper rash is most likely if you use cloth diapers that have been inadequately sterilized.

Self-help: Change your baby's diapers frequently and wash the diaper area thoroughly between each change. It is best to use disposable diapers, if possible, because these are certain to be sterile. If you continue to use cloth diapers, try not to put waterproof pants on your baby. Hiring a diaper service to clean the diapers may be helpful, since it is difficult to get rid of the ammonia that causes diaper rash by simple home laundering. Leave off your baby's diapers as often as possible to help the skin dry out and promote healing. Before putting on a clean diaper, apply a protective cream (see also *Caring for your baby's skin*, below). If these measures fail to clear up the diaper rash within 10 days, or if it starts to get worse, there is a possibility that the skin may have become infected by *Candida* (or thrush), a fungus that is often present in the bowel. In this case, consult your physician, who may prescribe a special cream and, possibly, medication to treat the infection.

Does your baby have spots or blotches anywhere on the body?

YES →

NO

A childhood infectious illness, such as chickenpox, is possible if a baby develops a rash and seems sick. See *Comparison of childhood infectious diseases* (p. 97) and consult your physician.

Consult your physician if you are unable to make a diagnosis from this chart.

Unexplained rashes in a healthy baby are usually due to minor skin irritations and are seldom any cause for concern. Consult your physician if the rash has not faded by the following day or your baby shows any signs of being sick.

CARING FOR YOUR BABY'S SKIN

A baby's skin is delicate and needs protection from severe cold or heat and strong sunlight (or it may become inflamed, dry and sore). Regular, careful washing is necessary to prevent skin infections and diaper rash.

Washing and bathing

A baby's skin should always be kept clean. Usually the best way to ensure this is to give your baby a daily bath. However, providing that you wash the diaper area thoroughly at each diaper change (see *Diapers*, right) and wipe away any excess spills elsewhere on your baby, less frequent bathing is adequate. When you bathe your baby, remember the following points:

- Make sure that the water is not too hot (check it using your elbow).
- Always hold your baby securely in the bath and, even when he or she can sit up unaided, never leave your baby in the bath unattended.
- Use a mild, unscented soap or baby bath solution. If your baby has dry skin, infantile eczema or seborrheic dermatitis, use emulsifying ointment and wash it away with plain water.
- When your baby's hair starts to grow thickly, wash it once a week with a mild shampoo.
- Dry your baby, using his or her own towel, making sure all moisture is removed from the skin folds.
- Talcum powder can be inhaled by the baby and is not recommended.

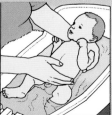
Hold your baby securely in the bath.

Diapers

Cloth diapers need careful washing and sterilizing and should be used with a "one-way" diaper liner to keep moisture away from the skin. Disposables are more convenient and are always sterile, but may hold less moisture than cloth diapers. Whichever you choose, change them regularly to prevent diaper rash.

Diaper changing

When you change your baby's diaper, wipe away all traces of urine and bowel movements with a clean washcloth and water or alcohol-free baby wipes. If your baby's skin is dry, lotion will help.

If possible, try to set aside some time at least once a day for your baby to be without diapers. Exposure to air helps the skin dry out thoroughly and helps prevent diaper rash.

If your baby has a sore bottom, try leaving the diapers off for long periods and let your baby lie in a warm room on a towel or diaper. This assists healing, as will the use of a diaper rash ointment containing zinc oxide. If your baby develops a fever or the rash persists, consult your physician.

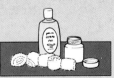
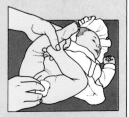
Use a clean washcloth moistened with water to clean your baby's bottom.

5 Excessive crying

Crying is a young baby's only means of communicating physical discomfort or emotional distress. All babies cry sometimes when they are hungry, wet, upset or in pain, and some babies often seem to cry for no obvious reason. Crying does not necessarily indicate a serious problem. Most parents learn to recognize the most common causes of their baby's crying. Consult this chart if your baby regularly cries more often than you think is normal, or if your baby suddenly starts to cry in an unusual way or for no apparent reason.

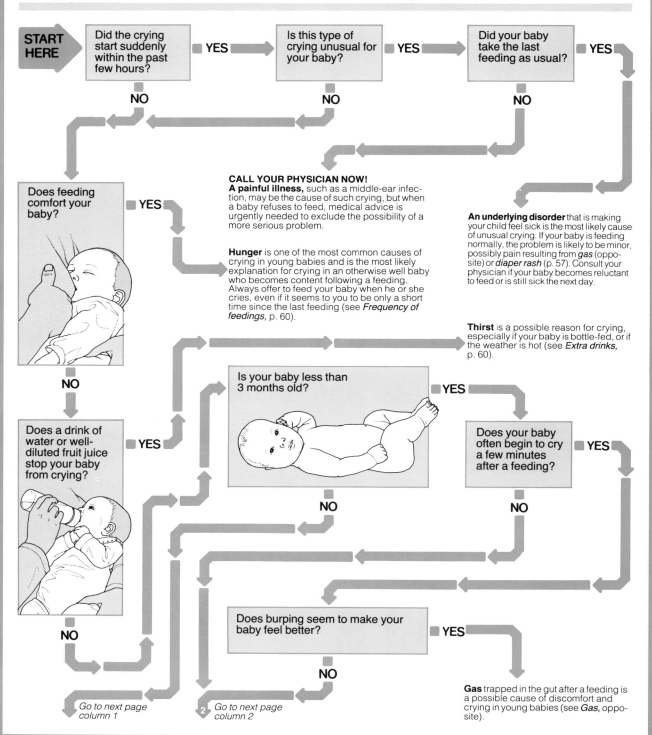

START HERE

Did the crying start suddenly within the past few hours?

YES → Is this type of crying unusual for your baby?

YES → Did your baby take the last feeding as usual?

YES →

NO ↓

Does feeding comfort your baby?

YES →

NO ↓

Does a drink of water or well-diluted fruit juice stop your baby from crying?

YES →

NO ↓

Is your baby less than 3 months old?

YES →

NO ↓

Does your baby often begin to cry a few minutes after a feeding?

YES →

NO ↓

Does burping seem to make your baby feel better?

YES →

NO ↓

CALL YOUR PHYSICIAN NOW!
A painful illness, such as a middle-ear infection, may be the cause of such crying, but when a baby refuses to feed, medical advice is urgently needed to exclude the possibility of a more serious problem.

Hunger is one of the most common causes of crying in young babies and is the most likely explanation for crying in an otherwise well baby who becomes content following a feeding. Always offer to feed your baby when he or she cries, even if it seems to you to be only a short time since the last feeding (see *Frequency of feedings,* p. 60).

An underlying disorder that is making your child feel sick is the most likely cause of unusual crying. If your baby is feeding normally, the problem is likely to be minor, possibly pain resulting from *gas* (opposite) or *diaper rash* (p. 57). Consult your physician if your baby becomes reluctant to feed or is still sick the next day.

Thirst is a possible reason for crying, especially if your baby is bottle-fed, or if the weather is hot (see *Extra drinks,* p. 60).

Gas trapped in the gut after a feeding is a possible cause of discomfort and crying in young babies (see *Gas,* opposite).

Go to next page column 1

2 *Go to next page column 2*

1 *Continued from previous page column 1*

2 *Continued from previous page column 2*

Does your baby seem content for most of the day but cry a great deal during the late afternoon and evening?

YES →

Evening (or 3-month) colic is the term often used to describe this common type of crying. It usually starts when a baby is about 6 weeks old and ceases after the age of 3 months. There are many possible explanations for this problem, including painful spasm of the intestines, tiredness and tension in the mother and a possible reduction in her milk supply at this time of day.

Self-help: There is no effective cure for evening colic. The main priority for parents is to find a way of minimizing the strain on themselves from a constantly crying baby. Try to find ways of preventing yourself from becoming too tired at the end of the day – for example, by taking an afternoon rest. Parents can take turns to give each other an evening off or you can sometimes ask a trusted babysitter to look after the baby. Discuss the problem with your physician, who may advise you on how to cope and may, in extreme cases, prescribe a medicine that helps your baby to settle down.

NO

Does your baby usually stop crying when picked up and given your full attention?

YES →

The need for attention and physical comfort is a common cause of crying. Some babies are quite happy when left alone for short times, but others need the constant reassurance of their parents' presence.

Self-help: Cuddle your baby as much as he or she seems to want. At this age there is no danger of "spoiling," and your baby will be happier as a result of an increased feeling of security. To enable you to get on with your everyday chores, you can try putting a young baby in a carrying sling while you go about the house. An older baby may be content if placed in a bouncing chair or infant seat propped up on some cushions where he or she can see you.

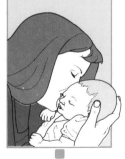

NO

Are you feeling tense or overtired OR has there been a recent major domestic upheaval?

YES →

Sensitivity to increased tension in the home and particularly in the mother can make a baby unsettled and more likely to cry.

Self-help: A baby will usually settle down to a new routine or in new surroundings within a week or so, although you will need to give more attention and reassurance than usual during this time. If you think that the cause of your baby's crying could be a reaction to tension in yourself, try to find ways of reducing any strain you are under. Discuss this with your physician, who may be able to suggest ways of helping. A crying baby is frustrating, and much child abuse starts when an overly tired parent must cope with an irritable baby. Seek advice from your physician or a child abuse hotline if you think you could lose your temper and become abusive.

NO

Consult your physician if you are unable to make a diagnosis from this chart.

GAS

Young babies often swallow air during feedings, especially those eager feeders who gulp greedily at the start of every feeding. Excess gas in the gut causes regurgitation of feedings and may be linked to discomfort and crying, so it is a good idea to spend a little time helping your baby to bring up gas after each feeding. Some of the best positions for burping are shown below.

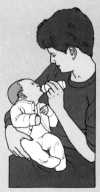

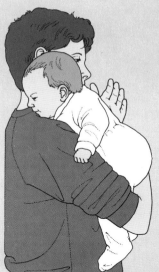

Positions for burping
When feeding your baby, make sure that he or she is supported in a semi-upright position (above). After feeding, help your baby to bring up gas by holding him or her against your shoulder (left), over your knee (below left) or on your lap (below).

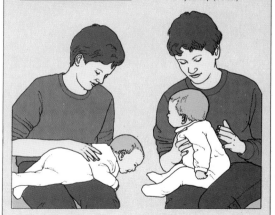

6 Feeding problems

Feeding problems are a common source of irritability and crying in young babies and of concern to their parents. Such problems may include a reluctance to feed, constant hungry crying, and swallowing too much air, leading to regurgitation. There may also be special problems for mothers who are breast-feeding. The diagnostic chart and the boxes on these pages deal with most of the common problems that may arise.

For children over one, see chart 39, Loss of appetite

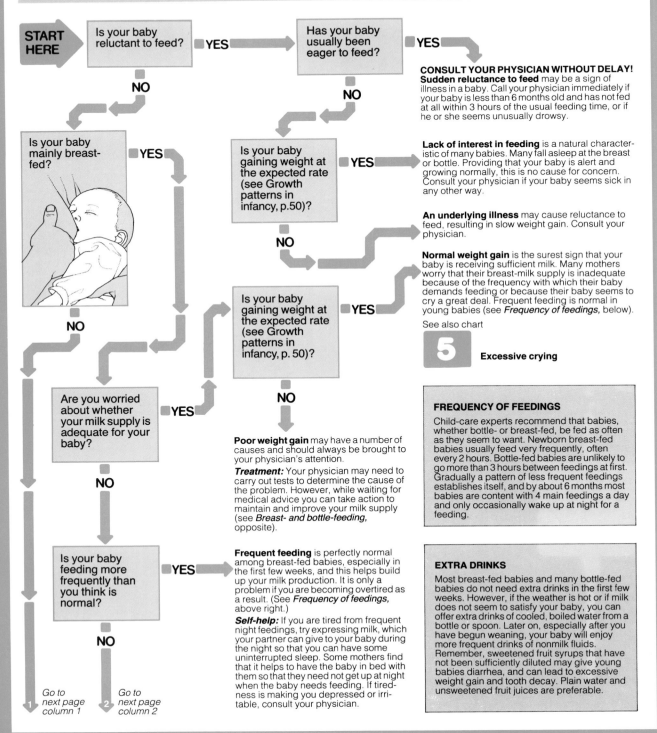

START HERE

Is your baby reluctant to feed? — YES → **Has your baby usually been eager to feed?** — YES →

NO ↓

CONSULT YOUR PHYSICIAN WITHOUT DELAY!
Sudden reluctance to feed may be a sign of illness in a baby. Call your physician immediately if your baby is less than 6 months old and has not fed at all within 3 hours of the usual feeding time, or if he or she seems unusually drowsy.

Is your baby mainly breast-fed? — YES →

NO ↓ (Has your baby... NO) ↓

Is your baby gaining weight at the expected rate (see Growth patterns in infancy, p.50)? — YES →

Lack of interest in feeding is a natural characteristic of many babies. Many fall asleep at the breast or bottle. Providing that your baby is alert and growing normally, this is no cause for concern. Consult your physician if your baby seems sick in any other way.

NO ↓

An underlying illness may cause reluctance to feed, resulting in slow weight gain. Consult your physician.

Is your baby gaining weight at the expected rate (see Growth patterns in infancy, p. 50)? — YES →

Normal weight gain is the surest sign that your baby is receiving sufficient milk. Many mothers worry that their breast-milk supply is inadequate because of the frequency with which their baby demands feeding or because their baby seems to cry a great deal. Frequent feeding is normal in young babies (see *Frequency of feedings*, below).

See also chart

5 **Excessive crying**

NO ↓

Are you worried about whether your milk supply is adequate for your baby? — YES →

NO ↓

Poor weight gain may have a number of causes and should always be brought to your physician's attention.
Treatment: Your physician may need to carry out tests to determine the cause of the problem. However, while waiting for medical advice you can take action to maintain and improve your milk supply (see *Breast- and bottle-feeding,* opposite).

Is your baby feeding more frequently than you think is normal? — YES →

NO ↓

Frequent feeding is perfectly normal among breast-fed babies, especially in the first few weeks, and this helps build up your milk production. It is only a problem if you are becoming overtired as a result. (See *Frequency of feedings,* above right.)
Self-help: If you are tired from frequent night feedings, try expressing milk, which your partner can give to your baby during the night so that you can have some uninterrupted sleep. Some mothers find that it helps to have the baby in bed with them so that they need not get up at night when the baby needs feeding. If tiredness is making you depressed or irritable, consult your physician.

1 Go to next page column 1

2 Go to next page column 2

FREQUENCY OF FEEDINGS

Child-care experts recommend that babies, whether bottle- or breast-fed, be fed as often as they seem to want. Newborn breast-fed babies usually feed very frequently, often every 2 hours. Bottle-fed babies are unlikely to go more than 3 hours between feedings at first. Gradually a pattern of less frequent feedings establishes itself, and by about 6 months most babies are content with 4 main feedings a day and only occasionally wake up at night for a feeding.

EXTRA DRINKS

Most breast-fed babies and many bottle-fed babies do not need extra drinks in the first few weeks. However, if the weather is hot or if milk does not seem to satisfy your baby, you can offer extra drinks of cooled, boiled water from a bottle or spoon. Later on, especially after you have begun weaning, your baby will enjoy more frequent drinks of nonmilk fluids. Remember, sweetened fruit syrups that have not been sufficiently diluted may give young babies diarrhea, and can lead to excessive weight gain and tooth decay. Plain water and unsweetened fruit juices are preferable.

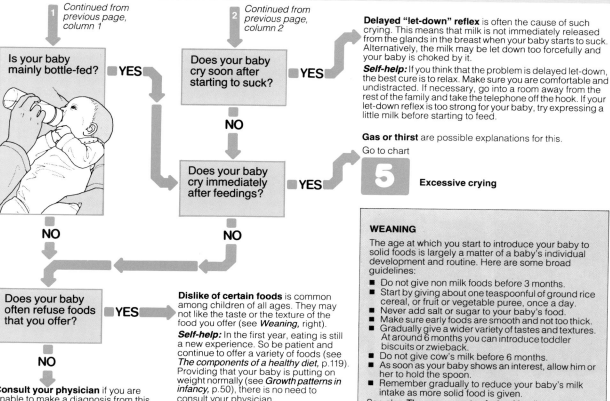

1 Continued from previous page, column 1

Is your baby mainly bottle-fed?

YES

2 Continued from previous page, column 2

Does your baby cry soon after starting to suck?

YES

Delayed "let-down" reflex is often the cause of such crying. This means that milk is not immediately released from the glands in the breast when your baby starts to suck. Alternatively, the milk may be let down too forcefully and your baby is choked by it.

Self-help: If you think that the problem is delayed let-down, the best cure is to relax. Make sure you are comfortable and undistracted. If necessary, go into a room away from the rest of the family and take the telephone off the hook. If your let-down reflex is too strong for your baby, try expressing a little milk before starting to feed.

NO

Does your baby cry immediately after feedings?

YES

Gas or thirst are possible explanations for this.

Go to chart

5

Excessive crying

NO

NO

Does your baby often refuse foods that you offer?

YES

Dislike of certain foods is common among children of all ages. They may not like the taste or the texture of the food you offer (see *Weaning,* right).

Self-help: In the first year, eating is still a new experience. So be patient and continue to offer a variety of foods (see *The components of a healthy diet,* p.119). Providing that your baby is putting on weight normally (see *Growth patterns in infancy,* p.50), there is no need to consult your physician.

NO

Consult your physician if you are unable to make a diagnosis from this chart.

WEANING

The age at which you start to introduce your baby to solid foods is largely a matter of a baby's individual development and routine. Here are some broad guidelines:

- Do not give non milk foods before 3 months.
- Start by giving about one teaspoonful of ground rice cereal, or fruit or vegetable puree, once a day.
- Never add salt or sugar to your baby's food.
- Make sure early foods are smooth and not too thick.
- Gradually give a wider variety of tastes and textures. At around 6 months you can introduce toddler biscuits or zwieback.
- Do not give cow's milk before 6 months.
- As soon as your baby shows an interest, allow him or her to hold the spoon.
- Remember gradually to reduce your baby's milk intake as more solid food is given.

See also *The components of a healthy diet,* p.119).

BREAST- and BOTTLE-FEEDING

Breast-feeding

All physicians agree that, when possible, breast-feeding is the best way to feed a baby. Breast milk contains all the nutrients a baby needs in the ideal proportions and in the most easily digested form. In addition, a baby who is breast-fed receives antibodies in the milk that protect against infection.

Although there are very few women who cannot or should not breast-feed their babies if they want to most early difficulties can be overcome with patience and determination. Some common breast-feeding problems are discussed below.

Sore nipples

Most new mothers experience some soreness in the first few days of breast-feeding. This normally gets better without special treatment, but here are some suggestions for minimizing discomfort:

- Ensure that your baby is latching on properly (see right).
- Prevent your breasts from becoming overfull (see right).
- Keep your nipples as dry as possible between feedings.
- If necessary, apply a bland, lanolin-based cream.

Consult your physician if the skin around the nipple becomes cracked or if pain continues throughout the feeding.

Maintaining your milk supply

Most mothers produce exactly the right amount of milk to meet their baby's needs. The following measures will ensure that your milk supply remains plentiful:

- Eat a nourishing diet (you may need 800 calories a day more than usual).
- Try not to become overtired – get some rest.
- Offer your baby a feeding whenever either of you feels the need.
- If you are temporarily unable to nurse, express milk at normal feeding times so that you can resume normal feeding later.
- Unless there is a special reason, avoid giving your baby supplementary bottles of formula; these will satisfy your baby's hunger but prevent your breasts from receiving the stimulation they need to produce more milk.

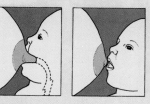

Latching on
When you put your baby to the breast, make sure that he or she takes the whole of the nipple and areola (colored area) into the mouth (far left); otherwise, your nipples may become sore. If your breasts are overfull, latching on may be difficult (left) and you should follow the advice below.

Engorged breasts

This is a common problem during the first few weeks of breast-feeding that can be uncomfortable for you and frustrating for your baby because it makes latching on difficult. Some suggestions:

- Encourage your baby to feed frequently.
- If latching on has become difficult for your baby, express a little milk from the nipple before each feeding.
- If your breasts are very full and your baby is not ready to feed, express some milk.

Consult your physician if your breasts become generally painful or red.

Bottle-feeding

For mothers who are unable or unwilling to breast feed, modern formulas provide a satisfactory alternative.

Making up the formula

If it is concentrated, formula should always be made up exactly according to the manufacturer's instructions. Ask your physician if you can use water straight from the tap or if you should boil and cool it first.

Washing feeding equipment

Bottle-fed babies are more susceptible to gastroenteritis than breast-fed babies because germs grow very easily in inadequately washed and rinsed bottles and utensils. Make sure you wash, rinse, and sterilize (boil) all your baby's feeding equipment thoroughly.

7 Vomiting in babies

Vomiting is the forceful throwing up of the contents of the stomach as a result of sudden contraction of the muscles around the stomach. Almost any minor upset can cause a baby to regurgitate, but persistent vomiting can be a sign of serious disease and needs prompt medical attention.

For children over 1 year, consult chart 37, Vomiting in children

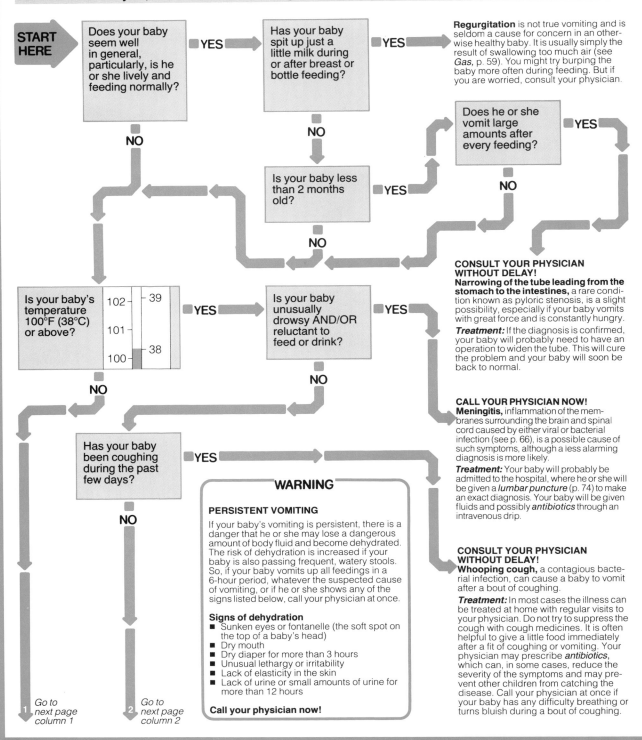

START HERE

Does your baby seem well in general, particularly, is he or she lively and feeding normally?

YES → **Has your baby spit up just a little milk during or after breast or bottle feeding?**

YES → **Regurgitation** is not true vomiting and is seldom a cause for concern in an otherwise healthy baby. It is usually simply the result of swallowing too much air (see *Gas*, p. 59). You might try burping the baby more often during feeding. But if you are worried, consult your physician.

NO

NO

Is your baby less than 2 months old?

YES

Does he or she vomit large amounts after every feeding?

YES

NO

NO

Is your baby's temperature 100°F (38°C) or above?

102 — 39
101 —
— 38
100 —

YES → **Is your baby unusually drowsy AND/OR reluctant to feed or drink?**

YES

NO

NO

CONSULT YOUR PHYSICIAN WITHOUT DELAY!
Narrowing of the tube leading from the stomach to the intestines, a rare condition known as pyloric stenosis, is a slight possibility, especially if your baby vomits with great force and is constantly hungry.

Treatment: If the diagnosis is confirmed, your baby will probably need to have an operation to widen the tube. This will cure the problem and your baby will soon be back to normal.

CALL YOUR PHYSICIAN NOW!
Meningitis, inflammation of the membranes surrounding the brain and spinal cord caused by either viral or bacterial infection (see p. 66), is a possible cause of such symptoms, although a less alarming diagnosis is more likely.

Treatment: Your baby will probably be admitted to the hospital, where he or she will be given a *lumbar puncture* (p. 74) to make an exact diagnosis. Your baby will be given fluids and possibly *antibiotics* through an intravenous drip.

Has your baby been coughing during the past few days?

YES

NO

CONSULT YOUR PHYSICIAN WITHOUT DELAY!
Whooping cough, a contagious bacterial infection, can cause a baby to vomit after a bout of coughing.

Treatment: In most cases the illness can be treated at home with regular visits to your physician. Do not try to suppress the cough with cough medicines. It is often helpful to give a little food immediately after a fit of coughing or vomiting. Your physician may prescribe *antibiotics*, which can, in some cases, reduce the severity of the symptoms and may prevent other children from catching the disease. Call your physician at once if your baby has any difficulty breathing or turns bluish during a bout of coughing.

WARNING

PERSISTENT VOMITING

If your baby's vomiting is persistent, there is a danger that he or she may lose a dangerous amount of body fluid and become dehydrated. The risk of dehydration is increased if your baby is also passing frequent, watery stools. So, if your baby vomits up all feedings in a 6-hour period, whatever the suspected cause of vomiting, or if he or she shows any of the signs listed below, call your physician at once.

Signs of dehydration
- Sunken eyes or fontanelle (the soft spot on the top of a baby's head)
- Dry mouth
- Dry diaper for more than 3 hours
- Unusual lethargy or irritability
- Lack of elasticity in the skin
- Lack of urine or small amounts of urine for more than 12 hours

Call your physician now!

1 Go to next page column 1

2 Go to next page column 2

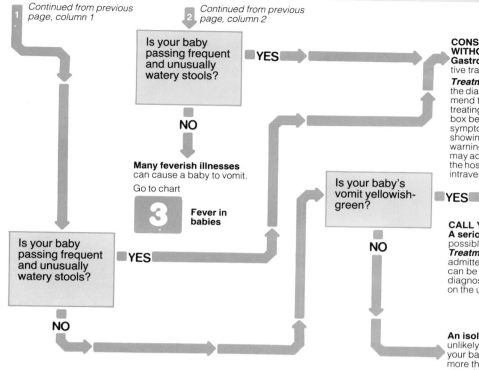

1 Continued from previous page, column 1

2 Continued from previous page, column 2

Is your baby passing frequent and unusually watery stools? **YES** →

NO ↓

Many feverish illnesses can cause a baby to vomit.

Go to chart **3** **Fever in babies**

Is your baby passing frequent and unusually watery stools? **YES**

NO ↓

Is your baby's vomit yellowish-green? **YES**

NO

CONSULT YOUR PHYSICIAN WITHOUT DELAY!
Gastroenteritis, infection of the digestive tract, is likely.

Treatment: If your physician confirms the diagnosis, he or she is likely to recommend that you follow the guidelines for treating gastroenteritis described in the box below. However, if your baby's symptoms are severe, or if he or she is showing signs of dehydration (see the warning box opposite), your physician may advise that your baby be admitted to the hospital, where fluids can be given by intravenous drip.

CALL YOUR PHYSICIAN NOW!
A serious abdominal condition is a possible cause of such symptoms.
Treatment: Your baby will probably be admitted to the hospital, where he or she can be properly examined and an exact diagnosis made. Treatment will depend on the underlying condition.

An isolated attack of vomiting is unlikely to be a sign of serious illness in your baby. However, if your baby vomits more than once in a day or seems sick, consult your physician.

TREATING GASTROENTERITIS (INFECTION OF THE STOMACH AND INTESTINES)

If your physician decides that your baby can be safely treated at home, he or she will probably recommend that you stop all milk and solids for at least 24 hours and gradually reintroduce a normal diet over the following days. Example schemes are described here. Instead of milk and other drinks you may be advised to give your baby a glucose solution.

Making up a glucose solution

Ready-to-use commercial glucose solutions are available, or you can make up your own by using 5 tablespoons of sugar to 1 quart of boiled water. Do not use for more than 24 hours without consulting your physician. Alternatively, you can use packets of glucose and mineral powder or ready-to-use mixtures of salt and sugar, available without a prescription at your pharmacy. A homemade mixture can be made by adding 3 tablespoons of sugar and ½ teaspoon of salt to 1 quart of water.

Baby's weight	Daily fluid intake
(pounds)	(ounces)
8 and under	16
9	18
10	20
11	22
12	24
13	26
14	28
15	30
16 – 17	33
18	36
19	38
20	40
21	42
22 and over	44

Calculating your baby's fluid needs

Babies with gastroenteritis need to receive a carefully regulated amount of fluid each day to prevent dehydration. To calculate an adequate amount for your baby, find his or her weight in the left-hand column of the table (below left) and then look across to the right-hand column to find an appropriate volume of fluid. No baby, regardless of weight, should receive less than ½ quart (16 oz) or more than 1½ quarts (48 oz).

Breast-fed babies

If your breast-fed baby has gastroenteritis, do not breast feed for the first 24 hours of the illness, but give the recommended amount of glucose solution. On each successive day reduce the amount of glucose solution you offer at each feeding by one fifth of the total recommended, and put your baby to the breast afterward. During the days of treatment you can relieve the discomfort of overfull breasts by expressing the excess breast milk.

Weaned babies

If your baby is already weaned, give no milk or dairy products for 5 days, but give the recommended amount of glucose solution for his or her weight. (Apple juice, jello or bouillon could also be given.) Give no solids on Day 1, but you can gradually introduce increased amounts of strained fruit or vegetables from Day 2 until Day 6, when you can resume your normal feeding routine. If your child's condition continues to improve in 24 to 28 hours, bananas, apple sauce and/or saltine crackers can be given, if introduced into the diet slowly.

Treatment scheme

While your baby is sick you must ensure that he or she drinks the correct amount of fluid for his or her weight each day (see **Calculating your baby's fluid needs**, above). While your baby is vomiting you will need to give fluids at frequent intervals (about every hour).

Bottle-fed babies

Day 1
Give no milk. Instead, give the glucose solution at regular intervals.

Day 2
Give your baby a mixture of 1 part made-up milk formula to 4 parts glucose solution at each feeding.

Day 3
Give a mixture of 2 parts milk formula to 3 parts glucose solution at each feeding.

Day 4
Give a mixture of 3 parts milk formula to 2 parts glucose solution at each feeding.

Day 5
Give a mixture of 4 parts milk formula to 1 part glucose solution at each feeding.

Day 6
Return to normal feeding.

Note: If at any time your baby's symptoms recur, go back to Day 1 and call your physician.

8 Diarrhea in babies

Diarrhea is the more frequent passage of runny, watery bowel movements than is usual for your baby. Remember, it is quite normal for a fully breast-fed baby to pass very soft bowel movements. However, if your baby has diarrhea, whatever the suspected cause, it is important to prevent dehydration (see below).

For children over 1 year, see chart 40, Diarrhea in children

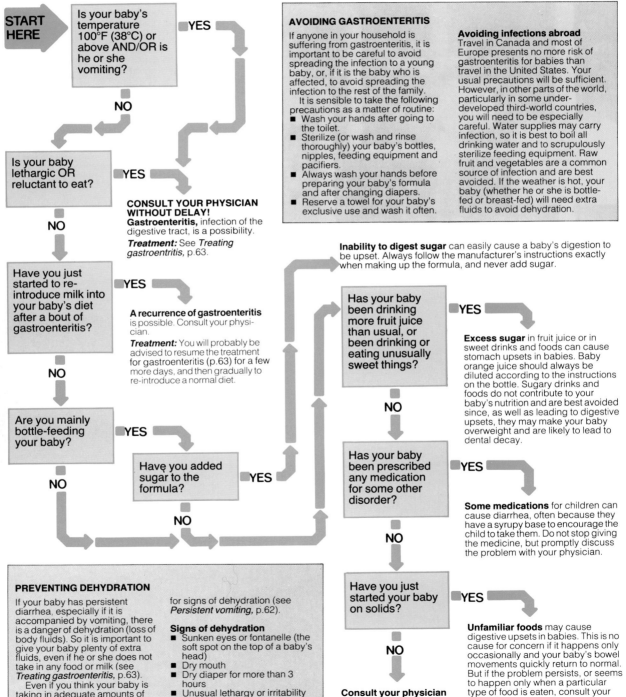

START HERE → Is your baby's temperature 100°F (38°C) or above AND/OR is he or she vomiting?

YES →

NO ↓

Is your baby lethargic OR reluctant to eat?

YES →

CONSULT YOUR PHYSICIAN WITHOUT DELAY!
Gastroenteritis, infection of the digestive tract, is a possibility.
Treatment: See *Treating gastroenteritis,* p.63.

NO ↓

Have you just started to re-introduce milk into your baby's diet after a bout of gastroenteritis?

YES →

A recurrence of gastroenteritis is possible. Consult your physician.
Treatment: You will probably be advised to resume the treatment for gastroenteritis (p.63) for a few more days, and then gradually to re-introduce a normal diet.

NO ↓

Are you mainly bottle-feeding your baby?

YES →

Have you added sugar to the formula?

YES →

NO ↓

AVOIDING GASTROENTERITIS

If anyone in your household is suffering from gastroenteritis, it is important to be careful to avoid spreading the infection to a young baby, or, if it is the baby who is affected, to avoid spreading the infection to the rest of the family.

It is sensible to take the following precautions as a matter of routine:
■ Wash your hands after going to the toilet.
■ Sterilize (or wash and rinse thoroughly) your baby's bottles, nipples, feeding equipment and pacifiers.
■ Always wash your hands before preparing your baby's formula and after changing diapers.
■ Reserve a towel for your baby's exclusive use and wash it often.

Avoiding infections abroad
Travel in Canada and most of Europe presents no more risk of gastroenteritis for babies than travel in the United States. Your usual precautions will be sufficient. However, in other parts of the world, particularly in some under-developed third-world countries, you will need to be especially careful. Water supplies may carry infection, so it is best to boil all drinking water and to scrupulously sterilize feeding equipment. Raw fruit and vegetables are a common source of infection and are best avoided. If the weather is hot, your baby (whether he or she is bottle-fed or breast-fed) will need extra fluids to avoid dehydration.

Inability to digest sugar can easily cause a baby's digestion to be upset. Always follow the manufacturer's instructions exactly when making up the formula, and never add sugar.

Has your baby been drinking more fruit juice than usual, or been drinking or eating unusually sweet things?

YES →

Excess sugar in fruit juice or in sweet drinks and foods can cause stomach upsets in babies. Baby orange juice should always be diluted according to the instructions on the bottle. Sugary drinks and foods do not contribute to your baby's nutrition and are best avoided since, as well as leading to digestive upsets, they may make your baby overweight and are likely to lead to dental decay.

NO ↓

Has your baby been prescribed any medication for some other disorder?

YES →

Some medications for children can cause diarrhea, often because they have a syrupy base to encourage the child to take them. Do not stop giving the medicine, but promptly discuss the problem with your physician.

NO ↓

Have you just started your baby on solids?

YES →

Unfamiliar foods may cause digestive upsets in babies. This is no cause for concern if it happens only occasionally and your baby's bowel movements quickly return to normal. But if the problem persists, or seems to happen only when a particular type of food is eaten, consult your physician.

NO ↓

Consult your physician if you are unable to make a diagnosis from this chart.

PREVENTING DEHYDRATION

If your baby has persistent diarrhea, especially if it is accompanied by vomiting, there is a danger of dehydration (loss of body fluids). So it is important to give your baby plenty of extra fluids, even if he or she does not take in any food or milk (see *Treating gastroenteritis,* p.63).

Even if you think your baby is taking in adequate amounts of fluid, you should be on the lookout for signs of dehydration (see *Persistent vomiting,* p.62).

Signs of dehydration
■ Sunken eyes or fontanelle (the soft spot on the top of a baby's head)
■ Dry mouth
■ Dry diaper for more than 3 hours
■ Unusual lethargy or irritability
■ Lack of elasticity in the skin

Children: all ages

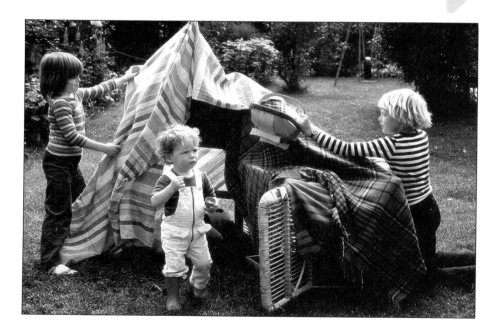

9 Feeling sick

A child may sometimes complain of feeling sick without giving you a clear idea of what exactly is the matter. Or you may suspect that your child is sick if he or she seems less lively or more irritable than usual. If this happens, you may be able to find a possible explanation for the problem by looking for specific signs of illness as described in this chart. If your child is under 2 years old, see the box below.

For unusual drowsiness, see chart 13, Drowsiness

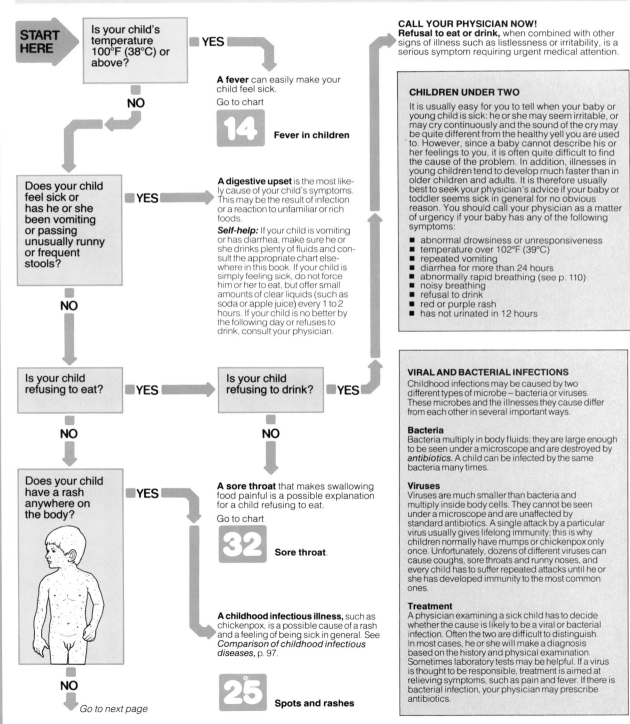

START HERE

Is your child's temperature 100°F (38°C) or above?

YES → A fever can easily make your child feel sick.

Go to chart

14 Fever in children

NO

Does your child feel sick or has he or she been vomiting or passing unusually runny or frequent stools?

YES → A digestive upset is the most likely cause of your child's symptoms. This may be the result of infection or a reaction to unfamiliar or rich foods.
Self-help: If your child is vomiting or has diarrhea, make sure he or she drinks plenty of fluids and consult the appropriate chart elsewhere in this book. If your child is simply feeling sick, do not force him or her to eat, but offer small amounts of clear liquids (such as soda or apple juice) every 1 to 2 hours. If your child is no better by the following day or refuses to drink, consult your physician.

NO

Is your child refusing to eat?

YES → **Is your child refusing to drink?**

YES →

NO

NO

Does your child have a rash anywhere on the body?

YES → A sore throat that makes swallowing food painful is a possible explanation for a child refusing to eat.

Go to chart

32 Sore throat.

A childhood infectious illness, such as chickenpox, is a possible cause of a rash and a feeling of being sick in general. See *Comparison of childhood infectious diseases,* p. 97.

25 Spots and rashes

NO

Go to next page

CALL YOUR PHYSICIAN NOW!
Refusal to eat or drink, when combined with other signs of illness such as listlessness or irritability, is a serious symptom requiring urgent medical attention.

CHILDREN UNDER TWO

It is usually easy for you to tell when your baby or young child is sick: he or she may seem irritable, or may cry continuously and the sound of the cry may be quite different from the healthy yell you are used to. However, since a baby cannot describe his or her feelings to you, it is often quite difficult to find the cause of the problem. In addition, illnesses in young children tend to develop much faster than in older children and adults. It is therefore usually best to seek your physician's advice if your baby or toddler seems sick in general for no obvious reason. You should call your physician as a matter of urgency if your baby has any of the following symptoms:

- abnormal drowsiness or unresponsiveness
- temperature over 102°F (39°C)
- repeated vomiting
- diarrhea for more than 24 hours
- abnormally rapid breathing (see p. 110)
- noisy breathing
- refusal to drink
- red or purple rash
- has not urinated in 12 hours

VIRAL AND BACTERIAL INFECTIONS

Childhood infections may be caused by two different types of microbe – bacteria or viruses. These microbes and the illnesses they cause differ from each other in several important ways.

Bacteria
Bacteria multiply in body fluids; they are large enough to be seen under a microscope and are destroyed by *antibiotics*. A child can be infected by the same bacteria many times.

Viruses
Viruses are much smaller than bacteria and multiply inside body cells. They cannot be seen under a microscope and are unaffected by standard antibiotics. A single attack by a particular virus usually gives lifelong immunity; this is why children normally have mumps or chickenpox only once. Unfortunately, dozens of different viruses can cause coughs, sore throats and runny noses, and every child has to suffer repeated attacks until he or she has developed immunity to the most common ones.

Treatment
A physician examining a sick child has to decide whether the cause is likely to be a viral or bacterial infection. Often the two are difficult to distinguish. In most cases, he or she will make a diagnosis based on the history and physical examination. Sometimes laboratory tests may be helpful. If a virus is thought to be responsible, treatment is aimed at relieving symptoms, such as pain and fever. If there is bacterial infection, your physician may prescribe antibiotics.

Continued from previous page

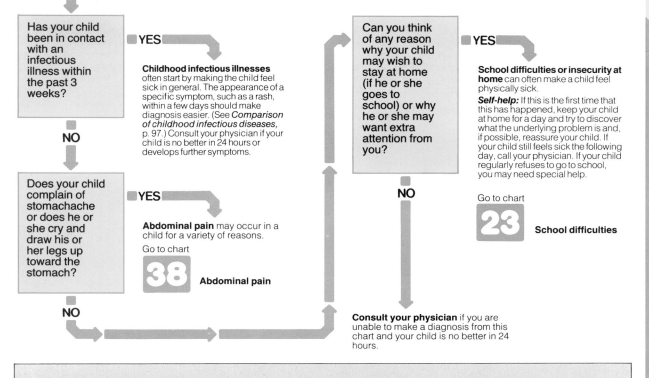

Has your child been in contact with an infectious illness within the past 3 weeks?

YES

Childhood infectious illnesses often start by making the child feel sick in general. The appearance of a specific symptom, such as a rash, within a few days should make diagnosis easier. (See *Comparison of childhood infectious diseases,* p. 97.) Consult your physician if your child is no better in 24 hours or develops further symptoms.

NO

Does your child complain of stomachache or does he or she cry and draw his or her legs up toward the stomach?

YES

Abdominal pain may occur in a child for a variety of reasons.

Go to chart

38 **Abdominal pain**

NO

Can you think of any reason why your child may wish to stay at home (if he or she goes to school) or why he or she may want extra attention from you?

YES

School difficulties or insecurity at home can often make a child feel physically sick.

Self-help: If this is the first time that this has happened, keep your child at home for a day and try to discover what the underlying problem is and, if possible, reassure your child. If your child still feels sick the following day, call your physician. If your child regularly refuses to go to school, you may need special help.

Go to chart

23 **School difficulties**

NO

Consult your physician if you are unable to make a diagnosis from this chart and your child is no better in 24 hours.

EXAMINATION BY THE PHYSICIAN

The examination that your physician performs on your sick child follows a methodical routine of assessment. The physician decides whether the child looks sick – in particular whether he or she is lively or apathetic.

Your physician then checks the pulse and breathing rates and examines the different body systems in turn.

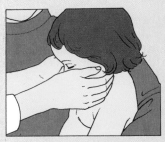

Lymph glands
The physician feels along the jaw (left) and in the armpits and groin for signs of swelling that may suggest infection.

Throat and mouth
The inside of the mouth and throat is examined for inflammation and spots using a wooden spatula and small flashlight (right).

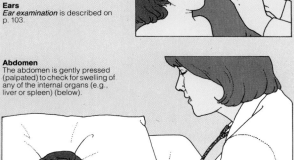

Heart and lungs
The health of heart and lungs are assessed by listening to the child's chest and back through a stethoscope (below).

Ears
Ear examination is described on p. 103.

Abdomen
The abdomen is gently pressed (palpated) to check for swelling of any of the internal organs (e.g., liver or spleen) (below).

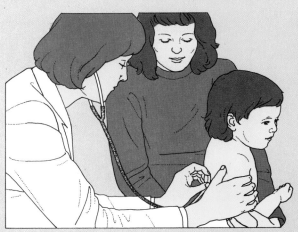

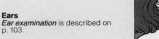

10 Slow growth

Many parents worry that their child is too short or too thin. Some children are naturally smaller than average as a result of heredity or other factors. However, serious growth disorders affecting general health are rare. The best way for you to avoid unnecessary anxiety is to keep a regular record of your child's height and weight so that you will know that your child is growing in proportion as well as at a normal rate (see the growth charts on pp. 300-301). Consult the diagnostic chart below only if your child's weight is increasing at a much slower rate than you would expect from his or her height, or if your child fails to grow in height as much as expected.

For children under 1 year, see chart 1, Slow weight gain

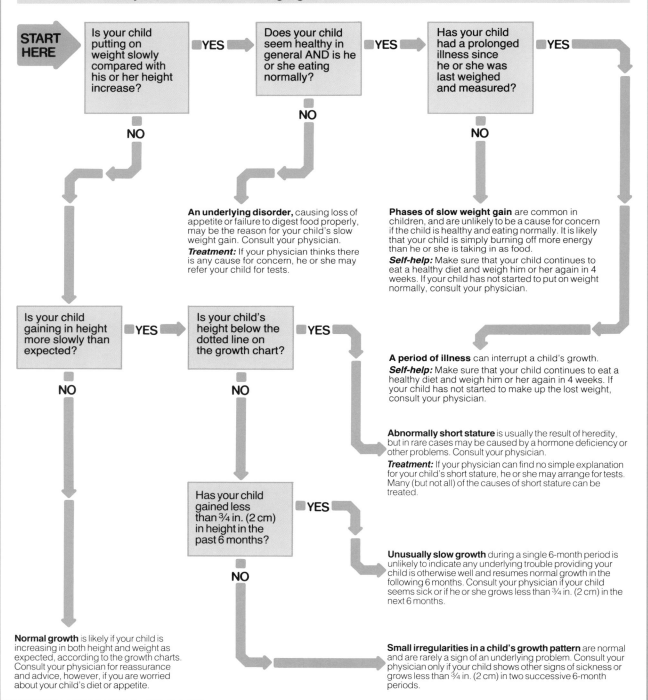

START HERE

Is your child putting on weight slowly compared with his or her height increase? — **YES** → **Does your child seem healthy in general AND is he or she eating normally?** — **YES** → **Has your child had a prolonged illness since he or she was last weighed and measured?** — **YES**

NO (from first box)

NO (from second box)

NO (from third box)

An underlying disorder, causing loss of appetite or failure to digest food properly, may be the reason for your child's slow weight gain. Consult your physician.
Treatment: If your physician thinks there is any cause for concern, he or she may refer your child for tests.

Phases of slow weight gain are common in children, and are unlikely to be a cause for concern if the child is healthy and eating normally. It is likely that your child is simply burning off more energy than he or she is taking in as food.
Self-help: Make sure that your child continues to eat a healthy diet and weigh him or her again in 4 weeks. If your child has not started to put on weight normally, consult your physician.

Is your child gaining in height more slowly than expected? — **YES** → **Is your child's height below the dotted line on the growth chart?** — **YES**

NO (gaining height box)

NO (height below box)

A period of illness can interrupt a child's growth.
Self-help: Make sure that your child continues to eat a healthy diet and weigh him or her again in 4 weeks. If your child has not started to make up the lost weight, consult your physician.

Abnormally short stature is usually the result of heredity, but in rare cases may be caused by a hormone deficiency or other problems. Consult your physician.
Treatment: If your physician can find no simple explanation for your child's short stature, he or she may arrange for tests. Many (but not all) of the causes of short stature can be treated.

Has your child gained less than ¾ in. (2 cm) in height in the past 6 months? — **YES**

NO (gained less box)

Unusually slow growth during a single 6-month period is unlikely to indicate any underlying trouble providing your child is otherwise well and resumes normal growth in the following 6 months. Consult your physician if your child seems sick or if he or she grows less than ¾ in. (2 cm) in the next 6 months.

Normal growth is likely if your child is increasing in both height and weight as expected, according to the growth charts. Consult your physician for reassurance and advice, however, if you are worried about your child's diet or appetite.

Small irregularities in a child's growth pattern are normal and are rarely a sign of an underlying problem. Consult your physician only if your child shows other signs of sickness or grows less than ¾ in. (2 cm) in two successive 6-month periods.

GROWTH PATTERNS IN CHILDHOOD

The growth charts on pp. 300–301 enable you to record your child's height and weight at regular intervals and to compare his or her progress with the standard growth rates for large, average and small children.

Usually, a child's growth will remain close to a standard curve for both height and weight throughout childhood. However, sometimes growth patterns can vary, as shown by the charts below.

Naturally slim
Some children are naturally slim. This is unlikely to be a cause for concern in a healthy child if both height and weight increase at a constant rate, and providing that the child's weight is only a little less than expected. The chart shown is that of a normal child who has always been light for his or her own height.

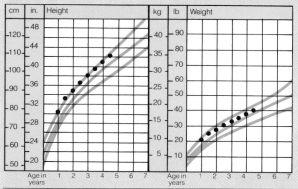

Losing excess weight
An overweight child may at first appear to be gaining insufficient weight as he or she slims down. The chart shows a child whose height is average, but whose weight was above average at 2 years. Over the next 2 years he or she gained little weight so that, by the age of 4, the child's weight was normal for his or her height.

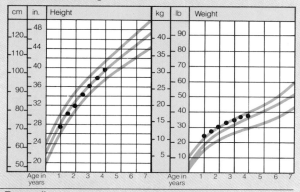

Too light
This chart shows a tall child whose weight is increasing much slower than normal, although he or she is growing in height as expected. If your child's weight is increasing at less than the normal rate, you should consult your physician.

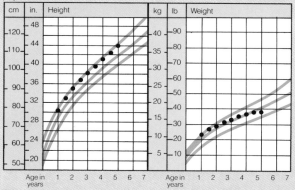

Too small
This chart shows both weight and height increasing at a much slower rate than is normal, even for a small child. If your child's growth chart looks like this, you should seek medical advice.

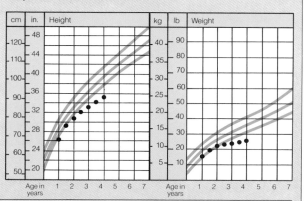

Overweight
The chart of a child who is overweight shows a normal rate of height increase – in this example the child is just below average height – but the weight increase curve is similar to that of a much taller child. If your child's growth chart looks like this, consult diagnostic chart 11, *Excessive weight gain*.

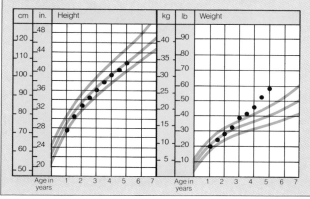

Late puberty
A child approaching puberty who is a late developer may appear to be growing more slowly than normal at an age when many of his or her contemporaries have reached a period of rapid growth. This is, however, no cause for concern; the child will usually make up for the delay later, as shown in this example. See also diagnostic chart 50, *Delayed puberty*.

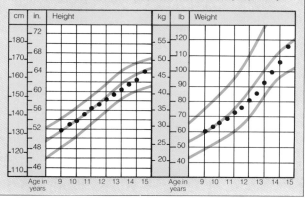

11 Excessive weight gain

Growing appreciation of the dangers of obesity in adults has led to an increasing awareness that the problem often starts in childhood, when eating habits are established. In addition, being overweight carries particular health risks for a child and may contribute to emotional and social problems as he or she gets older. It is therefore most important for parents to be alert to the possibility of excessive weight gain in their child. The appearance of a young baby is not always a reliable sign of obesity, as babies and toddlers are naturally chubby. The best way of ensuring that you quickly notice any weight problem in your child (whatever his or her age) is to keep a regular record of your child's growth (see the growth charts on pp. 300-301). If your child's weight-gain curve is rising more steeply than the curve for height, your child is probably becoming fat. Consult this diagnostic chart to find out what may be the reason.

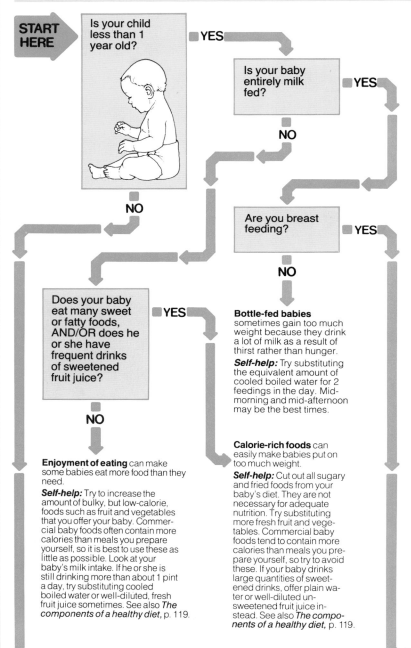

START HERE

Is your child less than 1 year old?

YES

Is your baby entirely milk fed?

YES

NO

Are you breast feeding?

YES

NO

NO

Does your baby eat many sweet or fatty foods, AND/OR does he or she have frequent drinks of sweetened fruit juice?

YES

NO

Bottle-fed babies sometimes gain too much weight because they drink a lot of milk as a result of thirst rather than hunger.

Self-help: Try substituting the equivalent amount of cooled boiled water for 2 feedings in the day. Mid-morning and mid-afternoon may be the best times.

Calorie-rich foods can easily make babies put on too much weight.

Self-help: Cut out all sugary and fried foods from your baby's diet. They are not necessary for adequate nutrition. Try substituting more fresh fruit and vegetables. Commercial baby foods tend to contain more calories than meals you prepare yourself, so try to avoid these. If your baby drinks large quantities of sweetened drinks, offer plain water or well-diluted unsweetened fruit juice instead. See also *The components of a healthy diet,* p. 119.

Enjoyment of eating can make some babies eat more food than they need.

Self-help: Try to increase the amount of bulky, but low-calorie, foods such as fruit and vegetables that you offer your baby. Commercial baby foods often contain more calories than meals you prepare yourself, so it is best to use these as little as possible. Look at your baby's milk intake. If he or she is still drinking more than about 1 pint a day, try substituting cooled boiled water or well-diluted, fresh fruit juice sometimes. See also *The components of a healthy diet,* p. 119.

CAUSES OF EXCESSIVE WEIGHT GAIN

The vast majority of children who become overweight do so because they regularly eat more food than they burn up to produce energy. The excess calories are then deposited under the skin as fat. Normally, children will adjust their intake of food according to their energy needs. However, the body's natural appetite-regulating mechanism can be upset by a number of factors.

Family overeating
The most common cause of obesity in children is habitual overeating in the family, so that the child loses touch with the body's real needs. The family may eat too many of the wrong foods (mainly sugar and fat) or may simply eat too much. So, if your child is overweight, look at yourself and the rest of the family; the chances are that you all weigh more than you should. In this case, the best way to help your child to slim down will be for the whole family to adopt healthier eating habits.

Enforced eating
A child who is brought up to finish everything on the plate, regardless of appetite, may also become overweight, because he or she will become used to eating more than necessary to please his or her parents.

Eating for comfort
Less commonly, a child may turn to eating in reaction to stress and anxiety. In this situation, food is used for comfort rather than to satisfy hunger, and over time the child may get into the habit of eating too much.

Medical causes
Medical problems that cause obesity are extremely rare and should be considered only if your child shows other signs of ill health or if genuine attempts at dieting fail.

Three golden rules for preventing your child from becoming overweight

- Make sure that the whole family is eating a healthy diet (see *The components of a healthy diet,* p. 119).
- Always be guided by your child's appetite and never force him or her to eat. He or she will not starve.
- Try to avoid giving or withholding food as a form of reward or punishment. This may give food emotional significance for your child, which can lead to eating problems in the future.

Breast-fed babies often gain weight quickly between 2 and 4 months. This is perfectly normal and no special action is necessary.

Go to next page

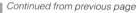
Continued from previous page

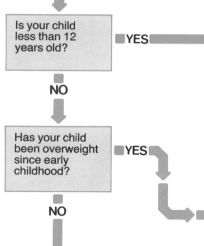

Is your child less than 12 years old?

YES

NO

Has your child been overweight since early childhood?

YES

NO

Family overeating is almost always the cause of excessive weight gain in this age group. See *Causes of excessive weight gain*, opposite.

Self-help: Suggestions for helping your child slim down are given below. Do not try to achieve a rapid weight loss or you will become overanxious about your child's eating habits and may transmit your anxiety to your child, creating additional problems. At this age, when children have plenty of growing to do before they reach adult size, concentrate simply on preventing additional weight gain, so that your child "stretches out" as he or she gets taller. If your child is severely overweight, discuss the problem with your physician, who will help you with diet advice, and may put you in contact with a self-help support group for overweight children.

Unhealthy eating habits established in early childhood are likely to persist into adolescence and adulthood unless action is taken.

Self-help: Your child probably realizes that he or she has a weight problem. Plenty of moral support from you is necessary to make any diet successful. This includes the cooperation of the whole family in eating sensibly. It is difficult for a child to lose weight if either parent is overeating. Look at the diet suggestions below and discuss the best methods of losing weight with your child. Your child's cooperation is essential; if you try to enforce a diet, he or she may only start to eat secretly. Crash dieting can be harmful physically and emotionally. Gradual weight loss is far more effective.

Sudden weight gain as a child approaches adolescence is common, particularly in girls. Slight weight gain may be the result of hormonal changes, but excessive weight gain is more likely to be the result of overeating, possibly as a result of emotional insecurity.

Self-help: If your child is only slightly overweight, no special action is necessary other than paying a little extra attention to providing a healthy diet. If your child has put on a lot of weight, try to find out why he or she is overeating. Does your child have any reason to feel insecure? Are there any problems in the family or at school? Tackling the underlying cause of any unhappiness as well as adopting a sensible reducing diet (see *How to help your child lose weight*, right) will help your child feel more self-confident.

THE DANGERS OF OBESITY IN CHILDHOOD

Dangers to health
The principal danger to physical health of obesity in childhood is that children who become fat are more likely to remain so and become fat adults, who in turn are at greater-than-average risk from disorders of the heart and circulation, and other problems. There are also risks to the health of the child. Some physicians believe that overweight children suffer from more chest infections than those who are slimmer. Tooth decay is more common in overweight children, who tend to eat more sugary foods than other children. A child who is overweight is likely to be less physically active than a slimmer child, making it more difficult to burn off the excess fat or to become physically fit in other ways.

Social and psychological risks
Although entirely unfair, a risk for obese children is that of social isolation. They are often the butt of other children's cruel ribbing, leading to much unhappiness. And, as these children approach adolescence, they will feel more self-conscious and less secure than other children at a time when self-confidence may be low in any case, and the need for social acceptance is at its greatest.

HOW TO HELP YOUR CHILD LOSE WEIGHT

Diet
The principal adjustment to your child's diet should be to cut out all foods that contain calories but few nutrients. Foods in this category include cakes, cookies, white bread and sweetened drinks. At mealtimes substitute fresh fruit for dessert, and encourage your child to drink plain water or unsweetened fruit juice instead of cola or pop. In many cases this change of diet alone is enough to help a child lose weight.

You should also look at the way you cook and serve food. Butter, margarine, oil and lard are all high in calories. So cut down on the amount of fat you use in cooking; grill or bake rather than fry. Do not coat vegetables in butter, and avoid heavy gravies and sauces. Spread butter and margarine very thinly on bread.

Replace the foods you have cut down on with plenty of fruit and vegetables. These will help satisfy hunger and supply vitamins without making your child fat.

The importance of exercise
The more physically active a child is, the easier it is to burn up excess fat.

Persuade your young child to walk rather than ride in a carriage or stroller, and encourage outdoor games that involve running or bicycling. An older child may need to be persuaded to take part in sports. Less competitive activities such as swimming, dancing and cycling may be more suitable for an overweight child.

Your support
For children to lose weight successfully, they must never be made to feel different or excluded. Adopt the diet suggestions for the whole family – it will do none of you any harm. Make exercise an enjoyable part of the family routine. Above all, never make your child feel that the diet is a form of punishment. Assure your child of your love no matter what, and you are far more likely to succeed.

You should be careful not to insist that your child be thin, especially if a girl. This may contribute to excessive dieting when she becomes a teenager. It is important that you are not extremely overweight – but this should not lead to the attitude that it is good to be underweight.

All the family can enjoy a healthy diet that helps your child to lose weight.

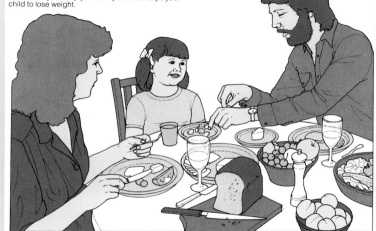

12 Sleeping problems

Most children over 1 year old will sleep through the night without interruption. The amount of sleep a child needs each night varies from about 9 to 12 hours according to age and individual requirements. Lack of sleep does not affect appetite, growth or development. However, refusal to go to bed at what you consider to be a reasonable time, and/or waking in the middle of the night, can be disruptive and sometimes distressing for the whole family. A number of factors may be responsible for such sleeping problems, including physical illness, emotional upset, nightmares and failure to establish a regular bedtime routine.

For children under 1 year, see chart 2, Waking at night

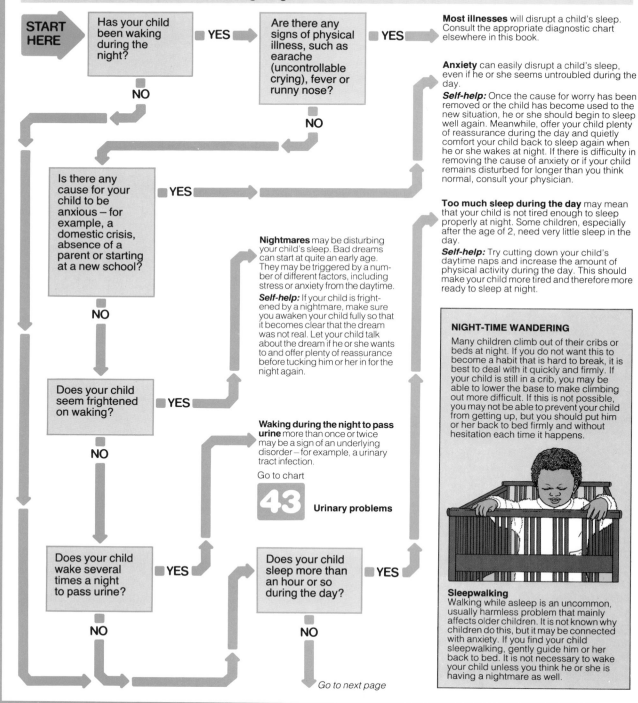

START HERE

Has your child been waking during the night?

YES ➡ Are there any signs of physical illness, such as earache (uncontrollable crying), fever or runny nose?

YES ➡ **Most illnesses** will disrupt a child's sleep. Consult the appropriate diagnostic chart elsewhere in this book.

NO

NO

Is there any cause for your child to be anxious – for example, a domestic crisis, absence of a parent or starting at a new school?

YES

Anxiety can easily disrupt a child's sleep, even if he or she seems untroubled during the day.
Self-help: Once the cause for worry has been removed or the child has become used to the new situation, he or she should begin to sleep well again. Meanwhile, offer your child plenty of reassurance during the day and quietly comfort your child back to sleep again when he or she wakes at night. If there is difficulty in removing the cause of anxiety or if your child remains disturbed for longer than you think normal, consult your physician.

Too much sleep during the day may mean that your child is not tired enough to sleep properly at night. Some children, especially after the age of 2, need very little sleep in the day.
Self-help: Try cutting down your child's daytime naps and increase the amount of physical activity during the day. This should make your child more tired and therefore more ready to sleep at night.

NO

Nightmares may be disturbing your child's sleep. Bad dreams can start at quite an early age. They may be triggered by a number of different factors, including stress or anxiety from the daytime.
Self-help: If your child is frightened by a nightmare, make sure you awaken your child fully so that it becomes clear that the dream was not real. Let your child talk about the dream if he or she wants to and offer plenty of reassurance before tucking him or her in for the night again.

Does your child seem frightened on waking?

YES

NIGHT-TIME WANDERING

Many children climb out of their cribs or beds at night. If you do not want this to become a habit that is hard to break, it is best to deal with it quickly and firmly. If your child is still in a crib, you may be able to lower the base to make climbing out more difficult. If this is not possible, you may not be able to prevent your child from getting up, but you should put him or her back to bed firmly and without hesitation each time it happens.

NO

Waking during the night to pass urine more than once or twice may be a sign of an underlying disorder – for example, a urinary tract infection.

Go to chart

43 **Urinary problems**

Does your child wake several times a night to pass urine?

YES ➡ Does your child sleep more than an hour or so during the day?

YES

NO

NO

Sleepwalking
Walking while asleep is an uncommon, usually harmless problem that mainly affects older children. It is not known why children do this, but it may be connected with anxiety. If you find your child sleepwalking, gently guide him or her back to bed. It is not necessary to wake your child unless you think he or she is having a nightmare as well.

Go to next page

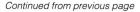
Continued from previous page

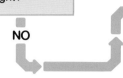
Does your child usually cry as soon as you leave the room at night?

YES

NO

Waking at night without obvious cause is usually the result of an irregular sleeping pattern. Your child may be in the habit of expecting attention from you during the night.

Self-help: To re-establish a regular sleeping rhythm, you will need to stick firmly to a plan such as the one described in the box on *Preventing and overcoming sleeping problems,* below. Your child will probably take up to 2 weeks to adjust to the new routine.

Fear of being left alone and a continuing need for the reassurance of your presence will often make a child reluctant to go to sleep at night.

Self-help: You will need to accustom your child gradually to the idea of going to sleep on his or her own each night. Try the suggestions for *Preventing and overcoming sleeping problems,* below. If you think your child may be frightened of the dark, leave a night-light on.

PREVENTING AND OVERCOMING SLEEPING PROBLEMS

Most children need to have a predictable bedtime ritual to help them settle down for the night. The suggestions made for establishing such a routine for babies under 1 year (see *Helping your baby sleep,* p. 52) also apply, on the whole, to older children. However, even if there is an established bedtime routine, many young children develop sleeping problems. A child may start to refuse to go to bed, or may regularly wake at night. This may be triggered by an upset to the routine, such as a holiday away from home or a stay at the hospital, but often may have no apparent cause. If your child has developed some bad sleeping habits, you will need to take steps to re-establish a more convenient pattern.

Refusal to go to sleep
If your child refuses to go to sleep and cries when put to bed for the night after the usual bedtime ritual, you can try one of the two "withdrawal" approaches that follow. Whichever method you choose, you will need to ensure total consistency from both parents; any exception to the rule will undermine the progress you have already made. Both methods are likely to involve prolonged periods of crying.

Sudden withdrawal
Once you have settled your child in the crib or bed, say goodnight and leave the room, and do not return when your child starts to cry. The first night your child may take an hour or more to go to sleep, but each successive night the period of crying should get shorter until, after a week or so, he or she should go to bed without a fuss. Your child will come to no harm from the crying, but many parents find this method too much of an ordeal.

Gradual withdrawal
Having put your child to bed, say goodnight, tell your child you will return in 10 minutes, and leave the room. In 10 minutes, return for a few moments to reassure your child that you are still there, say goodnight again, tell him or her that you will return in 20 minutes, and then leave. Repeat this, reducing the amount of time you spend in the room, until your child falls asleep. This may take several hours the first night but, if you persevere, the time should get shorter until after a week or two there is no further trouble.

Waking during the night
If your child has gotten into the habit of waking during the night, you can try a program of conditioning similar to the one described for refusal to go to sleep. If your child only whimpers in the night, do not go into the room at once; wait a few moments, he or she may still be half-asleep and will drift off again, if undisturbed. If your child is truly crying, you will need to go into the room to check that there is nothing wrong – for example, an earache or a nightmare. Once you are satisfied that all is well, give a drink of water if it is wanted, tuck your child in again, and say goodnight. Then leave the room as quickly and quietly as possible. After this you can either allow your child to cry himself or herself to sleep or return every 10 to 20 minutes or so as described under *gradual withdrawal,* above.

How your physician can help
If these suggestions do not work for your child, or if you are worn out by many sleepless nights, consult your physician. An older child who has difficulty falling asleep and wakes up early may be depressed. Never give your child sleeping drugs prescribed for an adult. These can be extremely dangerous for children.

Your child's bedroom
It is important to make your child's room as pleasant and as welcoming as possible, so that he or she is always happy to be left there at night (right).

Bedtime ritual
Most young children respond to a predictable bedtime ritual, such as a bath, always followed by a story, before turning the lights out (below).

Comforting objects
Many children become attached to a particular toy or to another comforting item, such as a blanket. Hugging this object will often encourage sleep (below right).

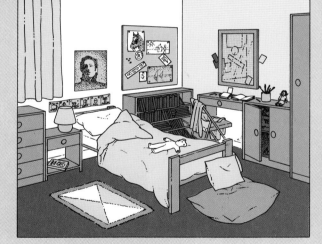

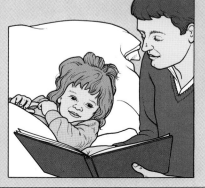

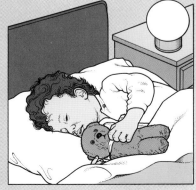

13 Drowsiness

Drowsiness (or excessive sleepiness) may be a child's natural response to lack of sleep or an unusually late night. In addition, a child who is sick – for example, with flu – is likely to sleep more than usual. Consult this chart if your child suddenly becomes unusually sleepy or unresponsive, or if he or she is difficult to arouse from sleep and you can find no obvious explanation. This is a serious symptom that should never be ignored.

START HERE

Does your child have one or more of the following symptoms?
- temperature of 100°F (38°C) or above
- vomiting without diarrhea
- reluctance to bend the head forward
- headache

YES

CALL YOUR PHYSICIAN NOW!
Meningitis (inflammation of the membranes surrounding the nervous system) or encephalitis (inflammation of the brain itself) may be present.

Treatment: Your child will probably be admitted to the hospital where he or she will be given a *lumbar puncture* (below right) to make an exact diagnosis and will also be given fluids and possibly *antibiotics* intravenously.

NO

Could your child have taken any of the following?
- drugs prescribed for an adult
- alcohol
- poisonous plants or berries

YES

EMERGENCY
GET MEDICAL HELP NOW!
Poisoning by any of these substances can cause a child to become drowsy. See *Poisoning* (p. 286) for first-aid advice.

NO

Go to chart

25 **Spots and rashes**

Does your child have a rash anywhere on the body?

YES

Has your child suffered a blow to the head within the past few days?

YES

NO

NO

Go to next page

EMERGENCY
GET MEDICAL HELP NOW!

A serious head injury, resulting in bleeding, may cause drowsiness.

Treatment: Your child will probably need to have an X-ray or *CT (computed tomography) scan* (p. 85) of the brain. If tests reveal bleeding inside the skull, an operation may be necessary.

LUMBAR PUNCTURE

A child with suspected meningitis will need to have a lumbar puncture to find out whether infection by viruses or bacteria is responsible for the disease. This test involves taking a sample of the fluid that surrounds the brain and spinal cord by using a needle at the base of the spinal cord. The area is numbed by local anesthetic before the needle is inserted, and most children suffer little discomfort.

The needle of the syringe is inserted between the backbones (vertebrae) at the base of the spinal cord to enable a sample of cerebrospinal fluid to be drawn off.

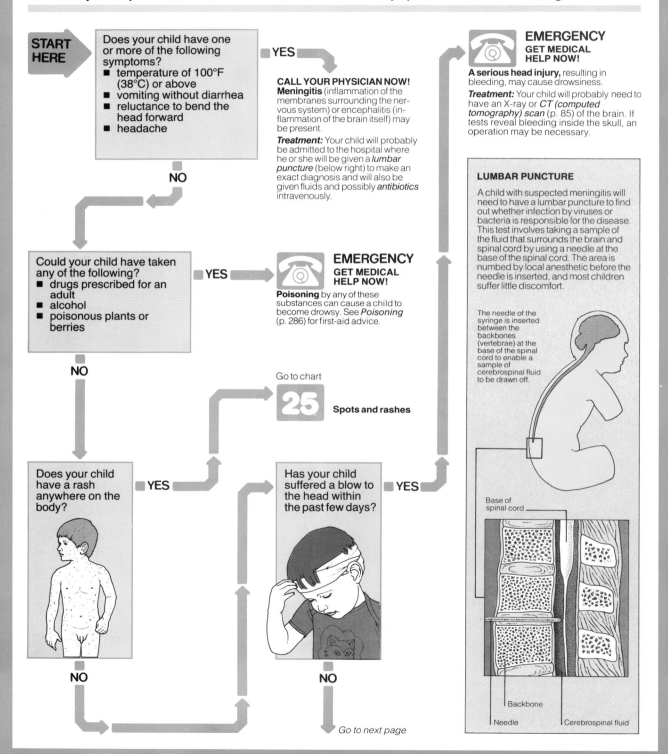

Base of spinal cord

Backbone

Needle

Cerebrospinal fluid

Continued from previous page

Does your child have diarrhea?

YES ► **CALL YOUR PHYSICIAN NOW!**
Dehydration as a result of persistent diarrhea is possible, especially if your child has been vomiting as well. This may originally have been caused by an infection of the digestive tract (gastroenteritis). (See chart 40, *Diarrhea in children.*)

Treatment: If your physician confirms the diagnosis of dehydration, your child will be admitted to the hospital, where fluids can be given intravenously.

NO

Has your child been unusually thirsty lately?

YES ► **Has your child been passing large amounts of urine?**

YES ► **CALL YOUR PHYSICIAN NOW!**
Too much sugar in the blood as a result of diabetes can cause drowsiness. Diabetes occurs when the body fails to make sufficient quantities of the hormone insulin, which helps convert sugar into energy.

Treatment: If your physician suspects this possibility, he or she will arrange for your child to be admitted to the hospital at once where tests will confirm the diagnosis. Your child will be given insulin injections and also fluids to reduce the level of sugar in the blood. If your child has diabetes, he or she will probably need injections of insulin for life.

NO

NO

Has your child lost weight AND/OR been unusually tired during the past few weeks?

YES ►

NO

Certain drugs, such as antihistamines given for allergic disorders, may cause mild drowsiness. Discuss the problem with your physician. If, however, your child becomes very drowsy and unresponsive, you should call your physician at once.

Is your child taking any medications prescribed by your physician?

YES ►

NO

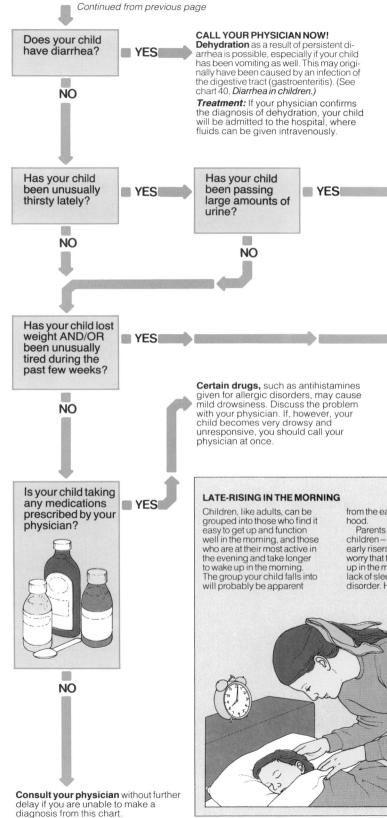

DROWSINESS AND DRUG AND ALCOHOL ABUSE IN OLDER CHILDREN

Parents of children over about 10 years of age should bear in mind the possibility of abuse of drugs (perhaps tranquilizers or marijuana), solvents (including glue and dry-cleaning fluids) or alcohol if the child has episodes of unusual sleepiness or lethargy over a period of days or weeks. Additional signs may include loss of appetite, red eyes, headaches or a falling off in school performance. There are, of course, a number of less worrisome explanations for such symptoms, such as a minor infection or temporary anxiety or depression. Whichever problem you suspect, your child's symptoms should be brought to your physician's attention.

See also *Smoking, alcohol and drug abuse,* p. 140.

LATE-RISING IN THE MORNING

Children, like adults, can be grouped into those who find it easy to get up and function well in the morning, and those who are at their most active in the evening and take longer to wake up in the morning. The group your child falls into will probably be apparent from the early years of childhood.

Parents of late-waking children – especially if they are early risers themselves – often worry that this reluctance to get up in the morning is a sign of lack of sleep or of a physical disorder. However, there is rarely any cause for concern if an otherwise healthy child who is alert and energetic for most of the rest of the day takes an hour or so to become fully awake in the morning. Enforcing an early bedtime when a child feels full of energy is unlikely to help the problem and may lead to unnecessary conflict.

When to consult your physician

While there is no cause for concern if a child is regularly sluggish in the mornings only, you should consult your physician in the following cases:
- If your child starts to become drowsy at other times of the day.
- If a normally early-waking child is unusually drowsy in the morning for no obvious reason.

Call your physician at once if you cannot rouse your child from sleep in the morning.

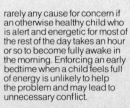

Consult your physician without further delay if you are unable to make a diagnosis from this chart.

14 Fever in children

A fever (above-normal body temperature) is usually caused by infection either by viruses or bacteria (p. 66). However, a child may also become feverish if allowed to become overheated – for example, as a result of playing too long in hot sunshine. A raised temperature will make a child's forehead feel hot and will cause increased sweating and a sick feeling. If you suspect that your child has a fever, take his or her temperature (see opposite). Consult this chart if the temperature reading is 100°F (38°C) or above.

For children under 1 year, see chart 3, Fever in babies

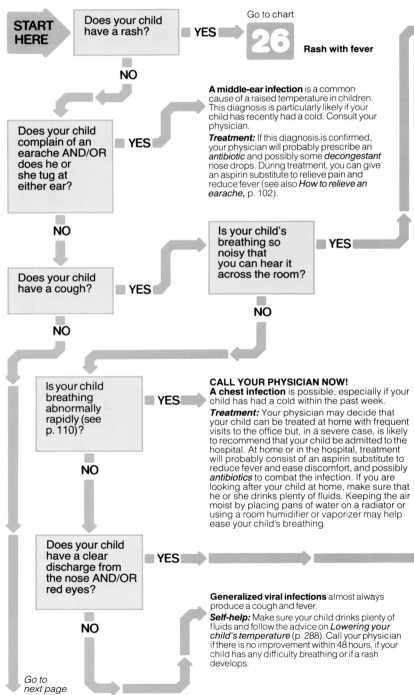

START HERE

Does your child have a rash?
YES → Go to chart **26** **Rash with fever**

NO

Does your child complain of an earache AND/OR does he or she tug at either ear?
YES →

NO

Does your child have a cough?
YES →

NO

Is your child breathing so noisy that you can hear it across the room?
YES →
NO

Is your child breathing abnormally rapidly (see p. 110)?
YES →

NO

Does your child have a clear discharge from the nose AND/OR red eyes?
YES →

NO

Go to next page

A middle-ear infection is a common cause of a raised temperature in children. This diagnosis is particularly likely if your child has recently had a cold. Consult your physician.

Treatment: If this diagnosis is confirmed, your physician will probably prescribe an *antibiotic* and possibly some *decongestant* nose drops. During treatment, you can give an aspirin substitute to relieve pain and reduce fever (see also *How to relieve an earache,* p. 102).

CALL YOUR PHYSICIAN NOW!
A chest infection is possible, especially if your child has had a cold within the past week.

Treatment: Your physician may decide that your child can be treated at home with frequent visits to the office but, in a severe case, is likely to recommend that your child be admitted to the hospital. At home or in the hospital, treatment will probably consist of an aspirin substitute to reduce fever and ease discomfort, and possibly *antibiotics* to combat the infection. If you are looking after your child at home, make sure that he or she drinks plenty of fluids. Keeping the air moist by placing pans of water on a radiator or using a room humidifier or vaporizer may help ease your child's breathing.

Generalized viral infections almost always produce a cough and fever.
Self-help: Make sure your child drinks plenty of fluids and follow the advice on *Lowering your child's temperature* (p. 288). Call your physician if there is no improvement within 48 hours, if your child has any difficulty breathing or if a rash develops.

EMERGENCY
GET MEDICAL HELP NOW!

Narrowing of the air passages caused by inflammation of the tissues resulting from infection is a possibility.

Treatment: While waiting for medical help, you may be able to ease your child's breathing by moistening the air with steam. Taking your child into a bathroom where you have turned on the hot water tap or shower to make steam is often effective. Your child may need to be admitted to the hospital, where oxygen and intravenous fluids will be given. Your child may also be given *antibiotics.*

FEVERISH CONVULSIONS

Young children (under 5) sometimes have convulsions when their temperatures rise too quickly. During such a convulsion, a child's arms and legs will shake uncontrollably and he or she may turn blue in the face. This may last for several minutes or sometimes longer.

What to do
Lay the child flat on his or her stomach with the head turned to the side. If there is vomiting, clean out the mouth with your finger. The convulsion will not damage your child's brain and it will stop by itself in a few minutes. If your child has a convulsion caused by fever, it *does not mean* that your child has epilepsy, and he or she may never have another convulsion. Some children, however, do have an underlying problem. Your physician may want to do more tests after your child recovers.

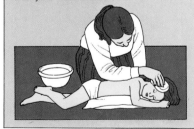

Measles often starts with a cough, fever, runny nose and/or inflamed eyes. The appearance of a red rash a few days later makes this diagnosis more likely, especially if your child has not been vaccinated against the disease (see *Comparison of childhood infectious diseases,* p. 97). Consult your physician.

Treatment: There is no specific treatment for measles. You will probably just be advised to keep your child's temperature down (see *Lowering your child's temperature,* p. 288). There is no need to darken your child's room as was once believed. Call your physician at once if your child develops an earache, has any difficulty breathing or becomes drowsy and difficult to wake. Full recovery normally takes about 10 days.

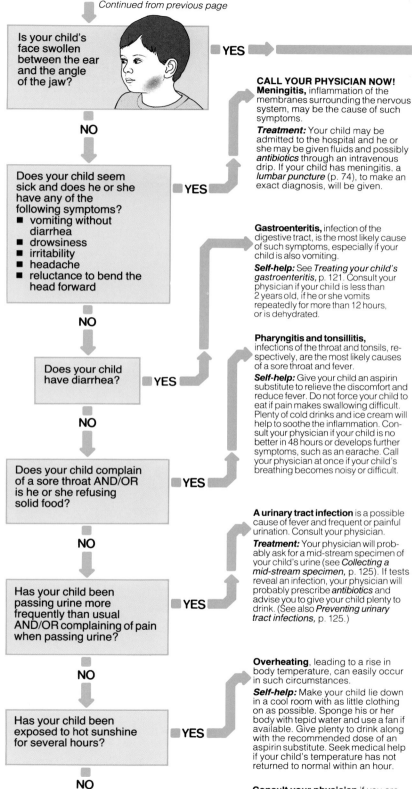

Continued from previous page

Is your child's face swollen between the ear and the angle of the jaw?

YES →

Mumps, a viral infection that mainly affects the salivary glands, is a possibility, especially if your child has been in contact with the disease within the past 3 weeks. (See *Comparison of childhood infectious diseases,* p. 97.) Consult your physician.

Treatment: Your physician will probably advise you to keep your child at home and give him or her an aspirin substitute and plenty of cold drinks to relieve the discomfort. Recovery normally takes 7 to 10 days.

NO ↓

Does your child seem sick and does he or she have any of the following symptoms?
- vomiting without diarrhea
- drowsiness
- irritability
- headache
- reluctance to bend the head forward

YES →

CALL YOUR PHYSICIAN NOW!
Meningitis, inflammation of the membranes surrounding the nervous system, may be the cause of such symptoms.

Treatment: Your child may be admitted to the hospital and he or she may be given fluids and possibly *antibiotics* through an intravenous drip. If your child has meningitis, a *lumbar puncture* (p. 74), to make an exact diagnosis, will be given.

NO ↓

Does your child have diarrhea?

YES →

Gastroenteritis, infection of the digestive tract, is the most likely cause of such symptoms, especially if your child is also vomiting.

Self-help: See *Treating your child's gastroenteritis,* p. 121. Consult your physician if your child is less than 2 years old, if he or she vomits repeatedly for more than 12 hours, or is dehydrated.

NO ↓

Does your child complain of a sore throat AND/OR is he or she refusing solid food?

YES →

Pharyngitis and tonsillitis, infections of the throat and tonsils, re-spectively, are the most likely causes of a sore throat and fever.

Self-help: Give your child an aspirin substitute to relieve the discomfort and reduce fever. Do not force your child to eat if pain makes swallowing difficult. Plenty of cold drinks and ice cream will help to soothe the inflammation. Con-sult your physician if your child is no better in 48 hours or develops further symptoms, such as an earache. Call your physician at once if your child's breathing becomes noisy or difficult.

NO ↓

Has your child been passing urine more frequently than usual AND/OR complaining of pain when passing urine?

YES →

A urinary tract infection is a possible cause of fever and frequent or painful urination. Consult your physician.

Treatment: Your physician will prob-ably ask for a mid-stream specimen of your child's urine (see *Collecting a mid-stream specimen,* p. 125). If tests reveal an infection, your physician will probably prescribe *antibiotics* and advise you to give your child plenty to drink. (See also *Preventing urinary tract infections,* p. 125.)

NO ↓

Has your child been exposed to hot sunshine for several hours?

YES →

Overheating, leading to a rise in body temperature, can easily occur in such circumstances.

Self-help: Make your child lie down in a cool room with as little clothing on as possible. Sponge his or her body with tepid water and use a fan if available. Give plenty to drink along with the recommended dose of an aspirin substitute. Seek medical help if your child's temperature has not returned to normal within an hour.

NO ↓

Consult your physician if you are unable to make a diagnosis from this chart.

TAKING YOUR CHILD'S TEMPERATURE

The best way to see if your child has a fever is to take the temperature using a clinical thermometer. For children under 7 years old, take a rectal temperature. (See *How to take a baby's temperature,* p. 55.) Older children can have their temperature taken by mouth.

Taking a temperature by mouth

1 Shake the thermometer with firm downward flicks of the wrist so that the mercury runs down into the bulb and reads well below the "normal" mark.

2 Place the bulb of the thermometer inside your child's mouth under the tongue. Let it remain in place for 3 minutes.

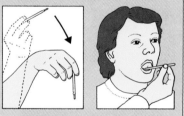

3 Remove the thermometer and turn it until you get a clear reading.

Using this method, you can consider your child feverish if his or her temperature is 100°F (38°C) or above. If your child's temperature rises above 102°F (39°C), whatever the suspected cause, call your physician at once.

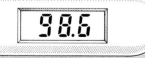

Digital thermometers
Digital thermometers, which display a numerical read-out, are also available for oral and under-the-arm temperatures.

FOREIGN TRAVEL

If your child develops a fever soon after a visit to a hot climate, be sure to tell your physician. Your child may have caught a disease that is rare in this country, one that your physician might not otherwise suspect.

15 Swollen glands

The term "swollen glands" usually refers to swelling (sometimes with tenderness) of one or more of the lymph glands (below right). In babies under 1 year, this is an unusual symptom that is difficult for the parent to diagnose. Consult your physician. In older children, the glands, especially those in the neck, often swell noticeably as a result of minor infections and this is rarely cause for concern. Persistent or generalized swelling of the glands, particularly if your child's color seems off, should be reported to your physician.

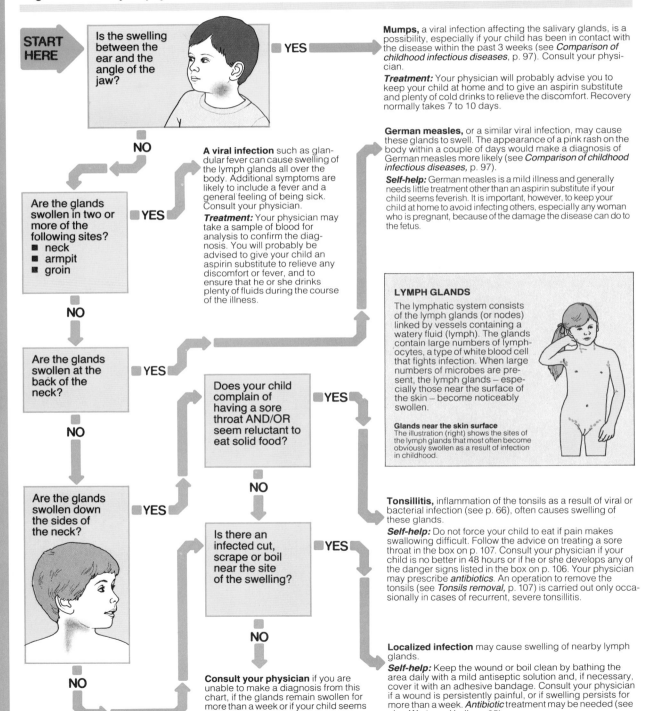

START HERE

Is the swelling between the ear and the angle of the jaw?

YES →

Mumps, a viral infection affecting the salivary glands, is a possibility, especially if your child has been in contact with the disease within the past 3 weeks (see *Comparison of childhood infectious diseases*, p. 97). Consult your physician.

Treatment: Your physician will probably advise you to keep your child at home and to give an aspirin substitute and plenty of cold drinks to relieve the discomfort. Recovery normally takes 7 to 10 days.

German measles, or a similar viral infection, may cause these glands to swell. The appearance of a pink rash on the body within a couple of days would make a diagnosis of German measles more likely (see *Comparison of childhood infectious diseases*, p. 97).

Self-help: German measles is a mild illness and generally needs little treatment other than an aspirin substitute if your child seems feverish. It is important, however, to keep your child at home to avoid infecting others, especially any woman who is pregnant, because of the damage the disease can do to the fetus.

NO ↓

Are the glands swollen in two or more of the following sites?
- neck
- armpit
- groin

YES →

A viral infection such as glandular fever can cause swelling of the lymph glands all over the body. Additional symptoms are likely to include a fever and a general feeling of being sick. Consult your physician.

Treatment: Your physician may take a sample of blood for analysis to confirm the diagnosis. You will probably be advised to give your child an aspirin substitute to relieve any discomfort or fever, and to ensure that he or she drinks plenty of fluids during the course of the illness.

NO ↓

Are the glands swollen at the back of the neck?

YES →

Does your child complain of having a sore throat AND/OR seem reluctant to eat solid food?

YES →

LYMPH GLANDS

The lymphatic system consists of the lymph glands (or nodes) linked by vessels containing a watery fluid (lymph). The glands contain large numbers of lymphocytes, a type of white blood cell that fights infection. When large numbers of microbes are present, the lymph glands – especially those near the surface of the skin – become noticeably swollen.

Glands near the skin surface
The illustration (right) shows the sites of the lymph glands that most often become obviously swollen as a result of infection in childhood.

NO ↓

NO ↓

Are the glands swollen down the sides of the neck?

YES →

Is there an infected cut, scrape or boil near the site of the swelling?

YES →

Tonsillitis, inflammation of the tonsils as a result of viral or bacterial infection (see p. 66), often causes swelling of these glands.

Self-help: Do not force your child to eat if pain makes swallowing difficult. Follow the advice on treating a sore throat in the box on p. 107. Consult your physician if your child is no better in 48 hours or if he or she develops any of the danger signs listed in the box on p. 106. Your physician may prescribe *antibiotics*. An operation to remove the tonsils (see *Tonsils removal*, p. 107) is carried out only occasionally in cases of recurrent, severe tonsillitis.

NO ↓

NO ↓

Consult your physician if you are unable to make a diagnosis from this chart, if the glands remain swollen for more than a week or if your child seems sick.

Localized infection may cause swelling of nearby lymph glands.

Self-help: Keep the wound or boil clean by bathing the area daily with a mild antiseptic solution and, if necessary, cover it with an adhesive bandage. Consult your physician if a wound is persistently painful, or if swelling persists for more than a week. *Antibiotic* treatment may be needed (see also *Warts and boils*, p. 95).

16 Itching

This diagnostic chart deals with itching that affects either the whole body or a particular area, such as the scalp or anus. A variety of disorders including allergies, contact with certain plants or chemicals, and certain infectious parasites may cause such irritation. Your child is likely to scratch. If unchecked, this may lead to the development of sore, infected areas, so it is important to deal with any disorder that produces itching.

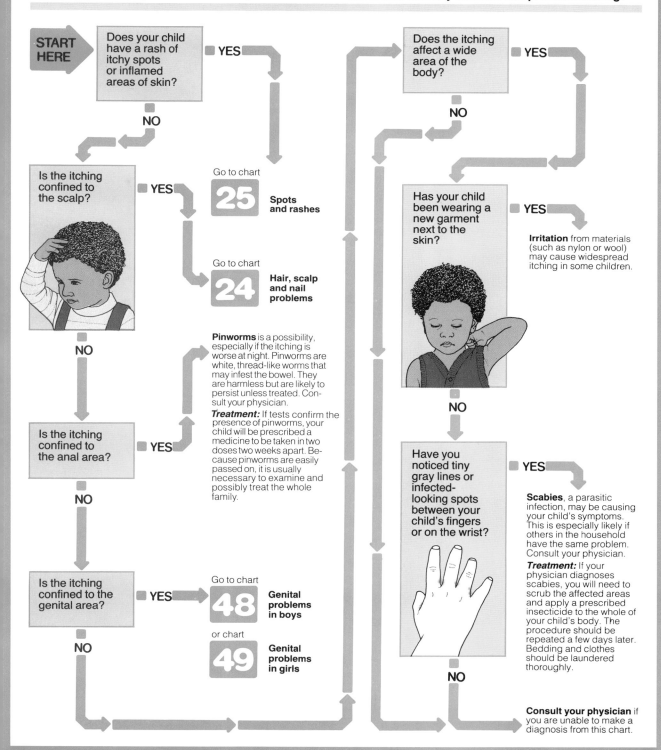

START HERE

Does your child have a rash of itchy spots or inflamed areas of skin?

YES → Go to chart **25** **Spots and rashes**

NO

Is the itching confined to the scalp?

YES → Go to chart **24** **Hair, scalp and nail problems**

NO

Is the itching confined to the anal area?

YES → **Pinworms** is a possibility, especially if the itching is worse at night. Pinworms are white, thread-like worms that may infest the bowel. They are harmless but are likely to persist unless treated. Consult your physician.
Treatment: If tests confirm the presence of pinworms, your child will be prescribed a medicine to be taken in two doses two weeks apart. Because pinworms are easily passed on, it is usually necessary to examine and possibly treat the whole family.

NO

Is the itching confined to the genital area?

YES → Go to chart **48** **Genital problems in boys**
or chart **49** **Genital problems in girls**

NO

Does the itching affect a wide area of the body?

YES →

NO

Has your child been wearing a new garment next to the skin?

YES → **Irritation** from materials (such as nylon or wool) may cause widespread itching in some children.

NO

Have you noticed tiny gray lines or infected-looking spots between your child's fingers or on the wrist?

YES → **Scabies**, a parasitic infection, may be causing your child's symptoms. This is especially likely if others in the household have the same problem. Consult your physician.
Treatment: If your physician diagnoses scabies, you will need to scrub the affected areas and apply a prescribed insecticide to the whole of your child's body. The procedure should be repeated a few days later. Bedding and clothes should be laundered thoroughly.

NO

Consult your physician if you are unable to make a diagnosis from this chart.

17 Fainting, dizzy spells and seizures

This chart deals with fainting, feelings of faintness and unsteadiness, dizzy spells and loss of consciousness including seizures and periods of "blankness." Many children feel faint from time to time and this is usually caused by anxiety or hunger, but frequent loss of consciousness or attacks during which a child suffers uncontrolled movements of the body or limbs is a sign of an underlying disorder.

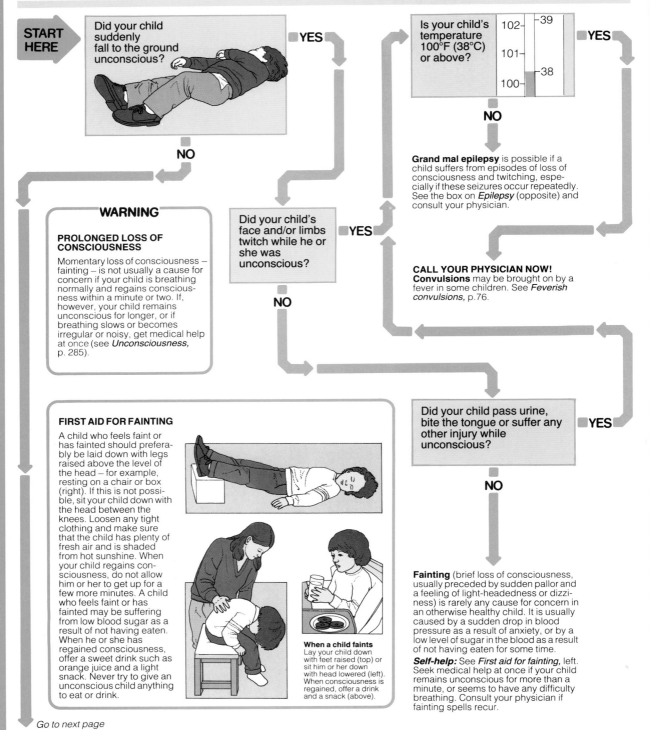

START HERE

Did your child suddenly fall to the ground unconscious?

YES

NO

Is your child's temperature 100°F (38°C) or above?

102— 101— 100—

—39 —38

YES

NO

WARNING

PROLONGED LOSS OF CONSCIOUSNESS

Momentary loss of consciousness – fainting – is not usually a cause for concern if your child is breathing normally and regains consciousness within a minute or two. If, however, your child remains unconscious for longer, or if breathing slows or becomes irregular or noisy, get medical help at once (see *Unconsciousness*, p. 285).

Did your child's face and/or limbs twitch while he or she was unconscious?

YES

NO

Grand mal epilepsy is possible if a child suffers from episodes of loss of consciousness and twitching, especially if these seizures occur repeatedly. See the box on *Epilepsy* (opposite) and consult your physician.

CALL YOUR PHYSICIAN NOW!
Convulsions may be brought on by a fever in some children. See *Feverish convulsions*, p.76.

FIRST AID FOR FAINTING

A child who feels faint or has fainted should preferably be laid down with legs raised above the level of the head – for example, resting on a chair or box (right). If this is not possible, sit your child down with the head between the knees. Loosen any tight clothing and make sure that the child has plenty of fresh air and is shaded from hot sunshine. When your child regains consciousness, do not allow him or her to get up for a few more minutes. A child who feels faint or has fainted may be suffering from low blood sugar as a result of not having eaten. When he or she has regained consciousness, offer a sweet drink such as orange juice and a light snack. Never try to give an unconscious child anything to eat or drink.

When a child faints
Lay your child down with feet raised (top) or sit him or her down with head lowered (left). When consciousness is regained, offer a drink and a snack (above).

Did your child pass urine, bite the tongue or suffer any other injury while unconscious?

YES

NO

Fainting (brief loss of consciousness, usually preceded by sudden pallor and a feeling of light-headedness or dizziness) is rarely any cause for concern in an otherwise healthy child. It is usually caused by a sudden drop in blood pressure as a result of anxiety, or by a low level of sugar in the blood as a result of not having eaten for some time.

Self-help: See *First aid for fainting,* left. Seek medical help at once if your child remains unconscious for more than a minute, or seems to have any difficulty breathing. Consult your physician if fainting spells recur.

Go to next page

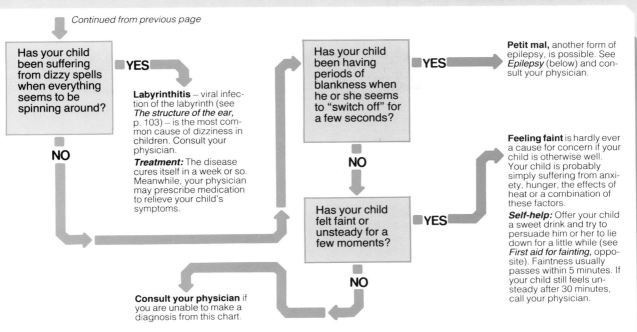

Continued from previous page

Has your child been suffering from dizzy spells when everything seems to be spinning around?

YES

Labyrinthitis – viral infection of the labyrinth (see *The structure of the ear*, p. 103) – is the most common cause of dizziness in children. Consult your physician.
Treatment: The disease cures itself in a week or so. Meanwhile, your physician may prescribe medication to relieve your child's symptoms.

NO

Has your child been having periods of blankness when he or she seems to "switch off" for a few seconds?

YES

Petit mal, another form of epilepsy, is possible. See *Epilepsy* (below) and consult your physician.

NO

Has your child felt faint or unsteady for a few moments?

YES

Feeling faint is hardly ever a cause for concern if your child is otherwise well. Your child is probably simply suffering from anxiety, hunger, the effects of heat or a combination of these factors.
Self-help: Offer your child a sweet drink and try to persuade him or her to lie down for a little while (see *First aid for fainting*, opposite). Faintness usually passes within 5 minutes. If your child still feels unsteady after 30 minutes, call your physician.

NO

Consult your physician if you are unable to make a diagnosis from this chart.

EPILEPSY

Epilepsy is the medical term for repeated loss or altered state of consciousness caused by abnormal electrical impulses in the brain. The underlying cause of the disorder is not known. The type and severity of symptoms may vary according to the nature of the abnormal impulses and the part of the brain affected. The two main forms of the disease are:

Grand mal
In the form of the disease known as grand mal, the child falls to the ground suddenly and may suffer injury during the fall. He or she remains unconscious for up to several minutes, often jerking the limbs or face uncontrollably. Gradually the movements stop and the child passes into normal sleep.

Petit mal
In petit mal epilepsy, the child loses full consciousness but does not fall to the ground. Such "absence attacks" last for 10 to 15 seconds, during which the child's face becomes vacant, and he or she stops speaking and does not hear what people are saying. Petit mal attacks often cease after adolescence.

Treatment
If your child has seizures that lead your physician to suspect a form of epilepsy, your child will probably be referred to a specialist (neurologist) for diagnosis and treatment. Diagnosis of the precise form of the disease and decisions about the best treatment for a child are usually made following *electroencephalography* (above right). Most forms of epilepsy are effectively controlled by drug treatment. The neurologist will advise you about any special precautions you will need to take with your child in regard to swimming, cycling and other activities, and will explain how to deal with the seizures. You should tell your child's teachers, and anyone else who has regular care of your child, about the disease and explain to them what to do during seizures.

Dealing with seizures
During a grand mal seizure your priorities are to prevent your child from inhaling vomit and from suffering any injury. At the first sign of a seizure place the child on his or her stomach with the head to one side. Move nearby objects away from jerking arms and legs, but do not try to restrain the child from moving. Never try to place anything in the mouth of a child having an attack. Once the involuntary movements have ceased, allow him or her to sleep undisturbed.
   A child having a petit mal seizure needs no special treatment and should be allowed to regain normal consciousness without interference.

Electroencephalography
Electroencephalography is a technique that enables physicians to monitor the electrical activity in the brain, and assists in the diagnosis of epilepsy and other conditions. A number of electrodes are placed on the scalp (right) and the signals that are picked up are recorded on paper. The procedure is not painful, but it may take some time and may therefore be tiresome for a young child.

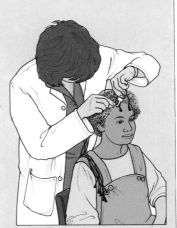

During a grand mal seizure
A child having a grand mal seizure should be gently turned on his or her stomach with the head to one side (below). Nearby objects likely to cause injury should be moved away.

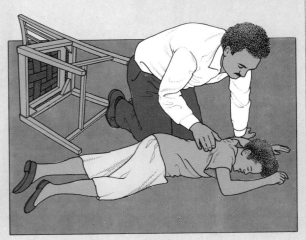

18 Headache

A headache can consist of pain on one or both sides of the head or forehead. It may vary from a dull ache to a sharp, stabbing pain. Children under the age of 3 are unlikely to complain of this symptom except as a direct result of injury. Headaches can be a symptom of a number of disorders, but they may also occur on their own, are most commonly due to muscle spasm and are usually easily cured by self-help measures.

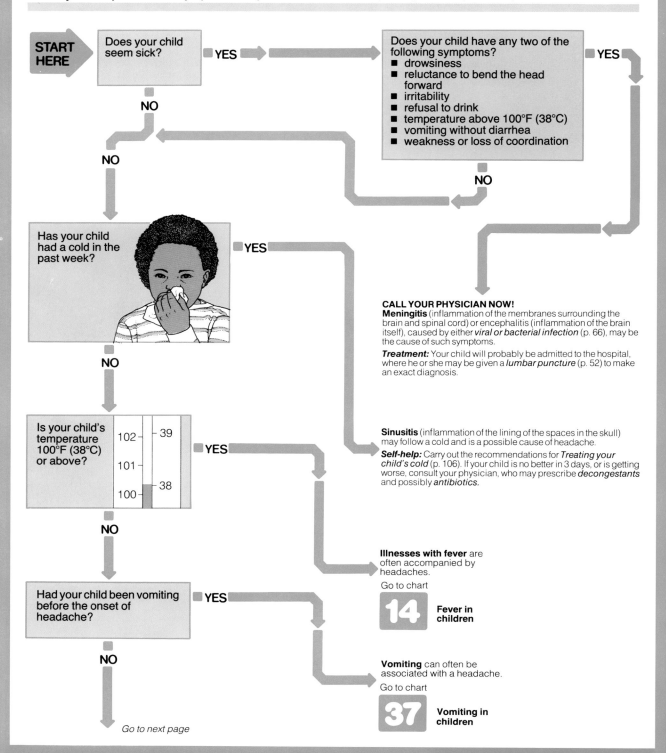

START HERE

Does your child seem sick? — **YES** →

Does your child have any two of the following symptoms?
- drowsiness
- reluctance to bend the head forward
- irritability
- refusal to drink
- temperature above 100°F (38°C)
- vomiting without diarrhea
- weakness or loss of coordination

YES

NO → **NO**

NO

Has your child had a cold in the past week? — **YES** →

NO

Is your child's temperature 100°F (38°C) or above?

102 — 39
101
100 — 38

YES →

NO

Had your child been vomiting before the onset of headache? — **YES** →

NO

Go to next page

CALL YOUR PHYSICIAN NOW!
Meningitis (inflammation of the membranes surrounding the brain and spinal cord) or encephalitis (inflammation of the brain itself), caused by either *viral or bacterial infection* (p. 66), may be the cause of such symptoms.

Treatment: Your child will probably be admitted to the hospital, where he or she may be given a *lumbar puncture* (p. 52) to make an exact diagnosis.

Sinusitis (inflammation of the lining of the spaces in the skull) may follow a cold and is a possible cause of headache.

Self-help: Carry out the recommendations for *Treating your child's cold* (p. 106). If your child is no better in 3 days, or is getting worse, consult your physician, who may prescribe *decongestants* and possibly *antibiotics*.

Illnesses with fever are often accompanied by headaches.
Go to chart

14 Fever in children

Vomiting can often be associated with a headache.
Go to chart

37 Vomiting in children

Continued from previous page

Does your child often have headaches?

YES → **Has your child had a headache every day this week?**

YES → **Frequent headaches** in a child should be brought to your physician's attention. They may be *migraines* (see below left), especially if other members of the family suffer from them, but your physician may want to rule out the possibility of a more serious underlying disorder.

NO

NO

The periodic syndrome is one term used to describe children's recurrent pains that may be of emotional origin.

Self-help: Although there may be no obvious physical cause for your child's headaches, the pain is nevertheless real. Follow the advice on *Relieving your child's headache* (below). Consult your physician if such measures fail to relieve the pain, if your child develops additional symptoms or if he or she seems sick. In addition, you should seek medical advice if the headaches start to occur increasingly often.

Did your child often suffer from unexplained abdominal pain when younger?

YES →

NO

Eyesight problems – for example, nearsightedness – may sometimes cause headaches after such activities. Consult your physician.

Treatment: Your physician will probably examine your child and may carry out a preliminary eye test (see *Eye testing*, p. 101). If your physician suspects a visual defect, your child will be referred for further eye tests, and may eventually need to wear eyeglasses.

Do headaches only seem to occur after your child has been reading or doing other close work?

YES →

NO

Migraine is the term used to describe recurrent, severe headaches that may be accompanied or preceded by additional symptoms, such as nausea, vomiting and/or visual disturbance. They are more common in adulthood, but may sometimes occur in children, particularly if a close relative also suffers from this type of headache. Consult your physician.

Treatment: If your physician confirms that your child is suffering from migraine, he or she will probably ask you about any factors that seem to trigger attacks. Certain foods, such as cheese and chocolate, are common causes of migraine. In addition, your physician may prescribe medication if normal self-help measures are ineffective (see *Relieving your child's headache*, right).

Are headaches usually accompanied by nausea or vomiting AND/OR has your child complained of any disturbance in vision before the onset of pain?

YES →

NO

RELIEVING YOUR CHILD'S HEADACHE

The vast majority of headaches in childhood can be treated simply at home in the following way:

- Give the recommended dose of an aspirin substitute.
- If your child is hungry, offer a light snack – for example, a glass of milk and a cookie.
- Allow your child to lie down in a cool, darkened room for a few hours.

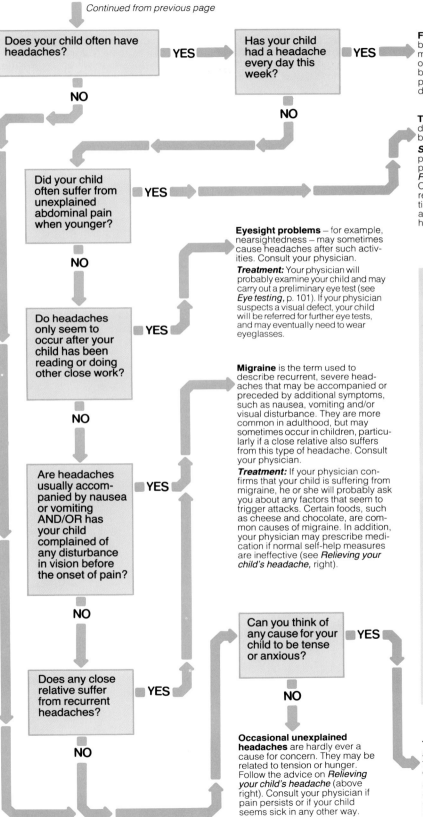

The earlier treatment is offered, the greater its effectiveness. Consult your physician if these measures fail to relieve a headache within 4 hours, or if your child seems sick.

Can you think of any cause for your child to be tense or anxious?

YES →

NO

Does any close relative suffer from recurrent headaches?

YES →

NO

Occasional unexplained headaches are hardly ever a cause for concern. They may be related to tension or hunger. Follow the advice on *Relieving your child's headache* (above right). Consult your physician if pain persists or if your child seems sick in any other way.

Tension headaches may be brought on by anxiety – for example, about schoolwork or family problems. Such headaches are generally no cause for concern.

Self-help: Follow the advice on *Relieving your child's headache* (above). Consult your physician if such measures fail to relieve the pain or if your child seems sick.

19 Clumsiness

Children differ greatly in their level of manual dexterity, physical coordination and agility. Some children naturally have more difficulty than others in carrying out delicate tasks (such as tying shoelaces) that require precise coordination between hand and eye. They may seem unable to prevent themselves from knocking things over. Such clumsiness is almost always present from birth and is most unlikely to be a sign of an underlying disorder. Occasionally, however, severe clumsiness or the sudden onset of clumsiness in a child who has previously been well coordinated may be the result of a nervous system or muscular disorder.

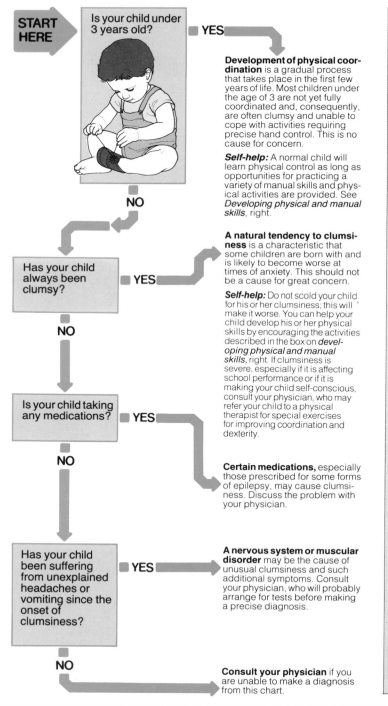

START HERE

Is your child under 3 years old? **YES**

Development of physical coordination is a gradual process that takes place in the first few years of life. Most children under the age of 3 are not yet fully coordinated and, consequently, are often clumsy and unable to cope with activities requiring precise hand control. This is no cause for concern.

Self-help: A normal child will learn physical control as long as opportunities for practicing a variety of manual skills and physical activities are provided. See *Developing physical and manual skills*, right.

NO

Has your child always been clumsy? **YES**

A natural tendency to clumsiness is a characteristic that some children are born with and is likely to become worse at times of anxiety. This should not be a cause for great concern.

Self-help: Do not scold your child for his or her clumsiness; this will make it worse. You can help your child develop his or her physical skills by encouraging the activities described in the box on *developing physical and manual skills*, right. If clumsiness is severe, especially if it is affecting school performance or if it is making your child self-conscious, consult your physician, who may refer your child to a physical therapist for special exercises for improving coordination and dexterity.

NO

Is your child taking any medications? **YES**

Certain medications, especially those prescribed for some forms of epilepsy, may cause clumsiness. Discuss the problem with your physician.

NO

Has your child been suffering from unexplained headaches or vomiting since the onset of clumsiness? **YES**

A nervous system or muscular disorder may be the cause of unusual clumsiness and such additional symptoms. Consult your physician, who will probably arrange for tests before making a precise diagnosis.

NO

Consult your physician if you are unable to make a diagnosis from this chart.

DEVELOPING PHYSICAL AND MANUAL SKILLS

Children learn to control their bodies from the first weeks of life. They soon learn skills such as following a moving object with the eyes and grasping a toy that is held out to them. Some children learn these skills more easily than others and are naturally more agile than their peers. However, throughout childhood, you can help your child develop muscular coordination and manual dexterity to the best of his or her abilities by giving as many chances as possible for varied physical activities.

Athletic skills
A toddler who is running, hopping and jumping is learning physical skills that will help him or her to be good at sports and games. Swimming is a particularly good form of exercise for less coordinated children. Ball games will help improve hand-and-eye coordination (see right) as well as provide opportunities for strenuous physical activity.

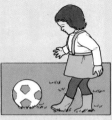

Moving to music
Dancing is not only fun for young children but teaches them to coordinate their body's movements with the rhythms of music. Disciplined forms of dancing, such as ballet, can also improve balance, physical grace and agility.

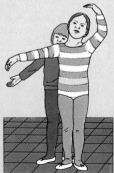

Coordinating hand and eye
Banging pegs into a frame with a hammer is a game that most toddlers enjoy (below right). It also helps to teach coordination between the hand and eye and will help your child learn more sophisticated manual tasks such as sewing and woodworking later on. Similarly, scribbling on crayons is an important stage in the development of the more delicate control needed for writing and drawing. Toys that are particularly good for hand-and-eye coordination include building blocks, puzzles with large pieces, and toy telephones.

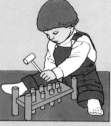

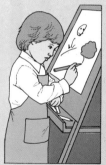

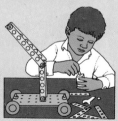

20 Confusion

Confused children may talk nonsense, appear dazed or agitated, or see and hear things that are not real. An **older child may mix up times, places and events. This is serious and requires medical attention.**

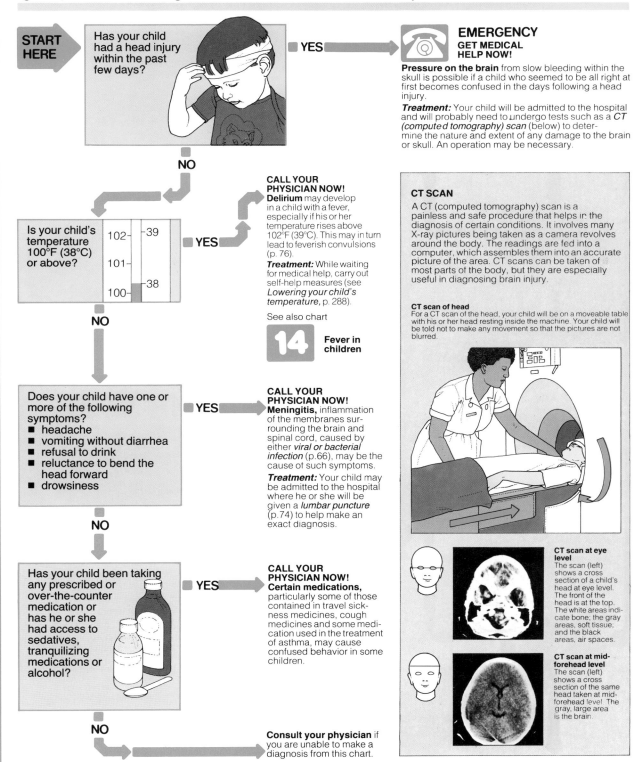

START HERE → **Has your child had a head injury within the past few days?** → **YES** →

EMERGENCY
GET MEDICAL HELP NOW!

Pressure on the brain from slow bleeding within the skull is possible if a child who seemed to be all right at first becomes confused in the days following a head injury.

Treatment: Your child will be admitted to the hospital and will probably need to undergo tests such as a *CT (computed tomography) scan* (below) to determine the nature and extent of any damage to the brain or skull. An operation may be necessary.

NO ↓

Is your child's temperature 100°F (38°C) or above?

102 — 39
101 —
100 — 38

YES →

CALL YOUR PHYSICIAN NOW!
Delirium may develop in a child with a fever, especially if his or her temperature rises above 102°F (39°C). This may in turn lead to feverish convulsions (p. 76).

Treatment: While waiting for medical help, carry out self-help measures (see *Lowering your child's temperature*, p. 288).

See also chart

14 Fever in children

NO ↓

Does your child have one or more of the following symptoms?
- headache
- vomiting without diarrhea
- refusal to drink
- reluctance to bend the head forward
- drowsiness

YES →

CALL YOUR PHYSICIAN NOW!
Meningitis, inflammation of the membranes surrounding the brain and spinal cord, caused by either *viral or bacterial infection* (p.66), may be the cause of such symptoms.

Treatment: Your child may be admitted to the hospital where he or she will be given a *lumbar puncture* (p.74) to help make an exact diagnosis.

NO ↓

Has your child been taking any prescribed or over-the-counter medication or has he or she had access to sedatives, tranquilizing medications or alcohol?

YES →

CALL YOUR PHYSICIAN NOW!
Certain medications, particularly some of those contained in travel sickness medicines, cough medicines and some medication used in the treatment of asthma, may cause confused behavior in some children.

NO ↓

Consult your physician if you are unable to make a diagnosis from this chart.

CT SCAN

A CT (computed tomography) scan is a painless and safe procedure that helps in the diagnosis of certain conditions. It involves many X-ray pictures being taken as a camera revolves around the body. The readings are fed into a computer, which assembles them into an accurate picture of the area. CT scans can be taken of most parts of the body, but they are especially useful in diagnosing brain injury.

CT scan of head
For a CT scan of the head, your child will be on a moveable table with his or her head resting inside the machine. Your child will be told not to make any movement so that the pictures are not blurred.

CT scan at eye level
The scan (left) shows a cross section of a child's head at eye level. The front of the head is at the top. The white areas indicate bone; the gray areas, soft tissue; and the black areas, air spaces.

CT scan at mid-forehead level
The scan (left) shows a cross section of the same head taken at mid-forehead level. The gray, large area is the brain.

21 Speech difficulties

Consult this chart if your child has any problem with his or her speech such as delay in starting to talk, lack of clarity, defects in pronunciation or stuttering. Most forms of speech difficulty resolve themselves in time without treatment. However, in some cases, a child's speech can be improved with therapy.

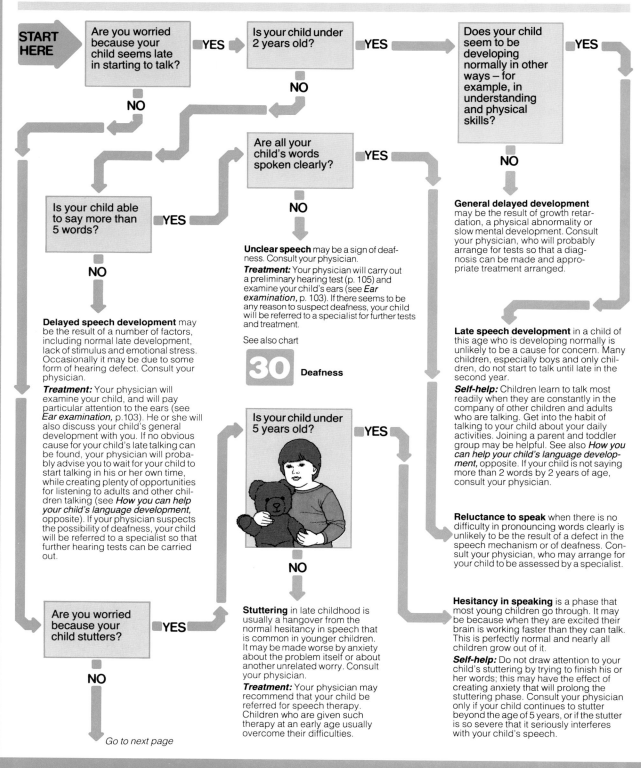

START HERE

Are you worried because your child seems late in starting to talk?

YES → Is your child under 2 years old?

YES → Does your child seem to be developing normally in other ways – for example, in understanding and physical skills?

NO (from first box) ↓

Is your child able to say more than 5 words?

YES → Are all your child's words spoken clearly?

YES →

NO (from "able to say more than 5 words") ↓

Delayed speech development may be the result of a number of factors, including normal late development, lack of stimulus and emotional stress. Occasionally it may be due to some form of hearing defect. Consult your physician.

Treatment: Your physician will examine your child, and will pay particular attention to the ears (see *Ear examination*, p.103). He or she will also discuss your child's general development with you. If no obvious cause for your child's late talking can be found, your physician will probably advise you to wait for your child to start talking in his or her own time, while creating plenty of opportunities for listening to adults and other children talking (see *How you can help your child's language development*, opposite). If your physician suspects the possibility of deafness, your child will be referred to a specialist so that further hearing tests can be carried out.

NO (from "Are all your child's words spoken clearly?") ↓

Unclear speech may be a sign of deafness. Consult your physician.

Treatment: Your physician will carry out a preliminary hearing test (p. 105) and examine your child's ears (see *Ear examination*, p. 103). If there seems to be any reason to suspect deafness, your child will be referred to a specialist for further tests and treatment.

See also chart

30 Deafness

NO (from "Is your child under 2 years old?") ↓

Is your child under 5 years old?

YES →

NO ↓

Stuttering in late childhood is usually a hangover from the normal hesitancy in speech that is common in younger children. It may be made worse by anxiety about the problem itself or about another unrelated worry. Consult your physician.

Treatment: Your physician may recommend that your child be referred for speech therapy. Children who are given such therapy at an early age usually overcome their difficulties.

General delayed development may be the result of growth retardation, a physical abnormality or slow mental development. Consult your physician, who will probably arrange for tests so that a diagnosis can be made and appropriate treatment arranged.

Late speech development in a child of this age who is developing normally is unlikely to be a cause for concern. Many children, especially boys and only children, do not start to talk until late in the second year.

Self-help: Children learn to talk most readily when they are constantly in the company of other children and adults who are talking. Get into the habit of talking to your child about your daily activities. Joining a parent and toddler group may be helpful. See also *How you can help your child's language development*, opposite. If your child is not saying more than 2 words by 2 years of age, consult your physician.

Reluctance to speak when there is no difficulty in pronouncing words clearly is unlikely to be the result of a defect in the speech mechanism or of deafness. Consult your physician, who may arrange for your child to be assessed by a specialist.

Hesitancy in speaking is a phase that most young children go through. It may be because when they are excited their brain is working faster than they can talk. This is perfectly normal and nearly all children grow out of it.

Self-help: Do not draw attention to your child's stuttering by trying to finish his or her words; this may have the effect of creating anxiety that will prolong the stuttering phase. Consult your physician only if your child continues to stutter beyond the age of 5 years, or if the stutter is so severe that it seriously interferes with your child's speech.

Are you worried because your child stutters?

YES →

NO ↓

Go to next page

Continued from previous page

Does your child have a lisp or another type of speech defect?

YES →

Is the defect so severe that strangers cannot easily understand what your child is saying OR is your child embarrassed about the problem?

YES →

Serious defects in pronunciation may be the result of a physical problem. Consult your physician.

Treatment: Your physician will examine your child, paying special attention to the mouth and ears, and may refer your child to a speech therapist for diagnosis and treatment. Many forms of speech defect can be corrected by speech therapy.

NO ↓

Consult your physician if you are unable to make a diagnosis from this chart.

NO ↓

Minor speech defects are common. In most cases children will gradually overcome their difficulties with various types of sound as they grow older. Trying to correct your child's speech is likely only to make your child anxious and self-conscious. Consult your physician if the speech defect starts to cause your child embarrassment or if it interferes with communication or school performance.

SPEECH DEVELOPMENT

The first year
Children begin to communicate well before they are ready to talk. From birth they listen to and enjoy the sound of their parents' voices and learn to associate such sounds with comfort and security. From about 2 months they are learning to make a variety of their own noises, including grunting, gurgling and cooing sounds. Such noises develop during the second half of the first year into recognizable syllables such as "ma," "da" and "ga." These words gradually become more complex until your child is babbling in long strings of syllables. By the end of the first year most children are able to understand a few simple words, phrases and commands, and have usually learned to say at least one recognizable word in its proper context.

The second year
During the early part of the second year a child's vocabulary increases rapidly, although much of a child's conversation is still babbling. Gradually, phrases of linked words joining names of people or objects to actions or commands appear – for example, "mommy go" or "doggie eat." At this stage, understanding of things that you say is also developing rapidly. And even though it may not yet be apparent in your child's speech, a broad base of vocabulary and grammatical structure is being built up.

The third year
The third year is a time during which a child consolidates and builds on the basic knowledge of vocabulary and grammar that was learned in the second year. An apparently never-ending stream of questions about the names of objects and what they do enlarges vocabulary and increases a child's confidence in using words. By the end of this year the majority of children understand most of what an adult says as long as it is not too complex or abstract, and can communicate their wants and thoughts and hold simple conversations about everyday subjects that interest them.

HOW YOU CAN HELP YOUR CHILD'S LANGUAGE DEVELOPMENT

Children learn to talk most readily when constantly exposed to the sound of voices, in particular those of their parents, from an early age. The following specific suggestions will help you ensure that your child receives plenty of stimulation and encouragement to learn to talk when he or she is ready:

- Get into the habit of talking to your child from birth.
- Look directly at your child when you speak, so that the expression on your face gives clues to the meaning of what you are saying.
- Use actions to help your child associate particular words with objects and events.
- Use simple books and nursery rhymes to extend your child's vocabulary and to build confidence by the repetition of familiar words and phrases.
- Provide plenty of opportunities for your child to mix with other children and adults.
- Try not to interrupt your child constantly to correct errors in grammar or pronunciation; this may undermine confidence. Instead, concentrate on providing a good example in the way you speak.

Do not worry if your child seems to be a little late in uttering his or her first words. Your child will nevertheless be listening to you talking and building up the groundwork of language. Most children who are late-talkers catch up with their early-talking contemporaries very quickly once they start.

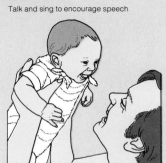
Talk and sing to encourage speech

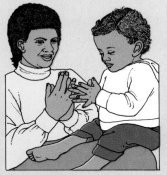
Word association helps understanding

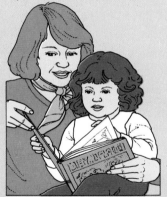
Repeated words in books build confidence

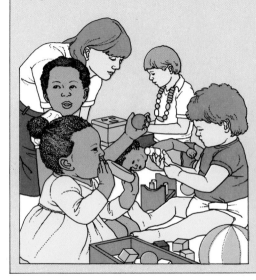
Playing with other children promotes communication skills

22 Behavior problems

Problems relating to your child's behavior can vary, and much depends on a parent's perception of what constitutes a problem. It is not possible to deal here with every aspect of childhood behavior problems. This chart covers some of the main areas that cause parents distress and worry. It will give you some idea when professional help, either from your family physician or from a child psychiatrist, may be advisable.

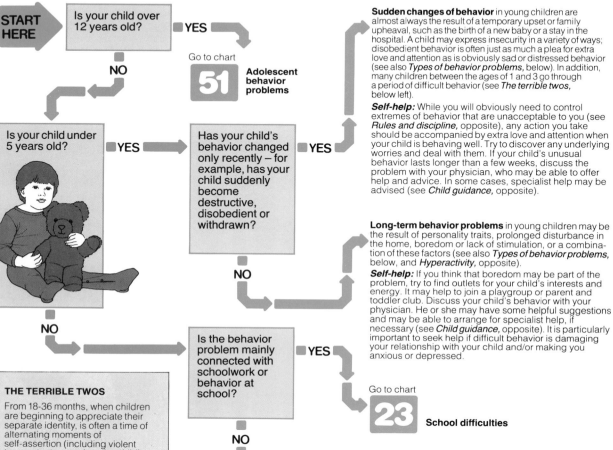

START HERE

Is your child over 12 years old?

YES — Go to chart **51** **Adolescent behavior problems**

NO

Is your child under 5 years old?

YES — **Has your child's behavior changed only recently – for example, has your child suddenly become destructive, disobedient or withdrawn?**

YES

NO

NO

Is the behavior problem mainly connected with schoolwork or behavior at school?

YES — Go to chart **23** **School difficulties**

NO

Sudden changes of behavior in young children are almost always the result of a temporary upset or family upheaval, such as the birth of a new baby or a stay in the hospital. A child may express insecurity in a variety of ways; disobedient behavior is often just as much a plea for extra love and attention as is obviously sad or distressed behavior (see also *Types of behavior problems,* below). In addition, many children between the ages of 1 and 3 go through a period of difficult behavior (see *The terrible twos,* below left).

Self-help: While you will obviously need to control extremes of behavior that are unacceptable to you (see *Rules and discipline,* opposite), any action you take should be accompanied by extra love and attention when your child is behaving well. Try to discover any underlying worries and deal with them. If your child's unusual behavior lasts longer than a few weeks, discuss the problem with your physician, who may be able to offer help and advice. In some cases, specialist help may be advised (see *Child guidance,* opposite).

Long-term behavior problems in young children may be the result of personality traits, prolonged disturbance in the home, boredom or lack of stimulation, or a combination of these factors (see also *Types of behavior problems,* below, and *Hyperactivity,* opposite).

Self-help: If you think that boredom may be part of the problem, try to find outlets for your child's interests and energy. It may help to join a playgroup or parent and toddler club. Discuss your child's behavior with your physician. He or she may have some helpful suggestions and may be able to arrange for specialist help, if necessary (see *Child guidance,* opposite). It is particularly important to seek help if difficult behavior is damaging your relationship with your child and/or making you anxious or depressed.

THE TERRIBLE TWOS

From 18-36 months, when children are beginning to appreciate their separate identity, is often a time of alternating moments of self-assertion (including violent temper tantrums when the child's wishes are frustrated), reckless adventuring and moments of increased dependency and insecurity (when he or she reverts to babyish habits or refuses to be separated from his or her parents). This type of behaviour can make the "terrible twos" a trying time for parents.

Dealing with tantrums

If your child has tantrums, it is essential to keep calm. If you can remain unmoved by your screaming child, pick up your child and hold him or her closely until he or she has calmed down. Showing sympathy without giving in to an impossible demand may nip a tantrum in the bud. But if you are upset by the tantrums, it is better to leave the room than to shout or display other signs of distress yourself. If frequent temper tantrums are making you feel anxious and unable to cope, consult your physician who may be able to offer constructive help.

TYPES OF BEHAVIOR PROBLEMS

Aggressiveness

Assertiveness may be a natural part of a child's personality, but excessively aggressive or violent behavior may be a response to worry, boredom or lack of parental attention.

Stealing

A child who steals may simply want something very badly or may do it for a thrill and to gain the admiration of friends. It is common for a child to steal as a result of insecurity to gain attention. Occasionally, a child may repeatedly steal objects of little value. This may be a sign of an emotional disturbance. Seek professional help.

Disobedience and rudeness

If your child persistently defies you, it may be a sign that the rules you have set up are too rigid and your child is using disobedience as a means of expressing independence. Or it may be that your child has not fully understood the reasons for the rules. Children may also use deliberate defiance and bad or insulting language as a means of gaining attention by provoking an angry reaction; such a response may be seen by them as preferable to no response at all (see *Rules and discipline,* opposite).

Withdrawal

Sudden withdrawal from social contact in a child who previously has enjoyed the company of others could be a sign of anxiety or depression. If this type of behavior persists, try to find out the cause and seek medical advice.

Go to next page

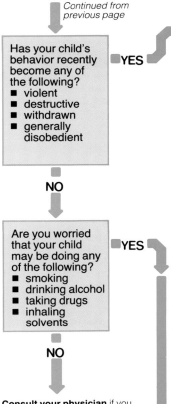

Continued from previous page

Has your child's behavior recently become any of the following?
- violent
- destructive
- withdrawn
- generally disobedient

YES

NO

Are you worried that your child may be doing any of the following?
- smoking
- drinking alcohol
- taking drugs
- inhaling solvents

YES

NO

Consult your physician if you are unable to find an explanation for your child's behavior on this chart, and if your child continues to behave in a worrisome way.

Has this change in behavior occurred following a family upset, such as the birth of a new baby or separation of the parents?

YES

NO

Difficult behavior that starts for no obvious reason may have a variety of underlying causes. There may be problems at school about which you are unaware – for example, bullying. Your child may be worried about some future event, or he or she may sense tension in the home. Alternatively, your child may be bored as a result of insufficient stimulation at school (see *Gifted children*, p.91) or lack of constructive activities in the home. You will know best which explanation is most likely in your child's case (see also *Types of behavior problems*, opposite).

Self-help: Try to channel your child's energies into demanding activities that he or she enjoys. These may include sports, family outings or creative pastimes such as painting and crafts. Discuss the problem with your child's teacher, who may suggest ways of adjusting schoolwork to meet your child's needs more closely. If you suspect that your child is worrying about something, try to find out what the trouble is so that you can offer reassurance. If these suggestions do not work, and if you are unable to control your child's behavior in the usual ways (see *Rules and discipline*, below), consult your physician, who may, if needed, arrange for specialist help (see *Child guidance*, below right).

Such activities are discussed in the box on *Smoking, alcohol and drug abuse*, p.140.

Insecurity and unhappiness can cause some children to misbehave. Bad behavior is a way for children to express anger with themselves or with others and is often a sign that a child needs extra reassurance and love (see *Types of behavior problems*, opposite).

Self-help: During this difficult time, you will need to be patient, but not overindulgent with your child. Continue to enforce your usual rules regarding behavior (see *Rules and discipline*, below left), but also make every effort to talk to your child about any underlying cause of insecurity. Offer plenty of reassurance. Try to set aside a regular time each day when you give your child your undivided attention. It is also a good idea to inform a child's teachers about any important changes in the home so that they will understand any temporary difficulties your child may have with schoolwork. If you find yourself unable to cope with your child's difficult behavior, or if you are worried that it seems to be persisting too long, consult your physician.

HYPERACTIVITY

Hyperactivity refers to excessively restless physical and mental activity in a child. A hyperactive child has a short attention span, is prone to temper tantrums, has apparently boundless energy and needs little sleep. Such behavior can be trying and requires patience and understanding.

Some physicians believe that hyperactivity is the result of brain damage so minimal that it cannot be detected by tests. The condition is thought to be the result of temperament, an allergy to certain foods or chemical food additives, or a marginal vitamin deficiency. It is also thought that the consumption of refined carbohydrates may be related to hyperactivity. However, other physicians view hyperactivity as one end of the spectrum of normal behavior. Treatment will depend on your physician, and may consist of counseling to encourage greater awareness and tolerance among family members — and offer ways to cope.

RULES AND DISCIPLINE

Most children benefit from a clearly understood system of rules setting out the bounds of acceptable behavior. Every family has its own standards of behavior and language; behavior that would not be tolerated in one family may be acceptable in another. As a parent you should be clear as to why you lay down certain rules; whether, for example, for reasons of safety or for consideration of the rights and feelings of others. And you should balance the advantages of adhering to certain rigid standards against the need for the occasional confrontation to enforce them. Wherever possible, try to allow your child scope for making independent decisions within the framework you lay down. Otherwise there is a danger of undermining initiative and self-confidence, or of provoking defiance to all your rules.

Punishment
Ideally, sanctions to enforce your wishes on your child should never be necessary. Your aim should be to avoid battles of will by using other, more positive, means of gaining your child's cooperation. Such means may include encouragement of good behavior through praise and reward, the use of example (particularly in relation to manners and language) and constant explanation of the reasons for any limitations you may want to impose. However, in the real world, every parent needs to use punishment occasionally, and, on the whole, children accept and respect this. The effectiveness of punishment largely depends on how you use it. The following guidelines may help:
- Always try to make the punishment appropriate to the seriousness of the misdemeanor. Where possible, make the punishment a form of reparation for the "crime."
- Any punishment should immediately follow the offense and should not be delayed until later.
- Never threaten a punishment that you know you will be unwilling to carry out; children can detect empty threats.
- Make sure that it is understood that punishment for a specific offense is not a sign that you have ceased to love your child. For many children, your anger is punishment in itself. A peacemaking hug and words of reassurance afterward are a good idea.
- Physical (corporal) punishment is generally an ineffective means of gaining a child's cooperation and can often lead to resentment that produces the opposite effect. However, the occasional spank is unlikely to do lasting damage. Seek advice from your physician if you find yourself unable to control your anger to the extent that you fear you may harm your child.

CHILD GUIDANCE

If your family physician feels that your child's persistent behavior problems could benefit from specialist help, he or she may suggest your child visit a child guidance clinic. This is a center specializing in the assessment of behavior problems in children so that the cause of the problem may be diagnosed accurately and appropriate treatment prescribed. Its staff may include a specialist in the treatment of emotional problems in childhood (child psychiatrist), specialists in child behavior and educational difficulties (educational psychologists) and, possibly, social workers to advise on practical difficulties that may contribute to, or arise out of, the child's problems.

Normally, on a first visit, the whole family will be asked to attend to discuss the problem with the clinic staff. On subsequent visits it may be necessary for the child to attend with only one parent. The child may participate in various activities such as play sessions or further discussions with the staff, depending on the child's age and the nature of the problem. This enables the staff to obtain a clear picture of the case and to advise on further action.

23 School difficulties

School difficulties fall into two main groups: those related principally to learning, whether of a specific subject or of schoolwork in general; and those more concerned with behavior, including classroom behavior and reluctance to go to school. Consult this chart if your child has any of these difficulties. Such problems may be the result of emotional difficulties, physical disorders or social factors, or they may arise out of a general problem of development. Most school difficulties benefit from discussions between parent and school staff, and it is often helpful to involve the family physician who has watched your child's development.

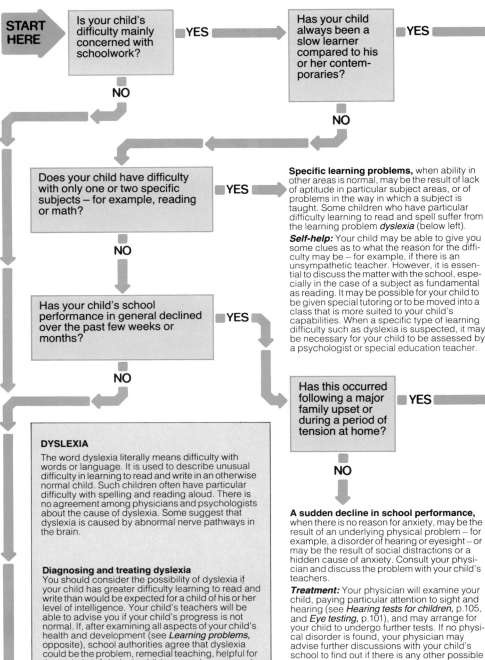

START HERE — Is your child's difficulty mainly concerned with schoolwork?

YES → Has your child always been a slow learner compared to his or her contemporaries?

YES →

Slow intellectual development may simply mean that your child acquires certain intellectual capabilities later than the average child. He or she is likely to catch up with his or her fast-learning friends during the next few years. Also, a child who has had emotional problems or who is of below-average intelligence may be expected to learn more slowly than average (see *Learning problems*, opposite).

Self-help: Discuss your child's progress with his or her teachers, who may be able to reassure you that your child's pace of learning is well within the normal range. It may be advisable in some cases for an intelligence test and a general physical examination to be carried out. Many children who are slow learners can be helped to catch up through remedial classes taught by specially trained teachers. However, in some cases, it may be advisable for a child to attend a special school.

NO

Does your child have difficulty with only one or two specific subjects – for example, reading or math?

YES →

Specific learning problems, when ability in other areas is normal, may be the result of lack of aptitude in particular subject areas, or of problems in the way in which a subject is taught. Some children who have particular difficulty learning to read and spell suffer from the learning problem *dyslexia* (below left).

Self-help: Your child may be able to give you some clues as to what the reason for the difficulty may be – for example, if there is an unsympathetic teacher. However, it is essential to discuss the matter with the school, especially in the case of a subject as fundamental as reading. It may be possible for your child to be given special tutoring or to be moved into a class that is more suited to your child's capabilities. When a specific type of learning difficulty such as dyslexia is suspected, it may be necessary for your child to be assessed by a psychologist or special education teacher.

NO

Has your child's school performance in general declined over the past few weeks or months?

YES →

NO

Has this occurred following a major family upset or during a period of tension at home?

YES →

NO

DYSLEXIA

The word dyslexia literally means difficulty with words or language. It is used to describe unusual difficulty in learning to read and write in an otherwise normal child. Such children often have particular difficulty with spelling and reading aloud. There is no agreement among physicians and psychologists about the cause of dyslexia. Some suggest that dyslexia is caused by abnormal nerve pathways in the brain.

Diagnosing and treating dyslexia

You should consider the possibility of dyslexia if your child has greater difficulty learning to read and write than would be expected for a child of his or her level of intelligence. Your child's teachers will be able to advise you if your child's progress is not normal. If, after examining all aspects of your child's health and development (see *Learning problems*, opposite), school authorities agree that dyslexia could be the problem, remedial teaching, helpful for the majority of dyslexic children, can be arranged.

A sudden decline in school performance, when there is no reason for anxiety, may be the result of an underlying physical problem – for example, a disorder of hearing or eyesight – or may be the result of social distractions or a hidden cause of anxiety. Consult your physician and discuss the problem with your child's teachers.

Treatment: Your physician will examine your child, paying particular attention to sight and hearing (see *Hearing tests for children,* p.105, and *Eye testing,* p.101), and may arrange for your child to undergo further tests. If no physical disorder is found, your physician may advise further discussions with your child's school to find out if there is any other possible cause of the difficulties. It may be necessary to make adjustments in your child's schoolwork arrangements.

Emotional insecurity almost always has an effect on a child's schoolwork.

Self-help: Resolution of the cause of worry usually brings about an improvement. It is usually a good idea to inform teachers about any home problems that may affect a child's schoolwork so that allowances can be made and, where necessary, extra help given. If your child's work does not improve following resolution of the underlying difficulty, or if you are unable to resolve the problem, consult your physician, who will be able to advise you on whether further specialist help is necessary.

Go to next page

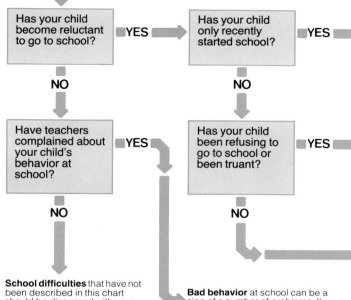

Continued from previous page

Has your child become reluctant to go to school? — YES → **Has your child only recently started school?** — YES →

Fear of school is very common in children just starting a new school (especially when starting a nursery or primary school) if a child has not been used to being away from home and family for long periods.

Self-help: In most cases, increasing familiarity with the school surroundings and growing interest in school activities will help your child overcome his or her misgivings. During the period of adjustment, try to reassure your child that being left at school is not a form of abandonment. Most nursery classes will allow parents to stay with their children for the first week or so. Make sure that there is no special cause for anxiety such as awkward bathroom facilities and try never to be late in picking your child up from school. If fear of school persists, discuss the problem with the school faculty, who may recommend professional advice.

NO ↓   NO ↓

Have teachers complained about your child's behavior at school? — YES → **Has your child been refusing to go to school or been truant?** — YES →

NO ↓   NO ↓

School difficulties that have not been described in this chart should be discussed with your child's teachers. Your physician's advice may also be helpful in some cases.

Bad behavior at school can be a sign of a number of problems. It could be that the level of schoolwork is too low, leading to boredom (see *Gifted children,* below left) or it may be too high, resulting in loss of interest and leading the child to use disruptive behavior to gain attention in class. It can also be the result of rejection of authority often linked to the emotional changes of adolescence (see chart 51, *Adolescent behavior problems*). In some cases, it may be the result of emotional disturbance.

Self-help: In cases of mild misbehavior it is often sufficient for your child to know that you are aware of the problem and invoke your usual forms of discipline (see *Rules and discipline,* p.89). However, it is also wise to discuss any possible causes of the problem with your child's teachers. Adjustments may need to be made in your child's schoolwork so that it meets your child's individual needs more closely. In cases of serious behavior problems, expert help through a *child guidance* professional (p.89) and, occasionally, special schools may be advisable.

Refusal to go to school is a sign that something is seriously wrong. It could be due to a problem at school such as bullying, a failure of the school to meet the child's individual needs, or it may be the result of the influence of friends at school. Occasionally, refusal to go to school is caused by anxiety about home life.

Self-help: To solve the problem of refusal to go to school, you are likely to need the help of the school authorities and possibly your physician, who may advise *child guidance* (p.89). The sooner the problem is tackled, the better. Make every effort to ensure that your child attends school and that the teachers concerned know that the problem exists so that unexplained absences from classes are not ignored. Meanwhile, try to discover the underlying cause of your child's refusal to go to school so that it can be dealt with as soon as possible.

Dislike of school can arise from a variety of factors. Your child may be having difficulties with schoolwork, or may be afraid of certain teachers or of other pupils.

Self-help: Dislike of school should be tackled promptly before it develops into the more serious problem of *refusal to go to school* (above). Try to find out from your child what the cause of the problem is and also discuss your child's feelings about school with his or her teachers so that they can look out for signs of a problem such as bullying or teasing. While you are trying to resolve the problem, do not keep your child at home unless advised to do so by the school; there is a danger that this may lead your child to stay away from school in the future. Depending on the underlying cause of the problem, it may be necessary for your child to change classes or to receive special tutoring.

GIFTED CHILDREN

Children who are unusually gifted, whether with an exceptional talent in one area or with a generally high level of intelligence, need special educational challenges from an early age. Without adequate stimulation, a gifted child may become unhappy, bored and/or disruptive.

You may suspect that your child is unusually gifted if he or she learns exceptionally quickly – especially if he or she reads voraciously and complains that school is boring. In this case you should discuss the matter with your child's teachers, who may arrange for your child to be assessed by an educational psychologist.

If your child is found to be exceptionally intelligent, the teachers may be able to devise a learning program that will challenge your child's intelligence adequately. Alternatively, education at a special school may be the best option. If your child has a special gift for music, for example, expert tutoring may be arranged.

Whatever educational program you choose for your child, you will need to remember that his or her emotional and social development is unlikely to be as advanced as his or her intellectual development. Your child should be encouraged to play with children of the same age and to join in sports and other recreational activities.

LEARNING PROBLEMS

In order to learn physical and intellectual skills at a normal rate, a child needs to have normal hearing, sight and intelligence. Impairment of any one of these faculties will lead to learning problems. In addition, a child's progress can be retarded by lack of sufficient stimulation in early childhood, by emotional upset, or by frequent absences from school.

Assessing the problem
Any child who is obviously having difficulty keeping pace with his or her contemporaries at school needs to be assessed by an educational psychologist. This can be arranged by the school authorities. The psychologist will carry out intelligence tests and may also arrange tests on hearing and vision. If a physi-

cal problem such as deafness is found, it may be treated by your family physician. If an emotional cause for the learning difficulty is suspected, referral to a *child guidance* specialist (see p.89) will probably be recommended. A child who seems to be of normal intelligence, but who has learning problems not caused by physical illness or emotional upset, may be suffering from a specific learning difficulty known as *dyslexia* (opposite). Such children, as well as those whose difficulty is caused by lower-than-average intelligence, may be helped by special remedial classes in a regular school. When intelligence is severely subnormal, it may be best for the child to be taught at a special school.

24 Hair, scalp and nail problems

Consult this diagnostic chart if your child has any problem affecting hair growth, including hair thinning and bald patches, or if your child's scalp is affected by itching or flaking. The most common causes of such problems are infection or parasitic infestation that, although not serious, require treatment.

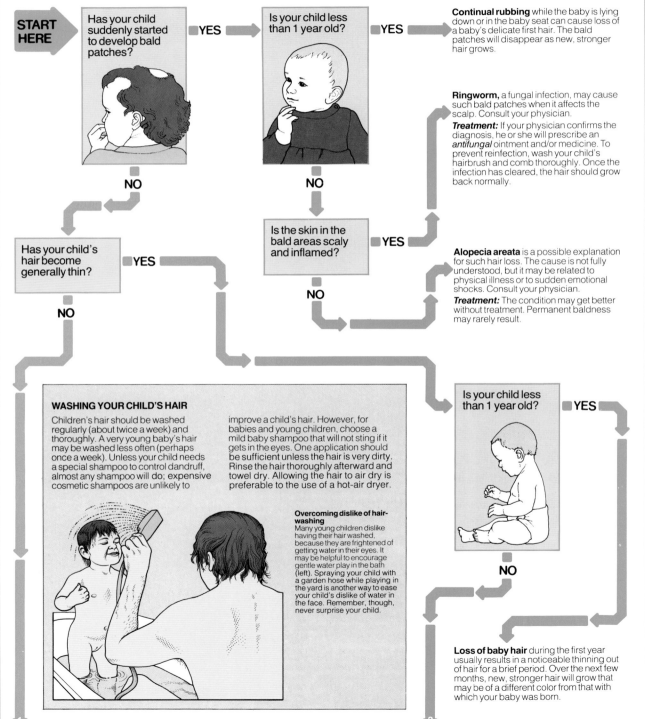

START HERE

Has your child suddenly started to develop bald patches?

— **YES** → Is your child less than 1 year old?

— **YES** → **Continual rubbing** while the baby is lying down or in the baby seat can cause loss of a baby's delicate first hair. The bald patches will disappear as new, stronger hair grows.

NO ↓ (from first question)

Has your child's hair become generally thin?

NO (from bald patches question, second path)

Is the skin in the bald areas scaly and inflamed?

— **YES** → **Ringworm,** a fungal infection, may cause such bald patches when it affects the scalp. Consult your physician.
Treatment: If your physician confirms the diagnosis, he or she will prescribe an *antifungal* ointment and/or medicine. To prevent reinfection, wash your child's hairbrush and comb thoroughly. Once the infection has cleared, the hair should grow back normally.

NO (skin scaly question)

Alopecia areata is a possible explanation for such hair loss. The cause is not fully understood, but it may be related to physical illness or to sudden emotional shocks. Consult your physician.
Treatment: The condition may get better without treatment. Permanent baldness may rarely result.

YES (hair become generally thin)

NO (hair become generally thin)

WASHING YOUR CHILD'S HAIR

Children's hair should be washed regularly (about twice a week) and thoroughly. A very young baby's hair may be washed less often (perhaps once a week). Unless your child needs a special shampoo to control dandruff, almost any shampoo will do; expensive cosmetic shampoos are unlikely to improve a child's hair. However, for babies and young children, choose a mild baby shampoo that will not sting if it gets in the eyes. One application should be sufficient unless the hair is very dirty. Rinse the hair thoroughly afterward and towel dry. Allowing the hair to air dry is preferable to the use of a hot-air dryer.

Overcoming dislike of hair-washing
Many young children dislike having their hair washed, because they are frightened of getting water in their eyes. It may be helpful to encourage gentle water play in the bath (left). Spraying your child with a garden hose while playing in the yard is another way to ease your child's dislike of water in the face. Remember, though, never surprise your child.

Is your child less than 1 year old?

— **YES** →

NO ↓

Loss of baby hair during the first year usually results in a noticeable thinning out of hair for a brief period. Over the next few months, new, stronger hair will grow that may be of a different color from that with which your baby was born.

Go to next page column 1

Go to next page column 2

Continued from previous
page column 1

Continued from previous
page column 2

Is your child's
scalp itchy?

YES

Does thorough
washing relieve
the itching for a
few days?

YES

Has your child
been taking any
medications
prescribed by
your physician?

YES

NO

NO

NO

Does your child
have greasy,
crusty patches on
the scalp?

YES

Head lice are a possibility, especially
if any of your child's friends are also
affected. Head lice are easily passed
from one person to another, and infestation is not the result of inadequate hair washing. Consult your
physician.

Treatment: The usual treatment for
head lice is to wash your child's hair
with a special shampoo that your
physician will prescribe. This will need
to be applied several times. After each
application, the hair can be combed
with a fine-tooth comb to remove the
eggs that remain stuck to the hair.

General thinning of the hair may be the result of
illness in the past few months or may occur for no
apparent reason.

Self-help: Other than ensuring that your child is
otherwise healthy and is receiving an adequate
diet (see *The components of a healthy diet*, p.119),
there is little you can do to encourage your child's
hair to grow more thickly. If your child's hair is long,
avoid tying it back tightly with elastic bands or
pulling it into tight styles. Use a soft nylon or bristle
brush because hard brushes may break the hair.
Your child's hair may appear thicker if cut in a short
style. If you are worried, consult your physician.

NO

Is your child's
scalp flaky?

YES

Cradle cap, a form of a harmless
condition called seborrheic dermatitis
(a type of eczema), is common in
babies under 1 year.

Self-help: If you find the crusts
unsightly, you can remove them by
rubbing your baby's scalp gently with
baby oil or petroleum jelly and then
washing the scalp to remove the
crusts. If cradle cap is extensive, your
physician may be able to prescribe a
special cream to control the condition.

Certain medications may cause temporary hair loss.
Discuss the problem with your physician.

NO

Consult your physician if you
are unable to make a diagnosis
from this chart.

Dandruff is the most likely cause of
flaking of the scalp (see *Dandruff,*
right).

Dandruff, which may sometimes be caused by
seborrheic dermatitis, a form of eczema, is the most
common cause of itching of the scalp. It is also likely
to lead to flaking of the scalp.

Self-help: Dandruff is best controlled by frequent use of
one of the many over-the-counter antidandruff shampoos.
If this is not effective, consult your physician, who will
prescribe another antidandruff shampoo, or a lotion to
apply to the scalp.

NAIL CARE

The nails of babies and children should always be kept short. In babies
this prevents accidental scratching and in older children helps to
prevent nail-biting and the spread of infection from dirt under the
fingernails. Always use blunt-ended scissors.

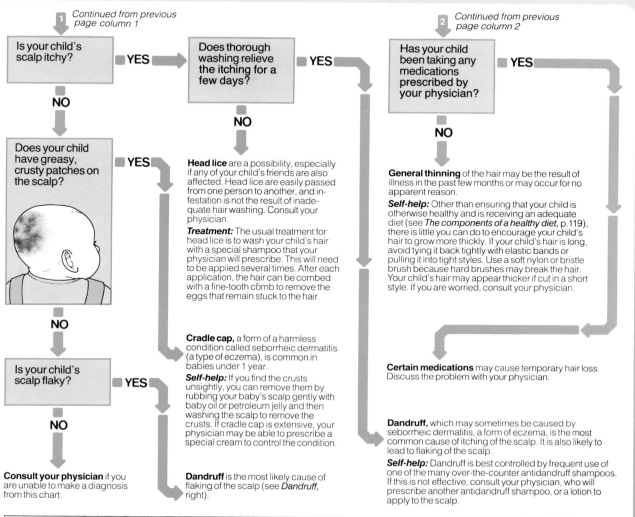

Fingernails
Fingernails should be
trimmed following the
shape of the finger tip.

Toenails
Toenails should be cut
straight across to
prevent ingrown
toenails.

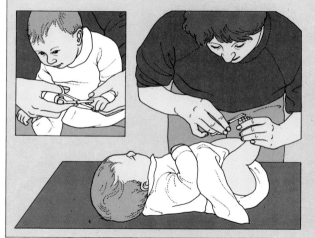

Nail-biting
Nail-biting is a habit that often develops in children of primary school
age. It may be copied from other children or arise as a nervous habit.
It presents no risk to health, but bitten nails are unsightly and, if bitten
down to the nail bed, may cause soreness.

If your child has a tendency to bite his or her nails, try to keep them
trimmed and smooth. Encourage your child to take pride in his or her
appearance. Buying a manicure set
and applying clear nail polish may
help. Bitter-tasting paint for the nails
is unlikely to have any effect and
may simply make your child
resentful.

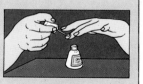

25 Spots and rashes

Spots and rashes in childhood are usually caused by inflammation of the skin as a result of infection, which may be localized, or part of a generalized illness or an allergic reaction. Most rashes that are not accompanied by a fever or a feeling of being sick are not a sign of serious illness but, if the rash is itchy or sore, you should consult your physician, who may be able to provide effective treatment.

For children under 1 year, see chart 4, Skin problems in babies

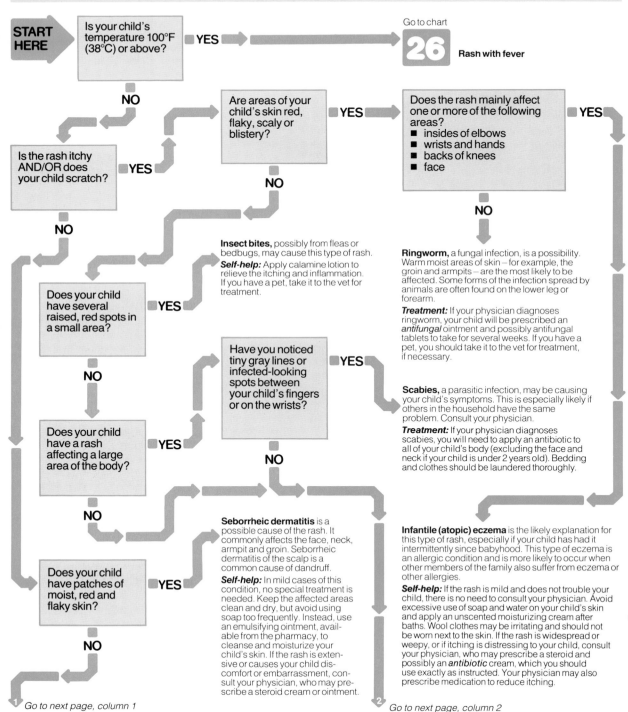

START HERE

Is your child's temperature 100°F (38°C) or above?

YES → Go to chart **26** Rash with fever

NO

Is the rash itchy AND/OR does your child scratch?

Are areas of your child's skin red, flaky, scaly or blistery? **YES** → Does the rash mainly affect one or more of the following areas?
- insides of elbows
- wrists and hands
- backs of knees
- face

YES

NO

YES

NO

NO

Does your child have several raised, red spots in a small area?

Insect bites, possibly from fleas or bedbugs, may cause this type of rash.
Self-help: Apply calamine lotion to relieve the itching and inflammation. If you have a pet, take it to the vet for treatment.

Ringworm, a fungal infection, is a possibility. Warm moist areas of skin – for example, the groin and armpits – are the most likely to be affected. Some forms of the infection spread by animals are often found on the lower leg or forearm.
Treatment: If your physician diagnoses ringworm, your child will be prescribed an *antifungal* ointment and possibly antifungal tablets to take for several weeks. If you have a pet, you should take it to the vet for treatment, if necessary.

YES

NO

Have you noticed tiny gray lines or infected-looking spots between your child's fingers or on the wrists?

YES

Does your child have a rash affecting a large area of the body?

YES

NO

Scabies, a parasitic infection, may be causing your child's symptoms. This is especially likely if others in the household have the same problem. Consult your physician.
Treatment: If your physician diagnoses scabies, you will need to apply an antibiotic to all of your child's body (excluding the face and neck if your child is under 2 years old). Bedding and clothes should be laundered thoroughly.

NO

Seborrheic dermatitis is a possible cause of the rash. It commonly affects the face, neck, armpit and groin. Seborrheic dermatitis of the scalp is a common cause of dandruff.
Self-help: In mild cases of this condition, no special treatment is needed. Keep the affected areas clean and dry, but avoid using soap too frequently. Instead, use an emulsifying ointment, available from the pharmacy, to cleanse and moisturize your child's skin. If the rash is extensive or causes your child discomfort or embarrassment, consult your physician, who may prescribe a steroid cream or ointment.

Infantile (atopic) eczema is the likely explanation for this type of rash, especially if your child has had it intermittently since babyhood. This type of eczema is an allergic condition and is more likely to occur when other members of the family also suffer from eczema or other allergies.
Self-help: If the rash is mild and does not trouble your child, there is no need to consult your physician. Avoid excessive use of soap and water on your child's skin and apply an unscented moisturizing cream after baths. Wool clothes may be irritating and should not be worn next to the skin. If the rash is widespread or weepy, or if itching is distressing to your child, consult your physician, who may prescribe a steroid and possibly an *antibiotic* cream, which you should use exactly as instructed. Your physician may also prescribe medication to reduce itching.

Does your child have patches of moist, red and flaky skin?

YES

NO

¹ Go to next page, column 1

² Go to next page, column 2

① Continued from previous page, column 1

② Continued from previous page, column 2

Does your child have a rash of pink spots that mainly affects the face and/or trunk?

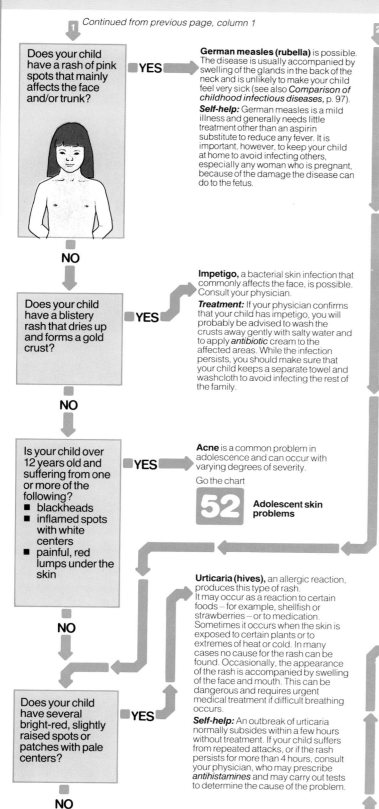

YES →

German measles (rubella) is possible. The disease is usually accompanied by swelling of the glands in the back of the neck and is unlikely to make your child feel very sick (see also *Comparison of childhood infectious diseases*, p. 97).

Self-help: German measles is a mild illness and generally needs little treatment other than an aspirin substitute to reduce any fever. It is important, however, to keep your child at home to avoid infecting others, especially any woman who is pregnant, because of the damage the disease can do to the fetus.

NO ↓

Does your child have a blistery rash that dries up and forms a gold crust?

YES →

Impetigo, a bacterial skin infection that commonly affects the face, is possible. Consult your physician.

Treatment: If your physician confirms that your child has impetigo, you will probably be advised to wash the crusts away gently with salty water and to apply *antibiotic* cream to the affected areas. While the infection persists, you should make sure that your child keeps a separate towel and washcloth to avoid infecting the rest of the family.

NO ↓

Is your child over 12 years old and suffering from one or more of the following?
- blackheads
- inflamed spots with white centers
- painful, red lumps under the skin

YES →

Acne is a common problem in adolescence and can occur with varying degrees of severity.

Go the chart

52 **Adolescent skin problems**

NO ↓

Does your child have several bright-red, slightly raised spots or patches with pale centers?

YES →

Urticaria (hives), an allergic reaction, produces this type of rash. It may occur as a reaction to certain foods – for example, shellfish or strawberries – or to medication. Sometimes it occurs when the skin is exposed to certain plants or to extremes of heat or cold. In many cases no cause for the rash can be found. Occasionally, the appearance of the rash is accompanied by swelling of the face and mouth. This can be dangerous and requires urgent medical treatment if difficult breathing occurs.

Self-help: An outbreak of urticaria normally subsides within a few hours without treatment. If your child suffers from repeated attacks, or if the rash persists for more than 4 hours, consult your physician, who may prescribe *antihistamines* and may carry out tests to determine the cause of the problem.

NO ↓

WARTS AND BOILS

Warts

A wart is a lump on the skin caused by virus infection. The most common type of wart is a hard, painless lump with a rough surface. Warts may occur singly, but more often several occur together. The hands are the most commonly affected area, but unraised warts called plantar warts often appear on the soles of the feet. Plantar warts may cause your child pain on walking.

Treatment

Warts need no treatment and will disappear on their own in time. However, if your child is embarrassed by unsightly warts, or has plantar warts, consult your physician, who may recommend treatment with a lotion painted onto the wart, or may refer your child to a clinic where the wart can be either burned or frozen off. Removal of warts by freezing does not cause scarring.

Boils

A boil occurs when a hair follicle (a pit in the skin from which a hair grows) becomes infected by bacteria, resulting in the collection of pus in the follicle. An inflamed lump with a white center develops under the skin. Eventually the boil bursts, releasing the pus, and the skin heals.

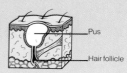

The formation of a boil
A boil forms when bacteria enter a hair follicle, causing pus to collect there.

Pus

Hair follicle

Treatment

A single boil usually heals without treatment. Adding a mild antiseptic to your child's bath water will help prevent the spread of infection. A warm, wet compress applied for 10 to 15 minutes twice a day will usually speed healing. When the boil bursts, carefully wipe away the pus with cotton soaked in an antiseptic solution and cover with an adhesive bandage. Consult your physician if your child has a large, painful boil, if several boils develop or if boils recur. Your physician may prescribe *antibiotics* or an antiseptic cream. Occasionally, a small cut is made in the center of a large boil to release the pus.

Certain medications may bring out a rash in susceptible children. Discuss the problem with your physician.

Is your child taking any medications?

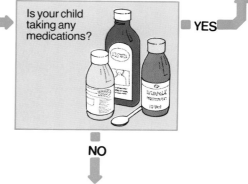

YES →

NO ↓

Consult your physician if you are unable to make a diagnosis from this chart.

26 Rash with fever

Consult this chart if your child develops a rash while having a fever. This combination of symptoms usually indicates a common infectious disease of childhood. These diseases are caused by viruses (see *Viral and* *bacterial infections,* p.66) and usually can be treated at home. In most cases, it is good for a child to get these infections out of the way. If your child is less than 1 year old, consult your physician to confirm the diagnosis.

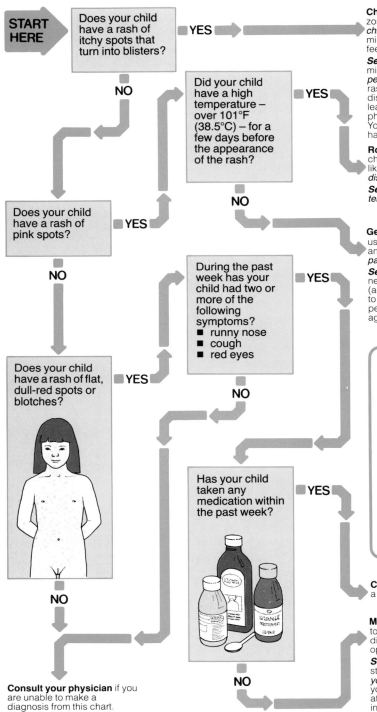

START HERE

Does your child have a rash of itchy spots that turn into blisters?

YES →

NO ↓

Did your child have a high temperature – over 101°F (38.5°C) – for a few days before the appearance of the rash?

YES →

NO ↓

Does your child have a rash of pink spots?

YES →

NO ↓

During the past week has your child had two or more of the following symptoms?
- runny nose
- cough
- red eyes

YES →

NO ↓

Does your child have a rash of flat, dull-red spots or blotches?

YES →

NO ↓

Has your child taken any medication within the past week?

YES →

NO ↓

Consult your physician if you are unable to make a diagnosis from this chart.

Chickenpox, an infection caused by the herpes varicella-zoster virus, is the likely diagnosis (see *Comparison of childhood infectious diseases,* opposite). This is usually a mild disease, although an older child or adolescent may feel sick for a few days.

Self-help: Give your child an aspirin substitute (acetaminophen) to reduce fever (see *Lowering your child's temperature,* p.288) and apply calamine lotion to soothe the rash. Never give aspirin. Your child should be discouraged from scratching the spots because this may lead to scarring. If itching is severe, consult your physician, who may prescribe medication to alleviate it. Your child is no longer contagious when all the blisters have turned to scabs.

Roseola infantum, a viral infection that commonly affects children between the ages of 6 months and 3 years, is a likely possibility (see *Comparison of childhood infectious diseases,* opposite).

Self-help: Follow the advice on *lowering your child's temperature,* p.288. Recovery normally takes about a week.

German measles (rubella) is possible. The disease is usually accompanied by swelling of the glands in the neck and is unlikely to make your child feel very sick (see *Comparison of childhood infectious diseases,* opposite).

Self-help: German measles is a mild illness and generally needs little treatment other than an aspirin substitute (acetaminophen) to reduce fever. It is important, however, to keep your child at home to avoid infecting others, especially any woman who is pregnant, because of the damage the disease can do to the unborn child.

WARNING

DANGER SIGNS

In the vast majority of cases, children recover from the childhood infectious diseases without special medical treatment and without experiencing complications or any long-term problems. However, in a small proportion of children, the viruses that produce these diseases may spread to the central nervous system, leading to encephalitis or meningitis or encouraging bacterial infection of the ears and lungs. Call your physician at once if your child develops any of the following danger signs in addition to the rash and raised temperature:

- unusual drowsiness
- refusal to drink
- earache
- abnormally fast breathing (see the box on p.110)
- noisy breathing
- severe headache

Certain medications, particularly *antibiotics,* may produce a rash in some children. Consult your physician.

Measles (rubeola) is a likely cause of such symptoms, even if your child has been vaccinated against the disease (see *Comparison of childhood infectious diseases,* opposite).

Self-help: There is no specific treatment for measles. Take steps to keep your child's temperature down (see *Lowering your child's temperature,* p.288). There is no need to darken your child's room as was once believed. Call your physician at once if your child develops any of the danger signs listed in the box above. Recovery takes about 10 days.

COMPARISON OF CHILDHOOD INFECTIOUS DISEASES

Disease	Symptoms	Visual signs	Typical course of illness
Measles (incubation period* 10–14 days)	Fever; cough; runny nose; red eyes; flat, dull-red spots and blotches that first appear on the face and behind the ears and later spread to the trunk and upper limbs. Infectious from onset of first symptoms until 4 days after the appearance of the rash.	Rash distribution	Symptoms: Cough; Runny nose/sore eyes; Rash. Temperature (102, 101, 100) over Days 1–9.
German measles (incubation period* 14–21 days)	Low fever; swollen glands in the neck; flat, pink spots that occur mainly on face and trunk at first. Infectious from 7 days before the rash appears until 4 days after.	Rash distribution; Swollen glands	Symptoms: Rash; Swollen glands. Temperature (102, 101, 100) over Days 1–9.
Chickenpox (incubation period* 7–21 days)	Fever; raised, red, itchy spots that turn into blisters and then scabs, mainly on face and trunk. Infectious from 5 days before the rash appears until all the spots have scabs.	Rash distribution	Symptoms: Spots/blisters; Scabs. Temperature (102, 101, 100) over Days 1–9.
Roseola infantum (incubation period* Variable)	High fever; flat, light-red rash on the trunk; swollen glands in the neck. Infectious for 5 days after the onset of symptoms.	Rash distribution; Swollen glands	Symptoms: Swollen glands; Rash. Temperature (102, 101, 100) over Days 1–9.
Mumps (incubation period* 14–28 days)	Swelling and tenderness of glands on one or both sides of the face; fever; sore throat. Infectious from 3 days before the glands swell until 7 days after the swelling has subsided.	Swollen glands	Symptoms: Swollen glands/sore throat. Temperature (102, 101, 100) over Days 1–9.

* Time between contact with the disease and the development of symptoms.

IMMUNIZATION

Your child can be given highly effective immunity against various infectious diseases by vaccination. Some vaccines contain living microbes in a harmless form and these give lasting protection. Vaccines made from dead microbes or from the toxins they produce have to be given several times for best results. In each case, the body is stimulated to produce substances known as antibodies to fight the disease. Immunization during childhood not only protects your child from disease, but helps to reduce the spread of disease in the community. Most forms of immunization carry little risk. However, some vaccinations may be dangerous for children who have had convulsions or if anyone in the family has suffered from convulsions. In these cases, certain vaccinations (such as for whooping cough) may not be advisable. Discuss this with your physician. In addition, you should not have your child vaccinated when he or she is sick. The table (right) shows a typical immunization schedule.

TYPICAL IMMUNIZATION SCHEDULE

Age	Disease	Method of vaccination
Birth	Hepatitis B	Injection
2 months	Diphtheria, tetanus, pertussis (DTP)	Combined injection
	Haemophilus influenzae type b (Hib)	Injection
	Hepatitis	Injection
	Poliomyelitis	Oral
4 months	Diphtheria, tetanus, pertussis	Combined injection
	Haemophilus influenzae type b	Injection
	Poliomyelitis	Oral
6 months	Diphtheria, tetanus, pertussis	Combined injection
	Hepatitis	Injection
	Haemophilus influenzae type b	Injection
15 months	Measles, mumps, rubella (German measles)	Combined injection
	Haemophilus influenzae type b	Injection
18 months	Diphtheria, tetanus, pertussis	Combined injection
	Poliomyelitis	Oral
4 – 6 years	Diphtheria, tetanus, pertussis	Combined injection
	Poliomyelitis	Oral
11 – 12 years	Measles, mumps, rubella	Combined injection
14 – 16 years	Diphtheria, tetanus Booster needed every 10 years throughout life	Combined injection

27 Eye problems

This charts deals with pain, itching, redness and/or discharge from one or both eyes. In children, such symptoms are most commonly the result of infection or local irritation and can often be treated at home without consulting your physician. However, you should seek immediate medical advice about any obvious injury to the eye or any foreign body in the eye that cannot be removed by simple first-aid measures.

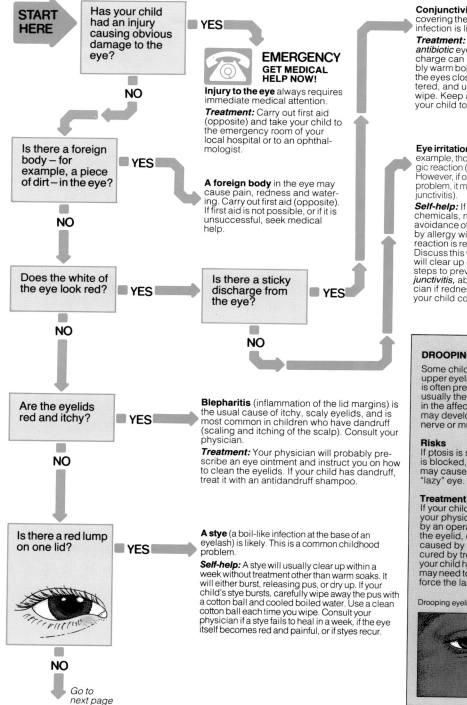

START HERE

Has your child had an injury causing obvious damage to the eye?

YES →

EMERGENCY GET MEDICAL HELP NOW!

Injury to the eye always requires immediate medical attention.
Treatment: Carry out first aid (opposite) and take your child to the emergency room of your local hospital or to an ophthalmologist.

NO ↓

Is there a foreign body – for example, a piece of dirt – in the eye?

YES →

A foreign body in the eye may cause pain, redness and watering. Carry out first aid (opposite). If first aid is not possible, or if it is unsuccessful, seek medical help.

NO ↓

Does the white of the eye look red?

YES →

Is there a sticky discharge from the eye?

YES →

NO ↓

NO ↓

Are the eyelids red and itchy?

YES →

Blepharitis (inflammation of the lid margins) is the usual cause of itchy, scaly eyelids, and is most common in children who have dandruff (scaling and itching of the scalp). Consult your physician.
Treatment: Your physician will probably prescribe an eye ointment and instruct you on how to clean the eyelids. If your child has dandruff, treat it with an antidandruff shampoo.

NO ↓

Is there a red lump on one lid?

YES →

A stye (a boil-like infection at the base of an eyelash) is likely. This is a common childhood problem.
Self-help: A stye will usually clear up within a week without treatment other than warm soaks. It will either burst, releasing pus, or dry up. If your child's stye bursts, carefully wipe away the pus with a cotton ball and cooled boiled water. Use a clean cotton ball each time you wipe. Consult your physician if a stye fails to heal in a week, if the eye itself becomes red and painful, or if styes recur.

NO ↓

Go to next page

Conjunctivitis (inflammation of the membrane covering the eye and lining the eyelids) caused by infection is likely. Consult your physician.
Treatment: Your physician will probably prescribe *antibiotic* eye drops or ointment. The sticky discharge can be gently bathed away with comfortably warm boiled water. Make sure your child keeps the eyes closed after the drops have been administered, and use a clean cotton ball each time you wipe. Keep a separate towel and washcloth for your child to prevent the spread of infection.

Eye irritation caused by fumes or chemicals (for example, those in swimming-pool water) or an allergic reaction (for example, to pollen) is possible. However, if other children in your area also have this problem, it may be due to viral infection (viral conjunctivitis).
Self-help: If you suspect irritation from fumes or chemicals, no treatment is needed other than avoidance of the irritant. Similarly, irritation caused by allergy will subside as soon as the cause of the reaction is removed, but this is not always possible. Discuss this with your physician. Viral conjunctivitis will clear up on its own, but you will need to take steps to prevent the spread of infection (see *Conjunctivitis,* above). In any case, consult your physician if redness persists for more than a week, or if your child complains of pain.

DROOPING EYELID

Some children have a permanently drooping upper eyelid, a condition known as ptosis. This is often present from birth, and in such cases is usually the result of weakness of the muscles in the affected eyelid. Occasionally, ptosis may develop later in childhood as a result of a nerve or muscle disorder.

Risks
If ptosis is so severe that the vision in that eye is blocked, and the condition is untreated, it may cause deterioration in the vision in the "lazy" eye.

Treatment
If your child has a drooping eyelid, consult your physician. The condition may be treated by an operation to strengthen the muscles of the eyelid, or by special glasses. Ptosis that is caused by a nerve or muscle disorder may be cured by treating the underlying condition. If your child has developed a lazy eye, he or she may need to wear a patch over the good eye to force the lazy eye to work harder.

Drooping eyelid in a child

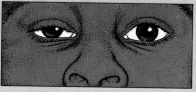

Continued from previous page

Does the eye produce tears even when your child is not crying?

YES →

Is your child less than 1 year old?

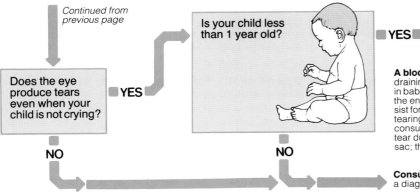

YES →

A blocked tear duct, which prevents tears from draining away normally, is possible. This is common in babies and may correct itself without treatment by the end of the first year. If tearing and redness persist for more than 2 weeks, consult your physician. If tearing alone persists for more than one month, consult your physician. He or she may massage the tear duct by firmly stroking downward over the tear sac; this often helps open the tear duct.

NO ↓   **NO** ↓

Consult your physician if you are unable to make a diagnosis from this chart.

FIRST AID FOR EYE INJURIES

If your child suffers an injury to the eye or eyelid, rapid action is essential (with the exception of a foreign body that has been successfully removed from the eye). As soon as you have carried out first aid, get your child to the emergency room of your local hospital or to an ophthalmologist by the fastest means possible.

Cuts to the eye or eyelid
Cover the injured eye with a clean pad (for example, a folded handkerchief) and hold the pad lightly in place with a bandage. Apply no pressure. Cover the other eye also to prevent movement of the eyeball. Seek medical help.

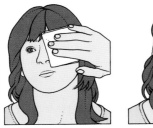

Blows to the eye area
Carry out first aid as for cuts to the eye or eyelid (above), but use a cold compress instead of a dry pad over the injured eye.

Corrosive chemicals in the eye
If your child spills any harsh chemical (for example, bleach) in the eye, immediately flood the eye with large quantities of cold, running water. Tilt your child's head with the injured eye downward so that the water runs from the inside outward. Keep the eyelids apart with your fingers (see below). When all traces of the chemical have been removed, lightly cover the eye with a clean pad and seek medical help.

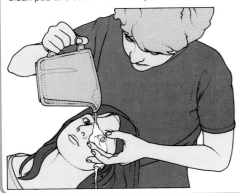

Foreign body in the eye
Never attempt to remove any of the following from your child's eye:

- an object that is embedded in the eyeball
- a chip of metal
- a particle over the colored part of the eye.

In any of these cases, cover both eyes as recommended for cuts to the eye or eyelid (left) and seek medical help.

Other foreign bodies – for example, specks of dirt or eyelashes floating on the white of the eye or inside the lids – may be removed as follows:

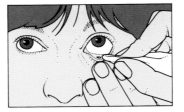   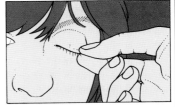

1 If you can see the particle on the white of the eye or inside the lower lid, pick it off using the moistened corner of a clean handkerchief or sterile cotton-tipped swab.

2 If you can see nothing, hold the lashes, pull the upper lid down over the lower lid and hold it for a moment. This may dislodge the particle.

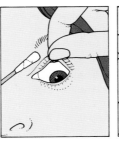   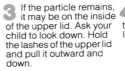   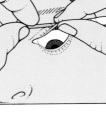   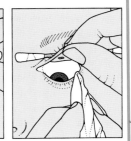

3 If the particle remains, it may be on the inside of the upper lid. Ask your child to look down. Hold the lashes of the upper lid and pull it outward and down.

4 Place a match or cotton-tipped swab over the upper lid and fold the lid back over it.

5 If the particle is now visible, pick it off with the corner of a handkerchief as in step 1.

If you do not succeed in removing the foreign body, lightly cover your child's injured eye and seek medical help at once.

28 Disturbed or impaired vision

Defects in vision in children are usually discovered at routine eye tests. But you may suspect that your child has a problem with his or her eyesight if he or she always holds books very close to the face. Or a teacher may notice that your child performs less well if he or she sits at the back of the classroom where it may be difficult to see the blackboard. Fortunately, disorders causing sudden or complete loss of vision are rare. Always consult your physician promptly about any problems with your child's eyesight.

START HERE

Has your child lost all or part of his or her vision? — YES → (see right)

NO ↓

Has your child been suffering from double vision? — YES → (see below)

NO ↓

Has your child had a recent head injury? — YES → (see EMERGENCY)

NO ↓ → CALL YOUR PHYSICIAN NOW!

**EMERGENCY
GET MEDICAL HELP NOW!**

Injury to the eye mechanism, or to part of the brain, is a possibility.

Treatment: Your child will probably be admitted to the hospital for examination by specialists. Tests such as a *CT (computed tomography) scan* (p. 85) may be necessary. Treatment will depend on the nature and extent of the damage.

CALL YOUR PHYSICIAN NOW!
Sudden loss of vision is always a serious symptom, even if it only lasts a few moments.

Treatment: Your physician will look at your child's eyes and may arrange for him or her to be examined by an ophthalmologist.

CONSULT YOUR PHYSICIAN WITHOUT DELAY!
An eye muscle problem is possible (see the box below).

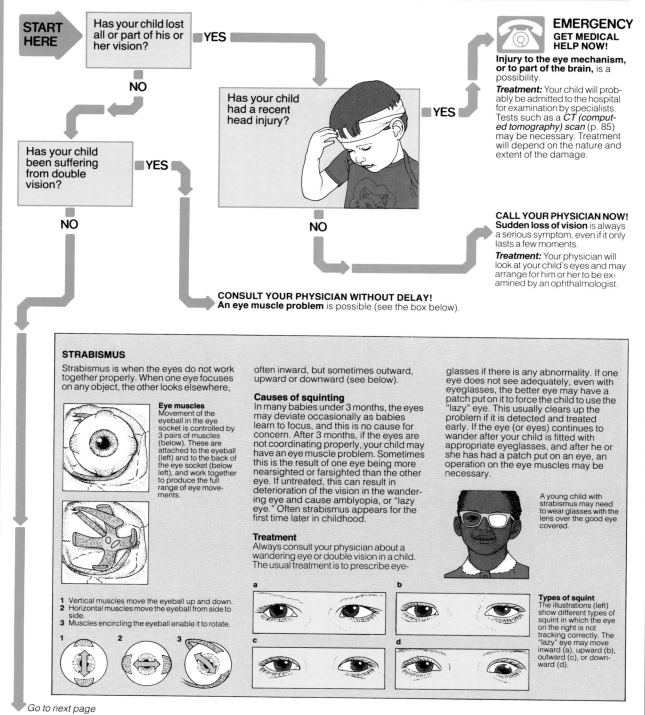

STRABISMUS

Strabismus is when the eyes do not work together properly. When one eye focuses on any object, the other looks elsewhere, often inward, but sometimes outward, upward or downward (see below).

Eye muscles
Movement of the eyeball in the eye socket is controlled by 3 pairs of muscles (below). These are attached to the eyeball (left) and to the back of the eye socket (below left), and work together to produce the full range of eye movements.

Causes of squinting
In many babies under 3 months, the eyes may deviate occasionally as babies learn to focus, and this is no cause for concern. After 3 months, if the eyes are not coordinating properly, your child may have an eye muscle problem. Sometimes this is the result of one eye being more nearsighted or farsighted than the other eye. If untreated, this can result in deterioration of the vision in the wandering eye and cause amblyopia, or "lazy eye." Often strabismus appears for the first time later in childhood.

Treatment
Always consult your physician about a wandering eye or double vision in a child. The usual treatment is to prescribe eye-glasses if there is any abnormality. If one eye does not see adequately, even with eyeglasses, the better eye may have a patch put on it to force the child to use the "lazy" eye. This usually clears up the problem if it is detected and treated early. If the eye (or eyes) continues to wander after your child is fitted with appropriate eyeglasses, and after he or she has had a patch put on an eye, an operation on the eye muscles may be necessary.

A young child with strabismus may need to wear glasses with the lens over the good eye covered.

1 Vertical muscles move the eyeball up and down.
2 Horizontal muscles move the eyeball from side to side.
3 Muscles encircling the eyeball enable it to rotate.

Types of squint
The illustrations (left) show different types of squint in which the eye on the right is not tracking correctly. The "lazy" eye may move inward (a), upward (b), outward (c), or downward (d).

Continued from previous page

Is your child's vision generally blurred? — **YES** →

NO ↓

Is either eye red and painful? — **YES** →

NO ↓

CONSULT YOUR PHYSICIAN WITHOUT DELAY!
Iritis (inflammation of the colored part of the eye) is possible, although uncommon in children. A less serious problem is more likely.

Treatment: If your physician diagnoses iritis, he or she will prescribe eye drops or ointment to reduce the inflammation and possibly medication to prevent damage to the lens. If your child has conjunctivitis, your physician may prescribe eye drops or ointment to counter infection. Your physician may perform a complete medical examination to find an underlying cause.

Could your child accidentally have taken medication prescribed for an adult? — **YES** →

NO ↓

CALL YOUR PHYSICIAN NOW!
Poisoning by certain drugs, in particular, quinine, may cause blurring of vision. See **Poisoning,** p.286.

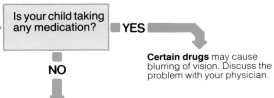

Is your child taking any medication? — **YES** →

NO ↓

Certain drugs may cause blurring of vision. Discuss the problem with your physician.

An error of refraction, which causes light to focus improperly, may cause blurred vision. The most common types of error in children are nearsightedness (difficulty in seeing far objects), farsightedness (difficulty in focusing on near objects) and astigmatism (distorted vision caused by uneven curvature of the front of the eye). Consult your physician.

Treatment: If your physician confirms the possibility of such a disorder, he or she will refer your child to an ophthalmologist for a full eye test. Your child may need to wear glasses.

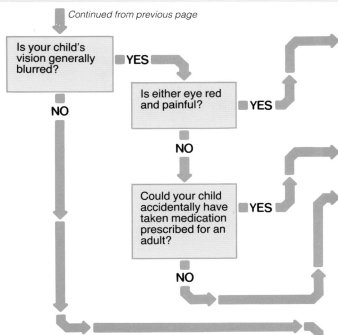

EYE TESTING

Your child's eyes and vision should be tested at regular intervals throughout childhood. In the preschool years your family physician will test your child's vision during routine visits.

When your child goes to school, his or her vision will be tested as part of a general medical examination. Most education authorities arrange for children to have several such examinations during their school years.

What happens

Your physician or ophthalmologist will test your child's ability to recognize objects at a distance. Each eye will be tested separately while the other is covered.

A child of school age will probably be asked to read letters of gradually diminishing size from a distance. Each eye will be tested separately with the other eye covered.

An eye examination by an ophthalmologist is recommended when a child is old enough to read or identify letters. If there is a family history of eye problems in childhood, an eye examination should be performed even earlier.

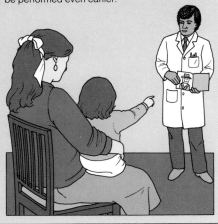

Does your child have difficulty seeing distant objects? — **YES** →

NO ↓

Nearsightedness is likely. This means that your child's eyes have difficulty focusing on distant objects. This type of defect is often inherited. Consult your physician.

Treatment: If your physician thinks that your child may be nearsighted, he or she will arrange for your child to have a full eye test by an ophthalmologist, who may prescribe glasses.

Has your child been seeing flashing lights or floating spots? — **YES** →

NO ↓

Has this happened on several past occasions AND does a severe headache normally follow? — **YES** →

NO ↓

Migraine headaches (recurrent severe headaches) may occasionally affect children. Consult your physician.

Treatment: If migraine is diagnosed, your physician may prescribe medication to take during attacks or to take (as a preventive measure) between attacks. Relaxing in a darkened room may also help your child's symptoms pass more quickly. See **Headache,** p.82.

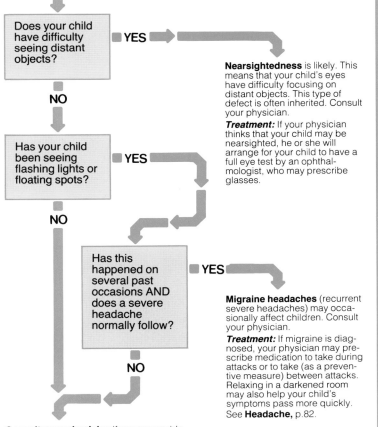

Consult your physician if you are unable to make a diagnosis from this chart.

29 Painful or irritated ear

Ear pain is common in babies and children (up to three attacks a year is usual) and can be distressing. A baby who is not old enough to tell you what the matter is may cry continuously or shriek loudly at intervals, and may pull at the affected ear. Earache is the most common explanation for waking at night in a baby who usually sleeps well. Most ear problems in childhood are due to infection and require medical attention.

START HERE

Does your child have an earache?

→ **YES** → **Does your child seem sick or feverish, AND/OR does he or she have a cold?** → **YES**

Infection of the middle ear is a possibility. This may have occurred as a result of germs traveling up the eustachian tube (see *The structure of the ear,* opposite). Consult your physician.

Treatment: If, after examining your child, the physician confirms that the middle ear is inflamed, he or she will probably prescribe *antibiotics.* During this treatment you can help to relieve the pain by following the self-help suggestions described below.

NO ↓

NO ↓

Does your child complain of itching in the ear, OR does he or she scratch the ear?

→ **YES**

Can you see a red lump inside the ear? → **YES**

A boil in the outer-ear canal can cause severe pain in a child. Consult your physician.

Treatment: If your physician confirms this diagnosis, he or she may prescribe ear drops or *antibiotics* taken by mouth or by injection. Lancing the boil may also help. The self-help suggestions below should help relieve the pain in the meantime.

NO ↓

NO ↓

Inflammation of the outer-ear canal is possible, especially if your child has been swimming in chlorinated water recently. Consult your physician.

Treatment: Ear drops will probably be prescribed to reduce inflammation and prevent infection.

Generalized infection of the outer-ear canal is probable. Consult your physician.

Treatment: If your child's outer ear is found to be infected, your physician will probably prescribe *antibiotic* ear drops to treat the infection and will recommend that you give your child an aspirin substitute for the pain (see *How to relieve earache,* below).

FIRST AID FOR A FOREIGN BODY IN THE EAR

Young children often cause ear problems by poking small objects, such as beads or beans, into their ears. If this happens, do not try to remove the object yourself unless it is very close to the entrance of the outer-ear canal and you are sure that you will do no damage to the delicate lining of the outer-ear canal or to the eardrum. If you are in any doubt, consult your physician or go to the emergency room of your local hospital.

Insect in the ear
If an insect gets into your child's ear, you can safely try to remove it by pouring warm olive, baby or mineral oil into the ear so that it floats out. As you pour, pull the lobe of the ear gently backwards and upwards to straighten the canal. If these measures do not remove the insect, consult your physician.

HOW TO RELIEVE EARACHE

Antibiotics may take up to 24 hours before helping to relieve the symptoms of an ear infection. During this time, you can help to relieve your child's earache by giving the recommended dose of syrup that contains an aspirin substitute or tablets (for an older child) every four hours, as needed. It may also be comforting to place a warm electric blanket or heating pad against the ear. Do not, however, put anything (a cotton ball, for example) inside the ear, as this may make the problem worse.

Remember, pain-relieving measures alone will not cure the underlying disorder. You should always seek your physician's advice about a persistent earache.

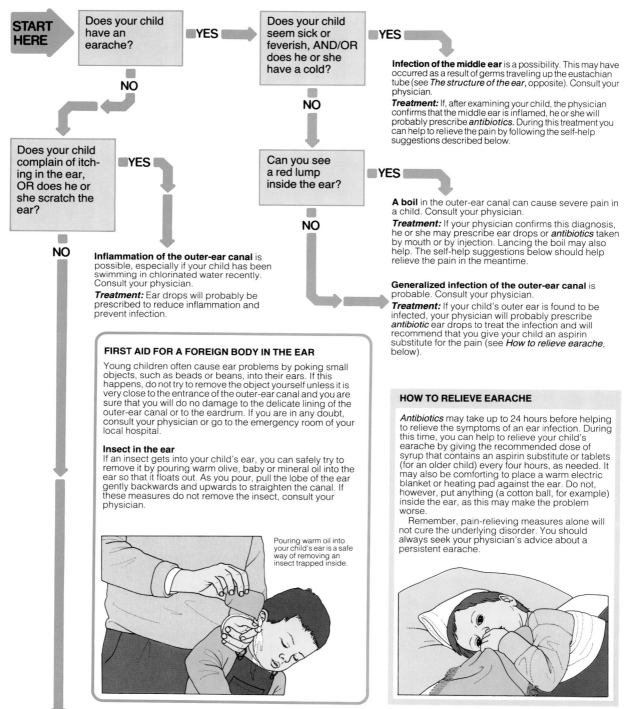

Pouring warm oil into your child's ear is a safe way of removing an insect trapped inside.

Go to next page

Continued from previous page

Is there a discharge from the affected ear? — **YES** → Does the pain become worse when you gently pull on your child's earlobe? — **YES** →

NO ↓

YES (from earlobe question):

Infection of the outer-ear canal may cause pain and discharge. Consult your physician.

Treatment: If your physician finds that your child's outer-ear canal is infected, he or she will probably advise you to gently clean away any discharge from the outer ear and may prescribe *antibiotic* ear drops.

NO ↓ (from earlobe question)

Infection of the middle ear may have caused your child's eardrum to rupture, producing pain and discharge. This is especially likely if your child has, or has recently had, a cold. Consult your physician.

Treatment: If your physician confirms this diagnosis, a course of *antibiotics* may be prescribed. Antibiotic ear drops to prevent infection of the outer-ear canal may also be prescribed and you will probably be advised to regularly clean away the discharge from the outer ear.

Did your child suddenly develop an earache during or immediately after air travel? — **YES** →

Barotrauma, in which the air pressure balance between the middle and outer ears is disrupted, is a possibility.

Self-help: To prevent barotrauma from occurring, encourage your child to suck and swallow during takeoff and landing. A baby can be fed by breast or bottle at these times and an older child can be offered hard candy to suck or gum to chew. Barotrauma is more likely to develop if your child has a stuffy nose, so it is best to avoid air travel, if possible, when your child has a cold. The symptoms of barotrauma normally clear up without treatment within a few hours. However, if the pain persists or your child seems otherwise sick, consult your physician.

NO ↓

Consult your physician if you are unable to make a diagnosis from this chart.

EAR EXAMINATION

Your child may need to have his or her ears examined because of ear problems or as part of a routine checkup. The physician uses an instrument called an otoscope to look inside the ear for abnormalities of the outer ear or of the eardrum. This is not usually painful, but a child with an ear infection may find the procedure uncomfortable. An older child can often be examined standing up, but a baby or young child can be examined sitting on your knee while you hold his or her head firmly against your chest to provide reassurance and to prevent the child from wriggling (below).

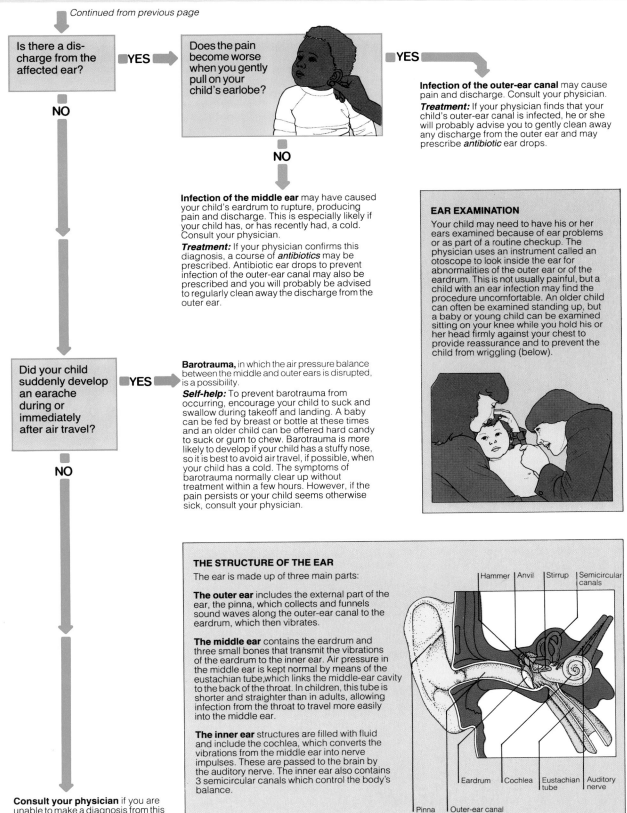

THE STRUCTURE OF THE EAR

The ear is made up of three main parts:

The outer ear includes the external part of the ear, the pinna, which collects and funnels sound waves along the outer-ear canal to the eardrum, which then vibrates.

The middle ear contains the eardrum and three small bones that transmit the vibrations of the eardrum to the inner ear. Air pressure in the middle ear is kept normal by means of the eustachian tube, which links the middle-ear cavity to the back of the throat. In children, this tube is shorter and straighter than in adults, allowing infection from the throat to travel more easily into the middle ear.

The inner ear structures are filled with fluid and include the cochlea, which converts the vibrations from the middle ear into nerve impulses. These are passed to the brain by the auditory nerve. The inner ear also contains 3 semicircular canals which control the body's balance.

Hammer | Anvil | Stirrup | Semicircular canals

Eardrum | Cochlea | Eustachian tube | Auditory nerve

Pinna | Outer-ear canal

30 Deafness

Deafness is often overlooked in a child, particularly if only one ear is affected. If you find that you are having to repeat things you say to your child, if he or she always needs to have the television or radio louder than you think necessary or if there is a sudden deterioration in school performance, you may suspect deafness.

Hearing problems in babies are usually detected by the physician during developmental checks or at other routine consultations, but you may be the first to notice that your baby is not responding to sounds or learning to speak as quickly as you think he or she should. This should always be brought to your physician's attention.

START HERE

Has the deafness come on recently?

— YES → **Does your child have, or has he or she recently had, an earache?** — YES →

Infection of the middle ear or of the outer-ear canal can cause pain and temporary deafness that may persist after the infection has cleared. Consult your physician.

Treatment: Your physician will examine your child's ear (see *Ear examination*, p. 103) and if he or she finds signs of infection may prescribe *antibiotics*, either as syrup (for middle-ear infections) or as ear drops (for outer-ear infections).

NO ↓   NO ↓

Did your child become deaf during or just after air travel? — YES →

Barotrauma, in which the air pressure balance between the middle and outer ears is disrupted, can lead to a temporary loss of hearing.

Self-help: To prevent barotrauma from occurring, encourage your child to suck and swallow during takeoff and landing. A baby can be fed by breast or bottle at these times and an older child can be offered a hard candy to suck or gum to chew. Barotrauma is more likely to develop if your child has a stuffy nose, so it is best to avoid air travel, if possible, when your child has a cold. The symptoms of barotrauma normally clear up without treatment within a few hours. However, if deafness persists, consult your physician.

NO ↓

Does your child have, or has he or she recently had, a cold AND/OR has he or she been sneezing? — YES →

Blockage of the eustachian tube (see *The structure of the ear,* p. 103) as a result of a cold or hay fever may account for your child's deafness. Consult your physician.

Treatment: Your physician may recommend that you simply wait for the ear to clear itself. If, however, the condition has persisted for some time, he or she may prescribe *decongestant* nose drops to clear the eustachian tube. If hay fever is the cause of the problem, your physician may also prescribe a medicine or spray to prevent the blockage from recurring.

NO ↓

Blockage of the outer-ear canal by wax, or perhaps by a foreign body, may be the cause of your child's deafness. Consult your physician.

Treatment: If your physician finds that your child's ears are blocked by wax, he or she will syringe or flush the wax out. The physician may first suggest you use wax-softening ear drops for a few days. If a foreign body is the cause of the trouble, your physician will remove it using the otoscope (see *Ear examination,* p. 103) or a syringe.

MYRINGOTOMY AND EAR TUBES

Myringotomy is a minor operation sometimes carried out in children when the eustachian tube, which runs between the middle ear and the back of the throat, may be blocked and the middle ear becomes filled with fluid. The operation may require a hospital stay but most often is done in a hospital or physician's office.

What happens
A small cut is made in the eardrum to allow the fluid to drain away. Usually a small plastic tube is then inserted into the hole to allow fluid to drain from the middle ear. In some cases, the adenoids may be removed at the same time (see *Adenoid removal,* p. 109). The tube usually stays in place for about six months, after which it drops out naturally. The hole in the eardrum then usually heals. While the tube is in place, it is important to avoid getting water in the ear canal.

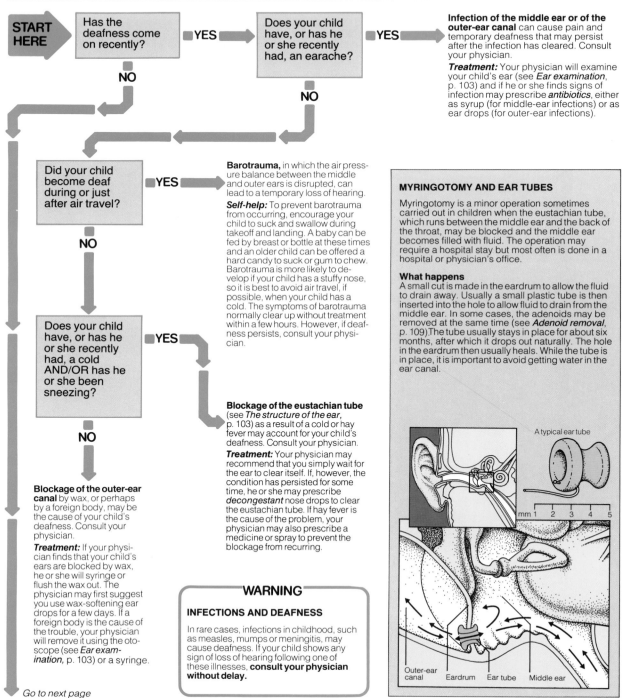

A typical ear tube

mm 1   2   3   4   5

Outer-ear canal   Eardrum   Ear tube   Middle ear

WARNING

INFECTIONS AND DEAFNESS

In rare cases, infections in childhood, such as measles, mumps or meningitis, may cause deafness. If your child shows any sign of loss of hearing following one of these illnesses, **consult your physician without delay.**

Go to next page

Continued from previous page

Did the onset of deafness follow an earache?

▶ **YES** ▶ **Serous otitis media,** accumulation of fluid in the middle ear, sometimes follows infection of the middle ear in children. Consult your physician.

Treatment: If your physician diagnoses middle-ear fluid, he or she may prescribe further *antibiotics* or medicine to reduce swelling of the tissues and disperse the fluid. If this does not work, or if the congestion is severe, your physician may recommend a myringotomy (a small cut in the eardrum) and the insertion of an ear tube (see opposite). In most cases, hearing is restored to normal.

NO ↓

Are you worried that your child has never been able to hear properly?

▶ **YES** ▶ **During pregnancy was there any possibility of contact or infection with German measles, OR was there any un-explained rash or fever?**

▶ **YES** ▶ **German measles during pregnancy** can cause deafness in the unborn child. Consult your physician.

Treatment: If your physician already knows that there was a possibility of German measles in pregnancy, it is likely that he or she is watching your child's progress carefully and would have noticed any hearing problems. However, if you are concerned about your child's hearing, explain your fears to your physician, who will be able to arrange for your child to have a hearing test. If your child is found to be deaf, you should receive advice from trained therapists on helping your child to talk and understand others.

NO ↓

Consult your physician if you are unable to make a diagnosis from this chart. The problem may simply be the result of wax blockage (see *Blockage of the outer-ear canal*, opposite).

NO

Congenital hearing defects are rare without a history of German measles or a family history of deafness. However, if you are worried about your child's hearing, discuss the problem with your physician, explaining the basis for your fears.

Treatment: Your physician will probably want to know about your child's general health and about the pregnancy, particularly whether any drugs were taken. If, after examining your child, he or she thinks there may be grounds for concern or, if you are not satisfied by his or her reassurances, your physician can arrange for your child to have a full hearing test.

HEARING TESTS FOR CHILDREN

All children should have their hearing tested at regular intervals during early childhood, ideally at 8 to 9 months, at 3 years and at 5 years. Preliminary hearing tests are carried out by your family physician and depend on the age of your child.

Under 6 months (below): The physician will make a sudden sound and look for a startled reaction.

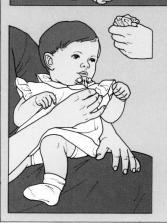

From 6 to 12 months (left): The best test is for one person to hold the baby's attention while another makes a soft sound (such as crinkling tissue paper) to distract the baby.

After 12 months: The physician will assess the child's reaction to quiet speech.

If the response to any of these tests gives your physician reason to suspect that your child may be deaf, he or she will be referred for special hearing tests, which can measure the response in the inner ear to sound, regardless of your child's age.

HEADPHONES AND LOUD MUSIC

Many older children and adolescents enjoy listening to loud music through headphones attached to a radio, stereo or portable tape player. However, parents should be aware of the potential danger to hearing that these present.

The risks
At normal volumes, headphones present no risk. But your child may be tempted to turn the volume up – for example, to exclude external noise – which could cause permanent hearing damage. The sound need not be painfully loud to damage hearing, so the fact that your child insists that the volume is not uncomfortably high is not a reliable way of judging what level is safe. A useful guideline is that if others in the room can hear the music when your child is wearing headphones, it is likely that the volume is too high. Portable tape players with headphones may also increase the risk of road accidents if used when walking or cycling in traffic because they reduce awareness of what is going on around you.

31 Runny or stuffed-up nose

Runny nose is probably the most common medical symptom in childhood. All children have a runny nose (usually accompanied by sneezing) at times, and, in most cases, the common cold, a virus, is responsible. A runny nose can be irritating for the parents and child, and a stuffy nose can be distressing for a baby, making sucking difficult, but neither symptom on its own is likely to be a sign of serious disease.

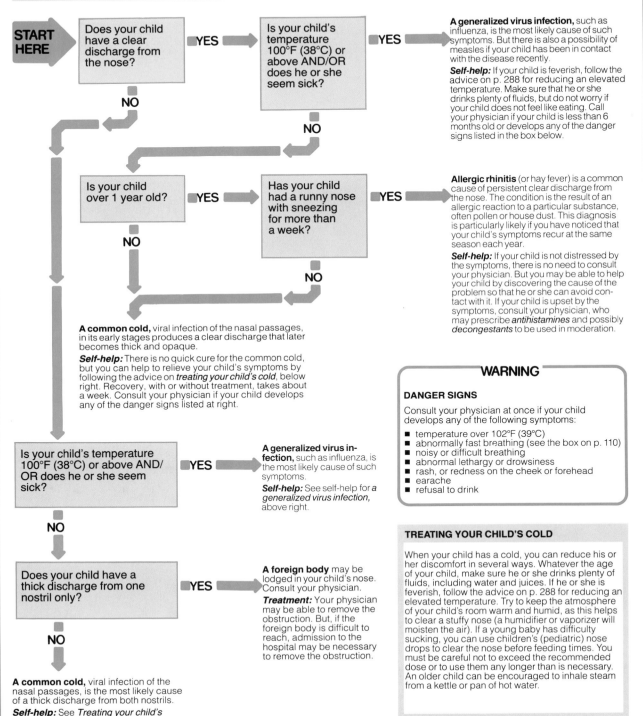

START HERE

Does your child have a clear discharge from the nose? — YES → **Is your child's temperature 100°F (38°C) or above AND/OR does he or she seem sick?** — YES →

A generalized virus infection, such as influenza, is the most likely cause of such symptoms. But there is also a possibility of measles if your child has been in contact with the disease recently.

Self-help: If your child is feverish, follow the advice on p. 288 for reducing an elevated temperature. Make sure that he or she drinks plenty of fluids, but do not worry if your child does not feel like eating. Call your physician if your child is less than 6 months old or develops any of the danger signs listed in the box below.

NO / NO

Is your child over 1 year old? — YES → **Has your child had a runny nose with sneezing for more than a week?** — YES →

Allergic rhinitis (or hay fever) is a common cause of persistent clear discharge from the nose. The condition is the result of an allergic reaction to a particular substance, often pollen or house dust. This diagnosis is particularly likely if you have noticed that your child's symptoms recur at the same season each year.

Self-help: If your child is not distressed by the symptoms, there is no need to consult your physician. But you may be able to help your child by discovering the cause of the problem so that he or she can avoid contact with it. If your child is upset by the symptoms, consult your physician, who may prescribe *antihistamines* and possibly *decongestants* to be used in moderation.

NO / NO

A common cold, viral infection of the nasal passages, in its early stages produces a clear discharge that later becomes thick and opaque.

Self-help: There is no quick cure for the common cold, but you can help to relieve your child's symptoms by following the advice on *treating your child's cold,* below right. Recovery, with or without treatment, takes about a week. Consult your physician if your child develops any of the danger signs listed at right.

Is your child's temperature 100°F (38°C) or above AND/OR does he or she seem sick? — YES →

A generalized virus infection, such as influenza, is the most likely cause of such symptoms.

Self-help: See self-help for *a generalized virus infection,* above right.

NO

Does your child have a thick discharge from one nostril only? — YES →

A foreign body may be lodged in your child's nose. Consult your physician.

Treatment: Your physician may be able to remove the obstruction. But, if the foreign body is difficult to reach, admission to the hospital may be necessary to remove the obstruction.

NO

A common cold, viral infection of the nasal passages, is the most likely cause of a thick discharge from both nostrils.

Self-help: See *Treating your child's cold,* right.

WARNING

DANGER SIGNS

Consult your physician at once if your child develops any of the following symptoms:

- temperature over 102°F (39°C)
- abnormally fast breathing (see the box on p. 110)
- noisy or difficult breathing
- abnormal lethargy or drowsiness
- rash, or redness on the cheek or forehead
- earache
- refusal to drink

TREATING YOUR CHILD'S COLD

When your child has a cold, you can reduce his or her discomfort in several ways. Whatever the age of your child, make sure he or she drinks plenty of fluids, including water and juices. If he or she is feverish, follow the advice on p. 288 for reducing an elevated temperature. Try to keep the atmosphere of your child's room warm and humid, as this helps to clear a stuffy nose (a humidifier or vaporizer will moisten the air). If a young baby has difficulty sucking, you can use children's (pediatric) nose drops to clear the nose before feeding times. You must be careful not to exceed the recommended dose or to use them any longer than is necessary. An older child can be encouraged to inhale steam from a kettle or pan of hot water.

32 Sore throat

Sore throat is a common symptom in childhood. An older child will usually tell you that his or her throat hurts; in the case of a younger child, your attention is most likely to be drawn to your child's reluctance to eat because of the pain caused by swallowing. Most sore throats that are due to viruses clear up within a few days, but, if you note any of the danger signs listed on the chart opposite, consult your physician.

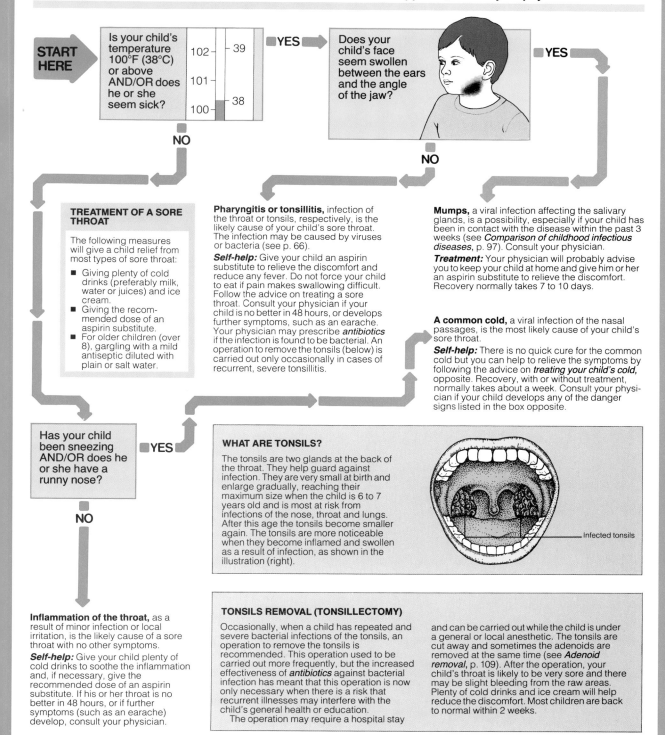

START HERE → Is your child's temperature 100°F (38°C) or above AND/OR does he or she seem sick?

102 — 39
101
100 — 38

YES → Does your child's face seem swollen between the ears and the angle of the jaw?

YES →

NO ↓

NO ↓

TREATMENT OF A SORE THROAT

The following measures will give a child relief from most types of sore throat:

- Giving plenty of cold drinks (preferably milk, water or juices) and ice cream.
- Giving the recommended dose of an aspirin substitute.
- For older children (over 8), gargling with a mild antiseptic diluted with plain or salt water.

Pharyngitis or tonsillitis, infection of the throat or tonsils, respectively, is the likely cause of your child's sore throat. The infection may be caused by viruses or bacteria (see p. 66).

Self-help: Give your child an aspirin substitute to relieve the discomfort and reduce any fever. Do not force your child to eat if pain makes swallowing difficult. Follow the advice on treating a sore throat. Consult your physician if your child is no better in 48 hours, or develops further symptoms, such as an earache. Your physician may prescribe *antibiotics* if the infection is found to be bacterial. An operation to remove the tonsils (below) is carried out only occasionally in cases of recurrent, severe tonsillitis.

Mumps, a viral infection affecting the salivary glands, is a possibility, especially if your child has been in contact with the disease within the past 3 weeks (see *Comparison of childhood infectious diseases*, p. 97). Consult your physician.

Treatment: Your physician will probably advise you to keep your child at home and give him or her an aspirin substitute to relieve the discomfort. Recovery normally takes 7 to 10 days.

A common cold, a viral infection of the nasal passages, is the most likely cause of your child's sore throat.

Self-help: There is no quick cure for the common cold but you can help to relieve the symptoms by following the advice on *treating your child's cold,* opposite. Recovery, with or without treatment, normally takes about a week. Consult your physician if your child develops any of the danger signs listed in the box opposite.

Has your child been sneezing AND/OR does he or she have a runny nose?

YES →

NO ↓

WHAT ARE TONSILS?

The tonsils are two glands at the back of the throat. They help guard against infection. They are very small at birth and enlarge gradually, reaching their maximum size when the child is 6 to 7 years old and is most at risk from infections of the nose, throat and lungs. After this age the tonsils become smaller again. The tonsils are more noticeable when they become inflamed and swollen as a result of infection, as shown in the illustration (right).

Infected tonsils

Inflammation of the throat, as a result of minor infection or local irritation, is the likely cause of a sore throat with no other symptoms.

Self-help: Give your child plenty of cold drinks to soothe the inflammation and, if necessary, give the recommended dose of an aspirin substitute. If his or her throat is no better in 48 hours, or if further symptoms (such as an earache) develop, consult your physician.

TONSILS REMOVAL (TONSILLECTOMY)

Occasionally, when a child has repeated and severe bacterial infections of the tonsils, an operation to remove the tonsils is recommended. This operation used to be carried out more frequently, but the increased effectiveness of *antibiotics* against bacterial infection has meant that this operation is now only necessary when there is a risk that recurrent illnesses may interfere with the child's general health or education.

The operation may require a hospital stay and can be carried out while the child is under a general or local anesthetic. The tonsils are cut away and sometimes the adenoids are removed at the same time (see *Adenoid removal*, p. 109). After the operation, your child's throat is likely to be very sore and there may be slight bleeding from the raw areas. Plenty of cold drinks and ice cream will help reduce the discomfort. Most children are back to normal within 2 weeks.

33 Coughing

Coughing, a normal reaction to irritation and congestion in the throat and lungs, is a noisy expulsion of air from the lungs. It is an unusual symptom in babies under 6 months, and can be a sign of a serious lung infection. In older children, the vast majority of cases are due to minor infec- tions of the nose and throat. Occasionally, a sudden cough can be a sign of a more serious blockage in the respiratory tract. You should call your physician at once if your child's breathing seems in any way abnormal between bouts of coughing.

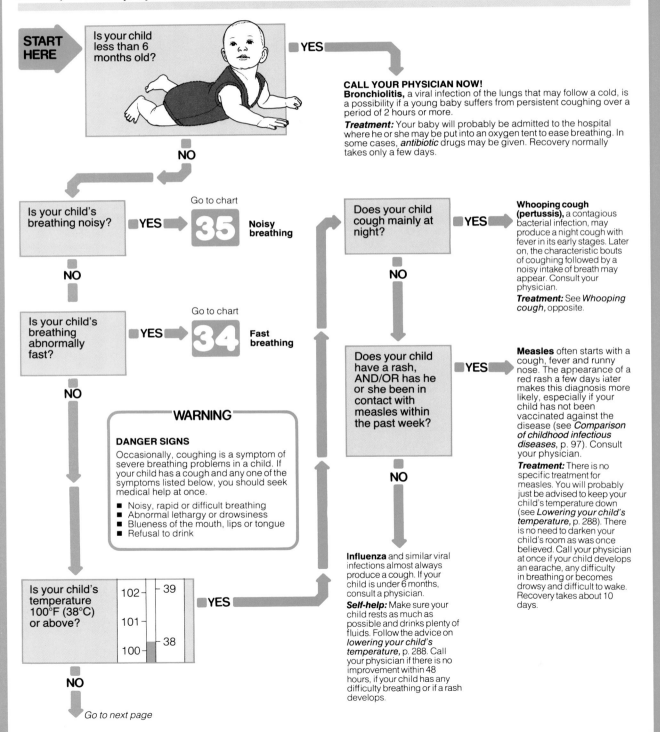

START HERE

Is your child less than 6 months old?

YES

CALL YOUR PHYSICIAN NOW!
Bronchiolitis, a viral infection of the lungs that may follow a cold, is a possibility if a young baby suffers from persistent coughing over a period of 2 hours or more.

Treatment: Your baby will probably be admitted to the hospital where he or she may be put into an oxygen tent to ease breathing. In some cases, ***antibiotic*** drugs may be given. Recovery normally takes only a few days.

NO

Is your child's breathing noisy? **YES** ➡ Go to chart **35** **Noisy breathing**

NO

Is your child's breathing abnormally fast? **YES** ➡ Go to chart **34** **Fast breathing**

NO

WARNING

DANGER SIGNS

Occasionally, coughing is a symptom of severe breathing problems in a child. If your child has a cough and any one of the symptoms listed below, you should seek medical help at once.

- Noisy, rapid or difficult breathing
- Abnormal lethargy or drowsiness
- Blueness of the mouth, lips or tongue
- Refusal to drink

Is your child's temperature 100°F (38°C) or above?

102	– 39
101	
100	– 38

YES

NO

Go to next page

Does your child cough mainly at night? **YES**

Whooping cough (pertussis), a contagious bacterial infection, may produce a night cough with fever in its early stages. Later on, the characteristic bouts of coughing followed by a noisy intake of breath may appear. Consult your physician.

Treatment: See *Whooping cough,* opposite.

NO

Does your child have a rash, AND/OR has he or she been in contact with measles within the past week? **YES**

Measles often starts with a cough, fever and runny nose. The appearance of a red rash a few days later makes this diagnosis more likely, especially if your child has not been vaccinated against the disease (see *Comparison of childhood infectious diseases*, p. 97). Consult your physician.

Treatment: There is no specific treatment for measles. You will probably just be advised to keep your child's temperature down (see *Lowering your child's temperature,* p. 288). There is no need to darken your child's room as was once believed. Call your physician at once if your child develops an earache, any difficulty in breathing or becomes drowsy and difficult to wake. Recovery takes about 10 days.

NO

Influenza and similar viral infections almost always produce a cough. If your child is under 6 months, consult a physician.

Self-help: Make sure your child rests as much as possible and drinks plenty of fluids. Follow the advice on *lowering your child's temperature,* p. 288. Call your physician if there is no improvement within 48 hours, if your child has any difficulty breathing or if a rash develops.

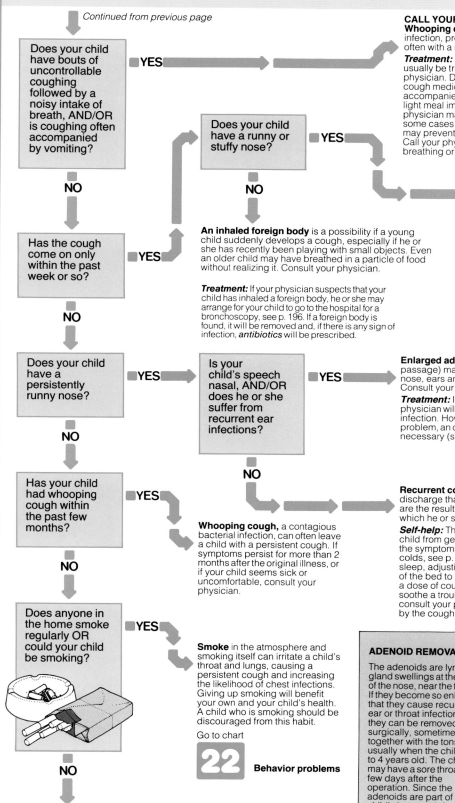

Continued from previous page

Does your child have bouts of uncontrollable coughing followed by a noisy intake of breath, AND/OR is coughing often accompanied by vomiting?

YES →

Does your child have a runny or stuffy nose?

YES →

NO ↓

NO ↓

Has the cough come on only within the past week or so?

YES →

An inhaled foreign body is a possibility if a young child suddenly develops a cough, especially if he or she has recently been playing with small objects. Even an older child may have breathed in a particle of food without realizing it. Consult your physician.

Treatment: If your physician suspects that your child has inhaled a foreign body, he or she may arrange for your child to go to the hospital for a bronchoscopy, see p. 196. If a foreign body is found, it will be removed and, if there is any sign of infection, *antibiotics* will be prescribed.

NO ↓

Does your child have a persistently runny nose?

YES →

Is your child's speech nasal, AND/OR does he or she suffer from recurrent ear infections?

YES →

NO ↓

NO ↓

Has your child had whooping cough within the past few months?

YES →

Whooping cough, a contagious bacterial infection, can often leave a child with a persistent cough. If symptoms persist for more than 2 months after the original illness, or if your child seems sick or uncomfortable, consult your physician.

NO ↓

Does anyone in the home smoke regularly OR could your child be smoking?

YES →

Smoke in the atmosphere and smoking itself can irritate a child's throat and lungs, causing a persistent cough and increasing the likelihood of chest infections. Giving up smoking will benefit your own and your child's health. A child who is smoking should be discouraged from this habit.

Go to chart

22 **Behavior problems**

NO ↓

Consult your physician if you are unable to make a diagnosis from this chart.

CALL YOUR PHYSICIAN NOW!
Whooping cough (pertussis), a contagious bacterial infection, produces this distinctive type of cough, often with a runny nose.

Treatment: In children over 1 year, pertussis can usually be treated at home with regular visits to the physician. Do not try to suppress the cough with cough medicines. If bouts of coughing are accompanied by vomiting, it is often helpful to give a light meal immediately after a coughing fit. Your physician may prescribe *antibiotics*, which can in some cases reduce the severity of the symptoms and may prevent other children from catching the disease. Call your physician at once if your child has difficulty in breathing or turns bluish during a bout of coughing.

A cold is often accompanied by a cough, which is a natural reaction to mucus dripping down the back of the throat. Coughing prevents the lungs from becoming congested.

Self-help: For the first day or so of a cold, it is best to keep your child at home in a warm, but not dry, atmosphere. A stuffy nose in an older child can often be eased by inhaling steam from a basin of hot water. If a young child has a severely stuffy nose, your physician may prescribe *decongestant* nose drops. For further information on treating colds, see p. 106.

Enlarged adenoids (glands at the back of the nasal passage) may be encouraging infection in your child's nose, ears and throat, creating an irritating discharge. Consult your physician.

Treatment: If the adenoids are enlarged, your physician will probably prescribe *antibiotics* to combat infection. However, if this treatment fails to cure the problem, an operation to remove the adenoids may be necessary (see *Adenoid removal*, below).

Recurrent colds can produce an irritating mucous discharge that causes the child to cough. Such colds are the result of the child being exposed to viruses to which he or she has not yet built up an immunity.

Self-help: There is little you can do to prevent your child from getting colds, but you can help to alleviate the symptoms. For general advice on the treatment of colds, see p. 106. If coughing is disturbing your child's sleep, adjusting the pitch of the bed (raising the head of the bed to promote drainage) may help. A drink and a dose of cough mixture before bedtime may also soothe a troublesome cough. There is no need to consult your physician unless your child is distressed by the cough or seems quite sick.

ADENOID REMOVAL (ADENOIDECTOMY)

The adenoids are lymph-gland swellings at the back of the nose, near the tonsils. If they become so enlarged that they cause recurrent ear or throat infections, they can be removed surgically, sometimes together with the tonsils, usually when the child is 3 to 4 years old. The child may have a sore throat for a few days after the operation. Since the adenoids are part of a child's immunodefense system, they should be removed only after careful consideration, which may include a second opinion.

Adenoids ⎯

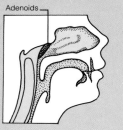

34 Fast breathing

A child's breathing is an important indicator for determining the seriousness of any problems affecting the windpipe or lungs. If your child's breathing is faster than the normal rate shown in the box below, there may be some cause for concern, especially if he or she is under 1 year or has additional symptoms, such as blueness of the mouth or excessive drowsiness, in which case you should get medical help at once.

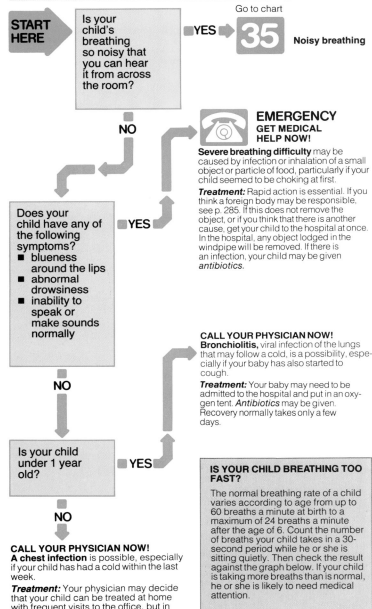

START HERE

Is your child's breathing so noisy that you can hear it from across the room?

YES ➡ Go to chart **35** Noisy breathing

NO

Does your child have any of the following symptoms?
- blueness around the lips
- abnormal drowsiness
- inability to speak or make sounds normally

NO

Is your child under 1 year old?

NO

YES (severe breathing)

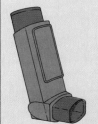

EMERGENCY
GET MEDICAL HELP NOW!

Severe breathing difficulty may be caused by infection or inhalation of a small object or particle of food, particularly if your child seemed to be choking at first.

Treatment: Rapid action is essential. If you think a foreign body may be responsible, see p. 285. If this does not remove the object, or if you think that there is another cause, get your child to the hospital at once. In the hospital, any object lodged in the windpipe will be removed. If there is an infection, your child may be given *antibiotics.*

YES

CALL YOUR PHYSICIAN NOW!
Bronchiolitis, viral infection of the lungs that may follow a cold, is a possibility, especially if your baby has also started to cough.

Treatment: Your baby may need to be admitted to the hospital and put in an oxygen tent. *Antibiotics* may be given. Recovery normally takes only a few days.

CALL YOUR PHYSICIAN NOW!
A chest infection is possible, especially if your child has had a cold within the last week.

Treatment: Your physician may decide that your child can be treated at home with frequent visits to the office, but in some cases he or she may recommend that your child be admitted to the hospital. In either case, treatment will probably consist of an aspirin substitute to reduce any fever and ease discomfort, and possibly *antibiotics* to fight the infection. If you are looking after your child at home; make sure that he or she drinks plenty of fluids. Keeping the air moist, by using a room humidifier, for example, may help to ease your child's breathing.

IS YOUR CHILD BREATHING TOO FAST?

The normal breathing rate of a child varies according to age from up to 60 breaths a minute at birth to a maximum of 24 breaths a minute after the age of 6. Count the number of breaths your child takes in a 30-second period while he or she is sitting quietly. Then check the result against the graph below. If your child is taking more breaths than is normal, he or she is likely to need medical attention.

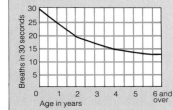

ALL ABOUT ASTHMA

In asthma the small airways in the lungs sometimes become narrowed by swelling of their walls and production of mucus. This partially obstructs the airflow in the lungs, causing difficulty in breathing. Asthma attacks can be triggered by an allergic reaction to a particular substance, such as house-dust mites, pollen or animal fur. However, attacks may also be triggered by infection, inhaling irritant substances or by physical or psychological distress.

Susceptibility to asthma often runs in families, and children who suffer from hay fever (allergic rhinitis) or eczema are more likely to develop asthma. Attacks of asthma are unusual in children under the age of 4 and often cease after puberty.

Symptoms
The main symptoms of asthma are attacks of wheezing and difficulty in breathing. The severity of these attacks can vary from slight wheezing to severe and distressing shortness of breath. Some children are rarely free from wheezing, while others may go many months in normal health between attacks. Severe attacks may be life-threatening and should always be taken seriously.

Treatment
Treatment will depend on the frequency and severity of the attacks. If your child has only occasional breathless attacks, your physician may prescribe a *bronchodilator* to use when the attacks occur or before exercise. However, if your child suffers from frequent attacks of asthma or often coughs at night, your physician may also prescribe medications to be taken regularly to prevent attacks.

An inhalant that sprays a bronchodilator drug into the lungs is prescribed for most asthmatic children.

Nowadays there is no need for the asthmatic child to be treated as an invalid. In fact, it has been shown that physical activity is beneficial, even if you have to increase the drug treatment to prevent attacks after exercise. Encourage your child to participate in sports such as swimming.

Preventing asthma attacks
If your child is asthmatic, you may be able to reduce the frequency of attacks by identifying, and then helping your child to avoid, the triggering factors. In many cases, however, there is no obvious cause. Your physician may help you by arranging skin tests in which a solution of the suspected allergen is put on or injected into the skin to see if it produces an allergic response. It may also be helpful to keep a diary of your child's activities, including what food he or she ate, or if, for example, he or she has attacks in the house, but not in the open country, or when staying with some friends, but not with others. All this information can give valuable clues to the cause of your child's asthma.

35 Noisy breathing

Many children wheeze slightly when they have a chest cold. This is no cause for concern, providing the child is not uncomfortable and is able to breathe easily. This chart deals only with breathing that is loud enough to be heard about 10 feet away. The sound produced may vary from loud wheezing and grunting to a harsh crowing noise that gets louder when the child breathes in. Except when a child has already diagnosed as having asthma and has home treatment available, such noisy breathing is always a serious symptom requiring swift, expert attention. In all cases you should be alert to any of the danger signs listed in the box below.

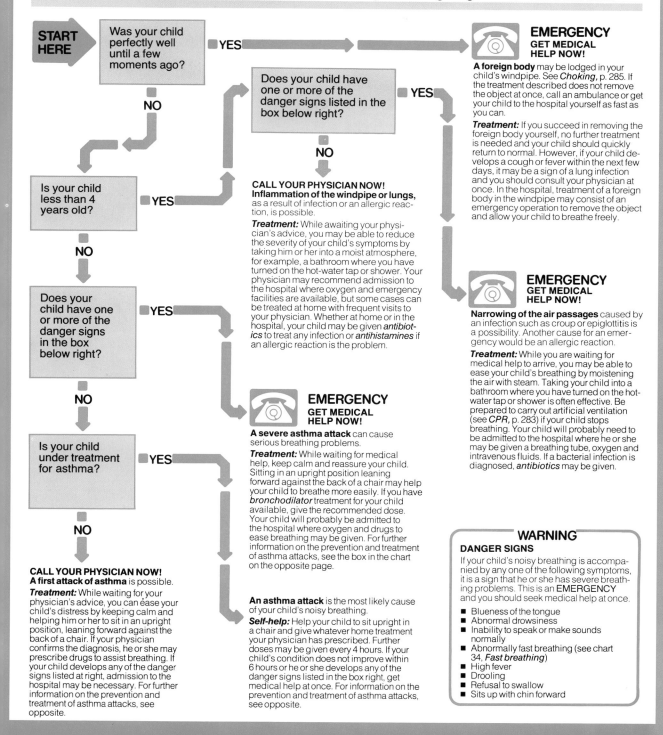

START HERE

Was your child perfectly well until a few moments ago?

YES →

EMERGENCY GET MEDICAL HELP NOW!

A foreign body may be lodged in your child's windpipe. See *Choking*, p. 285. If the treatment described does not remove the object at once, call an ambulance or get your child to the hospital yourself as fast as you can.

Treatment: If you succeed in removing the foreign body yourself, no further treatment is needed and your child should quickly return to normal. However, if your child develops a cough or fever within the next few days, it may be a sign of a lung infection and you should consult your physician at once. In the hospital, treatment of a foreign body in the windpipe may consist of an emergency operation to remove the object and allow your child to breathe freely.

NO

Is your child less than 4 years old?

YES →

Does your child have one or more of the danger signs listed in the box below right?

YES

NO

CALL YOUR PHYSICIAN NOW!
Inflammation of the windpipe or lungs, as a result of infection or an allergic reaction, is possible.

Treatment: While awaiting your physician's advice, you may be able to reduce the severity of your child's symptoms by taking him or her into a moist atmosphere, for example, a bathroom where you have turned on the hot-water tap or shower. Your physician may recommend admission to the hospital where oxygen and emergency facilities are available, but some cases can be treated at home with frequent visits to your physician. Whether at home or in the hospital, your child may be given *antibiotics* to treat any infection or *antihistamines* if an allergic reaction is the problem.

NO

Does your child have one or more of the danger signs in the box below right?

YES →

EMERGENCY GET MEDICAL HELP NOW!

Narrowing of the air passages caused by an infection such as croup or epiglottitis is a possibility. Another cause for an emergency would be an allergic reaction.

Treatment: While you are waiting for medical help to arrive, you may be able to ease your child's breathing by moistening the air with steam. Taking your child into a bathroom where you have turned on the hot-water tap or shower is often effective. Be prepared to carry out artificial ventilation (see *CPR*, p. 283) if your child stops breathing. Your child will probably need to be admitted to the hospital where he or she may be given a breathing tube, oxygen and intravenous fluids. If a bacterial infection is diagnosed, *antibiotics* may be given.

NO

EMERGENCY GET MEDICAL HELP NOW!

A severe asthma attack can cause serious breathing problems.

Treatment: While waiting for medical help, keep calm and reassure your child. Sitting in an upright position leaning forward against the back of a chair may help your child to breathe more easily. If you have *bronchodilator* treatment for your child available, give the recommended dose. Your child will probably be admitted to the hospital where oxygen and drugs to ease breathing may be given. For further information on the prevention and treatment of asthma attacks, see the box in the chart on the opposite page.

Is your child under treatment for asthma?

YES →

NO

CALL YOUR PHYSICIAN NOW!
A first attack of asthma is possible.

Treatment: While waiting for your physician's advice, you can ease your child's distress by keeping calm and helping him or her to sit in an upright position, leaning forward against the back of a chair. If your physician confirms the diagnosis, he or she may prescribe drugs to assist breathing. If your child develops any of the danger signs listed at right, admission to the hospital may be necessary. For further information on the prevention and treatment of asthma attacks, see opposite.

An asthma attack is the most likely cause of your child's noisy breathing.

Self-help: Help your child to sit upright in a chair and give whatever home treatment your physician has prescribed. Further doses may be given every 4 hours. If your child's condition does not improve within 6 hours or he or she develops any of the danger signs listed in the box right, get medical help at once. For information on the prevention and treatment of asthma attacks, see opposite.

WARNING

DANGER SIGNS

If your child's noisy breathing is accompanied by any one of the following symptoms, it is a sign that he or she has severe breathing problems. This is an EMERGENCY and you should seek medical help at once.

- Blueness of the tongue
- Abnormal drowsiness
- Inability to speak or make sounds normally
- Abnormally fast breathing (see chart 34, *Fast breathing*)
- High fever
- Drooling
- Refusal to swallow
- Sits up with chin forward

36 Toothache

Your child's teeth are just as much living structures as any other part of the body, despite their tough appearance. They are constantly under threat from our Western diet because of the high level of sugar we consume. Bacteria act on sugar to produce acids that attack enamel, the tooth's protective layer. When this happens, it is not long before bacterial destruction (decay) spreads down the root canal to the nerve, causing inflammation and pain. Any pain coming from your child's tooth, or from the teeth and gums in general, whether it is a dull throb or a sharp twinge, should be brought to your dentist's attention for investigation and treatment.

START HERE

Does your child have one or more of the following symptoms?
- continuous pain
- a tooth that feels long or high
- a tooth that feels loose
- a fever

YES

CONSULT YOUR DENTIST WITHOUT DELAY!
A tooth abscess is possible. This is formed when pus builds up in the bone and tissue near a tooth that has had a very deep filling or cavity, or one that has been injured.

Treatment: Two forms of treatment are common – root canal treatment or extraction. If the dentist feels the tooth can be saved, root canal may be performed. He or she will make an opening in the tooth to release the pus and relieve the pressure. Sometimes an emergency incision is made in the gum to relieve the swollen area. The dentist will then remove the diseased tissue from inside the tooth. Later, the tooth will be cleaned and a permanent filling will be placed in the tooth.

NO

Does he or she have repeated bouts of throbbing pain OR is the tooth extremely sensitive to both hot and cold stimuli and does the pain continue for several minutes after the stimulus is removed?

YES

Advanced dental decay, a very deep filling or an injury may have irreversibly inflamed the pulp (nerve) in the center of the tooth.

Treatment: The dentist will remove the decay and/or old filling. If the nerve is exposed, a root canal may be necessary to save the tooth, or an extraction may be needed. If the pulp is not visibly exposed, the dentist may try to soothe the inflamed pulp with a temporary, medicated filling. After a few weeks, the tooth will be re-evaluated for possible root canal treatment, an extraction, or a permanent filling.

NO

Has the dentist filled one or more of your child's teeth within the past few weeks?

YES

Does the tooth hurt only when he or she bites on it?

YES

NO

After a filling, especially a deep one, it is normal to have some sensitivity, especially to cold water or air. This sensitivity will be sharp, but will last for only a few seconds and then subside. If the sensitivity increases in intensity or duration, or if the tooth becomes sensitive to heat, consult your dentist for the possibility of irreversible pulp (nerve) damage.

NO

Go to next page

Go to next page

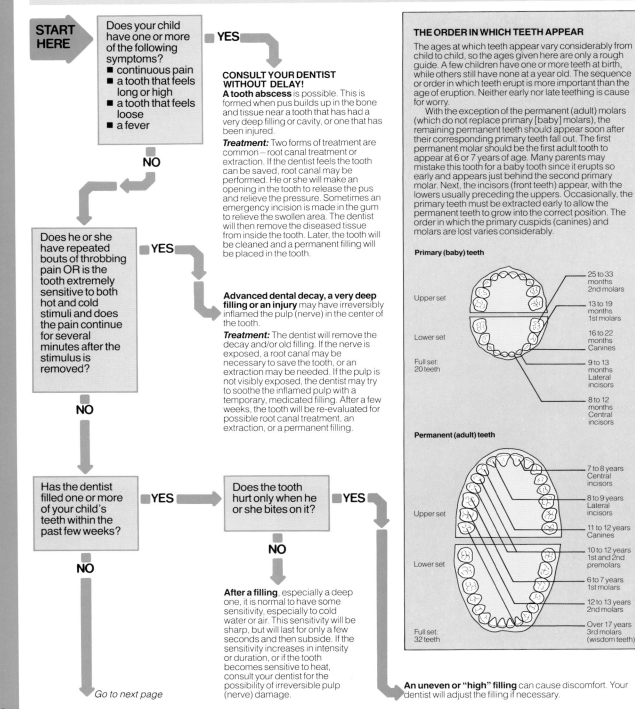

THE ORDER IN WHICH TEETH APPEAR

The ages at which teeth appear vary considerably from child to child, so the ages given here are only a rough guide. A few children have one or more teeth at birth, while others still have none at a year old. The sequence or order in which teeth erupt is more important than the age of eruption. Neither early nor late teething is cause for worry.

With the exception of the permanent (adult) molars (which do not replace primary [baby] molars), the remaining permanent teeth should appear soon after their corresponding primary teeth fall out. The first permanent molar should be the first adult tooth to appear at 6 or 7 years of age. Many parents may mistake this tooth for a baby tooth since it erupts so early and appears just behind the second primary molar. Next, the incisors (front teeth) appear, with the lowers usually preceding the uppers. Occasionally, the primary teeth must be extracted early to allow the permanent teeth to grow into the correct position. The order in which the primary cuspids (canines) and molars are lost varies considerably.

Primary (baby) teeth

Upper set

Lower set

Full set: 20 teeth

- 25 to 33 months 2nd molars
- 13 to 19 months 1st molars
- 16 to 22 months Canines
- 9 to 13 months Lateral incisors
- 8 to 12 months Central incisors

Permanent (adult) teeth

Upper set

Lower set

Full set: 32 teeth

- 7 to 8 years Central incisors
- 8 to 9 years Lateral incisors
- 11 to 12 years Canines
- 10 to 12 years 1st and 2nd premolars
- 6 to 7 years 1st molars
- 12 to 13 years 2nd molars
- Over 17 years 3rd molars (wisdom teeth)

An uneven or "high" filling can cause discomfort. Your dentist will adjust the filling if necessary.

Continued from previous page

Does the pain occur only when your child is eating something cold or sweet (ice cream or chocolate) AND does the pain go away after a few seconds?

YES →

Decay under an old filling, a cracked tooth or filling, or exposure of the root surface due to improper toothbrushing or gum disease may be the cause of the pain. Consult your dentist.

Treatment: Your dentist may recommend replacing an old filling or remove any decay. If the problem is sensitivity, the dentist may recommend a special desensitizing toothpaste, protective fluoride applications or bonding to seal over the sensitive root area.

NO ↓

Does the tooth hurt only when your child bites or chews on it?

YES →

A cracked filling or a cracked or fractured tooth is probably the cause of the pain. Consult your dentist.

Treatment: Your child may need to have the affected tooth crowned (capped) or have a root canal if the pain becomes more severe. The tooth may need to be extracted if the crack is too deep into the tooth. Pain may also be caused by acute sinus problems that make the upper back teeth ache and tender to bite on. If this is the case, your child may need to see a physician for further treatment.

NO ↓

Dental decay may have caused a hole (or cavity) in the tooth. Consult your dentist.

Treatment: Your dentist will probably clean out the affected tooth and put in a filling.

HOW TO RELIEVE YOUR CHILD'S TOOTHACHE

If the toothache is not too severe, a few home remedies may be helpful temporarily while you are waiting for professional help. Aspirin or an aspirin substitute should only be swallowed. Never place a tablet in the cheek next to a bothersome tooth. This can cause a "chemical burn" to the gum tissues. Oil of cloves applied to the aching tooth may also help.

OTHER DISEASES THAT CAUSE TOOTHACHES

Sinus problems
Often, since the roots of the upper back teeth are very near a sinus cavity, pressure on these roots from a sinus condition can simulate a dull toothache. Usually, several of these upper back teeth will hurt (not just one) when your child bites, and often he or she will experience an increased sensitivity to cold things (e.g., air or liquids). Your child may have a runny nose or congestion. When the condition clears up, the pain should subside. Consult your physician.

Periodontal disease
Periodontal disease is a common disease of the gums and other structures that support the teeth. The gums are usually red and swollen and bleed easily (especially with brushing). Pain does not frequently occur in the early stages of the disease. Treatment for early periodontal disease can range from calculus (tartar) removal by scaling the teeth to gum surgery. Young children may have early periodontal disease, which can be cleared up with thorough brushing and flossing each day.

PREVENTING DECAY

Fluoride
Fluoride is a naturally occurring mineral that has been shown to increase the tooth's resistance to acid attack, thereby lowering the risk of tooth decay. In many areas of the country, fluoride is added to the water supply. If you have a well or the amount of fluoride in your local water supply is low, your dentist may suggest that you give your child additional fluoride in the form of tablets or drops. Once the tooth erupts and appears in the mouth, giving fluoride in the form of toothpastes, rinses or topical applications can also be beneficial.

Diet
Sugar in the diet is the principal cause of tooth decay. Minimizing the amount, reducing the frequency and controlling the types of sweets (sticky sugars are worse than liquids) that your child eats are important steps in preventing tooth decay.

Nursing-bottle mouth
Never put an infant or young child to bed with a bottle filled with sweet liquids (juice, sugar water, milk or formula). These liquids pool around teeth and can cause serious decay, called "nursing-bottle mouth." If you feel you must give your child a bottle, fill it only with plain water or use a clean pacifier (one that is *not* dipped in any sweet liquid).

Cleaning your child's teeth
The goal of cleaning teeth is to remove the bacterial plaque (a sticky, colorless film that constantly forms, especially near the junction of the tooth and gum). Without plaque, there is no decay or periodontal disease.

You should ensure that your child's teeth are brushed and flossed thoroughly at least once a day. At first, clean your baby's teeth and gums using a clean, damp piece of gauze. You may find the best position to do this is with your baby sitting on your lap, held securely against your chest. Later on, develop your child's habit of brushing by encouraging the young child to help using a small toothbrush and a dab of toothpaste. But make sure that you follow this procedure with a thorough cleaning and rinsing. As for an infant, the proper position for cleaning a young child's teeth is from behind. When a child is 6 years old, he or she should be able to brush the teeth under supervision. Flossing can be done by the child, without supervision, when he or she is about 8 years old. A parent can check the effectiveness of the child's cleaning by using disclosing tablets or solutions to detect the remaining plaque.

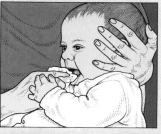

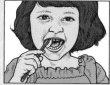

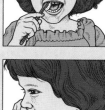

A baby should be held against your chest (left) while you clean the teeth and gums using toothpaste on cotton swabs or a piece of damp gauze.

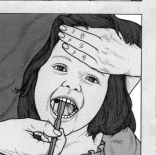

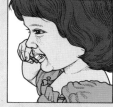

Using the toothbrush Teach your child to brush both the outer and inner surfaces of all the teeth, as well as the chewing surfaces. The brush should be angled 45° against the gums.

Sealants
Your child has natural deep grooves (pits or fissures) on the top surfaces of his or her back teeth. Your dentist may want to place a plastic resin in these grooves to help prevent decay.

37 Vomiting in children

Vomiting is the forceful throwing up of the contents of the stomach as a result of sudden contraction of the muscles around the stomach. In children, vomiting can be caused by almost any physical or emotional upset, but is most likely to be caused by an infection of the digestive tract. In rare cases, vomiting can be a symptom of a serious condition needing urgent medical attention, so you must always be on the lookout for the danger signs listed in the box below. Any child who is vomiting persistently needs to be given plenty of fluids to avoid dehydration (see What to do when your child vomits, opposite).

For children under 1 year, consult chart 7, Vomiting in babies

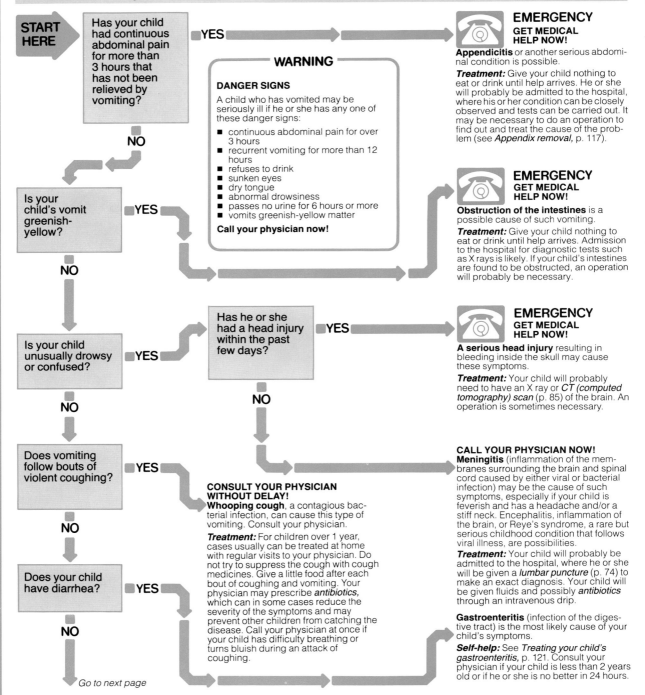

START HERE

Has your child had continuous abdominal pain for more than 3 hours that has not been relieved by vomiting?

YES →

EMERGENCY GET MEDICAL HELP NOW!
Appendicitis or another serious abdominal condition is possible.
Treatment: Give your child nothing to eat or drink until help arrives. He or she will probably be admitted to the hospital, where his or her condition can be closely observed and tests can be carried out. It may be necessary to do an operation to find out and treat the cause of the problem (see *Appendix removal,* p. 117).

NO ↓

WARNING

DANGER SIGNS

A child who has vomited may be seriously ill if he or she has any one of these danger signs:

- continuous abdominal pain for over 3 hours
- recurrent vomiting for more than 12 hours
- refuses to drink
- sunken eyes
- dry tongue
- abnormal drowsiness
- passes no urine for 6 hours or more
- vomits greenish-yellow matter

Call your physician now!

Is your child's vomit greenish-yellow?

YES →

EMERGENCY GET MEDICAL HELP NOW!
Obstruction of the intestines is a possible cause of such vomiting.
Treatment: Give your child nothing to eat or drink until help arrives. Admission to the hospital for diagnostic tests such as X rays is likely. If your child's intestines are found to be obstructed, an operation will probably be necessary.

NO ↓

Is your child unusually drowsy or confused?

YES → **Has he or she had a head injury within the past few days?**

YES →

EMERGENCY GET MEDICAL HELP NOW!
A serious head injury resulting in bleeding inside the skull may cause these symptoms.
Treatment: Your child will probably need to have an X ray or *CT (computed tomography) scan* (p. 85) of the brain. An operation is sometimes necessary.

NO ↓ (from head injury)

NO ↓ (from drowsy)

Does vomiting follow bouts of violent coughing?

YES →

CONSULT YOUR PHYSICIAN WITHOUT DELAY!
Whooping cough, a contagious bacterial infection, can cause this type of vomiting. Consult your physician.
Treatment: For children over 1 year, cases usually can be treated at home with regular visits to your physician. Do not try to suppress the cough with cough medicines. Give a little food after each bout of coughing and vomiting. Your physician may prescribe *antibiotics,* which can in some cases reduce the severity of the symptoms and may prevent other children from catching the disease. Call your physician at once if your child has difficulty breathing or turns bluish during an attack of coughing.

NO ↓

Does your child have diarrhea?

YES →

CALL YOUR PHYSICIAN NOW!
Meningitis (inflammation of the membranes surrounding the brain and spinal cord caused by either viral or bacterial infection) may be the cause of such symptoms, especially if your child is feverish and has a headache and/or a stiff neck. Encephalitis, inflammation of the brain, or Reye's syndrome, a rare but serious childhood condition that follows viral illness, are possibilities.
Treatment: Your child will probably be admitted to the hospital, where he or she will be given a *lumbar puncture* (p. 74) to make an exact diagnosis. Your child will be given fluids and possibly *antibiotics* through an intravenous drip.

Gastroenteritis (infection of the digestive tract) is the most likely cause of your child's symptoms.
Self-help: See *Treating your child's gastroenteritis,* p. 121. Consult your physician if your child is less than 2 years old or if he or she is no better in 24 hours.

NO ↓

Go to next page

Continued from previous page

Does your child have two or more of these symptoms?
- fever
- pain below the waist
- bed-wetting (when previously dry at night)
- pain on urination
- frequent urination
- foul-smelling urine

YES →

Urinary tract infection may be the cause of your child's vomiting. This diagnosis is more likely if your child is a girl (see *The structure of the urinary tract*, p. 125). Consult your physician.

Treatment: If your physician suspects a urinary tract infection, he or she will probably ask you to provide a sample of your child's urine for analysis (see *Collecting a mid-stream specimen*, p. 125). If tests confirm the diagnosis, the usual treatment is a course of *antibiotics*.

NO ↓

Did the vomiting occur while your child was very excited or before a possibly stressful event – for example, the first day at school?

YES →

Vomiting at times of emotional stress is common among children, and most parents learn to distinguish between this type of vomiting and a physical illness.

Self-help: Treat the vomiting sympathetically; your child is likely to be upset by it (see *What to do when your child vomits*, below). If you think that worry about a particular event has caused the vomiting, do not force your child to participate if you can avoid it. However, if the problem is related to school, you will need patience to help your child overcome his or her fears. Discussing the problem with the teacher or your physician may be useful.
See also chart

23 School difficulties

NO ↓

Is your child passing white stools and unusually dark urine?

YES →

Hepatitis (viral infection of the liver) is possible. Consult your physician.

Treatment: Your physician will probably advise you to give nothing to eat while vomiting and nausea persist. Instead, give frequent drinks of glucose solution (see *Treating gastroenteritis*, p. 63), possibly flavored with a little fruit juice. To prevent infection from spreading, you will need to keep your child's eating utensils and towels separate from those of the rest of the family. Your physician may recommend that other members of the family be immunized against the disease.

NO ↓

Occasional bouts of vomiting are normal during childhood and may often have no obvious physical cause.
Self-help: See *What to do when your child vomits*, below.

TRAVEL SICKNESS

Nausea and vomiting while traveling by car, sea or air are caused by disturbance to the balance mechanism of the inner ear by motion. Children's ears are particularly sensitive and this may be why they are especially prone to travel sickness. Most children become less susceptible to it as they get older. If your child is often travel sick, some of the following suggestions may help to prevent problems.

- Don't give heavy meals before or while traveling.
- Discourage your child from looking out of the car windows.
- Provide plenty of distractions, such as toys and games.
- Try to prevent your child from becoming overexcited.
- Keep at least one window of the car open.
- Allow frequent stops for your child to stretch his or her legs and get some fresh air.
- Travel at night when your child is more likely to sleep.
- Learn to recognize the signs of travel sickness (sudden pallor and quietness) and be prepared to stop.

WHAT TO DO WHEN YOUR CHILD VOMITS

A child who is vomiting may be frightened and upset and, above all, needs you to be calm and sympathetic. Your child may find it reassuring if you hold his or her forehead while he or she vomits. When the vomiting stops, give your child some water to rinse out the mouth and sponge his or her face. Give a change of clothes, if necessary. Then encourage him or her to lie down and sleep. If you think that your child may vomit again, have a bowl ready nearby.

If your child is vomiting persistently, you must make sure that he or she drinks plenty of fluids, especially if he or she has diarrhea as well (as in gastroenteritis). He or she should drink at least 1 quart (2 pints) a day of cold, clear fluids. This should preferably be a glucose solution (see *Treating gastroenteritis*, p. 63). It is better if this is taken in frequent, small sips, rather than in large quantities less often. While your child is feeling ill, give no solids or milk products.

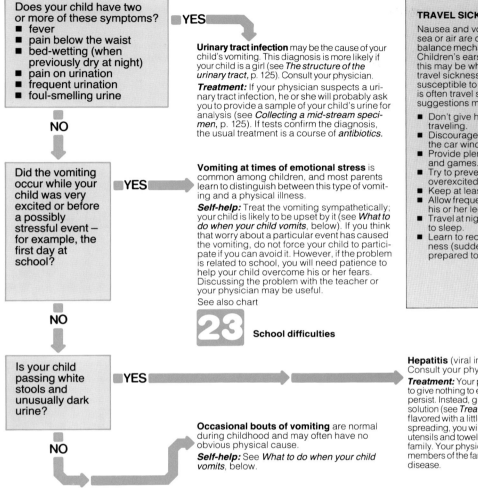

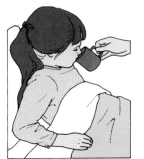

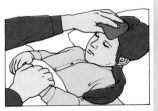

A hand held against the forehead while your child vomits (far left) is often comforting. After vomiting, a drink (left) and a face-wash (above) will make your child feel better.

38 Abdominal pain

Pain between the bottom of the rib cage and the groin in a child may have a wide variety of causes, both physical and emotional. Most stomachaches disappear on their own without treatment from a physician, but occasionally there is a serious physical cause, and you should be aware of the symptoms that may indicate such an illness so that you can feel confident in handling the far more likely minor conditions. The questions in this chart mainly concern children over the age of 2 because babies and toddlers are unlikely to complain of stomachache. However, if you suspect that your child under 2 has abdominal pain, consult your physician.

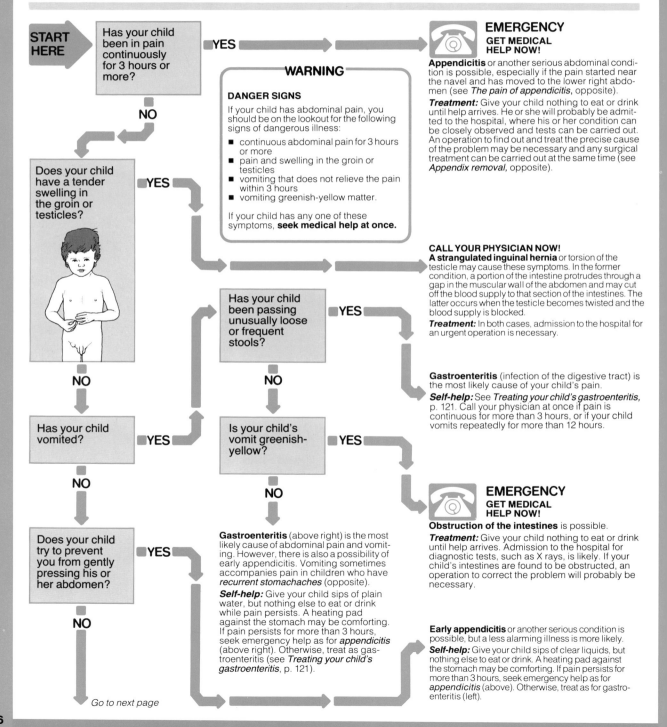

START HERE

Has your child been in pain continuously for 3 hours or more?

YES →

EMERGENCY GET MEDICAL HELP NOW!

Appendicitis or another serious abdominal condition is possible, especially if the pain started near the navel and has moved to the lower right abdomen (see *The pain of appendicitis*, opposite).

Treatment: Give your child nothing to eat or drink until help arrives. He or she will probably be admitted to the hospital, where his or her condition can be closely observed and tests can be carried out. An operation to find out and treat the precise cause of the problem may be necessary and any surgical treatment can be carried out at the same time (see *Appendix removal*, opposite).

NO ↓

WARNING

DANGER SIGNS

If your child has abdominal pain, you should be on the lookout for the following signs of dangerous illness:

- continuous abdominal pain for 3 hours or more
- pain and swelling in the groin or testicles
- vomiting that does not relieve the pain within 3 hours
- vomiting greenish-yellow matter.

If your child has any one of these symptoms, **seek medical help at once.**

Does your child have a tender swelling in the groin or testicles?

YES →

CALL YOUR PHYSICIAN NOW!
A strangulated inguinal hernia or torsion of the testicle may cause these symptoms. In the former condition, a portion of the intestine protrudes through a gap in the muscular wall of the abdomen and may cut off the blood supply to that section of the intestines. The latter occurs when the testicle becomes twisted and the blood supply is blocked.

Treatment: In both cases, admission to the hospital for an urgent operation is necessary.

Has your child been passing unusually loose or frequent stools?

YES →

Gastroenteritis (infection of the digestive tract) is the most likely cause of your child's pain.

Self-help: See *Treating your child's gastroenteritis*, p. 121. Call your physician at once if pain is continuous for more than 3 hours, or if your child vomits repeatedly for more than 12 hours.

NO ↓

Has your child vomited?

YES →

Is your child's vomit greenish-yellow?

YES →

EMERGENCY GET MEDICAL HELP NOW!
Obstruction of the intestines is possible.

Treatment: Give your child nothing to eat or drink until help arrives. Admission to the hospital for diagnostic tests, such as X rays, is likely. If your child's intestines are found to be obstructed, an operation to correct the problem will probably be necessary.

NO ↓

Does your child try to prevent you from gently pressing his or her abdomen?

YES →

Gastroenteritis (above right) is the most likely cause of abdominal pain and vomiting. However, there is also a possibility of early appendicitis. Vomiting sometimes accompanies pain in children who have *recurrent stomachaches* (opposite).

Self-help: Give your child sips of plain water, but nothing else to eat or drink while pain persists. A heating pad against the stomach may be comforting. If pain persists for more than 3 hours, seek emergency help as for *appendicitis* (above right). Otherwise, treat as gastroenteritis (see *Treating your child's gastroenteritis*, p. 121).

NO ↓

Early appendicitis or another serious condition is possible, but a less alarming illness is more likely.

Self-help: Give your child sips of clear liquids, but nothing else to eat or drink. A heating pad against the stomach may be comforting. If pain persists for more than 3 hours, seek emergency help as for *appendicitis* (above). Otherwise, treat as for gastroenteritis (left).

Go to next page

Continued from previous page

Does your child have pain below the waist AND two or more of the following symptoms?
- fever of 100°F (38°C) or above
- bed-wetting (when previously dry at night)
- pain on urination
- frequent urination
- foul-smelling urine

YES

Urinary tract infection may be the cause of your child's pain. This diagnosis is more likely if your child is a girl (see *The structure of the urinary tract*, p. 125). Consult your physician.

Treatment: If your physician suspects a urinary tract infection, he or she will probably want a sample of your child's urine for analysis (see *Collecting a mid-stream specimen*, p. 125). If tests confirm the diagnosis, the usual treatment is a course of *antibiotics*.

NO

Does your child have a cold or sore throat?

YES

Upper respiratory tract infections in children are often accompanied by abdominal pain. Look for any of the danger signs listed in the box opposite, but treat the cold or sore throat in the usual way (see *Treating your child's cold*, p. 106, and *Treatment of a sore throat*, p. 107).

NO

Did your child seem well before the onset of pain?

YES

Has your child had similar bouts of pain in the past few months?

YES

NO

NO

THE PAIN OF APPENDICITIS

Symptoms of appendicitis in children can vary considerably. But typically the pain starts in the center of the abdomen, near the navel, and moves toward the lower-right abdomen. If your child has this type of pain, you should be especially alert for any of the danger signs listed in the box opposite.

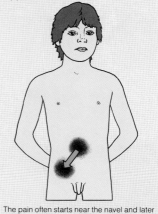

The pain often starts near the navel and later moves toward the lower-right abdomen.

Recurrent stomachaches are common in children. They may be the result of stress or insecurity, but often there is no obvious explanation.

Self-help: Take the symptoms seriously; although there is unlikely to be a physical cause, your child's pain is nevertheless real. Allow him or her to rest in bed with a heating pad. Do not force food on your child but make sure he or she drinks plenty of clear fluids. Remember that a child with recurrent stomachaches is just as likely to get a serious disease, such as appendicitis, as any other child, so be on the lookout for any of the danger signs listed in the box opposite. Call your physician if your child's symptoms differ from his or her usual stomachaches. If you have not already done so, discuss the problem with your physician, who will rule out the possibility of a physical disorder and try to help you discover any underlying emotional problems.

APPENDIX REMOVAL

Appendix removal (or appendectomy) is carried out in cases of appendicitis, when there is infection or inflammation of the appendix, a worm-shaped pouch that protrudes from the large intestine near where it meets the small intestine. The operation needs to be done as soon as symptoms suggest the possibility of appendicitis, because there is a danger that an inflamed appendix will burst, creating a dangerous generalized infection in the abdomen (peritonitis).

The operation itself is straightforward. Your child will be given a general anesthetic and an incision will be made in the abdomen. The appendix will then be removed. In most cases recovery is rapid and there are no after effects.

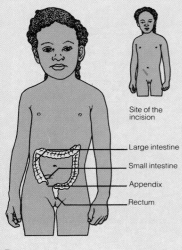

Site of the incision

Large intestine

Small intestine

Appendix

Rectum

The incision is made in the lower-right abdomen (above). The appendix is cut off at its base and removed (right).

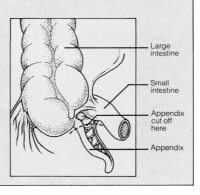

Large intestine

Small intestine

Appendix cut off here

Appendix

Unexplained abdominal pain is common in childhood. Give your child clear fluids only. A heating pad on the stomach may ease the pain. Look out for any of the danger signs in the box opposite and consult your physician if further symptoms develop, or if your child is still sick the following day.

39 Loss of appetite

Children's appetites are more closely governed by the body's energy requirements than are adult appetites. During active times children may consume large amounts, but when they use little energy they may have no appetite. A child who is growing rapidly is likely to eat much more than a child who is going through a phase of little growth. Some children naturally burn less

energy than others. Fluctuations in appetite are normal as long as your child is active and growing normally. Do not try to override the natural appetite-regulating mechanism by forcing your child to eat. However, be concerned if a child who has no appetite seems sick or is failing to grow at the expected rate (see *Growth patterns in childhood,* p. 69).

For children under 1 year, go to chart 6, Feeding problems

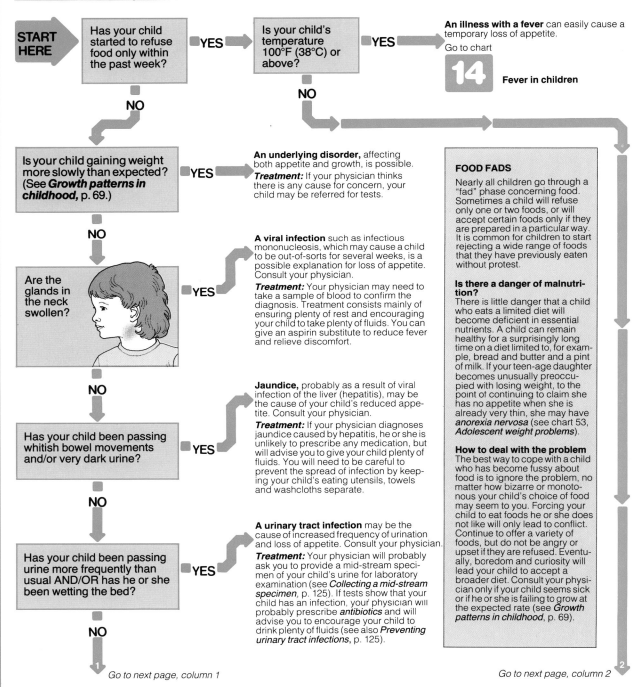

START HERE

Has your child started to refuse food only within the past week?

YES → **Is your child's temperature 100°F (38°C) or above?**

YES → **An illness with a fever** can easily cause a temporary loss of appetite.

Go to chart

14

Fever in children

NO

NO

Is your child gaining weight more slowly than expected? (See *Growth patterns in childhood,* p. 69.)

YES → **An underlying disorder,** affecting both appetite and growth, is possible.

Treatment: If your physician thinks there is any cause for concern, your child may be referred for tests.

NO

Are the glands in the neck swollen?

YES → **A viral infection** such as infectious mononucleosis, which may cause a child to be out-of-sorts for several weeks, is a possible explanation for loss of appetite. Consult your physician.

Treatment: Your physician may need to take a sample of blood to confirm the diagnosis. Treatment consists mainly of ensuring plenty of rest and encouraging your child to take plenty of fluids. You can give an aspirin substitute to reduce fever and relieve discomfort.

NO

Has your child been passing whitish bowel movements and/or very dark urine?

YES → **Jaundice,** probably as a result of viral infection of the liver (hepatitis), may be the cause of your child's reduced appetite. Consult your physician.

Treatment: If your physician diagnoses jaundice caused by hepatitis, he or she is unlikely to prescribe any medication, but will advise you to give your child plenty of fluids. You will need to be careful to prevent the spread of infection by keeping your child's eating utensils, towels and washcloths separate.

NO

Has your child been passing urine more frequently than usual AND/OR has he or she been wetting the bed?

YES → **A urinary tract infection** may be the cause of increased frequency of urination and loss of appetite. Consult your physician.

Treatment: Your physician will probably ask you to provide a mid-stream specimen of your child's urine for laboratory examination (see *Collecting a mid-stream specimen,* p. 125). If tests show that your child has an infection, your physician will probably prescribe *antibiotics* and will advise you to encourage your child to drink plenty of fluids (see also *Preventing urinary tract infections,* p. 125).

NO

FOOD FADS

Nearly all children go through a "fad" phase concerning food. Sometimes a child will refuse only one or two foods, or will accept certain foods only if they are prepared in a particular way. It is common for children to start rejecting a wide range of foods that they have previously eaten without protest.

Is there a danger of malnutrition?

There is little danger that a child who eats a limited diet will become deficient in essential nutrients. A child can remain healthy for a surprisingly long time on a diet limited to, for example, bread and butter and a pint of milk. If your teen-age daughter becomes unusually preoccupied with losing weight, to the point of continuing to claim she has no appetite when she is already very thin, she may have *anorexia nervosa* (see chart 53, *Adolescent weight problems*).

How to deal with the problem

The best way to cope with a child who has become fussy about food is to ignore the problem, no matter how bizarre or monotonous your child's choice of food may seem to you. Forcing your child to eat foods he or she does not like will only lead to conflict. Continue to offer a variety of foods, but do not be angry or upset if they are refused. Eventually, boredom and curiosity will lead your child to accept a broader diet. Consult your physician only if your child seems sick or if he or she is failing to grow at the expected rate (see *Growth patterns in childhood,* p. 69).

Go to next page, column 1

Go to next page, column 2

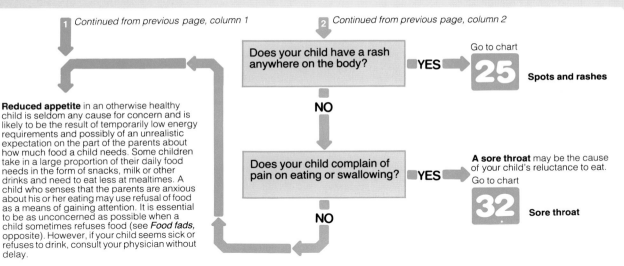

1 Continued from previous page, column 1

2 Continued from previous page, column 2

Does your child have a rash anywhere on the body? — **YES** → Go to chart **25** **Spots and rashes**

NO

Does your child complain of pain on eating or swallowing? — **YES** → **A sore throat** may be the cause of your child's reluctance to eat. Go to chart **32** **Sore throat**

NO

Reduced appetite in an otherwise healthy child is seldom any cause for concern and is likely to be the result of temporarily low energy requirements and possibly of an unrealistic expectation on the part of the parents about how much food a child needs. Some children take in a large proportion of their daily food needs in the form of snacks, milk or other drinks and need to eat less at mealtimes. A child who senses that the parents are anxious about his or her eating may use refusal of food as a means of gaining attention. It is essential to be as unconcerned as possible when a child sometimes refuses food (see *Food fads,* opposite). However, if your child seems sick or refuses to drink, consult your physician without delay.

THE COMPONENTS OF A HEALTHY DIET

A healthy diet is one that contains adequate amounts of each of the various nutrients that the body requires to function efficiently, to repair itself and, in the case of children, to grow. The main food categories and their nutritional values are listed in the table below. In western societies, dietary deficiencies in children are rare; the main risk is overnutrition, either in total calorie intake (see below), leading to obesity, or in consumption of unnecessarily large amounts of certain types of food such as fats and refined carbohydrates (for example, sugar or white flour). Providing a variety of different types of food will almost certainly ensure that your child is amply nourished. Even if your child becomes fussy about eating, malnutrition is most unlikely (see *Food fads,* opposite).

Food category	Diet advice
Proteins are used for growth, repair and replacement of body tissues. Animal products such as meat, fish, eggs, cheese and other milk products are high in protein, as are peas, beans and lentils.	Many animal products are also high in fat, so make a point of offering nonanimal sources of protein fairly often.
Carbohydrates are used for energy but when eaten in excess are stored in the body as fat. Foods containing a high proportion of carbohydrates include sugar, grain products and root vegetables.	When selecting carbohydrate foods, choose unrefined products such as whole-grain breads, which also contain fiber and other nutrients, in preference to sugar and refined cereals, which only provide energy or fat.
Fats (sometimes known as lipids) are a concentrated source of energy and provide more calories than any other food. They are found in animal products such as meat, eggs and butter, and also in certain plant products such as nuts, olives and vegetable oils.	Nutritionists recommend that intake of fats of all kinds be kept to a minimum.
Fiber is the indigestible residue of plant products that passes through the digestive system. While it contains no energy value or nutrients, it is essential for healthy bowel action.	To ensure adequate fiber intake, choose whole-grain products and serve plenty of fruit and vegetables.
Vitamins are complex chemical compounds that are needed by the body in tiny quantities. A child receiving a normal diet is unlikely to become deficient in any vitamin.	Vitamins may sometimes be destroyed by lengthy cooking, so offer uncooked vegetables and fruit regularly. Some physicians recommend vitamins for children under 5. While they are often unnecessary, they will do no harm and may reassure parents who are worried about whether their child is receiving an adequate diet.
Minerals and certain salts are needed in minute quantities. These include iron, potassium, calcium and sodium (found in table salt). A normal child is unlikely to suffer from shortages of such substances.	Too much salt in the diet may be harmful, so use as little as possible.
Calories are the units used to measure the amount of energy provided by food. If a child's diet contains more calories than necessary, the excess will be stored as fat. Conversely, if a child consumes fewer calories than are being burned up, he or she will use up fat reserves and become thin. Foods containing a high proportion of fats or carbohydrates are generally high in calories.	It is important that a child's diet contain enough, but not too many, calories. A child's natural appetite-regulating mechanism normally ensures that the correct amount of calories is eaten.

40 Diarrhea in children

Diarrhea is the passing of unusually runny bowel movements more frequently than is normal for your child. In older children diarrhea is unlikely to have a serious cause or to present any risk to health as long as you ensure that your child drinks plenty of fluids while diarrhea persists. The most common cause of diarrhea is infection of the digestive tract (gastroenteritis). In most cases, drugs are not effective; the best treatment is to allow the body to rid itself of the infection (see *Treating your child's gastroenteritis,* opposite).

For children under 1 year, see chart 8, Diarrhea in babies

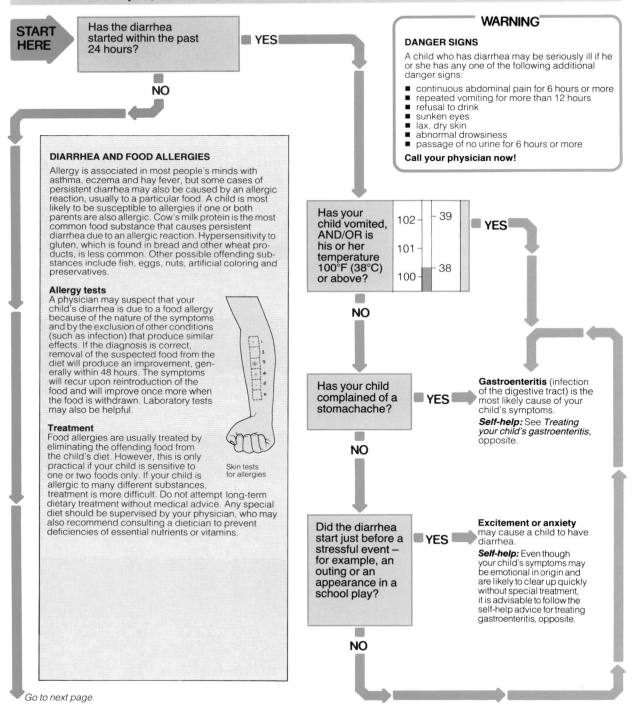

START HERE → Has the diarrhea started within the past 24 hours? → **YES**

NO

WARNING

DANGER SIGNS

A child who has diarrhea may be seriously ill if he or she has any one of the following additional danger signs:

- continuous abdominal pain for 6 hours or more
- repeated vomiting for more than 12 hours
- refusal to drink
- sunken eyes
- lax, dry skin
- abnormal drowsiness
- passage of no urine for 6 hours or more

Call your physician now!

DIARRHEA AND FOOD ALLERGIES

Allergy is associated in most people's minds with asthma, eczema and hay fever, but some cases of persistent diarrhea may also be caused by an allergic reaction, usually to a particular food. A child is most likely to be susceptible to allergies if one or both parents are also allergic. Cow's milk protein is the most common food substance that causes persistent diarrhea due to an allergic reaction. Hypersensitivity to gluten, which is found in bread and other wheat products, is less common. Other possible offending substances include fish, eggs, nuts, artificial coloring and preservatives.

Allergy tests

A physician may suspect that your child's diarrhea is due to a food allergy because of the nature of the symptoms and by the exclusion of other conditions (such as infection) that produce similar effects. If the diagnosis is correct, removal of the suspected food from the diet will produce an improvement, generally within 48 hours. The symptoms will recur upon reintroduction of the food and will improve once more when the food is withdrawn. Laboratory tests may also be helpful.

Treatment

Food allergies are usually treated by eliminating the offending food from the child's diet. However, this is only practical if your child is sensitive to one or two foods only. If your child is allergic to many different substances, treatment is more difficult. Do not attempt long-term dietary treatment without medical advice. Any special diet should be supervised by your physician, who may also recommend consulting a dietician to prevent deficiencies of essential nutrients or vitamins.

Skin tests for allergies

Has your child vomited, AND/OR is his or her temperature 100°F (38°C) or above?

102 — 39
101 —
100 — 38

YES

NO

Has your child complained of a stomachache? → **YES**

NO

Gastroenteritis (infection of the digestive tract) is the most likely cause of your child's symptoms.

Self-help: See *Treating your child's gastroenteritis,* opposite.

Did the diarrhea start just before a stressful event — for example, an outing or an appearance in a school play? → **YES**

NO

Excitement or anxiety may cause a child to have diarrhea.

Self-help: Even though your child's symptoms may be emotional in origin and are likely to clear up quickly without special treatment, it is advisable to follow the self-help advice for treating gastroenteritis, opposite.

Go to next page

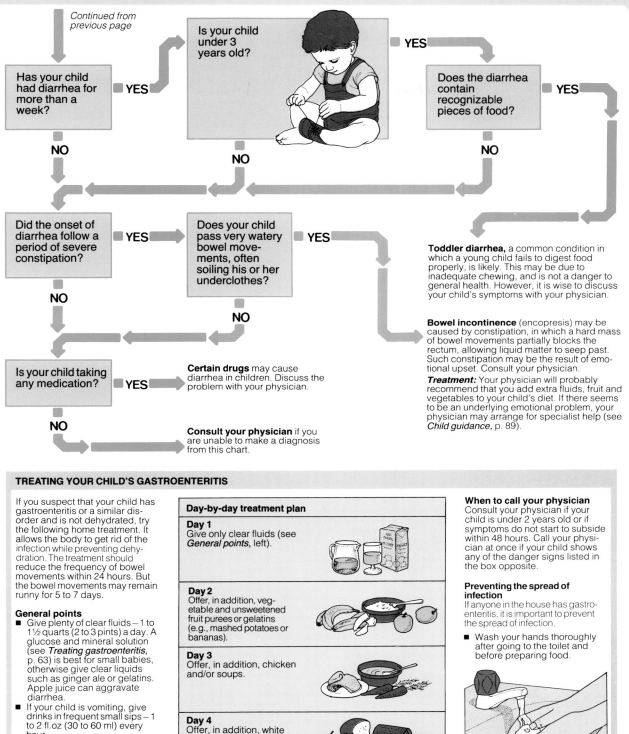

Continued from previous page

Has your child had diarrhea for more than a week?

YES →

Is your child under 3 years old?

YES →

Does the diarrhea contain recognizable pieces of food?

YES →

NO ↓ (Has your child had diarrhea)

NO ↓ (Is your child under 3 years old)

NO ↓ (Does the diarrhea contain recognizable pieces of food)

Did the onset of diarrhea follow a period of severe constipation?

YES →

Does your child pass very watery bowel movements, often soiling his or her underclothes?

YES →

NO ↓ (Did the onset of diarrhea)

NO ↓ (Does your child pass very watery bowel movements)

Is your child taking any medication?

YES →

Certain drugs may cause diarrhea in children. Discuss the problem with your physician.

NO ↓

Consult your physician if you are unable to make a diagnosis from this chart.

Toddler diarrhea, a common condition in which a young child fails to digest food properly, is likely. This may be due to inadequate chewing, and is not a danger to general health. However, it is wise to discuss your child's symptoms with your physician.

Bowel incontinence (encopresis) may be caused by constipation, in which a hard mass of bowel movements partially blocks the rectum, allowing liquid matter to seep past. Such constipation may be the result of emotional upset. Consult your physician.

Treatment: Your physician will probably recommend that you add extra fluids, fruit and vegetables to your child's diet. If there seems to be an underlying emotional problem, your physician may arrange for specialist help (see *Child guidance*, p. 89).

TREATING YOUR CHILD'S GASTROENTERITIS

If you suspect that your child has gastroenteritis or a similar disorder and is not dehydrated, try the following home treatment. It allows the body to get rid of the infection while preventing dehydration. The treatment should reduce the frequency of bowel movements within 24 hours. But the bowel movements may remain runny for 5 to 7 days.

General points
- Give plenty of clear fluids – 1 to 1½ quarts (2 to 3 pints) a day. A glucose and mineral solution (see *Treating gastroenteritis,* p. 63) is best for small babies, otherwise give clear liquids such as ginger ale or gelatins. Apple juice can aggravate diarrhea.
- If your child is vomiting, give drinks in frequent small sips – 1 to 2 fl.oz (30 to 60 ml) every hour.
- Give no milk products (milk, yogurt or cheese) for a week.
- If your older child has crampy diarrhea, a heating pad on the abdomen may be comforting.

Day-by-day treatment plan

Day 1
Give only clear fluids (see *General points*, left).

Day 2
Offer, in addition, vegetable and unsweetened fruit purees or gelatins (e.g., mashed potatoes or bananas).

Day 3
Offer, in addition, chicken and/or soups.

Day 4
Offer, in addition, white bread (spread with margarine, not butter), crackers, eggs, meat and/or fish.

Day 5
Resume a normal diet, but continue to exclude milk products for 2 more days.

When to call your physician
Consult your physician if your child is under 2 years old or if symptoms do not start to subside within 48 hours. Call your physician at once if your child shows any of the danger signs listed in the box opposite.

Preventing the spread of infection
If anyone in the house has gastroenteritis, it is important to prevent the spread of infection.

- Wash your hands thoroughly after going to the toilet and before preparing food.

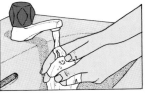

- Do not share towels, sponges or washcloths.

41 Constipation

There is no rule that says a child should have a bowel movement every day. Some children defecate a few times a day, others only once every 3 days. Both extremes are normal as long as your child is well and provided that the bowel movements are not so hard that they cause discomfort or straining. Temporary alterations in your child's normal bowel rhythms may be caused by a change in diet, minor illness or emotional stress.

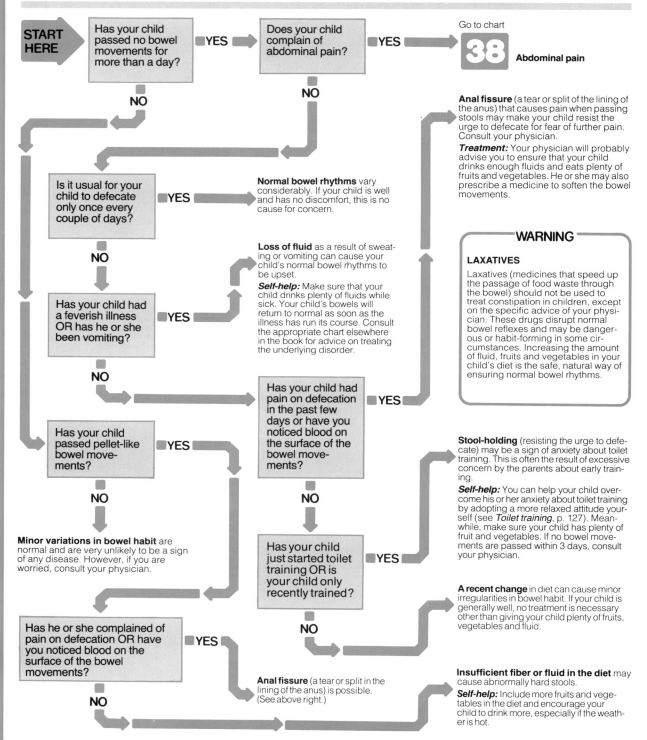

START HERE

Has your child passed no bowel movements for more than a day?

YES → Does your child complain of abdominal pain?

YES → Go to chart **38** Abdominal pain

NO

NO

Is it usual for your child to defecate only once every couple of days?

YES → **Normal bowel rhythms** vary considerably. If your child is well and has no discomfort, this is no cause for concern.

NO

Has your child had a feverish illness OR has he or she been vomiting?

YES → **Loss of fluid** as a result of sweating or vomiting can cause your child's normal bowel rhythms to be upset.
Self-help: Make sure that your child drinks plenty of fluids while sick. Your child's bowels will return to normal as soon as the illness has run its course. Consult the appropriate chart elsewhere in the book for advice on treating the underlying disorder.

NO

Has your child passed pellet-like bowel movements?

YES → Has your child had pain on defecation in the past few days or have you noticed blood on the surface of the bowel movements?

YES → **Anal fissure** (a tear or split of the lining of the anus) that causes pain when passing stools may make your child resist the urge to defecate for fear of further pain. Consult your physician.
Treatment: Your physician will probably advise you to ensure that your child drinks enough fluids and eats plenty of fruits and vegetables. He or she may also prescribe a medicine to soften the bowel movements.

NO

NO

Has your child just started toilet training OR is your child only recently trained?

YES → **Stool-holding** (resisting the urge to defecate) may be a sign of anxiety about toilet training. This is often the result of excessive concern by the parents about early training.
Self-help: You can help your child overcome his or her anxiety about toilet training by adopting a more relaxed attitude yourself (see *Toilet training*, p. 127). Meanwhile, make sure your child has plenty of fruit and vegetables. If no bowel movements are passed within 3 days, consult your physician.

Minor variations in bowel habit are normal and are very unlikely to be a sign of any disease. However, if you are worried, consult your physician.

NO

Has he or she complained of pain on defecation OR have you noticed blood on the surface of the bowel movements?

YES → **Anal fissure** (a tear or split in the lining of the anus) is possible. (See above right.)

NO

A recent change in diet can cause minor irregularities in bowel habit. If your child is generally well, no treatment is necessary other than giving your child plenty of fruits, vegetables and fluid.

Insufficient fiber or fluid in the diet may cause abnormally hard stools.
Self-help: Include more fruits and vegetables in the diet and encourage your child to drink more, especially if the weather is hot.

WARNING

LAXATIVES

Laxatives (medicines that speed up the passage of food waste through the bowel) should not be used to treat constipation in children, except on the specific advice of your physician. These drugs disrupt normal bowel reflexes and may be dangerous or habit-forming in some circumstances. Increasing the amount of fluid, fruits and vegetables in your child's diet is the safe, natural way of ensuring normal bowel rhythms.

42 Abnormal-looking bowel movements

Minor variations in the color of bowel movements are normal and are usually caused by a change in diet. Consult this chart only if there is a marked change in the appearance of your child's bowel movements. In most cases, the cause of the trouble is something that the child has eaten but, occasionally, there may be an underlying disorder that your physician should investigate. A sample of your child's bowel movements will assist in the diagnosis. Blood in the stools or on toilet paper should not be ignored.

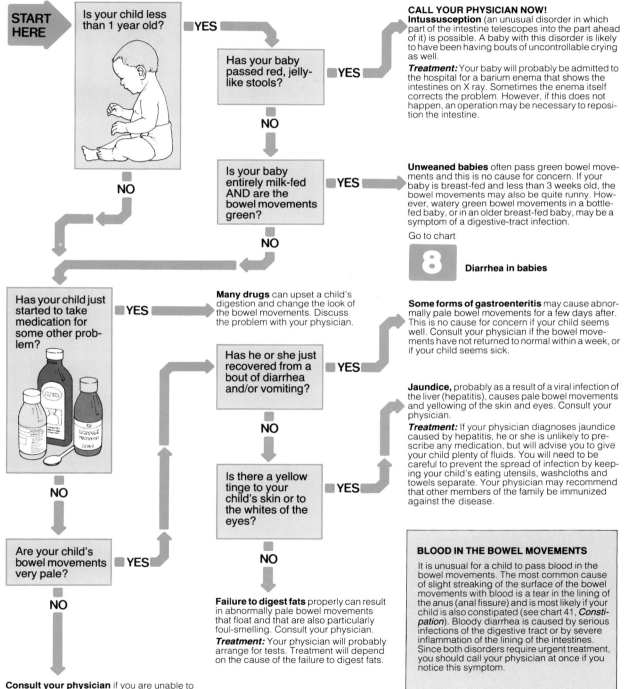

START HERE

Is your child less than 1 year old? — **YES**

Has your baby passed red, jelly-like stools? — **YES**

NO

CALL YOUR PHYSICIAN NOW!
Intussusception (an unusual disorder in which part of the intestine telescopes into the part ahead of it) is possible. A baby with this disorder is likely to have been having bouts of uncontrollable crying as well.

Treatment: Your baby will probably be admitted to the hospital for a barium enema that shows the intestines on X ray. Sometimes the enema itself corrects the problem. However, if this does not happen, an operation may be necessary to reposition the intestine.

Is your baby entirely milk-fed AND are the bowel movements green? — **YES**

NO

Unweaned babies often pass green bowel movements and this is no cause for concern. If your baby is breast-fed and less than 3 weeks old, the bowel movements may also be quite runny. However, watery green bowel movements in a bottle-fed baby, or in an older breast-fed baby, may be a symptom of a digestive-tract infection.

Go to chart

8 Diarrhea in babies

NO

Has your child just started to take medication for some other problem? — **YES**

Many drugs can upset a child's digestion and change the look of the bowel movements. Discuss the problem with your physician.

Has he or she just recovered from a bout of diarrhea and/or vomiting? — **YES**

Some forms of gastroenteritis may cause abnormally pale bowel movements for a few days after. This is no cause for concern if your child seems well. Consult your physician if the bowel movements have not returned to normal within a week, or if your child seems sick.

NO

NO

Is there a yellow tinge to your child's skin or to the whites of the eyes? — **YES**

Jaundice, probably as a result of a viral infection of the liver (hepatitis), causes pale bowel movements and yellowing of the skin and eyes. Consult your physician.

Treatment: If your physician diagnoses jaundice caused by hepatitis, he or she is unlikely to prescribe any medication, but will advise you to give your child plenty of fluids. You will need to be careful to prevent the spread of infection by keeping your child's eating utensils, washcloths and towels separate. Your physician may recommend that other members of the family be immunized against the disease.

Are your child's bowel movements very pale? — **YES**

NO

NO

Failure to digest fats properly can result in abnormally pale bowel movements that float and that are also particularly foul-smelling. Consult your physician.

Treatment: Your physician will probably arrange for tests. Treatment will depend on the cause of the failure to digest fats.

Consult your physician if you are unable to make a diagnosis from this chart.

BLOOD IN THE BOWEL MOVEMENTS

It is unusual for a child to pass blood in the bowel movements. The most common cause of slight streaking of the surface of the bowel movements with blood is a tear in the lining of the anus (anal fissure) and is most likely if your child is also constipated (see chart 41, *Constipation*). Bloody diarrhea is caused by serious infections of the digestive tract or by severe inflammation of the lining of the intestines. Since both disorders require urgent treatment, you should call your physician at once if you notice this symptom.

43 Urinary problems

Most children need to urinate more frequently than adults. This is because a child's bladder is smaller than that of an adult, and muscular control may be less well developed. In addition, children who drink large amounts are likely to need to pass urine more often than average. Consult this chart if your child has any pain when passing urine, if your child starts to urinate more frequently than usual without a noticeable increase in fluid intake, if your child needs to pass urine more than once an hour, if your child is passing small amounts of urine frequently or if your child has been waking several times during the night to pass urine.

For problems of bladder or bowel control, see chart 44, Toilet-training problems

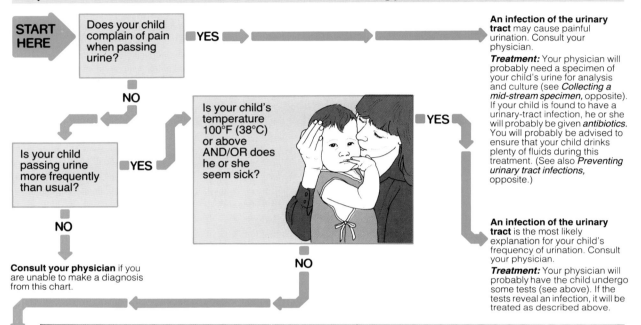

START HERE → Does your child complain of pain when passing urine?

YES → **An infection of the urinary tract** may cause painful urination. Consult your physician.

Treatment: Your physician will probably need a specimen of your child's urine for analysis and culture (see *Collecting a mid-stream specimen,* opposite). If your child is found to have a urinary-tract infection, he or she will probably be given *antibiotics*. You will probably be advised to ensure that your child drinks plenty of fluids during this treatment. (See also *Preventing urinary tract infections,* opposite.)

NO ↓

Is your child passing urine more frequently than usual?

YES → Is your child's temperature 100°F (38°C) or above AND/OR does he or she seem sick?

YES → **An infection of the urinary tract** is the most likely explanation for your child's frequency of urination. Consult your physician.

Treatment: Your physician will probably have the child undergo some tests (see above). If the tests reveal an infection, it will be treated as described above.

NO ↓ (temperature question)

NO ↓ (frequency question)

Consult your physician if you are unable to make a diagnosis from this chart.

ABNORMAL-LOOKING URINE

Color of urine	Possible causes	What action is necessary
Pink, red or smoky	There is a chance that there may be blood in the urine, possibly caused by infection or another disorder of the urinary tract. However, natural or artificial red food colorings can also pass into the urine.	Consult your physician without delay. He or she may need to take samples of urine and blood for analysis in order to make a firm diagnosis. Treatment will depend on the underlying problem.
Dark yellow or orange	Concentration of urine caused by low fluid intake, fever, diarrhea or vomiting can darken the urine.	This is no cause for concern. Your child's urine will return to its normal color as soon as the fluid intake is increased.
Clear and dark brown	Jaundice caused by hepatitis (liver infection) is a possibility, especially if your child's bowel movements are very pale, and the skin or eyes look yellow.	Consult your physician. He or she will take samples of urine and blood for analysis in order to make a firm diagnosis. Treatment will depend on the underlying problem.
Green or blue	Artificial coloring in food or medication is almost certainly the cause of this.	This is no cause for concern; the coloring will pass through without harmful effects.

Go to next page

Continued from previous page

When your child urinates, does he or she pass large volumes of urine? — YES → **Has your child lost any weight in the past few weeks AND/OR does he or she seem abnormally tired?** — YES →

CONSULT YOUR PHYSICIAN WITHOUT DELAY!
Diabetes may cause an increase in urination. This disorder occurs when the body fails to make sufficient quantities of the hormone insulin, which helps convert sugar into energy.

Treatment: Tests will reveal the presence of this disease. If diabetes is confirmed, your child may need to have regular injections of insulin for life.

NO ↓ NO ↓

Is your child taking any medications? — YES →

Certain drugs, in particular, some that are prescribed for *asthma* (see p. 110), may cause an increase in the frequency of urination. Discuss the problem with your physician.

Psychological stress may cause a child to urinate more often than usual. This may be partly because asking for frequent drinks is an effective way of gaining attention, or it may be that going to the toilet provides an escape from a possibly stressful situation – for example, school. However, you should consult your physician to rule out the possibility of an underlying disorder.

Treatment: Your physician will probably want a specimen of your child's urine (see *Collecting a mid-stream specimen,* below) to eliminate the possibility of infection. If no physical cause for the problem is found, your physician will advise you on how to overcome any underlying insecurity in your child.

NO ↓

Could your child be feeling insecure for any reason? — YES →

NO ↓

Consult your physician if you are unable to make a diagnosis from this chart.

THE STRUCTURE OF THE URINARY TRACT

The urinary tract consists of the 2 kidneys; the 2 tubes, called the ureters, leading from the kidneys to the bladder; the bladder itself; and the tube leading from the bladder to the outside, the urethra. Each kidney is supplied with blood from the renal artery. As blood passes through the tiny tubes in the cortex and medulla, waste products are filtered out in the form of urine. The filtered, purified blood is carried away via the renal vein.

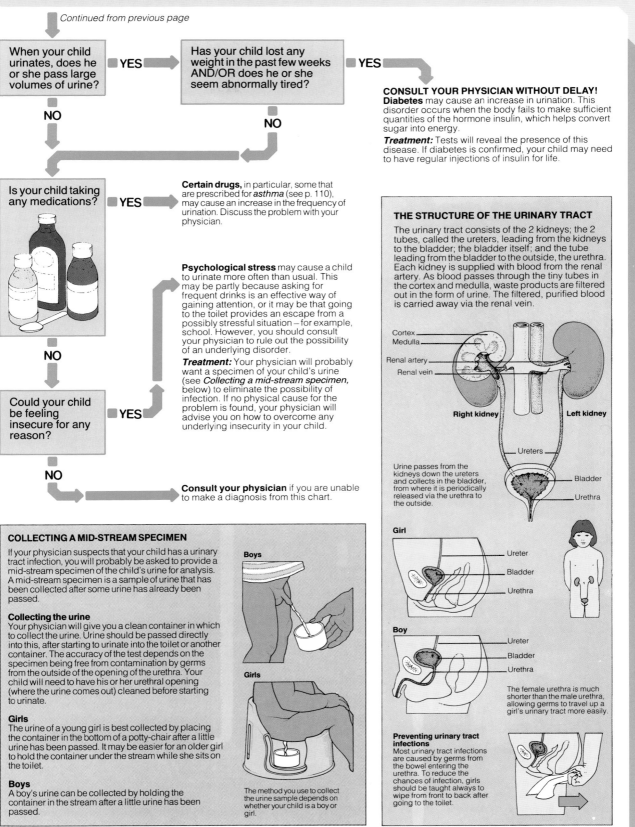

Cortex
Medulla
Renal artery
Renal vein

Right kidney   **Left kidney**

Ureters

Urine passes from the kidneys down the ureters and collects in the bladder, from where it is periodically released via the urethra to the outside.

Bladder
Urethra

Girl
Ureter
Bladder
Urethra

Boy
Ureter
Bladder
Urethra

The female urethra is much shorter than the male urethra, allowing germs to travel up a girl's urinary tract more easily.

Preventing urinary tract infections
Most urinary tract infections are caused by germs from the bowel entering the urethra. To reduce the chances of infection, girls should be taught always to wipe from front to back after going to the toilet.

COLLECTING A MID-STREAM SPECIMEN

If your physician suspects that your child has a urinary tract infection, you will probably be asked to provide a mid-stream specimen of the child's urine for analysis. A mid-stream specimen is a sample of urine that has been collected after some urine has already been passed.

Collecting the urine
Your physician will give you a clean container in which to collect the urine. Urine should be passed directly into this, after starting to urinate into the toilet or another container. The accuracy of the test depends on the specimen being free from contamination by germs from the outside of the opening of the urethra. Your child will need to have his or her urethral opening (where the urine comes out) cleaned before starting to urinate.

Girls
The urine of a young girl is best collected by placing the container in the bottom of a potty-chair after a little urine has been passed. It may be easier for an older girl to hold the container under the stream while she sits on the toilet.

Boys
A boy's urine can be collected by holding the container in the stream after a little urine has been passed.

Boys

Girls

The method you use to collect the urine sample depends on whether your child is a boy or girl.

44 Toilet-training problems

The neuromuscular function that results in gaining control over both the bladder and the bowels takes place over a span of about 3 years between the second and the fifth year. Few children have reliable control before the age of 2 years, and most do not have any problems apart from the occasional "accident" after the age of 5. Within this range, there are great variations in the order and in the timing at which an individual child masters the different skills of toilet training. Serious disorders causing delay or disruption of the development of bladder or bowel control are rare in normal children; most such problems resolve with time and patience. Consult this chart if you are concerned about your child's ability to control bladder or bowels.

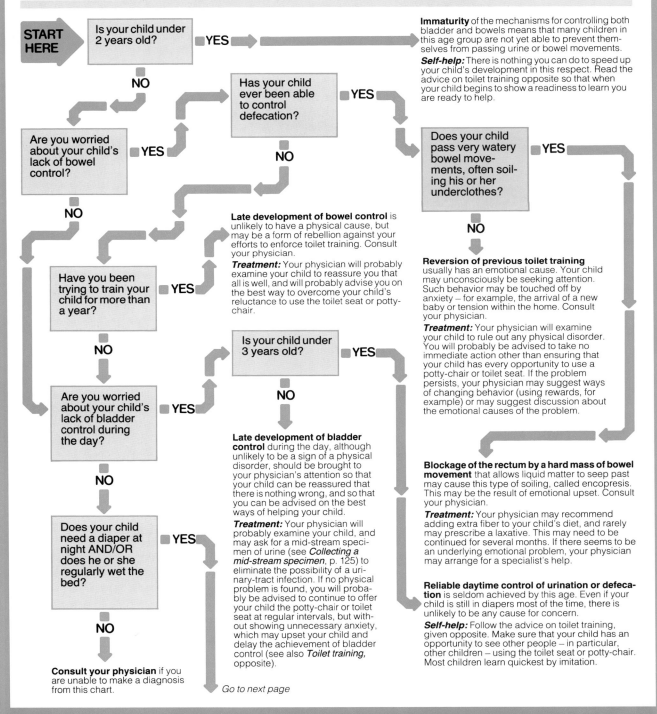

START HERE

Is your child under 2 years old?

NO / YES

Immaturity of the mechanisms for controlling both bladder and bowels means that many children in this age group are not yet able to prevent themselves from passing urine or bowel movements.

Self-help: There is nothing you can do to speed up your child's development in this respect. Read the advice on toilet training opposite so that when your child begins to show a readiness to learn you are ready to help.

Has your child ever been able to control defecation?

YES / NO

Are you worried about your child's lack of bowel control?

YES / NO

Does your child pass very watery bowel movements, often soiling his or her underclothes?

YES / NO

Late development of bowel control is unlikely to have a physical cause, but may be a form of rebellion against your efforts to enforce toilet training. Consult your physician.

Treatment: Your physician will probably examine your child to reassure you that all is well, and will probably advise you on the best way to overcome your child's reluctance to use the toilet seat or potty-chair.

Have you been trying to train your child for more than a year?

YES / NO

Is your child under 3 years old?

YES / NO

Reversion of previous toilet training usually has an emotional cause. Your child may unconsciously be seeking attention. Such behavior may be touched off by anxiety – for example, the arrival of a new baby or tension within the home. Consult your physician.

Treatment: Your physician will examine your child to rule out any physical disorder. You will probably be advised to take no immediate action other than ensuring that your child has every opportunity to use a potty-chair or toilet seat. If the problem persists, your physician may suggest ways of changing behavior (using rewards, for example) or may suggest discussion about the emotional causes of the problem.

Are you worried about your child's lack of bladder control during the day?

YES / NO

Late development of bladder control during the day, although unlikely to be a sign of a physical disorder, should be brought to your physician's attention so that your child can be reassured that there is nothing wrong, and so that you can be advised on the best ways of helping your child.

Treatment: Your physician will probably examine your child, and may ask for a mid-stream specimen of urine (see *Collecting a mid-stream specimen*, p. 125) to eliminate the possibility of a urinary-tract infection. If no physical problem is found, you will probably be advised to continue to offer your child the potty-chair or toilet seat at regular intervals, but without showing unnecessary anxiety, which may upset your child and delay the achievement of bladder control (see also *Toilet training*, opposite).

Does your child need a diaper at night AND/OR does he or she regularly wet the bed?

YES / NO

Blockage of the rectum by a hard mass of bowel movement that allows liquid matter to seep past may cause this type of soiling, called encopresis. This may be the result of emotional upset. Consult your physician.

Treatment: Your physician may recommend adding extra fiber to your child's diet, and rarely may prescribe a laxative. This may need to be continued for several months. If there seems to be an underlying emotional problem, your physician may arrange for a specialist's help.

Reliable daytime control of urination or defecation is seldom achieved by this age. Even if your child is still in diapers most of the time, there is unlikely to be any cause for concern.

Self-help: Follow the advice on toilet training, given opposite. Make sure that your child has an opportunity to see other people – in particular, other children – using the toilet seat or potty-chair. Most children learn quickest by imitation.

Consult your physician if you are unable to make a diagnosis from this chart.

Go to next page

Continued from previous page

| Has your child ever been dry at night for more than a week? | **▶ YES ▶** |

NO

| Is your child under 5 years old? | **▶ YES ▶** |

NO

Regular bed-wetting in an older child seldom has a physical cause. However, you should discuss the problem with your physician, who may be able to offer helpful advice.

Treatment: Most children are worried by their bed-wetting and need plenty of reassurance that they will soon learn to be dry at night. Try some of the suggestions for overcoming bed-wetting outlined in the box below.

A urinary tract infection may cause a child who has previously been reliably dry at night to start bed-wetting. Consult your physician.

Treatment: Your physician will probably ask you to provide a specimen of your child's urine for analysis and culture (see *Collecting a midstream specimen*, p. 125). If the tests reveal an infection, your child will probably be prescribed a course of *antibiotics*. You will probably be advised to ensure that your child has plenty of fluids during this treatment. If no infection is found, your physician will help you look into any possible emotional cause for the bed-wetting.

Lack of bladder control at night is common in children under 5, and is hardly ever a cause for concern. Even after this age, many children continue to wet their beds occasionally.

Self-help: The best way to help your child is to prevent yourself from showing anxiety. If you are still putting your child in diapers, continue to do so until they are often dry in the morning. If your child is out of diapers, but regularly wets the bed, try lifting your child onto the toilet seat before you go to bed at night. When accidents do occur, do not reprimand your child, but deal with the wet nightclothes and bedclothes without comment. Your child is probably as anxious as you to achieve night-time control, and will do so when ready.

THE DEVELOPMENT OF BLADDER AND BOWEL CONTROL

Control over passing urine and bowel movements depends on a child recognizing the sensation of a full bladder or rectum and then being able to hold onto or release the contents at will. Most children do not develop the capacity to do this until well into their second year. Most children learn reliable daytime control of bladder and bowel functions between the ages of 18 months and 3 years, although accidents, especially accidental urination, may occur from time to time. Control over urination at night usually develops between about 2½ and 3½ years of age, but regular bed-wetting is common up to age 5, and may happen occasionally until a child is older.

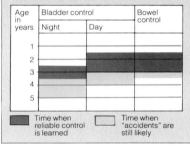

Age in years	Bladder control		Bowel control
	Night	Day	
1			
2			
3			
4			
5			

■ Time when reliable control is learned   □ Time when "accidents" are still likely

TOILET TRAINING

There is no single correct way of introducing your child to the use of the potty-chair or toilet. Much will depend on your child's level of development and personality, and on your family routine. The main thing for parents to remember is not to make the use of the toilet a cause for conflict or tension. Your child will master control of bladder and bowels when he or she is physiologically and mentally ready. Your job is simply to provide the conditions that will make the process of learning as relaxed and easy as possible.

The guide to toilet training below provides a basic structure. Use your own judgment to adapt it to your child's needs.

Gaining control by stages
1 Introductions
Buy a child's potty-chair when your child is about 18 months old. Explain what it is for, but don't expect your child to use it for some time. Allow your child to go without diapers during the day as often as possible so that he or she gets used to being without them. When your child has reached the stage of being able to control urination and bowel movements for several hours, you can start to suggest (but never insist) that he or she use the potty-chair occasionally. Once your child has started, move on to stage 2.

2 Becoming confident
Continue to encourage your child to use the potty-chair whenever he or she shows the need to urinate or defecate, but do not be upset when accidents occur. Conversely, do not be too effusive in your praise when your child succeeds in using the potty-chair properly. Gradually phase out the use of diapers until you are using them only at night.

3 Adult toilets and night-time control
Once your child is confident with the use of a potty-chair, you can introduce the use of the toilet. Buy a special child seat that fits inside the toilet seat to make your child feel more secure. Explain that the toilet can be used in the same way as a potty-chair. Alternate use of the potty-chair and toilet seat until your child feels equally at ease with both.

During this time look out for signs that your child is ready to go through the night without a diaper. Dry diapers on several mornings is probably the best indicator. When you decide to start leaving diapers off at night, prepare yourself mentally for the inevitable occasional wet beds. If your child's bed does not have a waterproof mattress, use a plastic undersheet. This will help you to be less concerned when your child does wet the bed. Some children can be helped to be dry at night by being lifted onto the toilet a few hours after bedtime. However, if this disturbs your child so that getting back to sleep after-

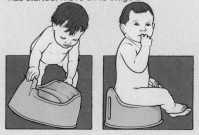

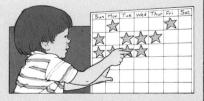

A child seat that fits inside the adult toilet seat and a step to help your child get up onto the toilet are useful aids when a child is graduating from potty-chair to adult toilet.

ward is difficult, it may not be worth the trouble. Restricting fluids in the evening is not usually an effective way of preventing bed-wetting.

Bed-wetting in an older child
Many children continue to wet their beds occasionally throughout childhood. This is seldom a cause for medical concern but, if a child frequently wets the bed, it can be distressing for parents and child. You may be able to help in the following ways:

■ **Recording dry nights** Give your child a calendar and encourage him or her to record (for example, by using a stick-on star) any dry nights. You can try offering a reward after an agreed number of stars (for example, 5 dry nights in a row). Wet nights should be ignored. Increasing numbers of stars will build up your child's confidence and will increase the incentive to master night time bladder control.

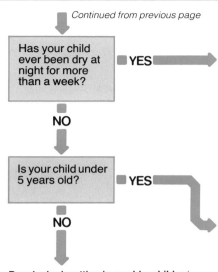

■ **Bed-wetting alarms** If record-keeping fails to help the problem, your physician may suggest the use of an alarm. This is a device fitted to a child's bed that causes an alarm to ring as soon as any urine is passed. This wakes the child so that he or she can get up to finish urinating in the potty-chair or toilet. This method has a high success rate.

45 Painful arm or leg

As soon as children start to walk, they become subject to frequent minor injuries as a result of falls, collisions and the straining of muscles. Pain in the arm or leg in childhood is usually the result of such injuries and is seldom serious enough to warrant medical attention.

Occasionally, however, an injury may result in a broken bone (or fracture) and this requires immediate medical treatment. Pain that occurs without obvious signs of injury should always be brought to your physician's attention if it lasts more than a day or so.

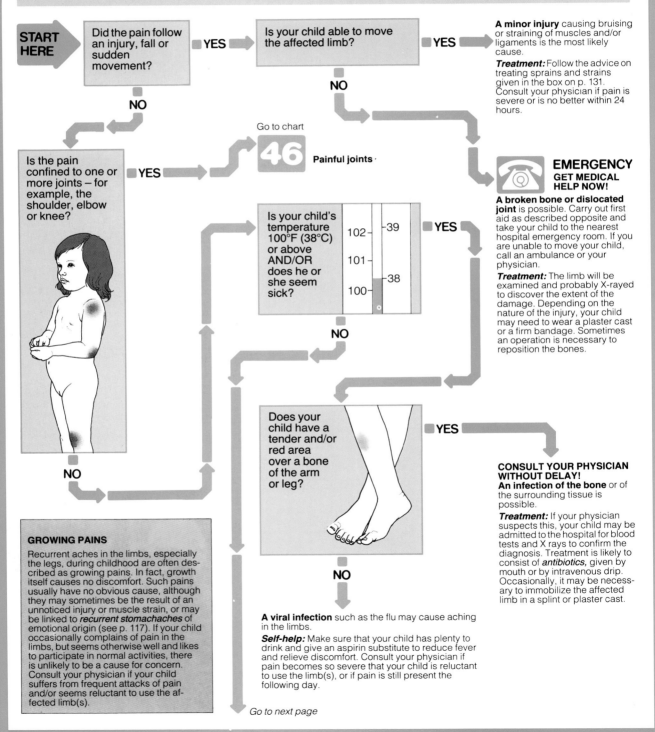

START HERE

Did the pain follow an injury, fall or sudden movement?

YES → **Is your child able to move the affected limb?**

YES → **A minor injury** causing bruising or straining of muscles and/or ligaments is the most likely cause.
Treatment: Follow the advice on treating sprains and strains given in the box on p. 131. Consult your physician if pain is severe or is no better within 24 hours.

NO (from "Did the pain follow...")

NO (from "able to move") →

Is the pain confined to one or more joints — for example, the shoulder, elbow or knee?

YES → Go to chart **46** **Painful joints**

NO ↓

EMERGENCY GET MEDICAL HELP NOW!
A broken bone or dislocated joint is possible. Carry out first aid as described opposite and take your child to the nearest hospital emergency room. If you are unable to move your child, call an ambulance or your physician.
Treatment: The limb will be examined and probably X-rayed to discover the extent of the damage. Depending on the nature of the injury, your child may need to wear a plaster cast or a firm bandage. Sometimes an operation is necessary to reposition the bones.

Is your child's temperature 100°F (38°C) or above AND/OR does he or she seem sick?

102	— 39
101	
100	— 38

YES →

NO ↓

Does your child have a tender and/or red area over a bone of the arm or leg?

YES →

CONSULT YOUR PHYSICIAN WITHOUT DELAY!
An infection of the bone or of the surrounding tissue is possible.
Treatment: If your physician suspects this, your child may be admitted to the hospital for blood tests and X rays to confirm the diagnosis. Treatment is likely to consist of *antibiotics,* given by mouth or by intravenous drip. Occasionally, it may be necessary to immobilize the affected limb in a splint or plaster cast.

NO ↓

A viral infection such as the flu may cause aching in the limbs.
Self-help: Make sure that your child has plenty to drink and give an aspirin substitute to reduce fever and relieve discomfort. Consult your physician if pain becomes so severe that your child is reluctant to use the limb(s), or if pain is still present the following day.

GROWING PAINS

Recurrent aches in the limbs, especially the legs, during childhood are often described as growing pains. In fact, growth itself causes no discomfort. Such pains usually have no obvious cause, although they may sometimes be the result of an unnoticed injury or muscle strain, or may be linked to *recurrent stomachaches* of emotional origin (see p. 117). If your child occasionally complains of pain in the limbs, but seems otherwise well and likes to participate in normal activities, there is unlikely to be a cause for concern. Consult your physician if your child suffers from frequent attacks of pain and/or seems reluctant to use the affected limb(s).

Go to next page

Continued from previous page

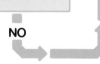

Has your child suffered from this type of pain on several occasions in the past?

YES

NO

Minor straining of the muscles or ligaments as a result of vigorous play is the most likely cause of pain in the arm or leg with no other symptoms. No special treatment is needed. Consult your physician if your child is reluctant to use the affected limb(s), if pain is present the following day, or if your child seems sick.

Recurrent limb pains are common in childhood and are generally no cause for concern (see *Growing pains,* opposite). Consult your physician if your child becomes reluctant to use the affected limb(s), if pain is still present the following day, or if your child seems sick.

FIRST AID FOR SUSPECTED BROKEN BONES AND DISLOCATED JOINTS

You may suspect that your child has broken a bone or dislocated a joint if he or she is unable to move the affected part, or if it looks misshapen.

General points
- If there is any bleeding from the wound, treat this first (see p. 284).
- Do not try to manipulate the bone or joint back into position yourself; this should only be carried out by a physician.
- While waiting for medical help, keep the child warm and be as calm as possible.
- Give nothing to eat or drink; a general anesthetic may be needed to reset the bone.
- If medical help is readily available, get assistance and then move the child as little as possible.
- If medical help may be some time arriving, or if you have to move the child, immobilize the limb in the most comfortable position by use of bandages and splints as described below.
- As soon as you have carried out first aid, summon medical help; or if your child can be moved (as in the case of an arm injury), take him or her to the emergency room of the local hospital.

Splints
A splint is a support used to immobilize an injured part of the body (usually an arm or a leg) to reduce pain and the likelihood of further damage. Always secure a splint in at least 2 places not too close to the injury – preferably on either side of it. Use wide lengths of material or bandages (not rope or string), and be careful not to tie these too tightly (you should be able to insert one finger between the bandage and limb). In an emergency you can make an improvised splint with a broom handle or rolled-up newspaper (see below). A pillow taped around an injured arm also makes a very effective splint.

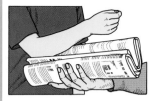

Improvising splints
A household object such as a rolled-up newspaper (left) can serve as a splint in an emergency. Make sure that you tie it securely in at least 2 places (below left) and make sure it is not too tight (below). You can provide additional support for an injured leg by securing it to the sound one with a well-padded splint in between (bottom).

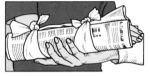

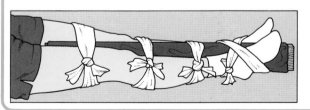

Arm injury
Gently place the injured arm in the bent position across the chest. Some padding should be placed between the arm and the chest (below left). Support the weight of the arm together with the padding in a sling along its length (below right). If the arm cannot be bent, use bandages to secure the arm to the side of the body. A splint (see below left) may provide increased support.

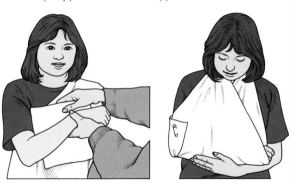

Shoulder, collarbone or elbow injury
Support the weight of the arm in a sling in the most comfortable position for the child.

Leg injury
Secure the injured leg to the sound one. If possible, place a well-padded splint (see bottom left) between them.

Knee injury
Support the joint in the most comfortable position for the child. If the knee is bent, apply a bandage extending well above and below the knee to support it in the bent position (below). If the knee is unable to bend, support the leg along its length from underneath using a board (or something similar) as a splint. Place padding between the knee and the splint, and around the heel.

Bandaging a knee injury
When an injured knee is most comfortable in the bent position, bandage it firmly but not too tightly to provide support. Take care to extend the bandage well above and below the injured knee (below).

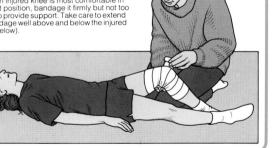

46 Painful joints

Pain in the joints – in particular, in those of the arm or leg – is almost always the result of injury or straining the muscles and ligaments surrounding a joint. Serious disorders causing pain in one or more joints are, fortunately, rare. However, such disorders need to be ruled out by your physician if pain is accompanied by generalized signs of being sick, or if your child suffers from persistent or recurrent pain.

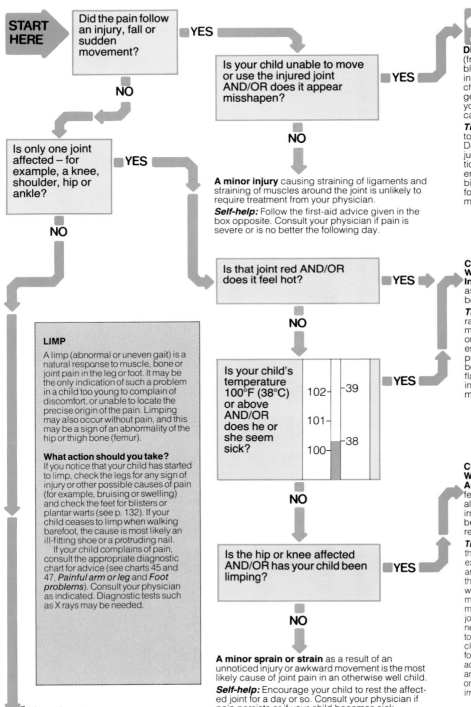

START HERE

Did the pain follow an injury, fall or sudden movement?

YES → **Is your child unable to move or use the injured joint AND/OR does it appear misshapen?** → **YES**

NO ↓

Is only one joint affected – for example, a knee, shoulder, hip or ankle?

YES →

NO ↓

A minor injury causing straining of ligaments and straining of muscles around the joint is unlikely to require treatment from your physician.
Self-help: Follow the first-aid advice given in the box opposite. Consult your physician if pain is severe or is no better the following day.

Is that joint red AND/OR does it feel hot? → **YES**

NO ↓

Is your child's temperature 100°F (38°C) or above AND/OR does he or she seem sick?

102 – 39
101 –
100 – 38

→ **YES**

NO ↓

Is the hip or knee affected AND/OR has your child been limping? → **YES**

NO ↓

A minor sprain or strain as a result of an unnoticed injury or awkward movement is the most likely cause of joint pain in an otherwise well child.
Self-help: Encourage your child to rest the affected joint for a day or so. Consult your physician if pain persists or if your child becomes sick.

EMERGENCY
GET MEDICAL HELP NOW!

Dislocation of the joint or a break (fracture) in a nearby bone is possible. Carry out first aid as described in the box on p. 129, and take your child to the nearest hospital emergency room or call your physician. If you are unable to move your child, call an ambulance.

Treatment: The joint will be X-rayed to discover the extent of the damage. Depending on the nature of the injury, the joint may need to be repositioned while your child is under general anesthesia, and may be immobilized by splints, casts or bandages for several weeks to allow torn ligaments and/or broken bones to heal.

CONSULT YOUR PHYSICIAN WITHOUT DELAY!
Inflammation of the joint, possibly as a result of bacterial infection, may be the cause of the pain.

Treatment: Your physician may arrange for a sample of fluid to be removed from the joint for tests. Tests on blood samples may also be necessary. If such tests confirm the presence of infection, your child will be given a course of *antibiotics.* If inflammation is not caused by infection, *anti-inflammatory* medication may be given.

CONSULT YOUR PHYSICIAN WITHOUT DELAY!
An abnormality of the hip or of the femur (thigh bone) is possible, although a condition known as irritable hip, in which the hip becomes painful for no obvious reason, is more likely.

Treatment: If your physician suspects the possibility of an abnormality after examining your child, he or she will arrange for an X ray of the affected hip. If this reveals such a disorder, your child will probably need to rest the hip as much as possible at first. Sometimes it may be necessary to immobilize the joint and, occasionally, surgery is needed. Later on, your child may need to do exercises to strengthen the muscles of the leg. If no cause of the pain is found, your physician will probably advise rest for about a week and avoidance of strenuous physical activity for one week more. This usually cures an irritable hip.

LIMP

A limp (abnormal or uneven gait) is a natural response to muscle, bone or joint pain in the leg or foot. It may be the only indication of such a problem in a child too young to complain of discomfort, or unable to locate the precise origin of the pain. Limping may also occur without pain, and this may be a sign of an abnormality of the hip or thigh bone (femur).

What action should you take?
If you notice that your child has started to limp, check the legs for any sign of injury or other possible causes of pain (for example, bruising or swelling) and check the feet for blisters or plantar warts (see p. 132). If your child ceases to limp when walking barefoot, the cause is most likely an ill-fitting shoe or a protruding nail.

If your child complains of pain, consult the appropriate diagnostic chart for advice (see charts 45 and 47, *Painful arm or leg* and *Foot problems*). Consult your physician as indicated. Diagnostic tests such as X rays may be needed.

Go to next page

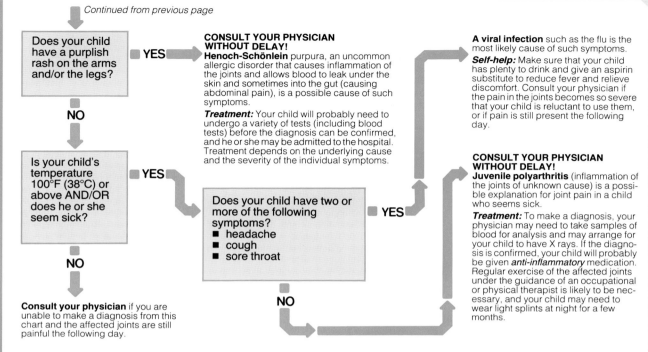

Continued from previous page

Does your child have a purplish rash on the arms and/or the legs?

YES →

CONSULT YOUR PHYSICIAN WITHOUT DELAY!
Henoch-Schönlein purpura, an uncommon allergic disorder that causes inflammation of the joints and allows blood to leak under the skin and sometimes into the gut (causing abdominal pain), is a possible cause of such symptoms.
Treatment: Your child will probably need to undergo a variety of tests (including blood tests) before the diagnosis can be confirmed, and he or she may be admitted to the hospital. Treatment depends on the underlying cause and the severity of the individual symptoms.

NO ↓

Is your child's temperature 100°F (38°C) or above AND/OR does he or she seem sick?

YES →

Does your child have two or more of the following symptoms?
■ headache
■ cough
■ sore throat

YES →

NO ↓

Consult your physician if you are unable to make a diagnosis from this chart and the affected joints are still painful the following day.

A viral infection such as the flu is the most likely cause of such symptoms.
Self-help: Make sure that your child has plenty to drink and give an aspirin substitute to reduce fever and relieve discomfort. Consult your physician if the pain in the joints becomes so severe that your child is reluctant to use them, or if pain is still present the following day.

CONSULT YOUR PHYSICIAN WITHOUT DELAY!
Juvenile polyarthritis (inflammation of the joints of unknown cause) is a possible explanation for joint pain in a child who seems sick.
Treatment: To make a diagnosis, your physician may need to take samples of blood for analysis and may arrange for your child to have X rays. If the diagnosis is confirmed, your child will probably be given **anti-inflammatory** medication. Regular exercise of the affected joints under the guidance of an occupational or physical therapist is likely to be necessary, and your child may need to wear light splints at night for a few months.

FIRST AID FOR SPRAINS AND STRAINS

A joint is said to be sprained when it is wrenched or twisted beyond its normal range of movement – in a fall, for example – tearing some or all of the ligaments that support it. Ankles are especially prone to this type of injury. The main symptoms, which may be indistinguishable from those of a minor strain, are pain, swelling and bruising. If your child is unable to move or put weight on the injured part, if it looks misshapen, or if pain affects parts of the limb other than the joints, a broken bone or dislocated joint is possible and you should carry out first aid as described on p. 129. In other cases, try the following first-aid treatment:

1 For the first 24 hours after the injury, cool the injured part (below left).

2 Support an injured joint or limb with a firm, but not tight, bandage (below right). An arm or wrist may be more comfortable in a sling.

3 Encourage your child to rest the injured part for a day or so. If it is a foot, leg or ankle that is injured, keep it raised whenever possible.

When to call your physician
If your child has a badly sprained ankle that is still painful the day after the injury, go to your physician, local hospital emergency room or urgent care center to have the joint firmly bandaged to prevent movement while the injury is healing. In this case, make sure that your child rests the joint for at least a week.

Cooling an injury
Applying cold to any injury that has caused pain, swelling and/or bruising will help reduce swelling and relieve pain. This is best done by use of an ice bag or a cloth bag filled with ice, but you can improvise using a cloth pad soaked in cold water or an unopened packet of frozen vegetables. After the first 24 hours, you should apply warmth to the affected part to speed healing.

Bruises
Bruising occurs when damage to a blood vessel near the surface of the skin causes blood to leak into the surrounding tissues. This produces the characteristic purplish-blue color of a bruise. Small bruises need no special treatment, but you can reduce the pain and severity of a large bruise by applying cold to the area immediately after the injury (see above).

1   2

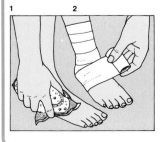

BACK PROBLEMS IN CHILDHOOD

In children, problems affecting the back are almost always related to injury resulting from awkward movements in sport or play, or from falls or unusual strain. Such injuries may cause pulled muscles, strained ligaments and bruising, leading to pain and stiffness. These symptoms usually disappear within a day or so without special treatment.

Serious back injuries
If your child suffers a major injury to the back – for example, a fall from a great height – **seek emergency help.** Do not attempt to move the child – this could lead to further damage. In addition, if your child suffers from any of the following symptoms in the days following an apparently minor back injury, call your physician at once.

■ Difficulty moving any limb
■ Loss of bladder or bowel control
■ Numbness or tingling in any limb

Persistent back pain
If your child has persistent back pain or stiffness for more than a day or two, whether or not he or she has suffered an injury, consult your physician.

Curvature of the spine
Some children are born with a sideways curvature of the spine (scoliosis) and this is usually noticed and treated in the first few years of life. However, some normal children develop such a curvature later on in childhood. This is particularly likely to occur in adolescence and affects girls more frequently than boys. It is important that curvature of the spine be assessed as soon as possible so that, if necessary, treatment by exercises, use of braces on the spine and/or surgery can be undertaken to correct the problem. If you notice that your child's spine has started to curve sideways, see your physician. Your physician will check the spine and, if necessary, send your child to a specialist for further assessment.

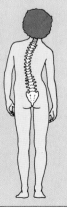

47 Foot problems

It is not unusual for a baby to be born with a foot or ankle that has been bent as a result of pressure within the uterus. The foot can be pressed gently into position and will correct itself over the following weeks. More serious malformations, such as club foot, will be noted by the physician at the first complete examination after birth and, if necessary, treatment will then be arranged. Consult this chart if your child develops any problem affecting one or both feet. Such problems may include pain, swelling, infection, injury, irritation or unusual appearance of the feet, such as flat feet or bent toes. Your physician will be able to offer advice.

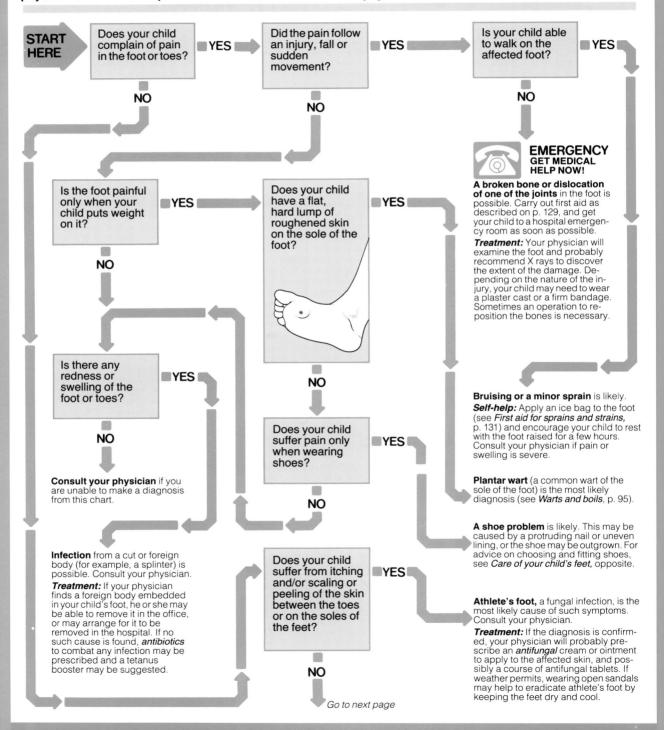

START HERE

Does your child complain of pain in the foot or toes? YES →

Did the pain follow an injury, fall or sudden movement? YES →

Is your child able to walk on the affected foot? YES →

NO ↓ NO ↓ NO ↓

Is the foot painful only when your child puts weight on it? YES →

Does your child have a flat, hard lump of roughened skin on the sole of the foot? YES →

NO ↓

Is there any redness or swelling of the foot or toes? YES →

NO ↓

Does your child suffer pain only when wearing shoes? YES →

NO ↓

Consult your physician if you are unable to make a diagnosis from this chart.

Does your child suffer from itching and/or scaling or peeling of the skin between the toes or on the soles of the feet? YES →

NO ↓

Go to next page

Infection from a cut or foreign body (for example, a splinter) is possible. Consult your physician.

Treatment: If your physician finds a foreign body embedded in your child's foot, he or she may be able to remove it in the office, or may arrange for it to be removed in the hospital. If no such cause is found, *antibiotics* to combat any infection may be prescribed and a tetanus booster may be suggested.

EMERGENCY GET MEDICAL HELP NOW!

A broken bone or dislocation of one of the joints in the foot is possible. Carry out first aid as described on p. 129, and get your child to a hospital emergency room as soon as possible.

Treatment: Your physician will examine the foot and probably recommend X rays to discover the extent of the damage. Depending on the nature of the injury, your child may need to wear a plaster cast or a firm bandage. Sometimes an operation to reposition the bones is necessary.

Bruising or a minor sprain is likely.
Self-help: Apply an ice bag to the foot (see *First aid for sprains and strains,* p. 131) and encourage your child to rest with the foot raised for a few hours. Consult your physician if pain or swelling is severe.

Plantar wart (a common wart of the sole of the foot) is the most likely diagnosis (see *Warts and boils,* p. 95).

A shoe problem is likely. This may be caused by a protruding nail or uneven lining, or the shoe may be outgrown. For advice on choosing and fitting shoes, see *Care of your child's feet,* opposite.

Athlete's foot, a fungal infection, is the most likely cause of such symptoms. Consult your physician.
Treatment: If the diagnosis is confirmed, your physician will probably prescribe an *antifungal* cream or ointment to apply to the affected skin, and possibly a course of antifungal tablets. If weather permits, wearing open sandals may help to eradicate athlete's foot by keeping the feet dry and cool.

Continued from previous page

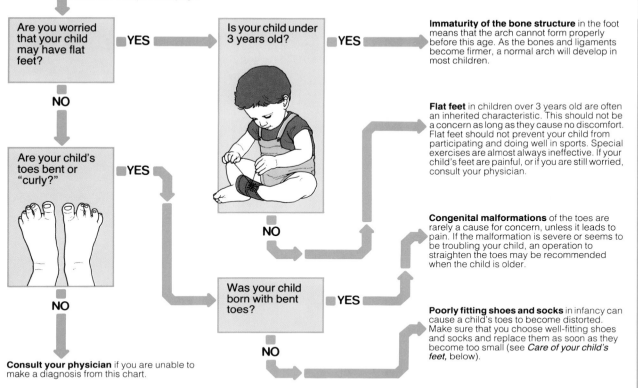

Are you worried that your child may have flat feet?

YES → **Is your child under 3 years old?**

YES → **Immaturity of the bone structure** in the foot means that the arch cannot form properly before this age. As the bones and ligaments become firmer, a normal arch will develop in most children.

NO ↓

Flat feet in children over 3 years old are often an inherited characteristic. This should not be a concern as long as they cause no discomfort. Flat feet should not prevent your child from participating and doing well in sports. Special exercises are almost always ineffective. If your child's feet are painful, or if you are still worried, consult your physician.

Are your child's toes bent or "curly?"

YES →

NO (under 3 years old) →

Congenital malformations of the toes are rarely a cause for concern, unless it leads to pain. If the malformation is severe or seems to be troubling your child, an operation to straighten the toes may be recommended when the child is older.

Was your child born with bent toes?

YES →

Poorly fitting shoes and socks in infancy can cause a child's toes to become distorted. Make sure that you choose well-fitting shoes and socks and replace them as soon as they become too small (see *Care of your child's feet*, below).

NO ↓

NO ↓

Consult your physician if you are unable to make a diagnosis from this chart.

CARE OF YOUR CHILD'S FEET

The bones in the foot are not fully formed until about 18 years of age (see right). Throughout childhood, and especially in the first 5 years of life, the bones and joints are soft and easily distorted by pressure from ill-fitting shoes and socks.

Baby feet
Young babies who are not yet walking should be left barefoot for as long as possible. If you need to cover your baby's feet to keep them warm, put on socks, soft bootees, or all-in-one suits that allow plenty of room for the toes to wriggle and stretch. Discard these as soon as the feet fill them.

When your child starts to walk, delay buying shoes until your child is steady on his or her feet and needs shoes for protection when walking outside. Allow your child to walk barefoot inside the house whenever possible.

Choosing and fitting your child's shoes
Well-fitting shoes in childhood are essential for healthy feet and toes in adult life. The main points to remember when choosing shoes for your child are listed below.

- Have your child's feet measured at regular intervals throughout childhood, at least every 3 months. More frequent measuring may be necessary at times of rapid growth.
- Where possible, go to a shop where the salespeople are trained to fit children's shoes.
- Choose shoes that are available in a variety of width fittings and that have adjustable fastenings over the instep.
- When you buy new shoes, make sure that there is about ¾ in. (2 cm) between the longest toe and the end of the shoe.
- Choose a style that has a straight inside edge and allows adequate room across the toes. Fashion shoes, especially those with raised heels, should be kept for special occasions only.
- If you can afford them, leather shoes are best but, even though they are expensive, do not be tempted to delay replacing them when they are outgrown. It is better to buy cheaper shoes that you can afford to replace more often.

1 year
5 years
18 years

- Remember that tight socks may also damage young feet, and you should take care to replace socks when they become too small.
- Shoes that are painful as soon as your child puts them on or after an hour or so are probably a poor fit and are likely to be damaging your child's feet.

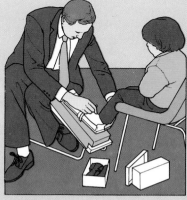
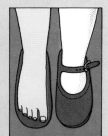
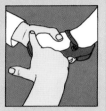

Fitting shoes
A salesperson will accurately measure the length and width (top left) of your child's foot and check that the shoes fit well, with about ¾ in. (2 cm), or a finger's width, to spare between the toes and the end of the shoes (top and bottom right).

Everyday care
When you wash your child's feet, be careful to dry them thoroughly, especially between the toes to reduce the likelihood of infections such as athlete's foot. Trim the toenails regularly (see *Nail care*, p. 93).

48 Genital problems in boys

Consult this chart if your son develops any pain or swelling within the scrotum (the supportive bag that encloses the testicles) or in the penis. In all cases you should consult your physician. Severe pain in the genital area is a matter of urgency. Medical attention should be sought immediately.

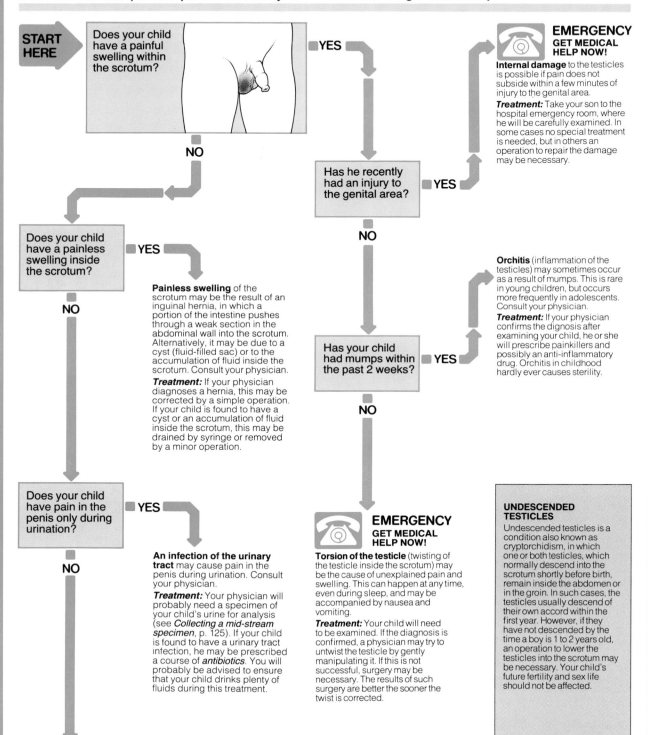

START HERE

Does your child have a painful swelling within the scrotum?

YES →

NO ↓

Has he recently had an injury to the genital area?

YES →

NO ↓

EMERGENCY
GET MEDICAL HELP NOW!

Internal damage to the testicles is possible if pain does not subside within a few minutes of injury to the genital area.

Treatment: Take your son to the hospital emergency room, where he will be carefully examined. In some cases no special treatment is needed, but in others an operation to repair the damage may be necessary.

Does your child have a painless swelling inside the scrotum?

YES →

NO ↓

Painless swelling of the scrotum may be the result of an inguinal hernia, in which a portion of the intestine pushes through a weak section in the abdominal wall into the scrotum. Alternatively, it may be due to a cyst (fluid-filled sac) or to the accumulation of fluid inside the scrotum. Consult your physician.

Treatment: If your physician diagnoses a hernia, this may be corrected by a simple operation. If your child is found to have a cyst or an accumulation of fluid inside the scrotum, this may be drained by syringe or removed by a minor operation.

Has your child had mumps within the past 2 weeks?

YES →

NO ↓

Orchitis (inflammation of the testicles) may sometimes occur as a result of mumps. This is rare in young children, but occurs more frequently in adolescents. Consult your physician.

Treatment: If your physician confirms the diagnosis after examining your child, he or she will prescribe painkillers and possibly an anti-inflammatory drug. Orchitis in childhood hardly ever causes sterility.

Does your child have pain in the penis only during urination?

YES →

NO ↓

An infection of the urinary tract may cause pain in the penis during urination. Consult your physician.

Treatment: Your physician will probably need a specimen of your child's urine for analysis (see *Collecting a mid-stream specimen*, p. 125). If your child is found to have a urinary tract infection, he may be prescribed a course of *antibiotics*. You will probably be advised to ensure that your child drinks plenty of fluids during this treatment.

EMERGENCY
GET MEDICAL HELP NOW!

Torsion of the testicle (twisting of the testicle inside the scrotum) may be the cause of unexplained pain and swelling. This can happen at any time, even during sleep, and may be accompanied by nausea and vomiting.

Treatment: Your child will need to be examined. If the diagnosis is confirmed, a physician may try to untwist the testicle by gently manipulating it. If this is not successful, surgery may be necessary. The results of such surgery are better the sooner the twist is corrected.

UNDESCENDED TESTICLES

Undescended testicles is a condition also known as cryptorchidism, in which one or both testicles, which normally descend into the scrotum shortly before birth, remain inside the abdomen or in the groin. In such cases, the testicles usually descend of their own accord within the first year. However, if they have not descended by the time a boy is 1 to 2 years old, an operation to lower the testicles into the scrotum may be necessary. Your child's future fertility and sex life should not be affected.

Go to next page

Continued from previous page

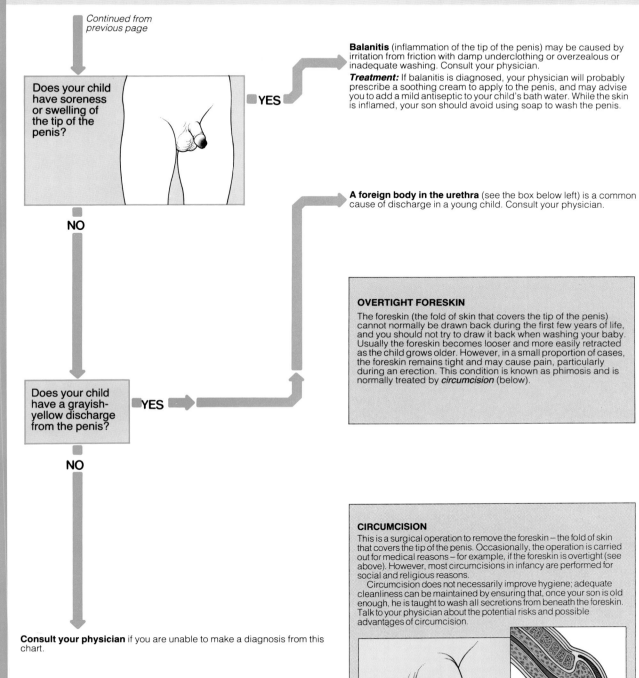

Does your child have soreness or swelling of the tip of the penis?

YES

Balanitis (inflammation of the tip of the penis) may be caused by irritation from friction with damp underclothing or overzealous or inadequate washing. Consult your physician.

Treatment: If balanitis is diagnosed, your physician will probably prescribe a soothing cream to apply to the penis, and may advise you to add a mild antiseptic to your child's bath water. While the skin is inflamed, your son should avoid using soap to wash the penis.

NO

A foreign body in the urethra (see the box below left) is a common cause of discharge in a young child. Consult your physician.

Does your child have a grayish-yellow discharge from the penis?

YES

NO

Consult your physician if you are unable to make a diagnosis from this chart.

OVERTIGHT FORESKIN

The foreskin (the fold of skin that covers the tip of the penis) cannot normally be drawn back during the first few years of life, and you should not try to draw it back when washing your baby. Usually the foreskin becomes looser and more easily retracted as the child grows older. However, in a small proportion of cases, the foreskin remains tight and may cause pain, particularly during an erection. This condition is known as phimosis and is normally treated by *circumcision* (below).

CIRCUMCISION

This is a surgical operation to remove the foreskin – the fold of skin that covers the tip of the penis. Occasionally, the operation is carried out for medical reasons – for example, if the foreskin is overtight (see above). However, most circumcisions in infancy are performed for social and religious reasons.

Circumcision does not necessarily improve hygiene; adequate cleanliness can be maintained by ensuring that, once your son is old enough, he is taught to wash all secretions from beneath the foreskin. Talk to your physician about the potential risks and possible advantages of circumcision.

Foreskin   Urethra   Glans

Site of the incision

The operation
The operation entails cutting away the foreskin at the base of the glans.

FOREIGN BODY IN THE URETHRA

Occasionally, a curious young child may push a small object into the urethral opening. If this is not promptly expelled during urination, it may lead to infection, which produces a grayish-yellow discharge from the penis. If you notice that your child has such a discharge, consult your physician. If there is a foreign body in the urethra, it may need to be removed by a minor operation under local anesthetic. Some children may require general anesthesia.

49 Genital problems in girls

The most common genital problem in young girls is itching and inflammation of the vulva – the external genital area. This may be caused by infection or by irritation from soaps or other substances, and may lead to pain during urination. You may also be worried because your child has an unusual vaginal discharge. Consult this diagnostic chart if you or your daughter notice any such problems.

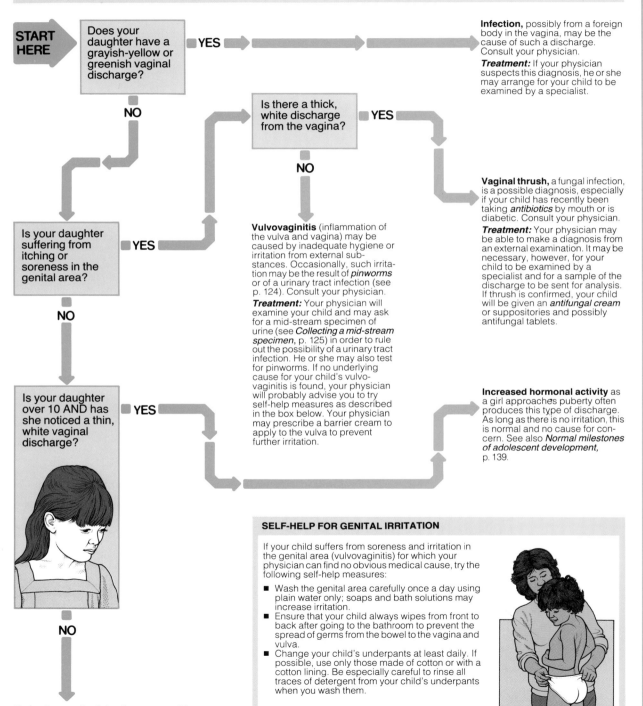

START HERE

Does your daughter have a grayish-yellow or greenish vaginal discharge?

YES →

Infection, possibly from a foreign body in the vagina, may be the cause of such a discharge. Consult your physician.

Treatment: If your physician suspects this diagnosis, he or she may arrange for your child to be examined by a specialist.

NO ↓

Is there a thick, white discharge from the vagina?

YES →

Vaginal thrush, a fungal infection, is a possible diagnosis, especially if your child has recently been taking *antibiotics* by mouth or is diabetic. Consult your physician.

Treatment: Your physician may be able to make a diagnosis from an external examination. It may be necessary, however, for your child to be examined by a specialist and for a sample of the discharge to be sent for analysis. If thrush is confirmed, your child will be given an *antifungal cream* or suppositories and possibly antifungal tablets.

NO ↓

Is your daughter suffering from itching or soreness in the genital area?

YES →

Vulvovaginitis (inflammation of the vulva and vagina) may be caused by inadequate hygiene or irritation from external substances. Occasionally, such irritation may be the result of *pinworms* or of a urinary tract infection (see p. 124). Consult your physician.

Treatment: Your physician will examine your child and may ask for a mid-stream specimen of urine (see *Collecting a mid-stream specimen*, p. 125) in order to rule out the possibility of a urinary tract infection. He or she may also test for pinworms. If no underlying cause for your child's vulvovaginitis is found, your physician will probably advise you to try self-help measures as described in the box below. Your physician may prescribe a barrier cream to apply to the vulva to prevent further irritation.

NO ↓

Is your daughter over 10 AND has she noticed a thin, white vaginal discharge?

YES →

Increased hormonal activity as a girl approaches puberty often produces this type of discharge. As long as there is no irritation, this is normal and no cause for concern. See also *Normal milestones of adolescent development*, p. 139.

NO ↓

Consult your physician if you are unable to make a diagnosis from this chart.

SELF-HELP FOR GENITAL IRRITATION

If your child suffers from soreness and irritation in the genital area (vulvovaginitis) for which your physician can find no obvious medical cause, try the following self-help measures:

- Wash the genital area carefully once a day using plain water only; soaps and bath solutions may increase irritation.
- Ensure that your child always wipes from front to back after going to the bathroom to prevent the spread of germs from the bowel to the vagina and vulva.
- Change your child's underpants at least daily. If possible, use only those made of cotton or with a cotton lining. Be especially careful to rinse all traces of detergent from your child's underpants when you wash them.

Children:
adolescents

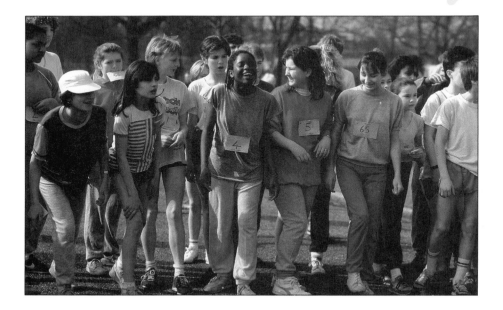

50 Delayed puberty

Puberty is the stage of development during which a child starts to undergo the physical changes that mark the transition into adulthood. Both sexes show a marked increase in height and weight and the apocrine sweat glands become active. In girls, physical changes include the development of breasts and pubic and underarm hair, as well as the onset of menstruation (monthly periods). Boys start to develop facial and other body hair, the voice deepens, the Adam's apple becomes apparent and the genitals become larger. The age at which a child reaches puberty is primarily a

matter of inheritance. A girl whose mother started her periods late is also likely to be a late developer. A boy who has been taller than average throughout childhood is likely to reach puberty sooner than shorter, lighter boys. In the overwhelming majority of cases, later-than-average onset of puberty is no cause for medical concern. Occasionally, however, delay in sexual development may be linked to an underlying condition that may influence hormone secretion. Consult this diagnostic chart if you are worried because your child seems abnormally late in reaching puberty.

GIRLS

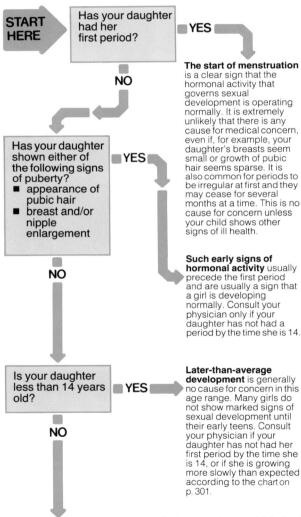

START HERE

Has your daughter had her first period?

YES

The start of menstruation is a clear sign that the hormonal activity that governs sexual development is operating normally. It is extremely unlikely that there is any cause for medical concern, even if, for example, your daughter's breasts seem small or growth of pubic hair seems sparse. It is also common for periods to be irregular at first and they may cease for several months at a time. This is no cause for concern unless your child shows other signs of ill health.

NO

Has your daughter shown either of the following signs of puberty?
■ appearance of pubic hair
■ breast and/or nipple enlargement

YES

Such early signs of hormonal activity usually precede the first period and are usually a sign that a girl is developing normally. Consult your physician only if your daughter has not had a period by the time she is 14.

NO

Is your daughter less than 14 years old?

YES

Later-than-average development is generally no cause for concern in this age range. Many girls do not show marked signs of sexual development until their early teens. Consult your physician if your daughter has not had her first period by the time she is 14, or if she is growing more slowly than expected according to the chart on p. 301.

NO

Delay in the onset of puberty is usually the result of a normal, inherited characteristic. However, it may also be caused by poor general health, certain forms of drug treatment and, in rare cases, hormonal or chromosomal (genetic) abnormalities. Consult your physician.

Treatment: Your physician will examine your daughter and may carry out an internal (vaginal) examination. He or she may also take a blood sample to assess the level of hormones and chromosomal characteristics. In most cases, your physician will be able to reassure you that all is well. Occasionally, it may be necessary to refer the child to a specialist for diagnosis and treatment with hormones.

BOYS

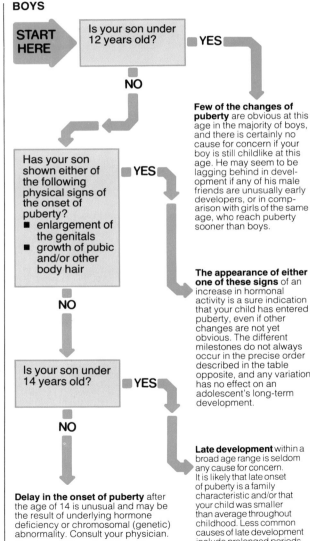

START HERE

Is your son under 12 years old?

YES

Few of the changes of puberty are obvious at this age in the majority of boys, and there is certainly no cause for concern if your boy is still childlike at this age. He may seem to be lagging behind in development if any of his male friends are unusually early developers, or in comparison with girls of the same age, who reach puberty sooner than boys.

NO

Has your son shown either of the following physical signs of the onset of puberty?
■ enlargement of the genitals
■ growth of pubic and/or other body hair

YES

The appearance of either one of these signs of an increase in hormonal activity is a sure indication that your child has entered puberty, even if other changes are not yet obvious. The different milestones do not always occur in the precise order described in the table opposite, and any variation has no effect on an adolescent's long-term development.

NO

Is your son under 14 years old?

YES

NO

Delay in the onset of puberty after the age of 14 is unusual and may be the result of underlying hormone deficiency or chromosomal (genetic) abnormality. Consult your physician.

Treatment: Your physician will examine your son and may arrange for blood tests so that hormone levels can be measured and chromosomal characteristics checked. If such tests reveal that your son is deficient in any hormone, supplements of that hormone will be prescribed. Such treatment ensures that puberty progresses normally.

Late development within a broad age range is seldom any cause for concern. It is likely that late onset of puberty is a family characteristic and/or that your child was smaller than average throughout childhood. Less common causes of late development include prolonged periods of illness in childhood and certain forms of drug treatment. Consult your physician only if your son shows no signs of puberty by the time he is 14 or if he is growing abnormally slowly according to the chart on p. 301.

NORMAL MILESTONES OF ADOLESCENT DEVELOPMENT

GIRLS

Aspect of development	Age at which change usually begins	Age at which rapid change usually ceases	Description of the changes	
Increase in height and weight	10–11	14–15	In childhood, growth continues at an average rate of 2 in. (5 cm) a year. One of the earliest signs of puberty is an increase in this rate up to a maximum of about 3 in. (8 cm) a year. The growth spurt may last for up to 4 years, but is most rapid in the first two years (see the growth chart on p. 301). There is a parallel increase in weight; the pelvis broadens and fat is deposited around the hips and thighs.	
Breast development	10–12	13–15	The first stage of breast development is usually the enlargement of the nipple and areola (the colored area surrounding the nipple). This is known as "budding." A year or so later the breasts themselves start to enlarge and the nipples and areola darken. Breast development normally ceases by the age of 15.	
Growth of pubic and underarm hair	pubic 10–11 underarm 12–13	pubic 14–15 underarm 15–16	Pubic hair normally first starts to appear as a light down around the external genital area. The hair gradually darkens and coarsens over the next 2 to 3 years and spreads to cover the pubic mound. Underarm hair appears 1 to 2 years after the emergence of pubic hair. The precise extent, color and thickness of body hair growth depends on inheritance and racial type.	
Development of apocrine sweat glands	12–13	15–16	Apocrine sweat glands produce a different type of sweat from that produced by the eccrine glands that are active all over the body from babyhood. Apocrine glands become active under the arms, in the groin and around the nipples during adolescence and produce a type of sweat that may lead to body odor if not regularly washed away.	
Onset of menstruation	First period (menarche) 11–14	Establishment of regular cycle 15–16	In the United States the average age for the occurrence of the menarche (first period) is 12 or 13. However, for some girls it is normal to start menstruating as early as 10 or as late as 17. It usually happens about 2 years after the start of the growth spurt and is unlikely to occur until a girl weighs at least 99 lb (45 kg). A girl may notice a thick, white, vaginal discharge in the year preceding the menarche. In the first few years following the menarche, periods are likely to be irregular and may cease altogether for several months.	

BOYS

Increase in height and weight	12–13	17–18	In childhood, growth continues at an average rate of 2 in. (5 cm) a year. One of the earliest signs of puberty is an increase in this rate up to a maximum of about 3 in. (8 cm) a year. The growth spurt may last for up to 4 years, but is most rapid in the first two years (see the growth chart on p. 300). There is a parallel increase in weight; the pelvis broadens and fat is deposited around the hips and thighs.	
Genital development and ejaculation	11–13	15–17	Hormonal activity at the start of puberty stimulates the development of the male sex glands, the testicles, leading to a noticeable increase in their size. The skin of the scrotum darkens and the penis lengthens and broadens. The ability to ejaculate seminal fluid usually develops within 2 years of such genital development.	
Growth of body and facial hair	11–15	15–19	The growth of hair in the genital (pubic) area normally starts first and is followed a year or so later by the growth of hair on the face, under the arms and, depending on inherited characteristics, in other areas of the body such as the legs, chest and abdomen.	
Development of apocrine sweat glands	13–15	17–18	Apocrine sweat glands produce a different type of sweat from that produced by the eccrine glands that are found all over the body from babyhood. Apocrine glands start to develop under the arms, in the groin and around the nipples during adolescence and produce a type of sweat that may lead to body odor if not regularly washed away.	
Deepening of the voice	13–15	16–17	The voice box (larynx) starts to enlarge and may develop into a noticeable "Adam's apple." The voice deepens ("breaks") within a year or so of such enlargement.	

EMOTIONAL DEVELOPMENT

The physical changes of puberty are accompanied by psychological changes that are also triggered by the secretion of sex hormones. In both boys and girls these hormones stimulate interest in sexuality. Rising levels of the male hormone testosterone are thought to play a part in the increased aggression and adventurousness typical of teenage boys. The increased output of hormones by the adrenal glands also influences behavior by increasing natural assertiveness, which helps to explain why teenagers have a tendency to be rebellious and argumentative.

Children whose physical development is delayed are also likely to be late maturers emotionally. This can sometimes cause social and psychological difficulties for the child, who must come to terms with being smaller, less physically developed and less assertive than most of his or her contemporaries.

51 Adolescent behavior problems

Adolescence, the transitional period between childhood and adulthood, is a time when difficult behavior and conflict with parents and other forms of authority are most likely to arise. The reasons for this may be partly physiological – the child is experiencing new and perhaps confusing feelings as a result of the hormonal activity that starts at puberty. However, there are also social and psychological factors present, including the need to develop both practical and emotional independence from the parents and to establish a separate identity. Few families with adolescent children escape arguments and misunderstandings – usually about dress, language or general conduct – but, providing that the parents are willing to allow sufficient flexibility while retaining a recognizable and affectionate family framework, family relationships are unlikely to suffer permanent damage. Most adolescent behavior problems can be successfully resolved within the family without the need for outside help. However, if you feel that any behavior problem is getting outside your control, to the extent that you fear that your adolescent may be endangering his or her health or risking conflict with the law, it is a good idea to discuss the problem with your physician. Although medical treatment is only rarely appropriate, your physician may put you in touch with relevant support services.

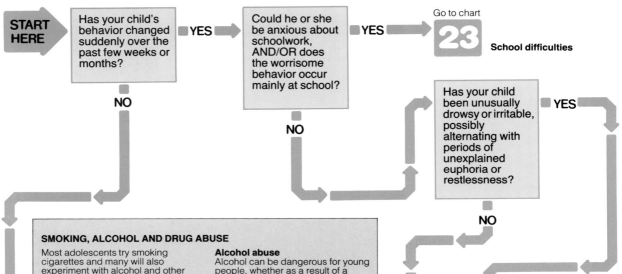

START HERE

Has your child's behavior changed suddenly over the past few weeks or months?

YES → **Could he or she be anxious about schoolwork, AND/OR does the worrisome behavior occur mainly at school?**

YES → Go to chart **23** School difficulties

NO ↓

NO ↓ **Has your child been unusually drowsy or irritable, possibly alternating with periods of unexplained euphoria or restlessness?**

YES →

NO ↓

SMOKING, ALCOHOL AND DRUG ABUSE

Most adolescents try smoking cigarettes and many will also experiment with alcohol and other drugs. Whether or not such experimentation develops into a major health risk for your child depends on a number of factors, including whether you smoke or drink regularly yourself, how prevalent the use of such substances is among your child's friends, and whether or not your child has an underlying emotional difficulty that may lead him or her to seek to escape through the use of drugs.

Cigarette smoking
Although smoking is unlikely to damage your child's health in the short term, it is one of the most serious risks to health in adult life. The habit is easily established in adolescence. It is therefore essential that parents make every effort to discourage smoking through their own example and by ensuring that their child is fully aware of the risks at an early age. Ominous warnings of lung cancer have little impact on teen behavior. Teens do respond, however, to the implication that smoking is a smelly, unattractive habit, which will lead to early wrinkles, bad breath and impaired athletic performance.

Alcohol abuse
Alcohol can be dangerous for young people, whether as a result of a single "binge" in which too much alcohol is drunk, or as a regular habit. If you drink, it is unreasonable to try to ban your teenager from drinking at all. However, you can ensure that he or she learns to drink sensibly by limiting alcoholic drinks to special occasions or small amounts at some mealtimes. Drinking to excess should always be clearly condemned.

Drug and solvent abuse
This is the problem that often causes parents the most worry. Arm yourself and your child with the facts about the dangers of drug-taking well before you think there may be any risk of your child being tempted to try any of these substances. Advice that is based on sound information is likely to be treated with greater respect than reactions based on instinctive fear of the problem. And an atmosphere in which a child feels free to talk about the subject may encourage your child to confide in you if he or she feels under pressure from friends to try drugs. Always consult your physician if you fear your child is taking drugs of any kind.

Drug abuse, drinking alcohol or inhaling solvents ("glue sniffing") are all possible explanations for this type of behavior, especially if your child always seems short of money and has any additional symptoms such as slurred speech, excessive sweating or abnormally large or small pupils.

Self-help: This is a worrisome problem that should always be tackled as soon as you suspect there may be any cause for concern. Talk to your child and try to find out whether or not your suspicions are correct. If your child admits to drinking or taking drugs of any kind, you will obviously try to convince him or her of the dangers of this type of behavior. If you are unable to do this because of difficulties in communication or because you do not feel sufficiently well-informed, consult your physician, who may be able to talk to your child more easily than you and will be able to offer sound advice. If your child denies drug-taking, it is also worthwhile seeking medical advice because this type of behavior may also indicate an underlying emotional problem (see also *Smoking, alcohol and drug abuse,* left).

▼1 *Go to next page column 1*

▼2 *Go to next page column 2*

1 Continued from previous page column 1

2 Continued from previous page column 2

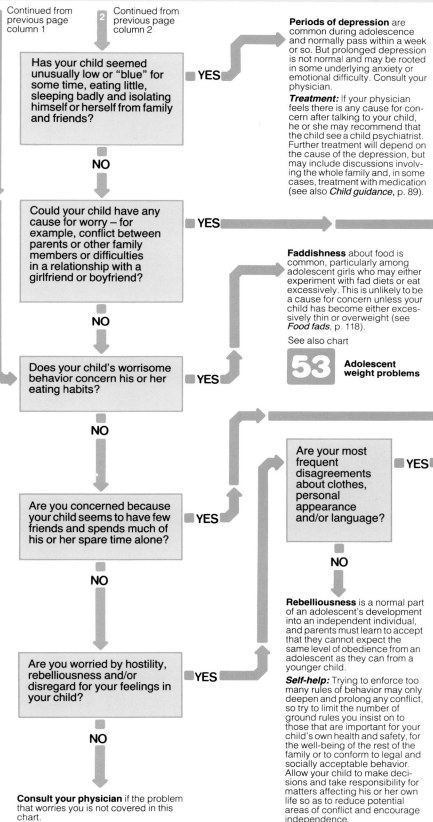

Has your child seemed unusually low or "blue" for some time, eating little, sleeping badly and isolating himself or herself from family and friends?

YES

Periods of depression are common during adolescence and normally pass within a week or so. But prolonged depression is not normal and may be rooted in some underlying anxiety or emotional difficulty. Consult your physician.

Treatment: If your physician feels there is any cause for concern after talking to your child, he or she may recommend that the child see a child psychiatrist. Further treatment will depend on the cause of the depression, but may include discussions involving the whole family and, in some cases, treatment with medication (see also *Child guidance*, p. 89).

Anxiety about a specific problem can cause an adolescent to behave out-of-character. Unusual behavior may include aggressiveness, sullenness, rudeness or, at the other end of the spectrum, child-ishness or overdependence on the parents.

Self-help: As with most adolescent behavior problems, you should start by discussing the matter directly with your child. You may be able to discover the cause of the problem and at the same time allay any fears or take practical steps to resolve a problem yourself. However, if you are unable to help your child or if you have difficulty discovering the reason for your child's changed behavior, consult your physician, who will be able to offer specific advice.

NO

Could your child have any cause for worry – for example, conflict between parents or other family members or difficulties in a relationship with a girlfriend or boyfriend?

YES

NO

Does your child's worrisome behavior concern his or her eating habits?

YES

Faddishness about food is common, particularly among adolescent girls who may either experiment with fad diets or eat excessively. This is unlikely to be a cause for concern unless your child has become either excessively thin or overweight (see *Food fads*, p. 118).

See also chart

53 **Adolescent weight problems**

Natural shyness or solitariness may be a normal part of your child's personality and this will not suddenly change during adolescence. However, if you suspect that there may be an underlying cause for your child's withdrawn behavior – for example, self-consciousness about a physical problem such as severe acne or being overweight – you should try to deal with it.

Self-help: If your child seems shy, try to ensure that he or she has plenty of opportunity to participate in activities that he or she enjoys, perhaps with the rest of the family or where your child has the chance to meet other young people who share similar interests. If your child has a skin or weight problem, consult chart 52, *Adolescent skin problems* or chart 53, *Adolescent weight problems.*

NO

Are you concerned because your child seems to have few friends and spends much of his or her spare time alone?

YES

Are your most frequent disagreements about clothes, personal appearance and/or language?

YES

NO

NO

Are you worried by hostility, rebelliousness and/or disregard for your feelings in your child?

YES

Rebelliousness is a normal part of an adolescent's development into an independent individual, and parents must learn to accept that they cannot expect the same level of obedience from an adolescent as they can from a younger child.

Self-help: Trying to enforce too many rules of behavior may only deepen and prolong any conflict, so try to limit the number of ground rules you insist on to those that are important for your child's own health and safety, for the well-being of the rest of the family or to conform to legal and socially acceptable behavior. Allow your child to make decisions and take responsibility for matters affecting his or her own life so as to reduce potential areas of conflict and encourage independence.

Looking and sounding like their contemporaries is important to most adolescents. It gives them a separate identity from their parents and the security of feeling that they belong to a group. Although extremes of dress or bad language can be distressing for parents, such behavior is rarely a cause for concern, providing that it does not lead, for example, to conflict in school. Every generation has its own hair and dress pattern; your adolescent is simply conforming to his or her friends' dress pattern. Accept this as a norm unless other behavioral problems, such as drug use, accompany the dress pattern.

Self-help: It is best to ignore such behavior if possible, only insisting that your child conform when it may cause offense to others. Most young people eventually learn to compromise between expressing themselves extremely in dress and language and the need in some circumstances to conform.

NO

Consult your physician if the problem that worries you is not covered in this chart.

52 Adolescent skin problems

The onset of adolescence often produces marked changes in the skin. Infantile eczema, which often affects younger children, may clear up altogether during adolescence. But another form of eczema may occur for the first time as a result of contact with certain metals or cosmetics, causing an itchy red rash. In addition, certain skin problems caused by infection or infestation may become more common as a result of close contact with other teenagers. However, the most noticeable skin changes during adolescence are caused by rising levels of sex hormones that encourage the sebaceous glands in the skin to produce increasing amounts of sebum – an oily substance that helps to lubricate and protect the skin. Not only does increased sebaceous activity give the skin an oily appearance, but it encourages the development of acne, the principal skin condition affecting adolescents. There are several types of acne and the condition may occur with varying degrees of severity. Consult this diagnostic chart if you are uncertain what, if any, treatment to advise for your adolescent's acne or oily skin. For other skin problems, see chart 25, Spots and rashes.

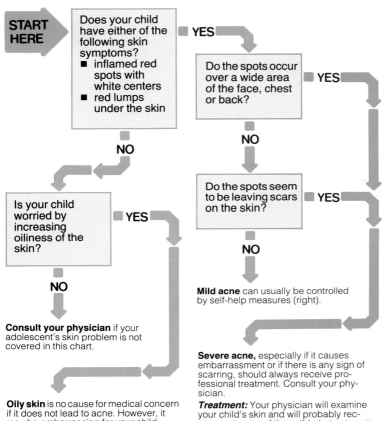

START HERE

Does your child have either of the following skin symptoms?
■ inflamed red spots with white centers
■ red lumps under the skin

YES

Do the spots occur over a wide area of the face, chest or back?

YES

NO

Do the spots seem to be leaving scars on the skin?

YES

NO

NO

Is your child worried by increasing oiliness of the skin?

YES

NO

Mild acne can usually be controlled by self-help measures (right).

Consult your physician if your adolescent's skin problem is not covered in this chart.

Oily skin is no cause for medical concern if it does not lead to acne. However, it may be embarrassing for your child.
Self-help: Regular washing with mild soap and water is normally all that is needed to keep oily skin under control. An astringent "skin-freshening" lotion may also be helpful.

Severe acne, especially if it causes embarrassment or if there is any sign of scarring, should always receive professional treatment. Consult your physician.

Treatment: Your physician will examine your child's skin and will probably recommend some of the self-help treatments described in the box at right. Depending on the severity with which your child is affected, your physician may refer your child to a skin specialist (dermatologist) and/or prescribe *antibiotics* or other forms of treatment.

ACNE

Acne is the name used to describe a group of related skin symptoms that mainly affects the face, chest and upper back. It is caused by blockage and infection of hair follicles in the skin and occurs principally during adolescence, when hormonal activity increases the production of sebum (natural skin oil), which makes the skin more susceptible to this disorder.

Symptoms
There are several main types of acne as follows:

Blackheads: See below left.

Pustules: Inflamed, raised spots that develop white centers. They are caused by bacterial activity in sebum that has collected in a hair follicle.

Cysts: Tender, inflamed lumps under the skin that are caused by scar tissue forming around an inflamed area under the skin. Cystic acne spots may leave permanent scars.

Self-help
Mild acne can usually be controlled using preparations that are available over-the-counter at your pharmacy.

Antibacterial skin-washing creams, lotions and soaps: These may help mild acne by reducing bacterial activity on the skin.

Sulfur or benzoyl peroxide preparations: These can help moderately severe acne, but should be used cautiously because they can make the skin sore.
Abrasives and keratolytics: These remove the top layer of skin, help to clear the blocked hair follicles that encourage acne and are good for getting rid of blackheads. However, these products should not be used too often or too vigorously. They may not be suitable if the skin is severely inflamed. In addition to these treatments, many people find that exposure to sunlight helps to reduce acne.

Professional treatment
When self-help measures are ineffective, or if acne is severe enough to cause embarrassment or scarring, your physician may prescribe one or more of the following treatments:
Keratolytics: These may be stronger than the over-the-counter preparations described but act in a similar way.
Antibiotics: These are given by mouth in low doses over an extended period. They help to counter bacterial activity in the skin and often produce a marked improvement in severe cases of acne.
Other drugs: Various drugs, including hormones and vitamin A derivatives, are sometimes prescribed for adults with severe acne, but your physician may be reluctant to prescribe them for those in their early teens.

BLACKHEADS

Blackheads (comedones) are tiny, black spots that principally occur around the nose and chin. They are caused by dead skin cells and sebum collecting in a hair follicle and becoming discolored by exposure to air. Blackheads may occur together with the more disfiguring forms of acne or on their own. If your adolescent is affected only by blackheads, treatment is unlikely to be necessary. However, if widespread blackheads are causing embarrassment, which is quite common for adolescents, they can be removed individually using a blackhead remover or by use of abrasives or keratolytic preparations (see *Acne,* right). Squeezing of blackheads by hand should be discouraged; this may lead to infection and abcess formation in the affected areas.

53 Adolescent weight problems

The rapid increase in height and the development of adult body proportions that occur in adolescence can lead a teenager to appear either too thin or too fat. Adolescence is also a time when young people are likely to be particularly sensitive about their appearance and worry unnecessarily about their figures. Girls are more likely than boys to be concerned about minor changes in weight. They are also much more likely to be affected by anorexia nervosa (see below), the most serious weight-related disorder of adolescence. However, although boys less commonly become seriously underweight, they are often overweight. In such cases, helpful and sympathetic advice from parents is just as important as for girls. The best way to determine whether or not your child's changing body shape indicates unhealthy weight gain or loss is to check that both weight and height are increasing at a parallel rate as indicated in the weight charts on pp. 300-301. Minor deviations from the standard growth curves are unlikely to be a cause for concern, but consult this chart if your child is significantly over 7 lb (3 kg) heavier or lighter than expected for his or her age and height.

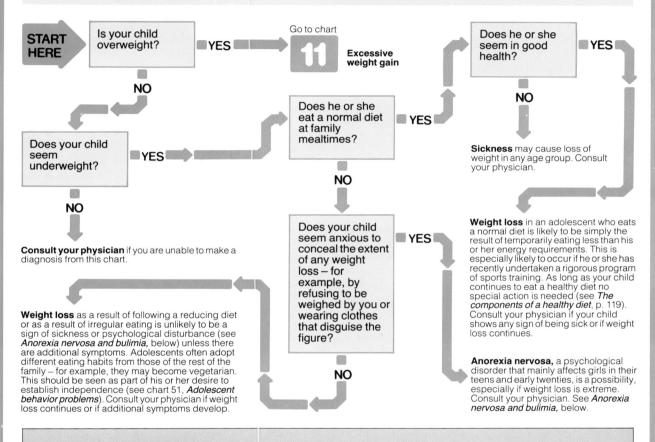

START HERE

Is your child overweight? — **YES** ▶ Go to chart **11** **Excessive weight gain**

NO

Does your child seem underweight? — **YES** ▶ **Does he or she eat a normal diet at family mealtimes?** — **YES** ▶

NO

Consult your physician if you are unable to make a diagnosis from this chart.

Does your child seem anxious to conceal the extent of any weight loss – for example, by refusing to be weighed by you or wearing clothes that disguise the figure? — **YES** ▶

NO

Weight loss as a result of following a reducing diet or as a result of irregular eating is unlikely to be a sign of sickness or psychological disturbance (see *Anorexia nervosa and bulimia,* below) unless there are additional symptoms. Adolescents often adopt different eating habits from those of the rest of the family – for example, they may become vegetarian. This should be seen as part of his or her desire to establish independence (see chart 51, *Adolescent behavior problems*). Consult your physician if weight loss continues or if additional symptoms develop.

Does he or she seem in good health? — **YES** ▶

NO

Sickness may cause loss of weight in any age group. Consult your physician.

Weight loss in an adolescent who eats a normal diet is likely to be simply the result of temporarily eating less than his or her energy requirements. This is especially likely to occur if he or she has recently undertaken a rigorous program of sports training. As long as your child continues to eat a healthy diet no special action is needed (see *The components of a healthy diet*, p. 119). Consult your physician if your child shows any sign of being sick or if weight loss continues.

Anorexia nervosa, a psychological disorder that mainly affects girls in their teens and early twenties, is a possibility, especially if weight loss is extreme. Consult your physician. See *Anorexia nervosa and bulimia,* below.

ANOREXIA NERVOSA AND BULIMIA

Anorexia nervosa is a psychological disturbance in which a person (often a teenage girl or young woman) refuses food because of an irrational fear of putting on weight. An anorectic convinces herself that she is too fat and that she has not lost enough weight even though she has. Many girls go through a temporary phase of excessive dieting, but of these only a few develop anorexia nervosa. The bulimia or binge-purge syndrome is a variant of anorexia nervosa. In the case of bulimia, a person eats or overeats and then induces vomiting and/or diarrhea (with the use of laxatives).

The signs of anorexia
The illness usually starts with normal dieting, but an anorectic eats less and less each day and, even if her figure becomes skeletal, she still sees herself as plump and is terrified of putting on weight. She may be reluctant to undress or weigh herself in front of others in order to conceal her weight loss. To avoid family pressure to eat sensibly she may hide food and throw it away. Or she may make herself vomit after meals. As weight loss progresses there may be hormonal disturbances that result in cessation of menstrual periods. She may also become depressed and withdrawn.

What action should you take?
If your adolescent has an unrealistic image of herself as being too fat and seems to be dieting excessively, although already very thin, you should discuss the matter with your physician. If, after examining your child, your physician thinks that she may be suffering from anorexia nervosa, he or she will probably arrange for treatment by a specialist in psychological disorders. In severe cases it may be necessary to admit your child to the hospital where food intake can be closely supervised.

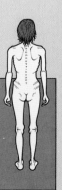

2 General medical: men and women

54 Feeling under the weather

Sometimes you may have a vague, generalized feeling of being sick without being able to locate a specific symptom such as pain. This may be the result of a minor infection or unhealthy life-style, but occasionally it may be a sign of a more serious underlying problem that requires medical treatment.

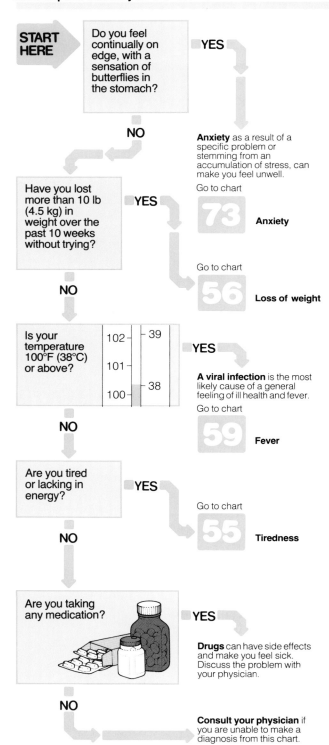

START HERE

Do you feel continually on edge, with a sensation of butterflies in the stomach?

YES → **Anxiety** as a result of a specific problem or stemming from an accumulation of stress, can make you feel unwell.
Go to chart
73 **Anxiety**

NO

Have you lost more than 10 lb (4.5 kg) in weight over the past 10 weeks without trying?

YES → Go to chart
56 **Loss of weight**

NO

Is your temperature 100°F (38°C) or above?

102 –	– 39
101 –	
	– 38
100 –	

YES → **A viral infection** is the most likely cause of a general feeling of ill health and fever.
Go to chart
59 **Fever**

NO

Are you tired or lacking in energy?

YES → Go to chart
55 **Tiredness**

NO

Are you taking any medication?

YES → **Drugs** can have side effects and make you feel sick. Discuss the problem with your physician.

NO

Consult your physician if you are unable to make a diagnosis from this chart.

THE EFFECTS OF ALCOHOL

The main immediate effect of alcohol is to dull the reactions of the brain. In small quantities, this can produce a pleasantly relaxed feeling but in larger amounts can lead to gross impairment of memory, judgment, coordination, and emotional reactions.

Alcohol also widens the blood vessels, making you feel temporarily warm. However, body heat is rapidly lost from the dilated blood vessels and this can lead to severe chilling (hypothermia).

After a heavy drinking session, you are likely to feel tired and nauseated, and may have a headache, as a result of dehydration and the damaging effect of alcohol on the stomach and intestines.

Long-term effects

Regular consumption of large amounts of alcohol can lead to the following serious health problems:

- Liver damage (which can lead to cirrhosis so that the body can no longer process nutrients or drugs) is almost inevitable.
- Addiction with accompanying social problems.
- Damage to the heart and pancreas.
- Malnutrition, stomach irritation, lowered resistance to disease, and irreversible brain or nervous system damage.

Maximum safe alcohol intake

Studies show that consumption of alcohol should be limited to a maximum of one or two drinks a day. Moderation is highly individual and depends on a variety of factors.

Women and alcohol

Excessive alcohol consumption has special dangers for women. It is now known that women are more susceptible than men to the harmful effects of alcohol on the liver. This is because of differences in the way their livers process alcohol. Apart from endangering their own health, women who drink during pregnancy risk damaging the fetus. Even small amounts of alcohol may increase the chance of a baby being born underweight and mentally retarded.

BLOOD ANALYSIS

Blood is the principal transport medium of the body. It carries oxygen, nutrients and other vital substances to the body tissues and carries waste products away. The blood is composed of three principal parts: red cells containing the red pigment (hemoglobin), which carries oxygen; the white cells (which fight infection) and platelets (which fight infection and seal damaged blood vessels); and the plasma, a yellowish fluid in which the blood cells, nutrients, chemicals and waste products are suspended.

Modern techniques for counting the numbers of different types of blood cells contained in a blood sample – a procedure known as a blood count – can help in the diagnosis of blood disorders. And examination of the chemicals in the plasma can give clues to diseases of many other parts of the body.

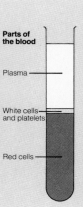

Parts of the blood

Plasma

White cells and platelets

Red cells

55 Tiredness

Consult this chart if you feel tired or lacking in energy during the day or if you spend more time asleep than you normally do. Lethargy is a common symptom of many disorders, some that require medical treatment. Sudden severe drowsiness is a serious symptom and requires prompt medical attention.

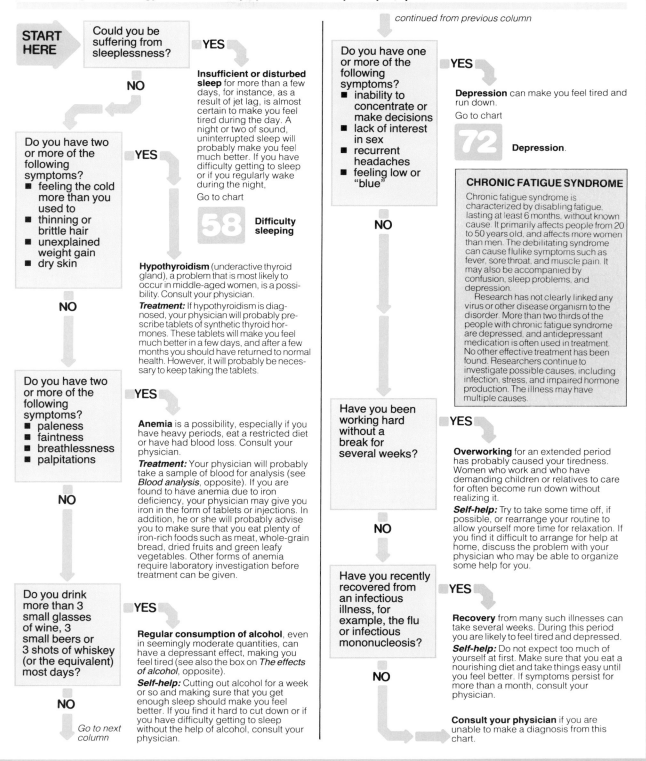

START HERE

Could you be suffering from sleeplessness?

YES

Insufficient or disturbed sleep for more than a few days, for instance, as a result of jet lag, is almost certain to make you feel tired during the day. A night or two of sound, uninterrupted sleep will probably make you feel much better. If you have difficulty getting to sleep or if you regularly wake during the night,

Go to chart

58 Difficulty sleeping

NO

Do you have two or more of the following symptoms?
- feeling the cold more than you used to
- thinning or brittle hair
- unexplained weight gain
- dry skin

YES

Hypothyroidism (underactive thyroid gland), a problem that is most likely to occur in middle-aged women, is a possibility. Consult your physician.

Treatment: If hypothyroidism is diagnosed, your physician will probably prescribe tablets of synthetic thyroid hormones. These tablets will make you feel much better in a few days, and after a few months you should have returned to normal health. However, it will probably be necessary to keep taking the tablets.

NO

Do you have two or more of the following symptoms?
- paleness
- faintness
- breathlessness
- palpitations

YES

Anemia is a possibility, especially if you have heavy periods, eat a restricted diet or have had blood loss. Consult your physician.

Treatment: Your physician will probably take a sample of blood for analysis (see *Blood analysis*, opposite). If you are found to have anemia due to iron deficiency, your physician may give you iron in the form of tablets or injections. In addition, he or she will probably advise you to make sure that you eat plenty of iron-rich foods such as meat, whole-grain bread, dried fruits and green leafy vegetables. Other forms of anemia require laboratory investigation before treatment can be given.

NO

Do you drink more than 3 small glasses of wine, 3 small beers or 3 shots of whiskey (or the equivalent) most days?

YES

Regular consumption of alcohol, even in seemingly moderate quantities, can have a depressant effect, making you feel tired (see also the box on *The effects of alcohol*, opposite).

Self-help: Cutting out alcohol for a week or so and making sure that you get enough sleep should make you feel better. If you find it hard to cut down or if you have difficulty getting to sleep without the help of alcohol, consult your physician.

NO

Go to next column

---

continued from previous column

Do you have one or more of the following symptoms?
- inability to concentrate or make decisions
- lack of interest in sex
- recurrent headaches
- feeling low or "blue"

YES

Depression can make you feel tired and run down.

Go to chart

72 Depression.

NO

CHRONIC FATIGUE SYNDROME

Chronic fatigue syndrome is characterized by disabling fatigue, lasting at least 6 months, without known cause. It primarily affects people from 20 to 50 years old, and affects more women than men. The debilitating syndrome can cause flulike symptoms such as fever, sore throat, and muscle pain. It may also be accompanied by confusion, sleep problems, and depression.

Research has not clearly linked any virus or other disease organism to the disorder. More than two thirds of the people with chronic fatigue syndrome are depressed, and antidepressant medication is often used in treatment. No other effective treatment has been found. Researchers continue to investigate possible causes, including infection, stress, and impaired hormone production. The illness may have multiple causes.

Have you been working hard without a break for several weeks?

YES

Overworking for an extended period has probably caused your tiredness. Women who work and who have demanding children or relatives to care for often become run down without realizing it.

Self-help: Try to take some time off, if possible, or rearrange your routine to allow yourself more time for relaxation. If you find it difficult to arrange for help at home, discuss the problem with your physician who may be able to organize some help for you.

NO

Have you recently recovered from an infectious illness, for example, the flu or infectious mononucleosis?

YES

Recovery from many such illnesses can take several weeks. During this period you are likely to feel tired and depressed.

Self-help: Do not expect too much of yourself at first. Make sure that you eat a nourishing diet and take things easy until you feel better. If symptoms persist for more than a month, consult your physician.

NO

Consult your physician if you are unable to make a diagnosis from this chart.

56 Loss of weight

Minor fluctuations in weight of only a few pounds, as a result of temporary changes in the amount of exercise you take or the amount of food you eat, are normal. However, more severe unintentional weight loss, especially when combined with loss of appetite or other symptoms, usually requires medical attention. Consult this chart if you have lost more than 10 lb (4.5 kg) in a period of 10 weeks or less, or if you have any of the signs of weight loss described in the box on the facing page.

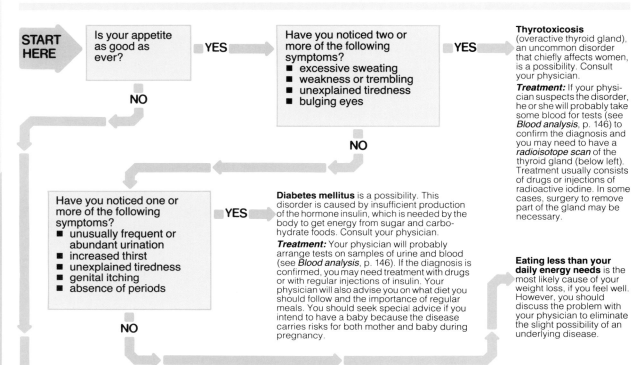

START HERE

Is your appetite as good as ever? — **YES** →

Have you noticed two or more of the following symptoms?
- excessive sweating
- weakness or trembling
- unexplained tiredness
- bulging eyes

— **YES** →

Thyrotoxicosis (overactive thyroid gland), an uncommon disorder that chiefly affects women, is a possibility. Consult your physician.

Treatment: If your physician suspects the disorder, he or she will probably take some blood for tests (see *Blood analysis*, p. 146) to confirm the diagnosis and you may need to have a *radioisotope scan* of the thyroid gland (below left). Treatment usually consists of drugs or injections of radioactive iodine. In some cases, surgery to remove part of the gland may be necessary.

NO (from appetite) ↓
NO (from symptoms) ↓

Have you noticed one or more of the following symptoms?
- unusually frequent or abundant urination
- increased thirst
- unexplained tiredness
- genital itching
- absence of periods

— **YES** →

Diabetes mellitus is a possibility. This disorder is caused by insufficient production of the hormone insulin, which is needed by the body to get energy from sugar and carbohydrate foods. Consult your physician.

Treatment: Your physician will probably arrange tests on samples of urine and blood (see *Blood analysis*, p. 146). If the diagnosis is confirmed, you may need treatment with drugs or with regular injections of insulin. Your physician will also advise you on what diet you should follow and the importance of regular meals. You should seek special advice if you intend to have a baby because the disease carries risks for both mother and baby during pregnancy.

Eating less than your daily energy needs is the most likely cause of your weight loss, if you feel well. However, you should discuss the problem with your physician to eliminate the slight possibility of an underlying disease.

NO ↓

RADIOISOTOPE SCAN

Physicians sometimes use this type of scan to find out whether and how a gland or organ is malfunctioning. A radioactive chemical is injected into the bloodstream and is absorbed by the organ being examined. This organ is then scanned with specialized equipment to determine whether or not the chemical is being absorbed evenly and normally. The result of the scan is shown either on photographs or on a television screen.

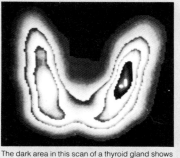

The dark area in this scan of a thyroid gland shows a possible thyroid nodule.

WEIGHT LOSS IN PREGNANCY

Many women lose some weight in the first 3 months of pregnancy, as a result mainly of loss of appetite, nausea and vomiting. This usually is not considered a problem unless you lose more than 8 lb (about 4 kg) or are extremely thin. In this case it is advisable to consult your physician, because it may mean that persistent vomiting is preventing you from obtaining adequate nourishment. Nausea and vomiting normally subside by the 12th week of pregnancy and by the 14th to 16th week you should begin to gain about 1 lb (about 0.5 kg) a week, until about the 38th week.

Abnormal weight loss
If you fail to gain weight at a satisfactory rate or if you lose weight after the first 3 months, you should consult your physician. He or she will ensure that you are eating properly and may arrange for tests, including urine and *blood analysis* (p. 146) and possibly an *ultrasound scan* (p. 276) to make sure that the placenta is functioning properly and that the fetus is developing normally. It is extremely important for you to get prenatal checkups throughout pregnancy so that a close watch may be kept on your weight gain and action taken when necessary.

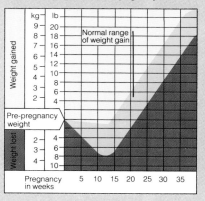

Pattern of weight gain and loss in pregnancy

Go to next page

Continued from previous page

Have you noticed one or more of these symptoms?
- recurrent bouts of diarrhea
- recurrent constipation
- recurrent abdominal pain
- blood in the stools
- recurrent nausea or vomiting

YES

CONSULT YOUR PHYSICIAN WITHOUT DELAY!
A digestive tract disorder may be causing your weight loss. Your intestines may be inflamed or you may have an ulcer, but there is also a possibility of a tumor, especially if you are over 40.

Treatment: Your physician will probably arrange for a variety of diagnostic tests. These may include analysis of samples of blood (p. 146) and bowel movements, *barium X rays* (p. 207) and possibly *sigmoidoscopy* (p. 216).

NO

Have you noticed two or more of the following symptoms?
- profuse sweating at night
- recurrent raised temperature
- general feeling of ill health
- persistent cough
- blood in phlegm

YES

CONSULT YOUR PHYSICIAN WITHOUT DELAY!
A chronic lung infection, such as tuberculosis or brucellosis, or another chronic infection, is possible.

Treatment: Your physician will probably take samples of blood and phlegm for analysis. You may also be given a *chest X ray* (p. 197) and a special skin test for tuberculosis. If you are found to have tuberculosis, you will be given a long course of special medications. With prompt treatment, symptomatic recovery in a few months is probable.

NO

Do you have one or more of the following symptoms?
- feeling low or "blue"
- difficulty sleeping
- lack of interest in sex
- inability to concentrate or make decisions

YES

Depression can sometimes cause a marked loss of appetite, leading to weight loss.

Go to chart

72 **Depression**.

NO

Consult your physician if you are unable to make a diagnosis from this chart.

SIGNS OF WEIGHT LOSS

If you lose weight without deliberately attempting to slim down, you should always take the matter seriously, especially if other symptoms suggest the possibility of illness. If you do not weigh yourself regularly, the following signs may indicate that you have lost weight:

- People remark on your changed appearance.
- Your cheeks become sunken.
- Your skirts or pants become loose around the waist.
- Your shirt collars become loose.
- You need a smaller bra size.

EXERCISE AND WEIGHT LOSS

For those who are overweight (see p. 150) exercise is a useful accompaniment to a planned reducing diet. While exercise alone will not solve a serious weight problem, it will boost the amount of energy (calories) you burn and will help tone up slack muscles. But if you are already thin, further weight loss may be unhealthy. It is therefore important for those involved in strenuous physical activity – for example, dancers and athletes – to ensure that they eat an adequate diet that takes account of their increased energy requirements.

If you increase your energy output without a corresponding increase in your intake of food, the body burns up fat reserves and the result is weight loss.

| Energy output |
| Energy (food) intake |
| Weight loss |

ANOREXIA NERVOSA

Anorexia is a psychological disturbance in which a person (most commonly a teenage girl or young woman) refuses food because of an irrational fear of putting on weight. An anorectic convinces herself that she is too fat, that she has not lost weight even though she has, and that there is nothing wrong with her even when she has lost an excessive amount of weight. Many young women go through a temporary phase of excessive dieting, but only a minority develop anorexia nervosa, which can lead to a dangerous loss of weight, hormonal disturbances and even death.

The signs of anorexia
The illness usually starts with normal dieting, but the anorectic eats less each day. She does this because she thinks that her arms or legs are still too fat. The less she eats, the less she wants to eat and, even if her figure becomes skeletal, she still sees herself as fat and is terrified of putting on weight. She may be reluctant to undress in front of others in order to conceal weight loss. To avoid family pressure to eat sensibly she may hide food and throw it away. Or she may eat a great deal of food and then make herself vomit after meals, a variation of anorexia known as bulimia. Anorectics often take large quantities of laxatives to keep their weight down.

As weight loss progresses, most anorectics cease to have periods. Skin may become sallow and a fine down may appear on the body. Without treatment, many anorectics become severely depressed and in some cases suicidal.

How you can help
If you know someone who has an unrealistic image of herself as being too fat and who seems to be dieting excessively, although already painfully thin, try to persuade her to consult a physician. While she may be unwilling to act on your advice, you should persevere until she does, because this can be a life-threatening condition.

An anorectic sees herself as overweight, even though in reality she is extremely thin.

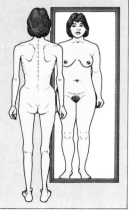

57 Overweight

Normally, fat accounts for no more than 25 percent of the weight of an adult woman. Any more than this is both unnecessary and unhealthy, increasing the risk of diseases such as diabetes, high blood pressure and arthritis. Most people reach their ideal weight in their teens and gradually gain a little weight as they get older, reaching their heaviest at about 50. Consult this chart if you weigh more than the healthy weight for your height shown in the charts on pages 302 and 303, or if you can pinch a fold of flesh that is more than an inch thick on your abdomen. In most cases, weight gain is due simply to eating more than you need and can be remedied by a balanced reducing diet, but occasionally there may be a medical reason for putting on weight.

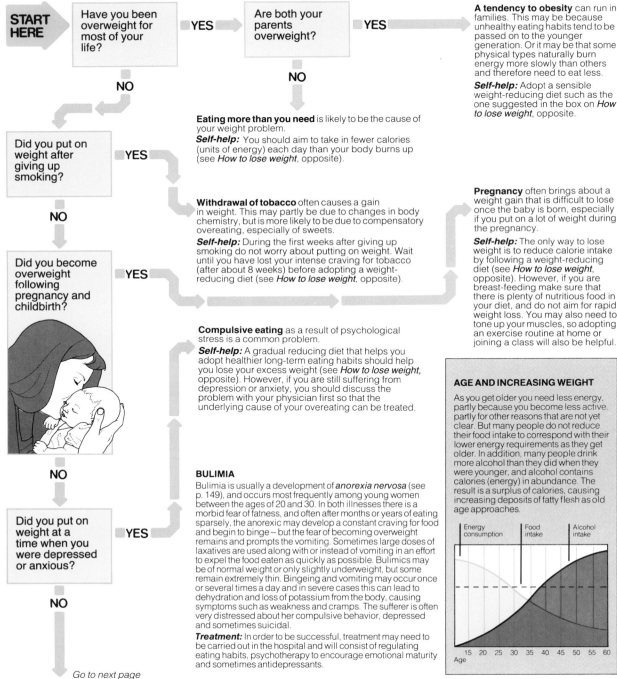

START HERE

Have you been overweight for most of your life?

YES

Are both your parents overweight?

YES

NO

NO

Did you put on weight after giving up smoking?

YES

NO

Did you become overweight following pregnancy and childbirth?

YES

NO

Did you put on weight at a time when you were depressed or anxious?

YES

NO

A tendency to obesity can run in families. This may be because unhealthy eating habits tend to be passed on to the younger generation. Or it may be that some physical types naturally burn energy more slowly than others and therefore need to eat less.

Self-help: Adopt a sensible weight-reducing diet such as the one suggested in the box on *How to lose weight*, opposite.

Eating more than you need is likely to be the cause of your weight problem.
Self-help: You should aim to take in fewer calories (units of energy) each day than your body burns up (see *How to lose weight*, opposite).

Withdrawal of tobacco often causes a gain in weight. This may partly be due to changes in body chemistry, but is more likely to be due to compensatory overeating, especially of sweets.
Self-help: During the first weeks after giving up smoking do not worry about putting on weight. Wait until you have lost your intense craving for tobacco (after about 8 weeks) before adopting a weight-reducing diet (see *How to lose weight*, opposite).

Pregnancy often brings about a weight gain that is difficult to lose once the baby is born, especially if you put on a lot of weight during the pregnancy.

Self-help: The only way to lose weight is to reduce calorie intake by following a weight-reducing diet (see *How to lose weight*, opposite). However, if you are breast-feeding make sure that there is plenty of nutritious food in your diet, and do not aim for rapid weight loss. You may also need to tone up your muscles, so adopting an exercise routine at home or joining a class will also be helpful.

Compulsive eating as a result of psychological stress is a common problem.
Self-help: A gradual reducing diet that helps you adopt healthier long-term eating habits should help you lose your excess weight (see *How to lose weight,* opposite). However, if you are still suffering from depression or anxiety, you should discuss the problem with your physician first so that the underlying cause of your overeating can be treated.

BULIMIA
Bulimia is usually a development of *anorexia nervosa* (see p. 149), and occurs most frequently among young women between the ages of 20 and 30. In both illnesses there is a morbid fear of fatness, and often after months or years of eating sparsely, the anorexic may develop a constant craving for food and begin to binge – but the fear of becoming overweight remains and prompts the vomiting. Sometimes large doses of laxatives are used along with or instead of vomiting in an effort to expel the food eaten as quickly as possible. Bulimics may be of normal weight or only slightly underweight, but some remain extremely thin. Bingeing and vomiting may occur once or several times a day and in severe cases this can lead to dehydration and loss of potassium from the body, causing symptoms such as weakness and cramps. The sufferer is often very distressed about her compulsive behavior, depressed and sometimes suicidal.

Treatment: In order to be successful, treatment may need to be carried out in the hospital and will consist of regulating eating habits, psychotherapy to encourage emotional maturity and sometimes antidepressants.

Go to next page

AGE AND INCREASING WEIGHT

As you get older you need less energy, partly because you become less active, partly for other reasons that are not yet clear. But many people do not reduce their food intake to correspond with their lower energy requirements as they get older. In addition, many people drink more alcohol than they did when they were younger, and alcohol contains calories (energy) in abundance. The result is a surplus of calories, causing increasing deposits of fatty flesh as old age approaches.

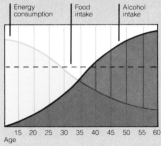

Energy consumption | Food intake | Alcohol intake

15 20 25 30 35 40 45 50 55 60
Age

Continued from previous page

Did the weight gain follow a change from a physically active life or strenuous job to a more sedentary life-style or work?

YES

NO

Energy requirements of the body vary according to the amount of exercise your daily routine involves. For instance, if you have a desk job, your average daily calorie requirement may be only 2,000 calories, but if you have a more active job you may require 2,500 calories.

Self-help: Adjusting your food intake to take account of your reduced energy requirements should help you to lose the weight you have put on. This may mean changing eating habits you have developed over many years and it may take a little while for you to become accustomed to your new diet. See *How to lose weight*, right, for some advice on a healthy reducing diet. You should also try to incorporate some physical exercise into your new routine to help keep your muscles firm and to assist weight loss.

Have you noticed two or more of the following symptoms since you began to put on weight?
- feeling the cold more than you used to
- thinning or brittle hair
- dry skin
- unexplained tiredness

YES

NO

Hypothyroidism (underactive thyroid gland) is a possibility. Consult your physician.

Treatment: If hypothyroidism is diagnosed, your physician will probably prescribe tablets of synthetic thyroid hormones. These tablets will help your body to burn up excess fat and after a few months you should have returned to your normal weight. However, it will probably be necessary to keep on taking the tablets indefinitely.

Are you taking any medications?

YES

NO

Certain drugs, particularly steroids prescribed for problems such as asthma or rheumatoid arthritis, can cause weight gain as a side effect. Discuss the problem with your physician.

Are you over 40 years old?

YES

NO

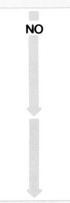

HOW TO LOSE WEIGHT

If you are fat, it is because your body is not using all the energy you feed it. To lose weight you must expend more energy than you take in, first by changing your diet, second by exercising more. It is best to avoid crash diets, which have no lasting effect because they do not encourage you to adopt healthy new habits. You will find it more helpful to follow this step-by-step diet, which is designed to help you change your eating habits over time.

1 Try to cut out, or at least cut down on, all foods in group 1, the sweet or rich foods. Reduce your daily alcohol intake to no more than two 12-oz cans of beer, two 6-oz glasses of wine or 2 shots (1.5 oz) of whiskey (or the equivalent). If you drink hard liquor, use low calorie mixers or unsweetened fruit juices. Eat normal portions of food from groups 2 and 3.

2 If you have not lost any weight after 2 weeks, stop having any group 1 foods, halve your helpings of group 2 foods and eat as much as you want from group 3. Cut down further on (or eliminate) your consumption of alcohol.

3 If you fail to lose weight after 2 more weeks, halve your helpings of group 3 foods and eat as little as possible from group 2. Consult your physician if you fail to lose weight after 4 more weeks.

Meat	Vegetables	Dairy foods	Fish	Other
Group 1 foods				
Visible fat on any meat Bacon Duck, goose Sausages, salami Pâtés		Butter Cream Ice cream		Thick gravies or sauces Fried food Sugar, candies Cakes, pies, cookies Puddings Canned fruits in syrup Dried fruits Nuts Jams, syrups Carbonated drinks Sherbets
Group 2 foods				
Lean beef Lamb Pork	Beans Lentils	Eggs Cheeses (other than cottage cheese) Whole milk	Oily fish (e.g., herring, mackerel, sardines, tuna packed in oil)	Pasta or rice Soups Breads, crackers Unsweetened cereals Margarine Polyunsaturated vegetable oils
Group 3 foods				
Poultry other than duck or goose (not including the skin)	Potatoes Vegetables (raw or lightly cooked) Clear or vegetable-only soups	Skim milk Yogurt Cottage cheese	Non oily fish (e.g., haddock, perch, cod) Shellfish (e.g., crab, shrimp) Tuna packed in water	Bran Fresh fruit Unsweetened fruit juice

Growing older is often accompanied by a gradual gain in weight. This is more than likely because you begin to exercise less at a time in your life when your body is beginning to take longer to burn up food.

Self-help: Reduce your food intake to correspond with your lower energy consumption (see *How to lose weight*, above).

Overeating is the likely cause of your excess weight.

Self-help: Follow the recommended reducing diet (see *How to lose weight,* above). If after a month you fail to lose weight, consult your physician, who will find out if the problem is due to any underlying disorder.

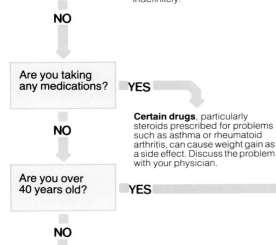

58 Difficulty sleeping

It is quite common to have an occasional night when you find it difficult to get to sleep and this need not be a cause for concern. Consult this chart if you regularly have difficulty falling asleep at night or if you wake during the night or early in the morning (a problem sometimes known as insomnia).

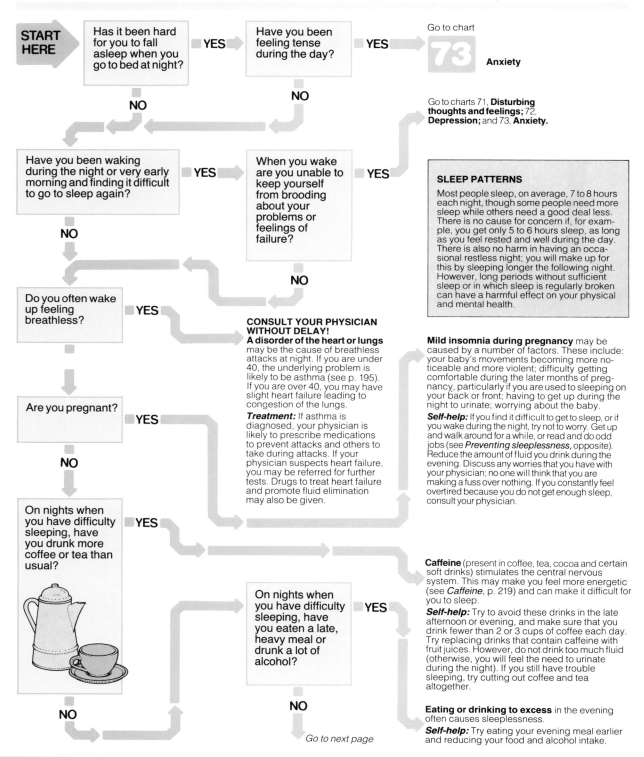

START HERE → Has it been hard for you to fall asleep when you go to bed at night?

YES → Have you been feeling tense during the day?

YES → Go to chart **73** **Anxiety**

NO (from "Has it been hard...")

NO (from "Have you been feeling tense...") → Go to charts 71, **Disturbing thoughts and feelings**; 72, **Depression**; and 73, **Anxiety**.

Have you been waking during the night or very early morning and finding it difficult to go to sleep again?

YES → When you wake are you unable to keep yourself from brooding about your problems or feelings of failure?

YES (to "Go to charts 71...")

NO (from "Have you been waking...")

NO (from "When you wake...")

Do you often wake up feeling breathless?

YES → **CONSULT YOUR PHYSICIAN WITHOUT DELAY!**
A disorder of the heart or lungs may be the cause of breathless attacks at night. If you are under 40, the underlying problem is likely to be asthma (see p. 195). If you are over 40, you may have slight heart failure leading to congestion of the lungs.

Treatment: If asthma is diagnosed, your physician is likely to prescribe medications to prevent attacks and others to take during attacks. If your physician suspects heart failure, you may be referred for further tests. Drugs to treat heart failure and promote fluid elimination may also be given.

NO

Are you pregnant?

YES →

NO

On nights when you have difficulty sleeping, have you drunk more coffee or tea than usual?

YES →

NO

On nights when you have difficulty sleeping, have you eaten a late, heavy meal or drunk a lot of alcohol?

YES →

NO

Go to next page

SLEEP PATTERNS

Most people sleep, on average, 7 to 8 hours each night, though some people need more sleep while others need a good deal less. There is no cause for concern if, for example, you get only 5 to 6 hours sleep, as long as you feel rested and well during the day. There is also no harm in having an occasional restless night; you will make up for this by sleeping longer the following night. However, long periods without sufficient sleep or in which sleep is regularly broken can have a harmful effect on your physical and mental health.

Mild insomnia during pregnancy may be caused by a number of factors. These include: your baby's movements becoming more noticeable and more violent; difficulty getting comfortable during the later months of pregnancy, particularly if you are used to sleeping on your back or front; having to get up during the night to urinate; worrying about the baby.

Self-help: If you find it difficult to get to sleep, or if you wake during the night, try not to worry. Get up and walk around for a while, or read and do odd jobs (see *Preventing sleeplessness*, opposite). Reduce the amount of fluid you drink during the evening. Discuss any worries that you have with your physician; no one will think that you are making a fuss over nothing. If you constantly feel overtired because you do not get enough sleep, consult your physician.

Caffeine (present in coffee, tea, cocoa and certain soft drinks) stimulates the central nervous system (see *Caffeine*, p. 219) and can make it difficult for you to sleep.

Self-help: Try to avoid these drinks in the late afternoon or evening, and make sure that you drink fewer than 2 or 3 cups of coffee each day. Try replacing drinks that contain caffeine with fruit juices. However, do not drink too much fluid (otherwise, you will feel the need to urinate during the night). If you still have trouble sleeping, try cutting out coffee and tea altogether.

Eating or drinking to excess in the evening often causes sleeplessness.
Self-help: Try eating your evening meal earlier and reducing your food and alcohol intake.

Continued from previous page

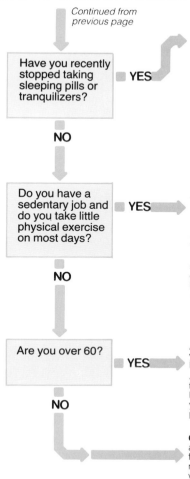

Have you recently stopped taking sleeping pills or tranquilizers?

YES

Drugs such as these can disrupt normal sleeping patterns, and it can take several weeks for your body to readjust after you stop taking them (see *Sleeping pills,* right).

Self-help: Try to be patient and resist the temptation to ask your physician to prescribe more pills to deal with your sleeping problem. Meanwhile, see *Preventing sleeplessness,* below. If you are still having difficulty sleeping after a month, discuss the problem with your physician.

NO

Do you have a sedentary job and do you take little physical exercise on most days?

YES

Lack of physical exercise during the day may mean that your body is not sufficiently tired to enable you to sleep easily. Also, stress and tension built up during the day may be making it difficult for you to relax.

Self-help: Try to get some form of strenuous exercise during the day or early evening. Not only will this help you sleep better, it will also improve your general health.

NO

Are you over 60?

YES

A declining need for sleep as you get older is quite normal as long as you continue to feel well.

Self-help: Try to find new activities to fill your extra waking hours. However, if lack of sleep is making you tired or irritable, consult your physician.

NO

Consult your physician if you are unable to make a diagnosis from this chart and if the self-help measures described below do not work.

SLEEPING PILLS

If you have difficulty sleeping at night, your physician may prescribe sleeping pills. These may be useful if you cannot sleep because of pain after an injury or during an illness, or at times of emotional stress – for example, following a bereavement.

What drugs are used?

There are two main types of drugs used to treat sleeplessness: antianxiety drugs and barbiturates. Both act in a similar way, but physicians usually prefer to prescribe an antianxiety drug because of the greater danger of overdose with barbiturates.

How do sleeping drugs work?

All sleeping drugs work by suppressing brain function in some way. This means that the sleep you get when taking a sleeping drug is not normal and may leave you less rested than after a natural night's sleep. This also means that if you suddenly stop taking sleeping pills after having used them regularly, you may sleep restlessly and have vivid dreams while your brain readjusts to normal *sleep patterns* (opposite).

Are sleeping pills dangerous?

Sleeping pills that are taken on your physician's advice and according to the dosage prescribed are unlikely to do you any harm. However, you may become dependent on these drugs if you take them regularly. If you wish to stop taking them, discuss this with your physician. In addition, you should consult your physician if you have difficulty waking up in the morning or if you find that your sleeping pills no longer work as effectively as before; you may need a change of drug.

People who take sleeping pills should always remember the following safety rules:

- Never take a larger dose than prescribed.
- Never drive or operate machinery before the effects of the sleeping drugs have worn off.
- Never take alcohol with these drugs; stop drinking at least 2 hours before taking a sleeping pill and do not start to drink until at least 8 hours afterward.
- Never give your sleeping pills to others, especially children.
- Never keep your tablets on your bedside table; there is a danger that you may accidentally take an additional dose when half asleep.

PREVENTING SLEEPLESSNESS

If you find that you cannot get to sleep as soon as you go to bed, try not to worry about it; this will only make matters worse. Even if you just relax or doze for a few hours you will probably be getting enough rest. The following self-help suggestions may help you get a good night's sleep:

- Try to do some form of physical exercise during the day so that your body needs rest because it is tired. A short, gentle stroll in the open air an hour or so before going to bed may also help.
- A full stomach generally is not conducive to sleep, but a warm, milky drink at bedtime may help you to feel sleepy.

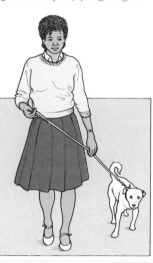

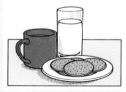

- Avoid heavy drinking.
- A warm bath is often relaxing. A shower may not be a good idea if it is too invigorating.
- Recreational reading, which is not associated with work or study, often makes people sleepy.
- Make sure that you are neither too hot nor too cold. Most people sleep best in a room temperature of 60 to 65°F.
- Make your environment as conducive to sleep as possible. Make sure that there are no irritating, dripping faucets or knocking radiators. A comfortable bed will help (see *Preventing backache,* p. 223).
- Sex may help you relax and fall asleep.

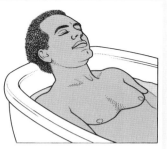

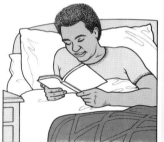

59 Fever

A fever (an abnormally high body temperature) can be a symptom of many diseases, but usually is a sign that your body is fighting infection. You may suspect that you have a fever if you feel hot or alternately hot, shivery and sweaty, and if you feel sick. To confirm that you have a fever, take your temperature as described below. Consult this chart if your temperature is 100°F (38°C) or above. Call your physician at once if your temperature rises above 104°F (40°C) or remains elevated for longer than 48 hours – whatever the suspected cause.

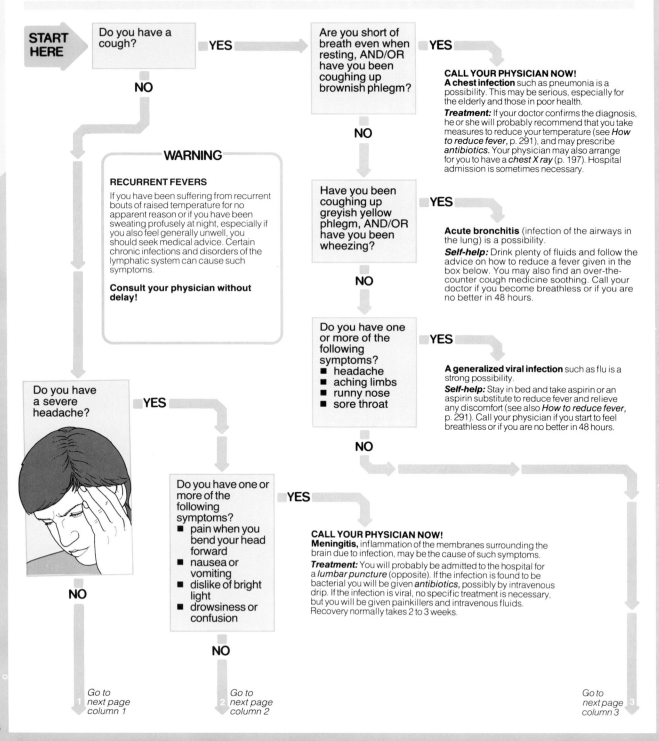

START HERE

Do you have a cough?
YES → **Are you short of breath even when resting, AND/OR have you been coughing up brownish phlegm?**
YES →
CALL YOUR PHYSICIAN NOW!
A chest infection such as pneumonia is a possibility. This may be serious, especially for the elderly and those in poor health.
Treatment: If your doctor confirms the diagnosis, he or she will probably recommend that you take measures to reduce your temperature (see *How to reduce fever*, p. 291), and may prescribe *antibiotics*. Your physician may also arrange for you to have a *chest X ray* (p. 197). Hospital admission is sometimes necessary.

NO ↓

Have you been coughing up greyish yellow phlegm, AND/OR have you been wheezing?
YES →
Acute bronchitis (infection of the airways in the lung) is a possibility.
Self-help: Drink plenty of fluids and follow the advice on how to reduce a fever given in the box below. You may also find an over-the-counter cough medicine soothing. Call your doctor if you become breathless or if you are no better in 48 hours.

NO ↓

Do you have one or more of the following symptoms?
■ headache
■ aching limbs
■ runny nose
■ sore throat
YES →
A generalized viral infection such as flu is a strong possibility.
Self-help: Stay in bed and take aspirin or an aspirin substitute to reduce fever and relieve any discomfort (see also *How to reduce fever*, p. 291). Call your physician if you start to feel breathless or if you are no better in 48 hours.

NO ↓

Cough NO ↓

WARNING

RECURRENT FEVERS

If you have been suffering from recurrent bouts of raised temperature for no apparent reason or if you have been sweating profusely at night, especially if you also feel generally unwell, you should seek medical advice. Certain chronic infections and disorders of the lymphatic system can cause such symptoms.

Consult your physician without delay!

Do you have a severe headache?
YES → **Do you have one or more of the following symptoms?**
■ pain when you bend your head forward
■ nausea or vomiting
■ dislike of bright light
■ drowsiness or confusion
YES →
CALL YOUR PHYSICIAN NOW!
Meningitis, inflammation of the membranes surrounding the brain due to infection, may be the cause of such symptoms.
Treatment: You will probably be admitted to the hospital for a *lumbar puncture* (opposite). If the infection is found to be bacterial you will be given *antibiotics*, possibly by intravenous drip. If the infection is viral, no specific treatment is necessary, but you will be given painkillers and intravenous fluids. Recovery normally takes 2 to 3 weeks.

NO ↓ (severe headache)

NO ↓ (symptoms)

Go to next page column 1

Go to next page column 2

Go to next page column 3

Continued from previous page, column 1

Continued from previous page, column 2

Continued from previous page, column 3

Do you have one or more of the following symptoms?
- aching limbs
- runny nose
- sore throat

YES → **A generalized viral infection** such as flu is a strong possibility.

Self-help: Stay in bed and take aspirin or an aspirin substitute to reduce fever and relieve any discomfort (see also *How to reduce fever*, p. 291). Call your physician if you start to feel breathless or if you are no better in 48 hours.

NO

Do you have a sore throat?

YES → Go to chart

86

Sore throat

NO

Have you recently returned from a stay in a hot country?

YES → **CONSULT YOUR PHYSICIAN WITHOUT DELAY!**
A tropical disease that is rare in this country – for example, malaria or typhoid – is a possibility.

Treatment: If your physician suspects such a disease after examining you, he or she may arrange for you to be admitted to hospital for tests. These may include *blood analysis* (p. 146) and tests on bowel movements. Treatment will depend on the eventual diagnosis.

NO

Do you have one or more of the following symptoms?
- pain in the small of the back
- abnormally frequent urination
- pain when passing urine
- pink or cloudy urine

YES → **CONSULT YOUR PHYSICIAN WITHOUT DELAY!**
An acute infection of the kidney or bladder may be the cause of this.

Treatment: Your physician will examine you and take a specimen of your urine and may prescribe *antibiotics*. He or she may also arrange for you to have a special X ray of the kidneys (see *Intravenous pyelography, men*, p. 238; *women*, p. 263) to try to find the underlying cause of the problem. Further treatment will depend on the results of the test.

NO

Have you spent most of the day in strong sunlight or in very hot conditions?

YES → **Exposure to heat** may have caused your temperature to rise. In most cases your temperature will return to normal after you have rested for an hour or so in a cool room. Call your physician at once if the fever continues to rise.

NO

Are you a woman?

YES → **Have you had a baby within the past 2 weeks?**

YES → **CALL YOUR PHYSICIAN NOW!**
Puerperal infection, although rare nowadays, is a possible cause of fever following childbirth. This occurs when the uterus and/or vagina become infected after delivery. If, however, you also have pain or redness in the breast, you may have a breast infection (see chart 146, *Breast-feeding problems*).

Treatment: If your physician thinks that you may have a puerperal infection, he or she may take a sample of discharge from your vagina for analysis. Treatment consists of a course of *antibiotics*.

NO

Do you have pain in the lower abdomen AND/OR have you had an unusually heavy or unpleasant-smelling vaginal discharge?

YES → **An infection of the fallopian tubes** (sometimes known as salpingitis) is a possible cause of such symptoms. Consult your physician.

Treatment: Your physician will probably give you a vaginal examination (p. 258), and will take a sample of vaginal discharge for analysis. If tests confirm the diagnosis you will probably be given a course of *antibiotics*.

NO

Consult your physician if you are unable to make a diagnosis from this chart and your temperature has not returned to normal within 48 hours, or if it rises again.

LUMBAR PUNCTURE

Lumbar puncture is a test that is used to diagnose disorders of the brain and nervous system, in particular, infections such as meningitis. A sample of the fluid that surrounds the brain and spinal cord is taken by syringe from the base of the spine for analysis. The area is first numbed by local anesthetic. Then a needle is inserted between the bones of the lower spine and a small amount of fluid is drawn off.

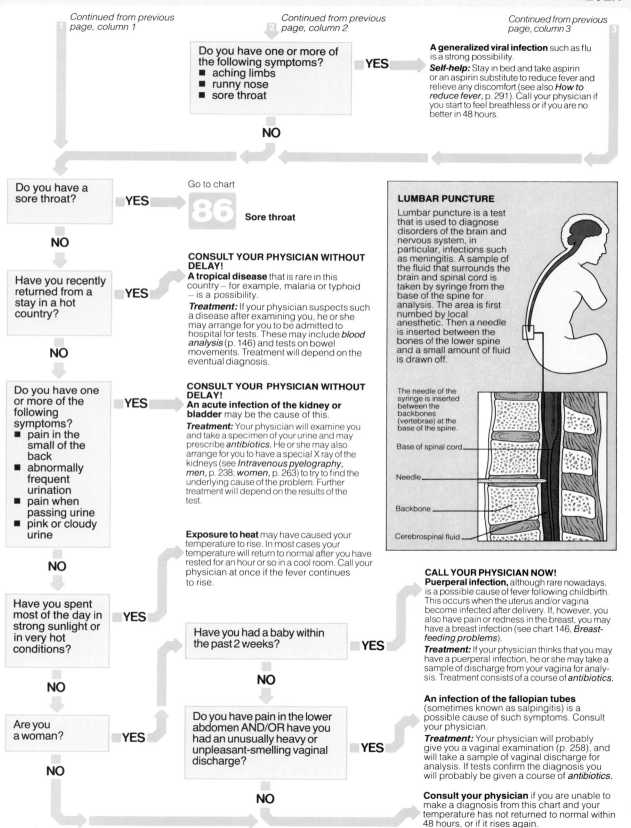

The needle of the syringe is inserted between the backbones (vertebrae) at the base of the spine.

Base of spinal cord

Needle

Backbone

Cerebrospinal fluid

60 Excessive sweating

Sweating is a natural mechanism for regulating body temperature and is the normal response to hot conditions or strenuous exercise. Some people naturally sweat more than others, so, if you have always sweated profusely, there is unlikely to be anything wrong. However, sweating that is not brought on by heat or exercise or that is more profuse than you are used to may be a sign of a number of medical conditions.

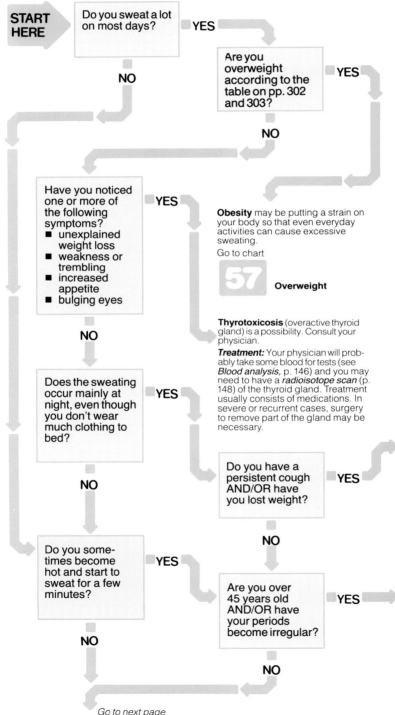

START HERE

Do you sweat a lot on most days? — **YES**

NO

Are you overweight according to the table on pp. 302 and 303? — **YES**

NO

Have you noticed one or more of the following symptoms?
- unexplained weight loss
- weakness or trembling
- increased appetite
- bulging eyes

YES

NO

Does the sweating occur mainly at night, even though you don't wear much clothing to bed? — **YES**

NO

Do you sometimes become hot and start to sweat for a few minutes? — **YES**

NO

Do you have a persistent cough AND/OR have you lost weight? — **YES**

NO

Are you over 45 years old AND/OR have your periods become irregular? — **YES**

NO

Obesity may be putting a strain on your body so that even everyday activities can cause excessive sweating.
Go to chart

57 **Overweight**

Thyrotoxicosis (overactive thyroid gland) is a possibility. Consult your physician.

Treatment: Your physician will probably take some blood for tests (see *Blood analysis*, p. 146) and you may need to have a *radioisotope scan* (p. 148) of the thyroid gland. Treatment usually consists of medications. In severe or recurrent cases, surgery to remove part of the gland may be necessary.

Go to next page

BODY ODOR

Sweat itself usually has no noticeable odor. However, if it remains on the skin for more than a few hours it may lead to body odor. This is caused by the activity of bacteria that live naturally on the surface of the skin. These flourish in the sweat, particularly that of the apocrine glands (see *Sweat glands,* opposite), which contains fats and proteins.

Preventing body odor
The most effective way to reduce body odor is to wash all over at least once a day. This will remove the stale sweat and control bacterial growth. Using an *antibacterial* soap, particularly in the areas where apocrine glands are located, will also be helpful.

Deodorants and antiperspirants
After washing, use a deodorant containing an antiperspirant, which prevents sweat from reaching the surface of the skin, under the arms. This will usually prevent body odor from building up during the day. Such deodorants may be bought in the form of a spray, a roll-on applicator or a cream. All are equally effective. However, some people may find that their skin becomes irritated by certain chemicals they contain, and you should change brands if this happens to you. Do not use a deodorant on broken skin.

Clothes
If sweat penetrates the fabric of your clothes, they may become a source of unpleasant odor. In addition, the bacteria that cause the odor may also in time damage the material. So, if you sweat a great deal, it is essential to wash clothes (especially those worn next to the skin) frequently.

CONSULT YOUR PHYSICIAN WITHOUT DELAY!
Tuberculosis (an infection that often starts in the lungs), or another chronic infectious disease, could be the cause of these symptoms.

Treatment: Your physician may arrange for you to have a special test for tuberculosis or a *chest X ray* (p. 197).If you are found to have tuberculosis, you will be given a long course of *antibiotics*. You may need to stay in the hospital until the infection is under control.

Hot flashes (sudden outbreaks of heat and sweating) are one of the most common symptoms of the onset of the menopause.

Self-help: Many women simply tolerate this unpleasant and sometimes embarrassing symptom, knowing that it will pass within a year or so. Remember that, although uncomfortable, hot flashes are rarely noticeable to anyone else. However, recent research has indicated that there are other good reasons to treat symptoms associated with menopause. Estrogen hormone replacements, for example, have been shown to reduce osteoporosis, or bone weakness.

Continued from previous page

Is your temperature 100°F (38°C) or above?

YES → **Sweating** is the normal response to fever.

Go to chart

59 **Fever**

NO ↓

Does the excessive sweating occur only during your periods?

YES → **Changes in the hormone balance** cause increased sweating during menstruation in some women. This is no cause for concern.

NO ↓

Did you notice the sweating after you had been drinking alcohol or taking large doses of aspirin?

YES → **Alcohol or aspirin** can cause increased sweating.

Self-help: If alcohol seems to be causing the problem, cut down on your drinking (see *The effects of alcohol,* p. 146). If aspirin taken for some other problem seems to be the cause of your sweating, ask your physician for advice.

NO ↓

Are you wearing clothes (or are your sleep clothes) made of nylon or other man-made materials?

YES → **Synthetic materials** often cause a noticeable increase in sweating. This is because they do not absorb moisture or allow your skin to breathe.

Self-help: Try wearing natural fibers, such as cotton or wool, as often as possible. In addition, make sure that your clothing is loose; this will increase the circulation of air and allow the sweat to evaporate more quickly.

NO ↓

Is the excessive sweating confined to your feet or hands?

YES → **A high concentration of sweat glands** on the hands and feet (see *Sweat glands,* left) makes these parts of the body react most noticeably to increases in temperature. This is no cause for concern.

Self-help: If your hands are sweaty, wash them frequently. The problem is likely to become worse if you worry, so try to relax. Make sure that you wash and dry your feet carefully at least once a day. It is best to avoid wearing shoes, hose and socks made of synthetic materials. If the problem is severe or causes embarrassment, consult your physician.

NO ↓

Do you notice the sweating only when you are anxious or excited?

YES → **Emotional stress** can easily cause an increase in sweating. This in itself is not a cause for concern, but, if it happens regularly or causes embarrassment, consult your physician.

Treatment: Your physician will advise you on the best methods of controlling the sweating. He or she will also discuss with you the possible causes of any underlying anxiety and may recommend medication (see also chart 73, *Anxiety*).

NO ↓

Are you in your teens?

YES → **The development of additional (apocrine) sweat glands during puberty** (see *Sweat glands,* left) usually causes an increase in sweating that is particularly noticeable under the arms. This is quite normal.

Self-help: There is no need to be embarrassed about any increased sweating. However, you will need to wash regularly and you may want to use an antiperspirant deodorant to reduce wetness and to prevent unpleasant body odor (see *Body odor,* opposite).

NO ↓

Consult your physician if you are unable to make a diagnosis from this chart and your excessive sweating continues to worry you. There is, however, not likely to be a serious cause for this symptom.

SWEAT GLANDS

Sweat glands are found under the skin all over the body and release moisture (sweat) through pores in the surface of the skin. There are two types of sweat glands – eccrine and apocrine glands – and these produce different kinds of sweat.

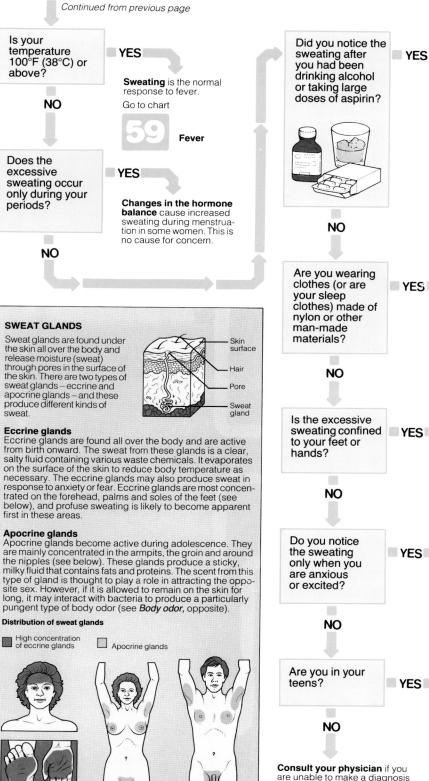

Skin surface
Hair
Pore
Sweat gland

Eccrine glands

Eccrine glands are found all over the body and are active from birth onward. The sweat from these glands is a clear, salty fluid containing various waste chemicals. It evaporates on the surface of the skin to reduce body temperature as necessary. The eccrine glands may also produce sweat in response to anxiety or fear. Eccrine glands are most concentrated on the forehead, palms and soles of the feet (see below), and profuse sweating is likely to become apparent first in these areas.

Apocrine glands

Apocrine glands become active during adolescence. They are mainly concentrated in the armpits, the groin and around the nipples (see below). These glands produce a sticky, milky fluid that contains fats and proteins. The scent from this type of gland is thought to play a role in attracting the opposite sex. However, if it is allowed to remain on the skin for long, it may interact with bacteria to produce a particularly pungent type of body odor (see *Body odor,* opposite).

Distribution of sweat glands

■ High concentration of eccrine glands   ☐ Apocrine glands

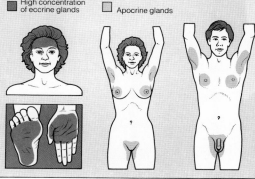

61 Itching

Itching (skin irritation that makes you want to scratch) is usually produced by contact with certain types of fabric or with a substance to which you are sensitive. Many skin disorders that produce a rash also cause itching.

Occasionally, itching is a sign of an underlying disease or of psychological stress. Irritation is likely to be most severe if you are hot or if your skin is dry, and is likely to be made worse by rubbing or scratching.

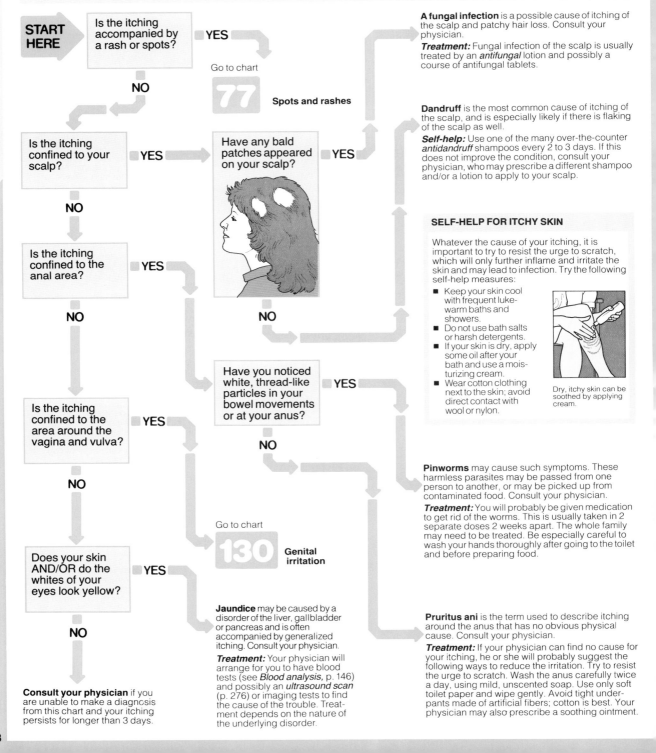

START HERE

Is the itching accompanied by a rash or spots?
YES → Go to chart **77** **Spots and rashes**
NO ↓

Is the itching confined to your scalp?
YES → **Have any bald patches appeared on your scalp?**
NO ↓

Is the itching confined to the anal area?
YES →
NO ↓

Have any bald patches appeared on your scalp?
YES →
NO ↓

Is the itching confined to the area around the vagina and vulva?
YES →
NO ↓

Have you noticed white, thread-like particles in your bowel movements or at your anus?
YES →
NO ↓
Go to chart **130** **Genital irritation**

Does your skin AND/OR do the whites of your eyes look yellow?
YES →
NO ↓

Consult your physician if you are unable to make a diagnosis from this chart and your itching persists for longer than 3 days.

A fungal infection is a possible cause of itching of the scalp and patchy hair loss. Consult your physician.
Treatment: Fungal infection of the scalp is usually treated by an *antifungal* lotion and possibly a course of antifungal tablets.

Dandruff is the most common cause of itching of the scalp, and is especially likely if there is flaking of the scalp as well.
Self-help: Use one of the many over-the-counter *antidandruff* shampoos every 2 to 3 days. If this does not improve the condition, consult your physician, who may prescribe a different shampoo and/or a lotion to apply to your scalp.

SELF-HELP FOR ITCHY SKIN

Whatever the cause of your itching, it is important to try to resist the urge to scratch, which will only further inflame and irritate the skin and may lead to infection. Try the following self-help measures:

- Keep your skin cool with frequent luke-warm baths and showers.
- Do not use bath salts or harsh detergents.
- If your skin is dry, apply some oil after your bath and use a mois-turizing cream.
- Wear cotton clothing next to the skin; avoid direct contact with wool or nylon.

Dry, itchy skin can be soothed by applying cream.

Pinworms may cause such symptoms. These harmless parasites may be passed from one person to another, or may be picked up from contaminated food. Consult your physician.
Treatment: You will probably be given medication to get rid of the worms. This is usually taken in 2 separate doses 2 weeks apart. The whole family may need to be treated. Be especially careful to wash your hands thoroughly after going to the toilet and before preparing food.

Jaundice may be caused by a disorder of the liver, gallbladder or pancreas and is often accompanied by generalized itching. Consult your physician.
Treatment: Your physician will arrange for you to have blood tests (see *Blood analysis*, p. 146) and possibly an *ultrasound scan* (p. 276) or imaging tests to find the cause of the trouble. Treatment depends on the nature of the underlying disorder.

Pruritus ani is the term used to describe itching around the anus that has no obvious physical cause. Consult your physician.
Treatment: If your physician can find no cause for your itching, he or she will probably suggest the following ways to reduce the irritation. Try to resist the urge to scratch. Wash the anus carefully twice a day, using mild, unscented soap. Use only soft toilet paper and wipe gently. Avoid tight under-pants made of artificial fibers; cotton is best. Your physician may also prescribe a soothing ointment.

62 Lumps and swellings

Consult this chart if you notice one or more swollen areas or lumps beneath the surface of the skin. In most cases such swellings are the result of enlargement of the lymph glands, which is a natural response to the presence of infection. You should always consult your doctor about a painful or persistent swelling.

For lumps and swellings in the breasts see chart 124, or in the testicles see chart 115.

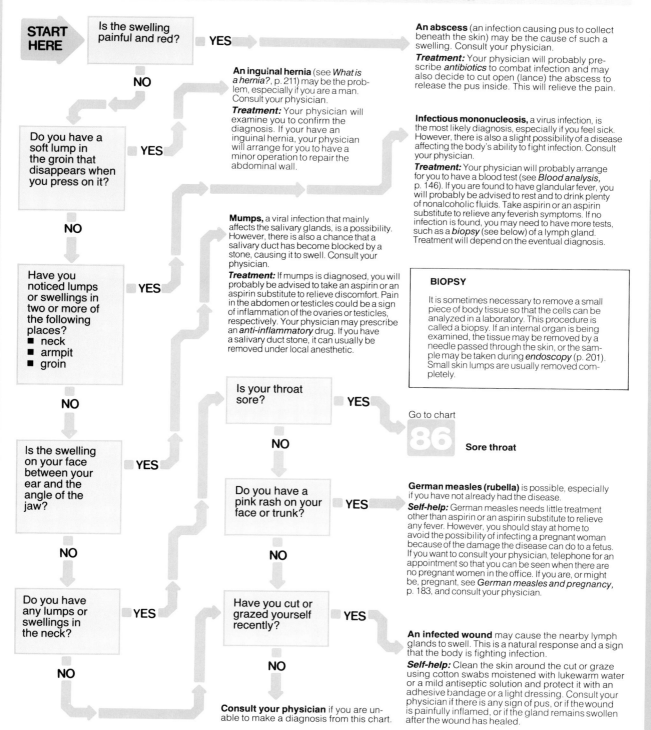

START HERE

Is the swelling painful and red?

YES →

NO

Do you have a soft lump in the groin that disappears when you press on it?

YES →

NO

Have you noticed lumps or swellings in two or more of the following places?
■ neck
■ armpit
■ groin

YES →

NO

Is the swelling on your face between your ear and the angle of the jaw?

YES →

NO

Do you have any lumps or swellings in the neck?

YES →

NO

An inguinal hernia (see *What is a hernia?*, p. 211) may be the problem, especially if you are a man. Consult your physician.
Treatment: Your physician will examine you to confirm the diagnosis. If you have an inguinal hernia, your physician will arrange for you to have a minor operation to repair the abdominal wall.

Mumps, a viral infection that mainly affects the salivary glands, is a possibility. However, there is also a chance that a salivary duct has become blocked by a stone, causing it to swell. Consult your physician.
Treatment: If mumps is diagnosed, you will probably be advised to take an aspirin or an aspirin substitute to relieve discomfort. Pain in the abdomen or testicles could be a sign of inflammation of the ovaries or testicles, respectively. Your physician may prescribe an *anti-inflammatory* drug. If you have a salivary duct stone, it can usually be removed under local anesthetic.

Is your throat sore?

YES →

NO

Do you have a pink rash on your face or trunk?

YES →

NO

Have you cut or grazed yourself recently?

YES →

NO

Consult your physician if you are unable to make a diagnosis from this chart.

An abscess (an infection causing pus to collect beneath the skin) may be the cause of such a swelling. Consult your physician.
Treatment: Your physician will probably prescribe *antibiotics* to combat infection and may also decide to cut open (lance) the abscess to release the pus inside. This will relieve the pain.

Infectious mononucleosis, a virus infection, is the most likely diagnosis, especially if you feel sick. However, there is also a slight possibility of a disease affecting the body's ability to fight infection. Consult your physician.
Treatment: Your physician will probably arrange for you to have a blood test (see *Blood analysis,* p. 146). If you are found to have glandular fever, you will probably be advised to rest and to drink plenty of nonalcoholic fluids. Take aspirin or an aspirin substitute to relieve any feverish symptoms. If no infection is found, you may need to have more tests, such as a *biopsy* (see below) of a lymph gland. Treatment will depend on the eventual diagnosis.

BIOPSY

It is sometimes necessary to remove a small piece of body tissue so that the cells can be analyzed in a laboratory. This procedure is called a biopsy. If an internal organ is being examined, the tissue may be removed by a needle passed through the skin, or the sample may be taken during *endoscopy* (p. 201). Small skin lumps are usually removed completely.

Go to chart

86

Sore throat

German measles (rubella) is possible, especially if you have not already had the disease.
Self-help: German measles needs little treatment other than aspirin or an aspirin substitute to relieve any fever. However, you should stay at home to avoid the possibility of infecting a pregnant woman because of the damage the disease can do to a fetus. If you want to consult your physician, telephone for an appointment so that you can be seen when there are no pregnant women in the office. If you are, or might be, pregnant, see *German measles and pregnancy,* p. 183, and consult your physician.

An infected wound may cause the nearby lymph glands to swell. This is a natural response and a sign that the body is fighting infection.
Self-help: Clean the skin around the cut or graze using cotton swabs moistened with lukewarm water or a mild antiseptic solution and protect it with an adhesive bandage or a light dressing. Consult your physician if there is any sign of pus, or if the wound is painfully inflamed, or if the gland remains swollen after the wound has healed.

63 Faintness and fainting

Fainting – a brief loss of consciousness – is usually preceded by a sensation of lightheadedness or dizziness, and you may be pale and suddenly feel cold or clammy. Such feelings of faintness may sometimes occur on their own without loss of consciousness. Faintness is usually the result of a sudden drop in blood pressure – as a result, for example, of an emotional shock – or it may be caused by an abnormally low level of sugar in the blood. Isolated episodes of fainting with no other symptoms are hardly ever a cause for concern but, if you suffer repeated fainting attacks or have additional symptoms, you should seek medical advice.

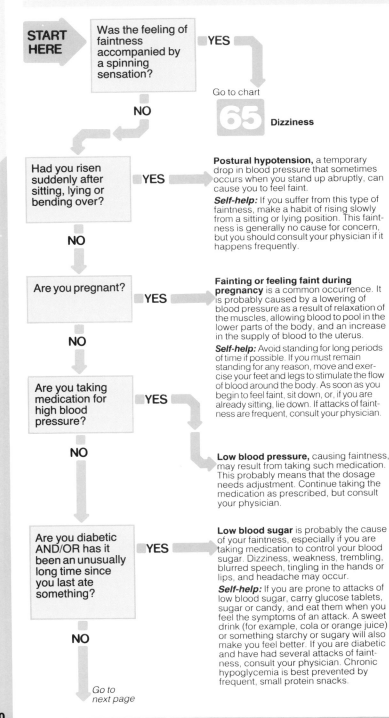

START HERE

Was the feeling of faintness accompanied by a spinning sensation?

YES → Go to chart **65** Dizziness

NO ↓

Had you risen suddenly after sitting, lying or bending over?

YES → **Postural hypotension,** a temporary drop in blood pressure that sometimes occurs when you stand up abruptly, can cause you to feel faint.
Self-help: If you suffer from this type of faintness, make a habit of rising slowly from a sitting or lying position. This faintness is generally no cause for concern, but you should consult your physician if it happens frequently.

NO ↓

Are you pregnant?

YES → **Fainting or feeling faint during pregnancy** is a common occurrence. It is probably caused by a lowering of blood pressure as a result of relaxation of the muscles, allowing blood to pool in the lower parts of the body, and an increase in the supply of blood to the uterus.
Self-help: Avoid standing for long periods of time if possible. If you must remain standing for any reason, move and exercise your feet and legs to stimulate the flow of blood around the body. As soon as you begin to feel faint, sit down, or, if you are already sitting, lie down. If attacks of faintness are frequent, consult your physician.

NO ↓

Are you taking medication for high blood pressure?

YES → **Low blood pressure,** causing faintness, may result from taking such medication. This probably means that the dosage needs adjustment. Continue taking the medication as prescribed, but consult your physician.

NO ↓

Are you diabetic AND/OR has it been an unusually long time since you last ate something?

YES → **Low blood sugar** is probably the cause of your faintness, especially if you are taking medication to control your blood sugar. Dizziness, weakness, trembling, blurred speech, tingling in the hands or lips, and headache may occur.
Self-help: If you are prone to attacks of low blood sugar, carry glucose tablets, sugar or candy, and eat them when you feel the symptoms of an attack. A sweet drink (for example, cola or orange juice) or something starchy or sugary will also make you feel better. If you are diabetic and have had several attacks of faintness, consult your physician. Chronic hypoglycemia is best prevented by frequent, small protein snacks.

NO ↓

Go to next page

WARNING

PROLONGED LOSS OF CONSCIOUSNESS

Momentary loss of consciousness – fainting – is not usually a cause for concern if the person is breathing normally and regains consciousness within a minute or two. If someone in your presence remains unconscious for longer, or if breathing slows or becomes irregular or noisy, get medical help at once. While waiting for medical help to arrive, place the person on her stomach as shown.

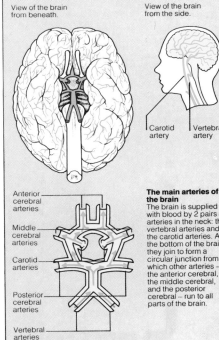

HOW BLOOD FLOWS TO THE BRAIN

The brain is more dependent on a constant supply of oxygenated blood that any other organ in the body. Temporary interruption in this supply is likely to cause the brain to malfunction, and more serious disruption to the blood flow may cause lasting damage to brain cells.

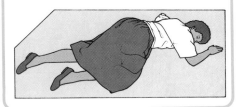

View of the brain from beneath.

View of the brain from the side.

Carotid artery   Vertebral artery

Anterior cerebral arteries

Middle cerebral arteries

Carotid arteries

Posterior cerebral arteries

Vertebral arteries

The main arteries of the brain
The brain is supplied with blood by 2 pairs of arteries in the neck: the vertebral arteries and the carotid arteries. At the bottom of the brain they join to form a circular junction from which other arteries – the anterior cerebral, the middle cerebral, and the posterior cerebral – run to all parts of the brain.

Continued from previous page

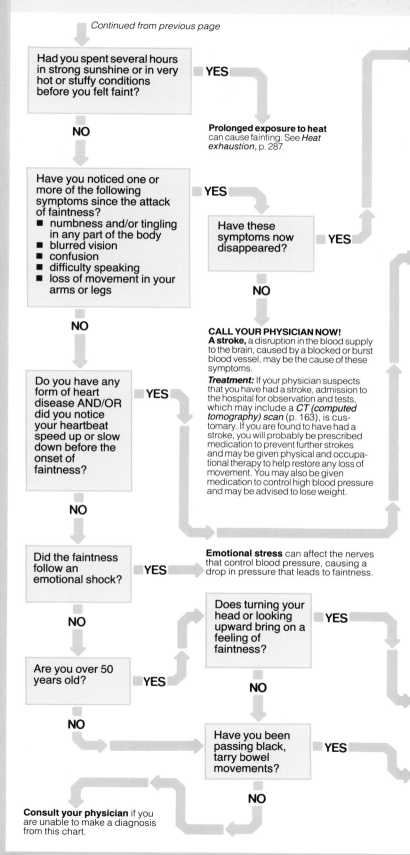

Had you spent several hours in strong sunshine or in very hot or stuffy conditions before you felt faint?

YES →

Prolonged exposure to heat can cause fainting. See *Heat exhaustion*, p. 287.

NO ↓

Have you noticed one or more of the following symptoms since the attack of faintness?
- numbness and/or tingling in any part of the body
- blurred vision
- confusion
- difficulty speaking
- loss of movement in your arms or legs

YES →

Have these symptoms now disappeared?

YES →

CALL YOUR PHYSICIAN NOW!
A transient ischemic attack – a temporary interruption in the blood supply to the brain, sometimes linked to a narrowing of the arteries (see *How blood flows to the brain,* opposite) – may have caused your symptoms.

Treatment: If your physician suspects that this is the problem, you will probably be referred to a specialist for tests. At a later stage, you may need to undergo *angiography* (p. 227) of the arteries. You may be prescribed medication to control high blood pressure, if you have it, and further medication to prevent the formation of blood clots. Surgery may be necessary in some cases.

NO ↓

CALL YOUR PHYSICIAN NOW!
A stroke, a disruption in the blood supply to the brain, caused by a blocked or burst blood vessel, may be the cause of these symptoms.

Treatment: If your physician suspects that you have had a stroke, admission to the hospital for observation and tests, which may include a *CT (computed tomography) scan* (p. 163), is customary. If you are found to have had a stroke, you will probably be prescribed medication to prevent further strokes and may be given physical and occupational therapy to help restore any loss of movement. You may also be given medication to control high blood pressure and may be advised to lose weight.

NO ↓

Do you have any form of heart disease AND/OR did you notice your heartbeat speed up or slow down before the onset of faintness?

YES →

CALL YOUR PHYSICIAN NOW!
An Adams-Stokes attack (sudden alteration of the heart rhythm) could have caused the fainting. Such attacks may be a sign of an underlying disorder of heart rate or rhythm.

Treatment: If your physician suspects the possibility of such a disorder, he or she will arrange for you to undergo *electrocardiography* (p. 219). If this shows abnormal heart rhythms, you will probably be prescribed medication to regulate the heart's activity.

NO ↓

Did the faintness follow an emotional shock?

YES →

Emotional stress can affect the nerves that control blood pressure, causing a drop in pressure that leads to faintness.

NO ↓

Are you over 50 years old?

YES →

Does turning your head or looking upward bring on a feeling of faintness?

YES →

Cervical osteoarthritis, a disorder of the bones and joints in the neck, can cause feelings of faintness. Consult your physician.
Treatment: See *Cervical osteoarthritis,* p. 224.

NO ↓

NO ↓

Have you been passing black, tarry bowel movements?

YES →

CALL YOUR PHYSICIAN NOW!
Bleeding in the digestive tract, perhaps from a stomach ulcer, is a possibility.

Treatment: Your physician will probably arrange for you to have tests, such as *endoscopy* (p. 201), a *biopsy* (p. 159) of the stomach lining and a *barium X ray* (p. 207). These tests should reveal the underlying cause of your symptoms.

NO ↓

Consult your physician if you are unable to make a diagnosis from this chart.

FIRST AID

Dealing with faintness
If you feel faint, lie down with your legs raised or, if this is not possible, sit with your head between your knees until you feel better.

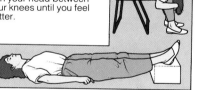

Dealing with fainting
To help someone who has fainted, check that breathing is normal. Lay the person on his or her back with legs raised as high as possible above the level of the head. Hold the legs up, or rest them on a chair. Loosen any tight clothing (e.g., collar or waistband) and make sure that the person gets plenty of fresh air. If you are indoors, open the windows to allow air to circulate. If you are outdoors, make sure that the person is in the shade. When the person regains consciousness, it is important that he or she remain lying down for a few minutes before attempting to get up.

64 Headache

From time to time nearly everyone suffers from headaches that develop gradually and clear up after a few hours, leaving no aftereffects. Headaches like this are unlikely to be a sign of any disorder and are usually caused by factors such as tension, tiredness, excessive consumption of alcohol or staying in an overheated or smoke-filled atmosphere. However, a headache that is severe, lasts for more than 24 hours, or recurs several times during one week should be brought to your physician's attention.

START HERE

Is your temperature 100°F (38°C) or above?

YES ▸

NO ▾

Many illnesses with fever may cause a headache.

Go to chart

59 Fever

Have you injured your head within the past few days?

YES ▸

Bruising of the brain, or a more serious form of injury, may be the cause of your symptoms. A headache following a minor head injury will probably disappear within a few hours. You should, however, consult your physician to rule out the possibility of more serious damage to the brain or skull if the pain persists for more than a day or so. If you passed out, even for a few seconds, or if you were confused, lost your memory of the accident, or have had recurrent headaches or vomited, seek medical help at once.

Treatment: In most cases, no treatment is necessary and your physician will probably advise you to take over-the-counter painkillers to ease the headache. If your physician suspects that you have suffered some internal damage, he or she will advise you to go to the hospital, where you will be fully examined and tests such as a skull X ray can be carried out. You may be admitted to the hospital and, if necessary, further investigations, including a *CT (computed tomography) scan* (opposite), may be performed to determine the extent and nature of the injury. If bleeding inside the skull or fracture of the skull is diagnosed, surgery may be needed.

NO ▾

Is your vision blurred and/or do you have eye pain?

YES ▸

NO ▾

Have you felt nauseated or been vomiting?

YES ▸

Did the headache develop before the onset of nausea or vomiting?

YES ▸

Go to next page column 2

A headache often follows an attack of vomiting.

Go to chart

94 Vomiting

NO ▾

Go to next page column 1

NO ▾

RELIEVING HEADACHE

Most minor headaches can be relieved by the following self-help measures:

- Take the recommended dose of aspirin or an aspirin substitute.
- Take a warm bath to relieve tension.
- Rest in a quiet, darkened room.

Consult your physician if such measures fail to reduce the pain, or if pain is still present the following day.

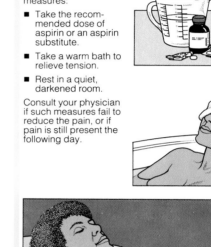

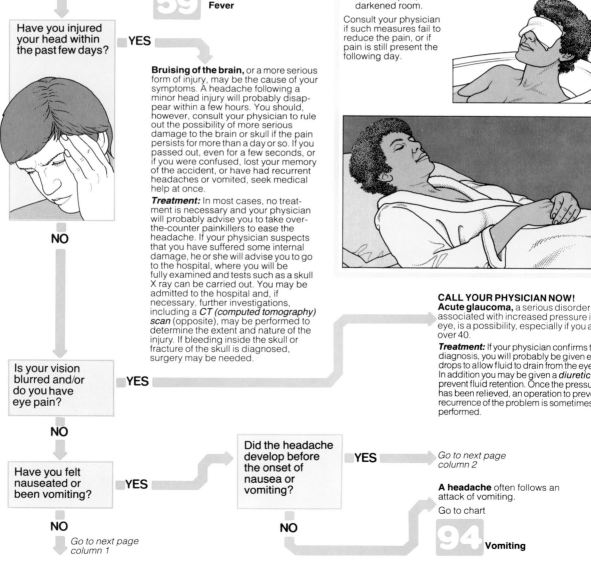

CALL YOUR PHYSICIAN NOW!
Acute glaucoma, a serious disorder associated with increased pressure in the eye, is a possibility, especially if you are over 40.

Treatment: If your physician confirms the diagnosis, you will probably be given eye drops to allow fluid to drain from the eye. In addition you may be given a *diuretic* to prevent fluid retention. Once the pressure has been relieved, an operation to prevent a recurrence of the problem is sometimes performed.

Continued from previous page, column 1

1

Continued from previous page, column 2

2

Do you have a stuffy nose?

YES

Sinusitis (inflammation of the membranes lining the air spaces in the skull) may be the cause of this problem, although it is possible that you have a common cold.

Self-help: Stay inside in a warm and humid atmosphere and take aspirin or an aspirin substitute to relieve the discomfort. If you are no better in 48 hours, consult your physician, who may prescribe *antibiotics* and *decongestants*.

NO

Did the headache occur after you had been reading or doing other close work?

YES

Muscle strain in your neck as a result of poor posture or tension from concentration is the likely cause of your headache (see *Eyestrain*, p. 184).

Self-help: In order to prevent the problem from recurring, make sure that when you read you are not sitting in an awkward position or in poor light. Periodic rest from whatever you are doing for a few minutes of relaxation will also help. If headaches recur, consult your physician, who may recommend that you have an *eye test* (p. 186).

NO

Are you sleeping poorly AND/OR are you feeling tense or under stress?

YES

Tension headaches are often caused by psychological stress.

Go to chart

73 **Anxiety**

NO

Are you currently taking any medication AND/OR are you taking a birth-control pill?

YES

Certain medications can cause headaches as a side effect. Discuss the problem with your physician. If you are taking the pill and have recurrent headaches, your physician may suggest that you use an alternative form of contraception.

See also chart

136 **Choosing a contraceptive method**

NO

Consult your physician if you are unable to make a diagnosis from this chart and if the headache persists overnight or if you develop other symptoms.

Have you suddenly begun to have a severe, throbbing pain in one or both temples?

YES

CONSULT YOUR PHYSICIAN WITHOUT DELAY!
Temporal arteritis, inflammation of the arteries of the head, is a possibility, especially if you are over 50. Urgent treatment may be needed to prevent this condition from affecting your eyesight.

Treatment: Your physician will probably prescribe medication to reduce the inflammation and it may be necessary for you to have regular blood tests to confirm that the treatment is effective.

NO

Was your vision disturbed in any way before the onset of pain?

YES

Migraine, a recurrent, severe headache that usually occurs on one side of the head, but may occasionally be on both sides, may be the explanation for your symptoms. Migraines often occur before or during menstruation. They may also be brought on by different "trigger" factors such as stress, eating cheese or chocolate, or drinking red wine. Consult your physician.

Treatment: You may find that the pain can be eased by self-help measures (see *Relieving headache,* opposite). It will also help if you can discover what causes your migraines. Your physician may offer medication if self-help measures are not effective or if the attacks recur.

NO

CONSULT YOUR PHYSICIAN WITHOUT DELAY!
Unexplained headaches, especially if severe and accompanied by additional symptoms such as nausea and vomiting, should always be brought to your physician's attention.

CT SCAN

A CT (computed tomography) scan is a safe and painless procedure that helps in the diagnosis of certain conditions. It involves hundreds of tiny X-ray pictures being taken as a camera revolves around the body. The readings are fed into a computer, which assembles them into an accurate picture of the area. CT scans can be taken of most parts of the body, but they are especially used to diagnose brain disorders.

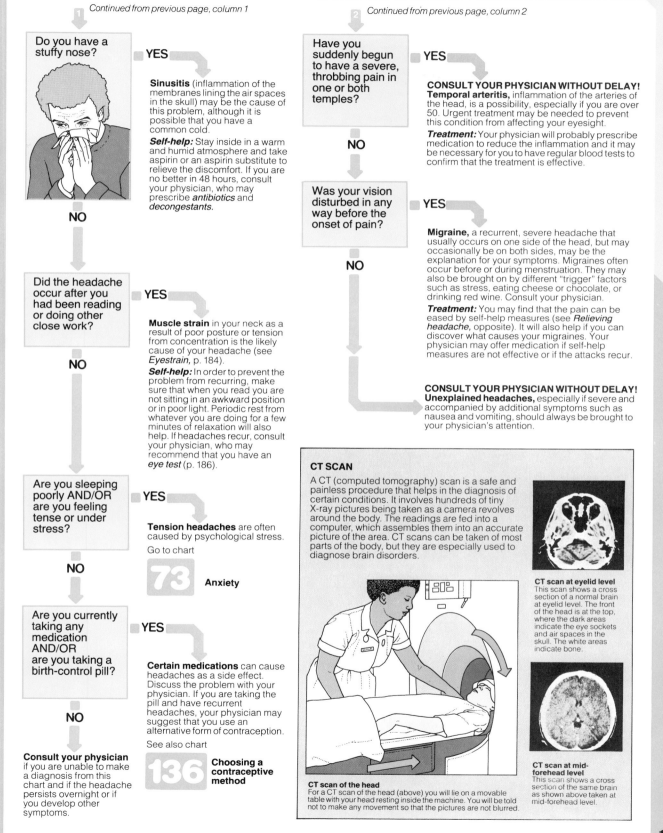

CT scan at eyelid level
This scan shows a cross section of a normal brain at eyelid level. The front of the head is at the top, where the dark areas indicate the eye sockets and air spaces in the skull. The white areas indicate bone.

CT scan at mid-forehead level
This scan shows a cross section of the same brain as shown above taken at mid-forehead level.

CT scan of the head
For a CT scan of the head (above) you will lie on a movable table with your head resting inside the machine. You will be told not to make any movement so that the pictures are not blurred.

65 Dizziness

Dizziness is a feeling of unsteadiness or that everything around you is spinning. This usually occurs when you have been spinning around – for example, on a merry-go-round. If you feel dizzy for no reason, it may be a symptom of an underlying disorder and should be brought to your physician's attention.

START HERE

Have you noticed one or more of the following symptoms since you felt dizzy?
- difficulty speaking
- temporary total or partial loss of vision in one or both eyes
- weakness in your arms or legs
- numbness and/or tingling in any part or your body

YES →

Have all your symptoms now disappeared?

YES →

CALL YOUR PHYSICIAN NOW!
A transient ischemic attack – a temporary interruption in the blood supply to the brain, sometimes linked to a narrowing of the arteries (see *How blood flows to the brain*, p. 160) – may have caused your symptoms.

Treatment: If your physician suspects that this is the problem, you will probably need to have tests, including *electrocardiography* (p. 219). At a later stage, you may need to undergo *angiography* (p. 227) or *ultrasound scanning* (p. 276) of the arteries. Treatment consists of taking steps to reduce factors that may contribute to narrowing of the arteries. These are discussed in the box on *coronary heart disease* (p. 221). You may also be prescribed medication to control high blood pressure, if you have it, and further medication to prevent the formation of blood clots. Surgery may be necessary in some cases.

NO

CALL YOUR PHYSICIAN NOW!
A stroke, a disruption in the blood supply to the brain caused by a blocked or burst blood vessel, may be the cause of these symptoms.

Treatment: If your physician suspects that you have had a stroke, admission to the hospital for observation and tests, which may include a *CT (computed tomography) scan* (p.163) is customary. If you are found to have had a stroke, you will probably be prescribed medication to prevent further strokes and may be given therapy to help restore any loss of movement. You may also be given medication to help control high blood pressure and may be advised to lose weight.

NO

Have you been vomiting AND/OR finding it difficult to keep your balance?

YES →

NO

Labyrinthitis, inflammation of the part of the inner ear that is responsible for maintaining balance (see *How you keep your balance*, right) due to viral infection, may cause these symptoms. Consult your physician.

Treatment: Your physician will examine your ears. If labyrinthitis is diagnosed, you will probably be prescribed tranquilizers to alleviate your symptoms and you will be advised to rest quietly in bed for a week or so. Most cases clear up within 3 weeks.

Have you noticed some loss of hearing AND/OR noises in the ear?

YES →

NO

Ménière's disease may be the problem. This disorder occurs when there is an increase in the amount of fluid in the labyrinth (see *How to keep your balance*, right). Ménière's disease is most common in middle age. Consult your physician.

Treatment: Your physician will probably arrange for you to undergo tests in the hospital to confirm the diagnosis. If you are found to have Ménière's disease, you will probably be given medication to reduce the amount of fluid in the labyrinth. You may be advised to cut down on your intake of salt to reduce frequency of further attacks. Occasionally, an operation is recommended.

Does turning your head or looking upwards bring on dizziness?

YES →

NO

Cervical osteoarthritis, a disorder of the bones and joints in the neck that may cause pressure on nearby nerves and blood vessels, may be the cause of this, especially if you are over 50. Consult your physician.

Treatment: Your physician may arrange for you to have an X ray of your neck. If he or she thinks that your dizziness is due to this disorder, you may be given a collar to wear for about 3 months to reduce the mobility of your neck and to relieve pressure on the nerves and blood vessels. Aspirin or an aspirin substitute can be taken to relieve any discomfort.

Consult your physician if you are unable to make a diagnosis from this chart.

HOW YOU KEEP YOUR BALANCE
The brain relies on information from the inner ear (or labyrinth) for balance as well as hearing. The acoustic nerve sends messages about your movements to the brain, where they are coordinated with other information from your eyes, limbs and muscles, to assess your exact position so that your body can make adjustments to keep balanced.

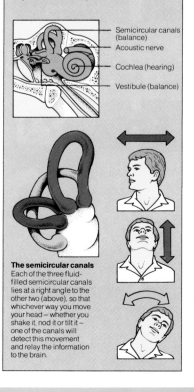

Semicircular canals (balance)
Acoustic nerve
Cochlea (hearing)
Vestibule (balance)

The semicircular canals
Each of the three fluid-filled semicircular canals lies at a right angle to the other two (above), so that whichever way you move your head – whether you shake it, nod it or tilt it – one of the canals will detect this movement and relay the information to the brain.

66 Numbness or tingling

It is normal to experience numbness or tingling if you are cold, sitting in an awkward position or sleeping on an arm. The feeling disappears as soon as you move around and is rarely a circulation problem. Numbness or tingling that occurs without apparent cause may need medical treatment.

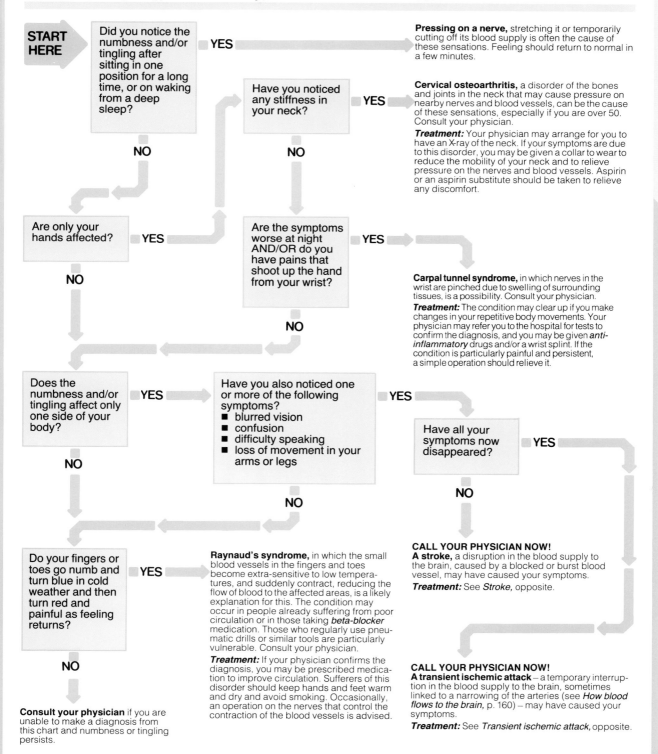

START HERE

Did you notice the numbness and/or tingling after sitting in one position for a long time, or on waking from a deep sleep?

YES → **Pressing on a nerve,** stretching it or temporarily cutting off its blood supply is often the cause of these sensations. Feeling should return to normal in a few minutes.

NO ↓

Have you noticed any stiffness in your neck?

YES → **Cervical osteoarthritis,** a disorder of the bones and joints in the neck that may cause pressure on nearby nerves and blood vessels, can be the cause of these sensations, especially if you are over 50. Consult your physician.
Treatment: Your physician may arrange for you to have an X-ray of the neck. If your symptoms are due to this disorder, you may be given a collar to wear to reduce the mobility of your neck and to relieve pressure on the nerves and blood vessels. Aspirin or an aspirin substitute should be taken to relieve any discomfort.

NO ↓

Are only your hands affected? → YES

Are the symptoms worse at night AND/OR do you have pains that shoot up the hand from your wrist?

YES → **Carpal tunnel syndrome,** in which nerves in the wrist are pinched due to swelling of surrounding tissues, is a possibility. Consult your physician.
Treatment: The condition may clear up if you make changes in your repetitive body movements. Your physician may refer you to the hospital for tests to confirm the diagnosis, and you may be given *anti-inflammatory* drugs and/or a wrist splint. If the condition is particularly painful and persistent, a simple operation should relieve it.

NO ↓

Does the numbness and/or tingling affect only one side of your body? → YES

Have you also noticed one or more of the following symptoms?
■ blurred vision
■ confusion
■ difficulty speaking
■ loss of movement in your arms or legs

YES → **Have all your symptoms now disappeared?**

YES → **CALL YOUR PHYSICIAN NOW!**
A stroke, a disruption in the blood supply to the brain, caused by a blocked or burst blood vessel, may have caused your symptoms.
Treatment: See *Stroke,* opposite.

NO ↓

NO ↓

Do your fingers or toes go numb and turn blue in cold weather and then turn red and painful as feeling returns?

YES → **Raynaud's syndrome,** in which the small blood vessels in the fingers and toes become extra-sensitive to low temperatures, and suddenly contract, reducing the flow of blood to the affected areas, is a likely explanation for this. The condition may occur in people already suffering from poor circulation or in those taking *beta-blocker* medication. Those who regularly use pneumatic drills or similar tools are particularly vulnerable. Consult your physician.
Treatment: If your physician confirms the diagnosis, you may be prescribed medication to improve circulation. Sufferers of this disorder should keep hands and feet warm and dry and avoid smoking. Occasionally, an operation on the nerves that control the contraction of the blood vessels is advised.

CALL YOUR PHYSICIAN NOW!
A transient ischemic attack – a temporary interruption in the blood supply to the brain, sometimes linked to a narrowing of the arteries (see *How blood flows to the brain,* p. 160) – may have caused your symptoms.
Treatment: See *Transient ischemic attack,* opposite.

NO ↓

Consult your physician if you are unable to make a diagnosis from this chart and numbness or tingling persists.

67 Twitching and trembling

Consult this chart if you experience any involuntary or uncontrolled movements of any part of your body. Such movements may range from slight occasional twitching of an eyelid or the corner of your mouth to persistent trembling or shaking – for example, of the hands, arms or head. In many cases, such movements are no cause for concern, being simply the result of tiredness, stress or an inherited tendency. Occasionally, however, twitching and trembling may be caused by problems that require medical treatment, such as excessive consumption of alcohol or a disorder of the thyroid gland. Involuntary movements that are accompanied by weakness of the affected part of the body should be brought to your physician's attention.

START HERE

Is your trouble confined to brief, flickering movements of one small part of the body – your eyelid, for example?

YES →

Tiredness or tension can often cause such minor twitching. This in itself is most unlikely to be a cause for concern.

NO ↓

Have you been suffering from trembling or shaking movements of any part of the body?

YES →

Are you over 55 AND is the trembling worse when the affected part of the body is at rest?

YES →

Parkinson's disease may cause such trembling. This is a disorder of nerve centers in the brain that control body coordination. Consult your physician.

Treatment: If your physician confirms the diagnosis, he or she will probably want to see you every few months to monitor the progress of your condition. In mild cases, specific treatment may not be necessary but, if trembling is severe, you may be offered drugs to relieve your symptoms.

NO ↓

Have you just cut down your alcohol intake after a period of heavy drinking?

YES →

Sudden withdrawal of alcohol can lead to uncontrolled shaking. This is a sign that you have become dangerously dependent on alcohol. Consult your physician at once (see also *The effects of alcohol*, p. 146).

Treatment: Your physician will advise you on the best way of controlling your drinking and may prescribe drugs to relieve unpleasant withdrawal symptoms. You may also be advised to contact a self-help group for alcoholics, such as Alcoholics Anonymous.

NO ↓

Have you drunk more than 5 cups of coffee or 10 cups of tea within the past 12 hours?

YES →

Caffeine poisoning in a mild form is a possibility (see *Caffeine*, p.219).

Self-help: Drink no more coffee or tea for the next few hours and your body should return to normal. If you regularly suffer from such symptoms after drinking coffee or tea, or if you have trouble sleeping, it may be advisable to cut down permanently on your regular caffeine intake.

NO ↓

Have you noticed two or more of the following symptoms?
- excessive sweating
- unexplained tiredness
- bulging eyes
- unexplained weight loss

YES →

Thyrotoxicosis (overactive thyroid gland) may cause trembling and shaking. Consult your physician.

Treatment: Your physician will probably take some blood for tests (see *Blood analysis*, p.146) and you may need to have a *radioisotope scan* (left) of the thyroid gland. Treatment usually consists of drugs, radioactive iodine or surgery to remove part of the gland.

NO ↓

A tendency to tremble or shake may be inherited. The symptoms may be brought on by stress or anxiety. Consult your physician.

Treatment: Your physician will probably check your general health to reassure you that nothing is wrong. If necessary, he or she may prescibe an *anti-anxiety* drug to relieve your symptoms.

NO ↓

Consult your physician if you are unable to make a diagnosis from this chart.

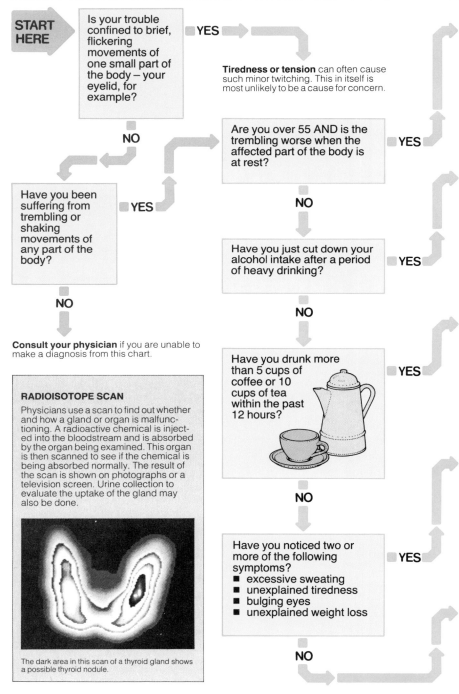

RADIOISOTOPE SCAN
Physicians use a scan to find out whether and how a gland or organ is malfunctioning. A radioactive chemical is injected into the bloodstream and is absorbed by the organ being examined. This organ is then scanned to see if the chemical is being absorbed normally. The result of the scan is shown on photographs or a television screen. Urine collection to evaluate the uptake of the gland may also be done.

The dark area in this scan of a thyroid gland shows a possible thyroid nodule.

68 Pain in the face

Consult this chart if you have pain or discomfort that is limited to the area of the face and/or forehead. Facial pain may be dull and throbbing or sharp and stabbing. It is usually caused by infection or inflammation of the underlying tissues. Although it may be distressing, it is not often a sign of a serious disorder.

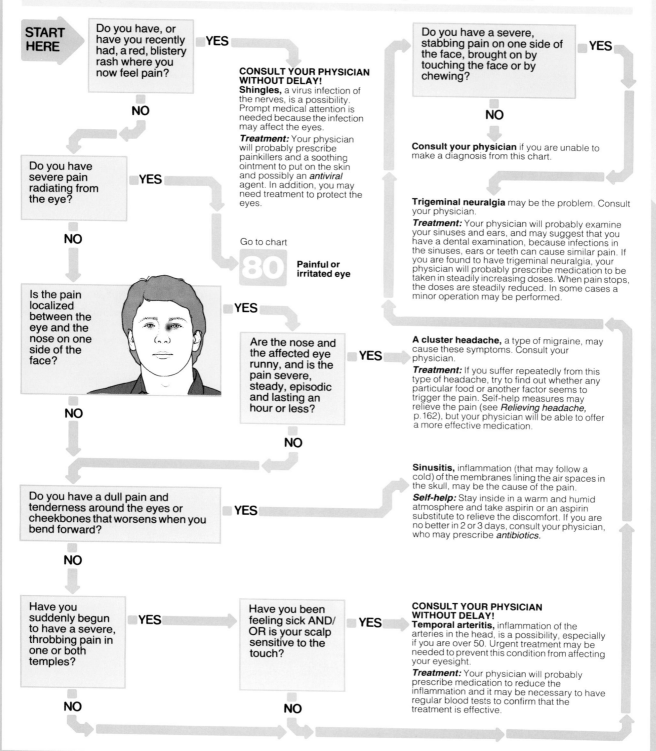

START HERE

Do you have, or have you recently had, a red, blistery rash where you now feel pain?

YES →

NO ↓

Do you have severe pain radiating from the eye?

YES →

NO ↓

Is the pain localized between the eye and the nose on one side of the face?

YES →

NO ↓

Do you have a dull pain and tenderness around the eyes or cheekbones that worsens when you bend forward?

YES →

NO ↓

Have you suddenly begun to have a severe, throbbing pain in one or both temples?

YES →

NO ↓

Are the nose and the affected eye runny, and is the pain severe, steady, episodic and lasting an hour or less?

YES →

NO ↓

Have you been feeling sick AND/OR is your scalp sensitive to the touch?

YES →

NO ↓

Do you have a severe, stabbing pain on one side of the face, brought on by touching the face or by chewing?

YES →

NO ↓

CONSULT YOUR PHYSICIAN WITHOUT DELAY!
Shingles, a virus infection of the nerves, is a possibility. Prompt medical attention is needed because the infection may affect the eyes.

Treatment: Your physician will probably prescribe painkillers and a soothing ointment to put on the skin and possibly an *antiviral* agent. In addition, you may need treatment to protect the eyes.

Go to chart

80 **Painful or irritated eye**

Consult your physician if you are unable to make a diagnosis from this chart.

Trigeminal neuralgia may be the problem. Consult your physician.

Treatment: Your physician will probably examine your sinuses and ears, and may suggest that you have a dental examination, because infections in the sinuses, ears or teeth can cause similar pain. If you are found to have trigeminal neuralgia, your physician will probably prescribe medication to be taken in steadily increasing doses. When pain stops, the doses are steadily reduced. In some cases a minor operation may be performed.

A cluster headache, a type of migraine, may cause these symptoms. Consult your physician.

Treatment: If you suffer repeatedly from this type of headache, try to find out whether any particular food or another factor seems to trigger the pain. Self-help measures may relieve the pain (see *Relieving headache,* p.162), but your physician will be able to offer a more effective medication.

Sinusitis, inflammation (that may follow a cold) of the membranes lining the air spaces in the skull, may be the cause of the pain.

Self-help: Stay inside in a warm and humid atmosphere and take aspirin or an aspirin substitute to relieve the discomfort. If you are no better in 2 or 3 days, consult your physician, who may prescribe *antibiotics.*

CONSULT YOUR PHYSICIAN WITHOUT DELAY!
Temporal arteritis, inflammation of the arteries in the head, is a possibility, especially if you are over 50. Urgent treatment may be needed to prevent this condition from affecting your eyesight.

Treatment: Your physician will probably prescribe medication to reduce the inflammation and it may be necessary to have regular blood tests to confirm that the treatment is effective.

69 Forgetfulness and confusion

We all suffer from mild forgetfulness and, to a lesser extent, confusion from time to time. Often such "absent-mindedness" happens because we are tense or preoccupied. This is no cause for concern. However, if confusion comes on suddenly or if forgetfulness and confusion are so severe that they disrupt everyday life, there may be an underlying medical disorder. This chart deals with sudden or severe confusion or forgetfulness that you are aware of in yourself or in a relative or friend who may not be aware of the problem. Remember that loss of memory for recent events is a natural aging phenomenon. Its onset occurs at different ages.

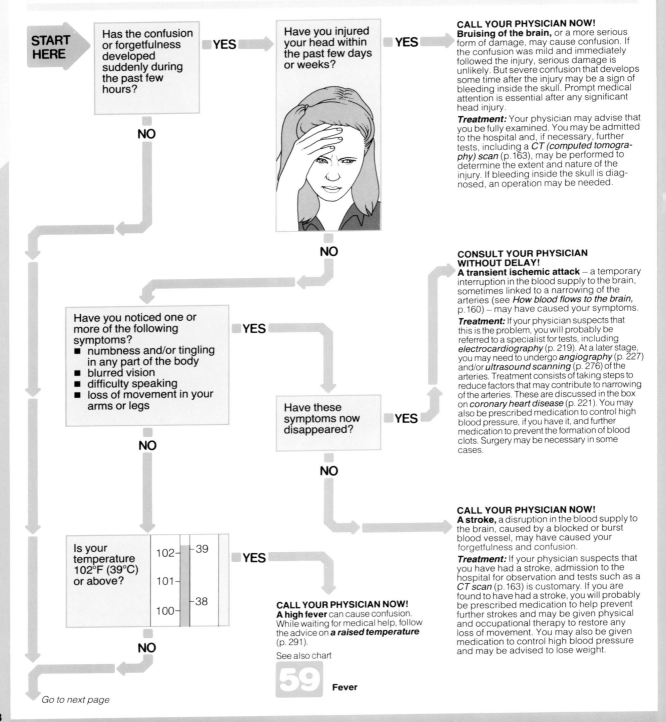

START HERE

Has the confusion or forgetfulness developed suddenly during the past few hours?

YES →

Have you injured your head within the past few days or weeks?

YES →

CALL YOUR PHYSICIAN NOW!
Bruising of the brain, or a more serious form of damage, may cause confusion. If the confusion was mild and immediately followed the injury, serious damage is unlikely. But severe confusion that develops some time after the injury may be a sign of bleeding inside the skull. Prompt medical attention is essential after any significant head injury.

Treatment: Your physician may advise that you be fully examined. You may be admitted to the hospital and, if necessary, further tests, including a *CT (computed tomography) scan* (p.163), may be performed to determine the extent and nature of the injury. If bleeding inside the skull is diagnosed, an operation may be needed.

NO (head injury)

NO

Have you noticed one or more of the following symptoms?
■ numbness and/or tingling in any part of the body
■ blurred vision
■ difficulty speaking
■ loss of movement in your arms or legs

YES →

Have these symptoms now disappeared?

YES →

CONSULT YOUR PHYSICIAN WITHOUT DELAY!
A transient ischemic attack – a temporary interruption in the blood supply to the brain, sometimes linked to a narrowing of the arteries (see *How blood flows to the brain,* p.160) – may have caused your symptoms.

Treatment: If your physician suspects that this is the problem, you will probably be referred to a specialist for tests, including *electrocardiography* (p. 219). At a later stage, you may need to undergo *angiography* (p. 227) and/or *ultrasound scanning* (p. 276) of the arteries. Treatment consists of taking steps to reduce factors that may contribute to narrowing of the arteries. These are discussed in the box on *coronary heart disease* (p. 221). You may also be prescribed medication to control high blood pressure, if you have it, and further medication to prevent the formation of blood clots. Surgery may be necessary in some cases.

NO

NO

Is your temperature 102°F (39°C) or above?

102–	–39
101–	
100–	–38

YES →

CALL YOUR PHYSICIAN NOW!
A stroke, a disruption in the blood supply to the brain, caused by a blocked or burst blood vessel, may have caused your forgetfulness and confusion.

Treatment: If your physician suspects that you have had a stroke, admission to the hospital for observation and tests such as a *CT scan* (p.163) is customary. If you are found to have had a stroke, you will probably be prescribed medication to help prevent further strokes and may be given physical and occupational therapy to restore any loss of movement. You may also be given medication to control high blood pressure and may be advised to lose weight.

CALL YOUR PHYSICIAN NOW!
A high fever can cause confusion. While waiting for medical help, follow the advice on *a raised temperature* (p. 291).

See also chart

59 **Fever**

NO

Go to next page

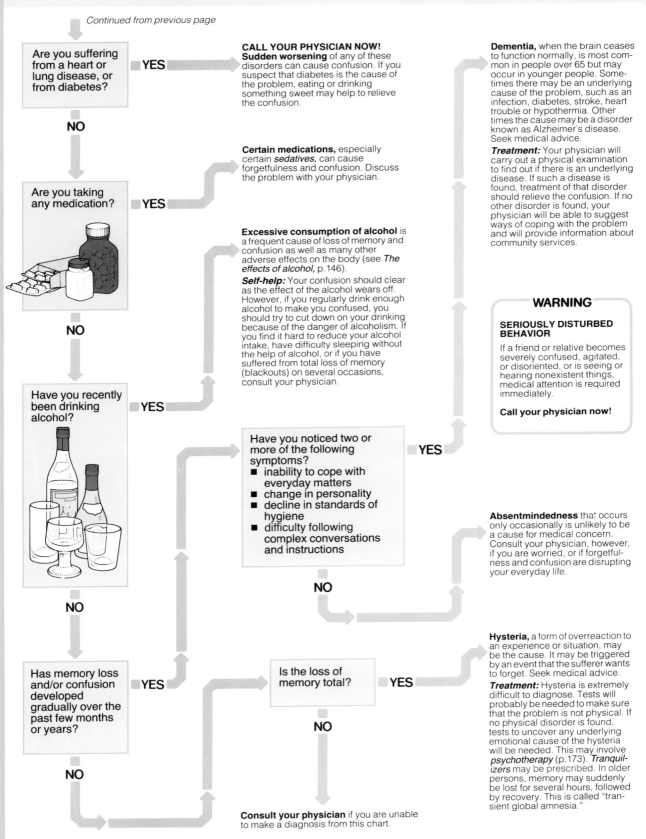

Continued from previous page

Are you suffering from a heart or lung disease, or from diabetes?

YES → **CALL YOUR PHYSICIAN NOW!**
Sudden worsening of any of these disorders can cause confusion. If you suspect that diabetes is the cause of the problem, eating or drinking something sweet may help to relieve the confusion.

NO

Are you taking any medication?

YES → **Certain medications,** especially certain *sedatives,* can cause forgetfulness and confusion. Discuss the problem with your physician.

NO

Have you recently been drinking alcohol?

YES → **Excessive consumption of alcohol** is a frequent cause of loss of memory and confusion as well as many other adverse effects on the body (see *The effects of alcohol,* p.146).
Self-help: Your confusion should clear as the effect of the alcohol wears off. However, if you regularly drink enough alcohol to make you confused, you should try to cut down on your drinking because of the danger of alcoholism. If you find it hard to reduce your alcohol intake, have difficulty sleeping without the help of alcohol, or if you have suffered from total loss of memory (blackouts) on several occasions, consult your physician.

NO

Has memory loss and/or confusion developed gradually over the past few months or years?

YES →

NO

Have you noticed two or more of the following symptoms?
- inability to cope with everyday matters
- change in personality
- decline in standards of hygiene
- difficulty following complex conversations and instructions

YES →

NO

Is the loss of memory total?

YES →

NO

Consult your physician if you are unable to make a diagnosis from this chart.

Dementia, when the brain ceases to function normally, is most common in people over 65 but may occur in younger people. Sometimes there may be an underlying cause of the problem, such as an infection, diabetes, stroke, heart trouble or hypothermia. Other times the cause may be a disorder known as Alzheimer's disease. Seek medical advice.
Treatment: Your physician will carry out a physical examination to find out if there is an underlying disease. If such a disease is found, treatment of that disorder should relieve the confusion. If no other disorder is found, your physician will be able to suggest ways of coping with the problem and will provide information about community services.

Absentmindedness that occurs only occasionally is unlikely to be a cause for medical concern. Consult your physician, however, if you are worried, or if forgetfulness and confusion are disrupting your everyday life.

Hysteria, a form of overreaction to an experience or situation, may be the cause. It may be triggered by an event that the sufferer wants to forget. Seek medical advice.
Treatment: Hysteria is extremely difficult to diagnose. Tests will probably be needed to make sure that the problem is not physical. If no physical disorder is found, tests to uncover any underlying emotional cause of the hysteria will be needed. This may involve *psychotherapy* (p.173). *Tranquilizers* may be prescribed. In older persons, memory may suddenly be lost for several hours, followed by recovery. This is called "transient global amnesia."

WARNING

SERIOUSLY DISTURBED BEHAVIOR

If a friend or relative becomes severely confused, agitated, or disoriented, or is seeing or hearing nonexistent things, medical attention is required immediately.

Call your physician now!

---

70 Difficulty speaking

Consult this chart if you have difficulty finding, using or defining words, or if your speech becomes slurred or unclear. Such speech difficulties may be related to disorders or medication affecting the speech centers in the brain or they may be due to a disorder affecting the movement of the mouth or tongue.

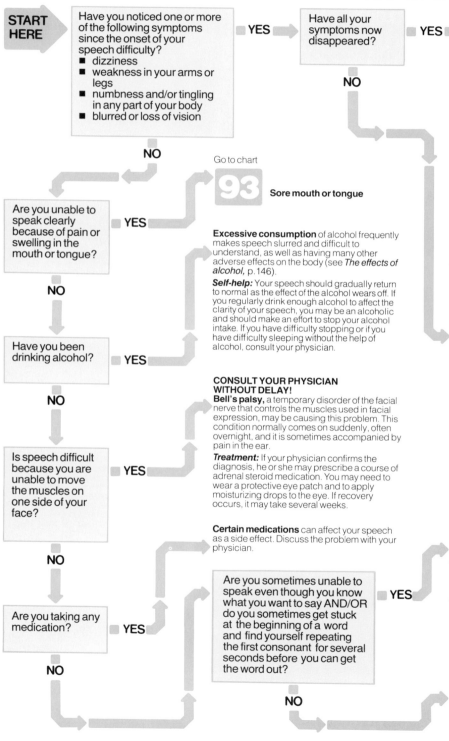

START HERE

Have you noticed one or more of the following symptoms since the onset of your speech difficulty?
- dizziness
- weakness in your arms or legs
- numbness and/or tingling in any part of your body
- blurred or loss of vision

YES →

Have all your symptoms now disappeared?

YES →

NO

NO

Go to chart

93 Sore mouth or tongue

Are you unable to speak clearly because of pain or swelling in the mouth or tongue?

YES

NO

Excessive consumption of alcohol frequently makes speech slurred and difficult to understand, as well as having many other adverse effects on the body (see *The effects of alcohol,* p.146).
Self-help: Your speech should gradually return to normal as the effect of the alcohol wears off. If you regularly drink enough alcohol to affect the clarity of your speech, you may be an alcoholic and should make an effort to stop your alcohol intake. If you have difficulty stopping or if you have difficulty sleeping without the help of alcohol, consult your physician.

Have you been drinking alcohol?

YES

NO

CONSULT YOUR PHYSICIAN WITHOUT DELAY!
Bell's palsy, a temporary disorder of the facial nerve that controls the muscles used in facial expression, may be causing this problem. This condition normally comes on suddenly, often overnight, and it is sometimes accompanied by pain in the ear.
Treatment: If your physician confirms the diagnosis, he or she may prescribe a course of adrenal steroid medication. You may need to wear a protective eye patch and to apply moisturizing drops to the eye. If recovery occurs, it may take several weeks.

Is speech difficult because you are unable to move the muscles on one side of your face?

YES

NO

Certain medications can affect your speech as a side effect. Discuss the problem with your physician.

Are you taking any medication?

YES

NO

Are you sometimes unable to speak even though you know what you want to say AND/OR do you sometimes get stuck at the beginning of a word and find yourself repeating the first consonant for several seconds before you can get the word out?

YES

NO

CALL YOUR PHYSICIAN NOW!
A transient ischemic attack – a temporary interruption in the blood supply to the brain, sometimes linked to a narrowing of the arteries (see *How blood flows to the brain,* p.160) – may have caused your symptoms.

Treatment: If your physician suspects that this is the problem, you will probably be referred to a specialist for tests, including *electrocardiography* (p. 219). At a later stage, you may need to undergo *angiography* (p. 227) and/or an *ultrasound scan* (p. 276) of the arteries. Treatment consists of taking steps to reduce factors that may contribute to narrowing of the arteries. These are discussed in the box on *coronary heart disease* (p. 221). You may also be prescribed medication to control high blood pressure, if you have it, and further medication to prevent the formation of blood clots. Surgery may be necessary in some cases.

CALL YOUR PHYSICIAN NOW!
A stroke, a disruption in the blood supply to the brain, caused by a blocked or burst blood vessel, may be the cause of these symptoms.

Treatment: If your physician suspects that you have had a stroke, admission to the hospital for observation and tests, which may include a *CT (computed tomography) scan* (p.163), is customary. If you are found to have had a stroke, you will probably be prescribed medication to help prevent further strokes and may be given speech therapy to help overcome your speech difficulty. Physical and occupational therapy will probably be ordered also. You may also be given medication to control high blood pressure and may be advised to lose weight.

Stuttering may be brought on or made worse by anxiety, particularly if you had this trouble in early childhood.
Self-help: Many stutterers find that their speech improves if they try to relax and speak more slowly. If your stutter is so severe that it makes communication difficult, consult your physician, who may refer you to a speech therapist.

CONSULT YOUR PHYSICIAN WITHOUT DELAY!
Unexplained difficulty speaking may be an early sign of an underlying disorder of the brain or nervous system, and early treatment is important.

71 Disturbing thoughts and feelings

Consult this chart if you begin to have thoughts and feelings that worry you or that seem to you or to others to be abnormal or unhealthy. Such feelings may include aggressive or sexual thoughts and unfamiliar or uncontrolled emotions. If your thoughts and feelings continue to worry you, whatever your particular problem, talk to your physician, who may be able to help you put your feelings into proper context and offer treatment where appropriate. Simply talking about your problem may make you feel better.

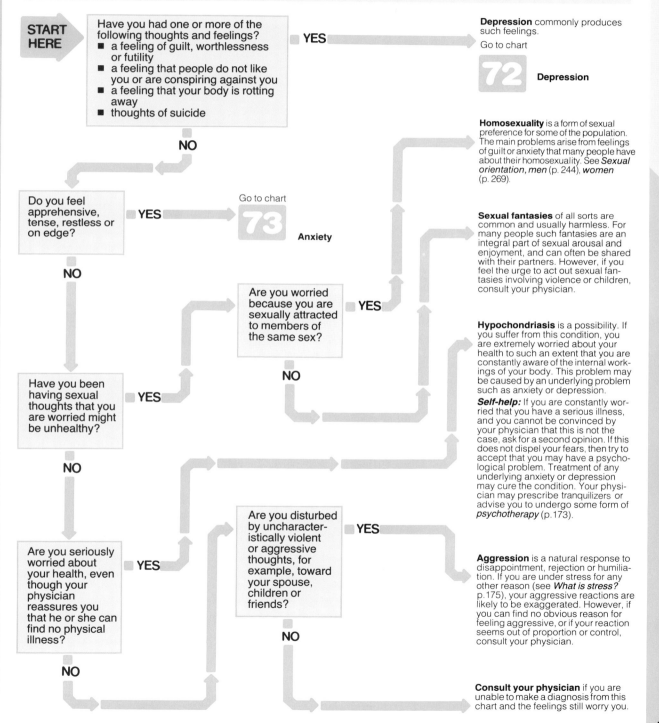

START HERE

Have you had one or more of the following thoughts and feelings?
- a feeling of guilt, worthlessness or futility
- a feeling that people do not like you or are conspiring against you
- a feeling that your body is rotting away
- thoughts of suicide

YES — **Depression** commonly produces such feelings.

Go to chart

72 **Depression**

NO

Do you feel apprehensive, tense, restless or on edge?

YES — Go to chart

73 **Anxiety**

NO

Have you been having sexual thoughts that you are worried might be unhealthy?

YES — Are you worried because you are sexually attracted to members of the same sex?

YES — **Homosexuality** is a form of sexual preference for some of the population. The main problems arise from feelings of guilt or anxiety that many people have about their homosexuality. See *Sexual orientation, men* (p. 244), *women* (p. 269).

NO — **Sexual fantasies** of all sorts are common and usually harmless. For many people such fantasies are an integral part of sexual arousal and enjoyment, and can often be shared with their partners. However, if you feel the urge to act out sexual fantasies involving violence or children, consult your physician.

NO

Are you seriously worried about your health, even though your physician reassures you that he or she can find no physical illness?

YES — **Hypochondriasis** is a possibility. If you suffer from this condition, you are extremely worried about your health to such an extent that you are constantly aware of the internal workings of your body. This problem may be caused by an underlying problem such as anxiety or depression.

Self-help: If you are constantly worried that you have a serious illness, and you cannot be convinced by your physician that this is not the case, ask for a second opinion. If this does not dispel your fears, then try to accept that you may have a psychological problem. Treatment of any underlying anxiety or depression may cure the condition. Your physician may prescribe tranquilizers or advise you to undergo some form of *psychotherapy* (p.173).

Are you disturbed by uncharacteristically violent or aggressive thoughts, for example, toward your spouse, children or friends?

YES — (leads up to Aggression / Hypochondriasis section)

NO

Aggression is a natural response to disappointment, rejection or humiliation. If you are under stress for any other reason (see *What is stress?* p.175), your aggressive reactions are likely to be exaggerated. However, if you can find no obvious reason for feeling aggressive, or if your reaction seems out of proportion or control, consult your physician.

NO

Consult your physician if you are unable to make a diagnosis from this chart and the feelings still worry you.

72 Depression

Most people have minor ups and downs in mood, feeling particularly good one day but low the next. This is often due to an identifiable cause, and quickly passes. More severe depression, characterized by feelings of futility and guilt and often with physical symptoms such as headache, insomnia, lack of appetite, loss of weight, constipation and delusion, is sometimes brought on by some major event, such as bereavement, divorce or becoming unemployed. Some people, however, are prone to repeated attacks of depression that have no apparent cause. Also, there are certain times when we are more susceptible to depression – for instance, during adolescence, after having a baby, at middle age and at retirement.

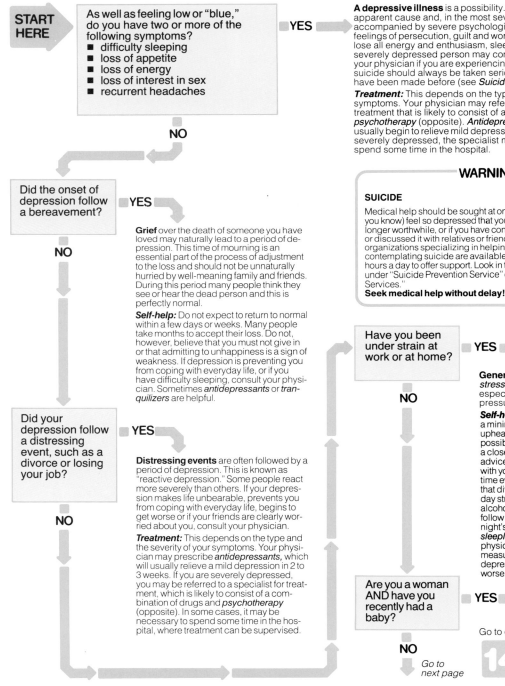

START HERE

As well as feeling low or "blue," do you have two or more of the following symptoms?
- difficulty sleeping
- loss of appetite
- loss of energy
- loss of interest in sex
- recurrent headaches

YES

A depressive illness is a possibility. This often develops with no apparent cause and, in the most severe cases, it may be accompanied by severe psychological symptoms such as feelings of persecution, guilt and worthlessness. Some sufferers lose all energy and enthusiasm, sleep poorly and wake early. A severely depressed person may contemplate suicide. Consult your physician if you are experiencing these feelings. A threat of suicide should always be taken seriously, even if such threats have been made before (see *Suicide*, below).

Treatment: This depends on the type and severity of your symptoms. Your physician may refer you to a specialist for treatment that is likely to consist of a combination of drugs and *psychotherapy* (opposite). *Antidepressants,* if prescribed, usually begin to relieve mild depression in 2 or 3 weeks. If you are severely depressed, the specialist may recommend that you spend some time in the hospital.

NO

Did the onset of depression follow a bereavement?

YES

Grief over the death of someone you have loved may naturally lead to a period of depression. This time of mourning is an essential part of the process of adjustment to the loss and should not be unnaturally hurried by well-meaning family and friends. During this period many people think they see or hear the dead person and this is perfectly normal.

Self-help: Do not expect to return to normal within a few days or weeks. Many people take months to accept their loss. Do not, however, believe that you must not give in or that admitting to unhappiness is a sign of weakness. If depression is preventing you from coping with everyday life, or if you have difficulty sleeping, consult your physician. Sometimes *antidepressants* or *tranquilizers* are helpful.

NO

WARNING

SUICIDE

Medical help should be sought at once if you (or someone you know) feel so depressed that you think that life is no longer worthwhile, or if you have contemplated suicide or discussed it with relatives or friends. Voluntary organizations specializing in helping people who are contemplating suicide are available on the telephone 24 hours a day to offer support. Look in the telephone book under "Suicide Prevention Service" or "Mental Health Services."
Seek medical help without delay!

Did your depression follow a distressing event, such as a divorce or losing your job?

YES

Distressing events are often followed by a period of depression. This is known as "reactive depression." Some people react more severely than others. If your depression makes life unbearable, prevents you from coping with everyday life, begins to get worse or if your friends are clearly worried about you, consult your physician.

Treatment: This depends on the type and the severity of your symptoms. Your physician may prescribe *antidepressants,* which will usually relieve a mild depression in 2 to 3 weeks. If you are severely depressed, you may be referred to a specialist for treatment, which is likely to consist of a combination of drugs and *psychotherapy* (opposite). In some cases, it may be necessary to spend some time in the hospital, where treatment can be supervised.

NO

Have you been under strain at work or at home?

YES

Generalized stress (see *What is stress?* p. 175) may be the cause, especially if you have felt under pressure for a long period.

Self-help: Try to keep stress to a minimum by avoiding major upheavals in your life as much as possible. Discuss your feelings with a close friend and listen to his or her advice about how you might cope with your problems. Devote some time every day to physical relaxation that diverts your mind from day-to-day strain and worry. Keep your alcohol consumption down. Also, follow the advice on getting a good night's sleep (see *Preventing sleeplessness* (p. 153). Consult your physician if you feel that the self-help measures are not working, or if your depression seems to be getting worse.

NO

Are you a woman AND have you recently had a baby?

YES

Go to chart

Depression after childbirth

NO

Go to next page

Continued from previous page

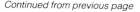

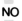

Are you a woman AND do you feel depressed or irritable in the days before your period?

YES

NO

Premenstrual syndrome (PMS) is a common occurrence. It can vary from anything as mild as a feeling of moderate unhappiness to a depression so severe that it affects all bodily functions. It is often accompanied by increased irritability, aggression and physical symptoms such as a slight increase in weight, lower abdominal pain, bloated stomach and swollen ankles, which make matters worse (see *The menstrual cycle*, p. 253). If your symptoms are severe enough to interfere with your day-to-day routine, consult your physician.

Treatment: Your physician will reassure you and advise you to keep premenstrual days as nonstressful as possible. He or she may also prescribe drugs to counteract the physical symptoms (see *Treatment of menstrual problems*, p. 255).

Have you recently recovered from an infectious illness, such as the flu or infectious mononucleosis?

YES

NO

Infectious illnesses are often followed by a period of depression.

Self-help: Do not try to return to your normal routine too quickly after you have had such an illness. Make sure that you eat well and get plenty of sleep to allow your strength to build up. If your depression lasts longer than 2 weeks, consult your physician, who may prescribe an *antidepressant*.

Have you been drinking alcohol every day for a prolonged period?

YES

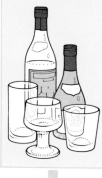

NO

Regular consumption of alcohol, even in seemingly moderate amounts over a period of time, has a depressive effect on the body and mind, and this may persist on days when you have had no alcohol (see *The effects of alcohol*, p. 146).

Self-help: Your depression should clear if you stop drinking alcohol. If you find it difficult to cut down on the amount of alcohol you drink, or your depression persists or begins to get worse, consult your physician.

Emotional instability in the years surrounding the menopause may be the cause of your depression. Social and psychological factors such as fear of approaching old age and curtailment of opportunities for advancement in your job may contribute to depression. A further complication is the hormonal upheaval that takes place at this age, sometimes with unpleasant symptoms such as hot flashes and dryness or itching of the vagina (see *The menopause*, p. 252).

Are you between 40 and 55 years old?

YES

Self-help: Try to accept that the menopause is a natural fact of life. Discuss your feelings with your partner or with friends in a similar position. You may find it helpful to find new interests – for example, starting a job, if you have not been working, or taking up a new hobby. Maintain your physical health by ensuring that you do not become overweight (see *How to lose weight*, p. 151) and exercise regularly (see *Fitness and exercise*, p. 36). If these measures do not work, or if your depression is so severe that you cannot cope, consult your physician, who will examine you to make sure that there is no underlying disorder. He or she may recommend hormone replacement therapy (see *The menopause*, p. 252) and, possibly, an *antidepressant*.

NO

Are you currently taking any medication?

YES

NO

Certain drugs, especially sedatives, can cause depression. Discuss the problem with your physician.

Consult your physician if you are unable to find a cause for your depression from this chart.

PSYCHOTHERAPY

Psychotherapy is the treatment of psychological problems by a therapist who encourages you to talk about your feelings and fears, and who can provide expert help and advice. This process may range from talking about your troubles with your own physician, to an extended course of psychoanalysis with a psychiatrist. The more common forms of psychotherapy are described here. Many therapists combine one or more of these forms along with medication.

Group therapy

This involves a number of sessions during which the therapist guides a discussion among a group of people with a problem in common. The advantage of group psychotherapy is that the members of the group gain strength from knowing that other people have the same problem and that they can learn from each other's experiences. There is also a certain amount of group pressure to develop a healthier attitude to personal problems and group support for this attitude to continue.

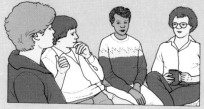

Behavior therapy

This is usually used in the treatment of specific phobias, such as fear of flying, or fear of dogs or spiders. In one form of behavior therapy known as desensitization, the sufferer is gradually helped by the therapist to overcome the fear. For example, in the case of fear of flying, the therapist encourages you to imagine the events associated with the flight – taking a bus to the airport, waiting in the terminal, dealing with the ticket agent, boarding, and finally sitting on the plane while it taxis on the runway, takes off and lands. Later, when you actually come to fly, you will feel as though you have been through it before and it will hold no fear for you.

Another method, called flooding, involves a confrontation, under the supervision of your therapist, with the object of your fears in an extreme form – for example, a confrontation with a dog as treatment for fear of dogs. Experiencing the worst imaginable degree of exposure helps you to realize that all along there has been no real danger involved and that your fear has been exaggerated. Both methods should be attempted only under the guidance of a trained therapist.

Psychoanalysis

This form of psychotherapy, based on the belief that much human behavior is determined by early childhood conflicts, was developed in the late 19th and early 20th centuries. Psychoanalysis involves a series of meetings with a psychoanalyst during which he or she will encourage you to talk at will. He or she may ask occasional questions to guide the direction of your thoughts. By listening to your recollections, thoughts and feelings, he or she may be able to pinpoint the root of your problem and, through discussion, enable you to reach a better understanding of yourself and help you reconcile any internal conflicts.

73 Anxiety

If you are suffering from anxiety, you will feel tense and unable to concentrate, think clearly or sleep well. Some people have headaches, chest pains, palpitations, backache, abdominal distress and a general feeling of tired- ness. This is often a natural reaction to a stressful situation and is only temporary. Other people, however, suffer from anxiety that comes on without apparent cause and persists for long periods.

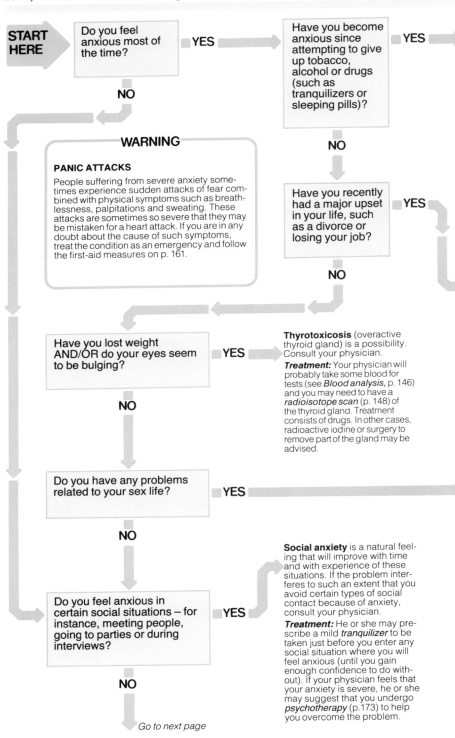

START HERE

Do you feel anxious most of the time?
YES →
NO ↓

Have you become anxious since attempting to give up tobacco, alcohol or drugs (such as tranquilizers or sleeping pills)?
YES →
NO ↓

Sudden withdrawal of these substances may precipitate feelings of anxiety. Consult your physician.
Treatment: Your physician will advise you on the best way to deal with your addiction and monitor your progress. He or she may prescribe a short course of medication to help alleviate anxiety during the withdrawal period. In order to reduce the possibility of you reverting to addiction, it may be necessary for you to undergo some form of ***psychotherapy*** (p. 173). Your physician will be able to put you in touch with one of the many self-help organizations that exist, where you will be able to talk about your problems with people in the same position. This way you will gain strength from hearing about how other people have coped with the same problem.

WARNING

PANIC ATTACKS

People suffering from severe anxiety sometimes experience sudden attacks of fear combined with physical symptoms such as breathlessness, palpitations and sweating. These attacks are sometimes so severe that they may be mistaken for a heart attack. If you are in any doubt about the cause of such symptoms, treat the condition as an emergency and follow the first-aid measures on p. 161.

Have you recently had a major upset in your life, such as a divorce or losing your job?
YES →
NO ↓

Stress, as a result of this major upset, is probably making you feel anxious (see *What is stress?* opposite).
Self-help: It is important to minimize your general stress level if you have recently suffered a major upset in your life (for instance, if you have just been divorced, changed jobs or are taking on new responsibilities). Make sure that you eat regular meals and do not drink too much alcohol — otherwise, your body may be put under more strain (see *The effects of stress,* opposite). If your anxiety becomes so severe that you feel that you can no longer cope with everyday life, consult your physician.

Have you lost weight AND/OR do your eyes seem to be bulging?
YES →
NO ↓

Thyrotoxicosis (overactive thyroid gland) is a possibility. Consult your physician.
Treatment: Your physician will probably take some blood for tests (see *Blood analysis,* p. 146) and you may need to have a *radioisotope scan* (p. 148) of the thyroid gland. Treatment consists of drugs. In other cases, radioactive iodine or surgery to remove part of the gland may be advised.

Do you have any problems related to your sex life?
YES →
NO ↓

Anxiety about sex is a common occurrence. Possible causes of worry may include fear of pregnancy or of contracting a sexually transmitted disease. Or you may be concerned about a specific sex problem such as pain during intercourse or a difficulty affecting your partner.
Self-help: If you have a regular partner, discuss your feelings. Talking about sex openly is often the best way to solve and alleviate feelings of anxiety. It is important that you be aware of your partner's feelings and vice versa. If this does not help because you are unable to communicate satisfactorily with each other, or you do not have a regular partner with whom you can talk, consult your physician, who will be able to offer helpful advice or possibly refer you for *sex counseling* (p. 268). For diagnosis of specific sex problems, see *Special problems: men, women,* pp. 233-272.

Do you feel anxious in certain social situations — for instance, meeting people, going to parties or during interviews?
YES →
NO ↓

Social anxiety is a natural feeling that will improve with time and with experience of these situations. If the problem interferes to such an extent that you avoid certain types of social contact because of anxiety, consult your physician.
Treatment: He or she may prescribe a mild *tranquilizer* to be taken just before you enter any social situation where you will feel anxious (until you gain enough confidence to do without). If your physician feels that your anxiety is severe, he or she may suggest that you undergo *psychotherapy* (p.173) to help you overcome the problem.

Go to next page

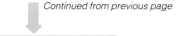

Continued from previous page

Do you feel anxious only when confronted with specific objects of fear or if you are prevented from doing things in your usual way?

YES →

NO →

A phobia or compulsive disorder may cause your anxiety. A phobia is an irrational fear of a specific object or situation. For instance, you may have a fear of enclosed spaces (claustrophobia). If you have a compulsive disorder, you feel an irresistible need to behave in a certain fashion, even though you may know that it is unreasonable. For example, you may feel that you have to walk to work on the same side of the street and, if prevented from doing so, you worry about it. Consult your physician.

Treatment: Your physician will try to discover the underlying cause of the problem and may be able to reassure you that your worries and fears are understandable but that it is possible to come to terms with them. He or she may decide that *antidepressants* or *tranquilizers* will help. If your symptoms are severe, he or she may refer you for *psychotherapy* (p. 173).

Consult your physician if you are unable to make a diagnosis from this chart and unexplained feelings of anxiety persist.

WHAT IS STRESS?

Stress refers to physical or mental demands that require an increased response from the body. Stress can be caused by changes in daily routine, including changes for the better – getting married or having a baby – as well as for the worse – losing a job or getting divorced. The greater the change, the more stress you will suffer. A single major event such as the death of a close relative may, on its own, equal the stress resulting from an accumulation of smaller changes such as a change in job responsibilities, a move to a new house or a vacation overseas.

The effects of stress

A certain amount of stress can be beneficial when it excites and stimulates the body and improves performance. However, as stress levels continue to rise, helpful stimulation becomes replaced by fatigue and, if stress is not reduced, may increase susceptibility to physical and mental illness. Everybody has a different level of toler-

ance to stress; some people never seem to suffer harmful effects from seemingly high levels of stress in their lives, while others can cope with only a few changes at a time without becoming anxious, depressed or physically ill.

Some of the most common disorders that may be caused by or made worse by stress are:

- Mental and emotional problems, including anxiety and depression
- Asthma
- Mouth ulcers
- Angina and some other heart conditions
- Stomach or duodenal ulcers
- Ulcerative colitis; irritable bowel (see p. 210)
- Stuttering
- Skin problems, including eczema and psoriasis
- Cessation of periods
- Certain forms of hair loss

RELAXATION TECHNIQUES

Some people manage to remain relaxed and easygoing no matter how much strain they are under at work or at home. Others become tense and worried as a result of even minor stresses (see *What is stress?* above). If you are one of the latter type, learning to relax may help mitigate the harmful effects of stress and enable you to cope with problems more easily. Try practicing some of the simple relaxation techniques described below once or twice a day. See also *Preventing sleeplessness* (p. 153).

Breathing exercises

Try taking deep rather than shallow breaths. To develop the habit, sit or lie in a comfortable position and breathe deeply and slowly for one minute, counting the number of breaths you take. Try to reduce your breathing rate so that you take half as many breaths as you normally do during a minute. Try this twice daily.

Meditation

Meditation involves emptying the mind of all distractions, thoughts and worries. Try the following method:

1 Find a quiet part of the house and sit in a comfortable chair with your eyes closed.

2 Without moving your lips, repeat a word silently to yourself, paying attention only to this action. Do not choose a word that has any emotional overtones. If your mind wanders, do not fight this new train of thought but continue to focus your attention on the unspoken sound of the word. (Some people find it easier to concentrate on something visual – a door knob or a vase of flowers – rather than a word).

3 Do this for 5 minutes twice a day for a week, then gradually increase the meditation period until you can manage about 20 minutes at each session.

Muscle relaxation exercises
Try these exercises each evening or at other times if you feel tense. Wear comfortable clothes that enable you to move freely.

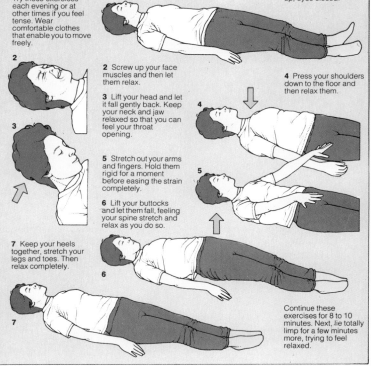

1 Lie on the floor, face up, eyes closed.

2 Screw up your face muscles and then let them relax.

3 Lift your head and let it fall gently back. Keep your neck and jaw relaxed so that you can feel your throat opening.

4 Press your shoulders down to the floor and then relax them.

5 Stretch out your arms and fingers. Hold them rigid for a moment before easing the strain completely.

6 Lift your buttocks and let them fall, feeling your spine stretch and relax as you do so.

7 Keep your heels together, stretch your legs and toes. Then relax completely.

Continue these exercises for 8 to 10 minutes. Next, lie totally limp for a few minutes more, trying to feel relaxed.

74 Hair and scalp problems

Hair grows over the whole surface of the human body, except the palms and soles, and grows especially thickly on the head, in the armpits and in the genital area. Your hair color and type are inherited, but your hair's condition may be affected by your overall health, your diet and the environment. This chart pinpoints common problems affecting hair on the head and the condition of the scalp.

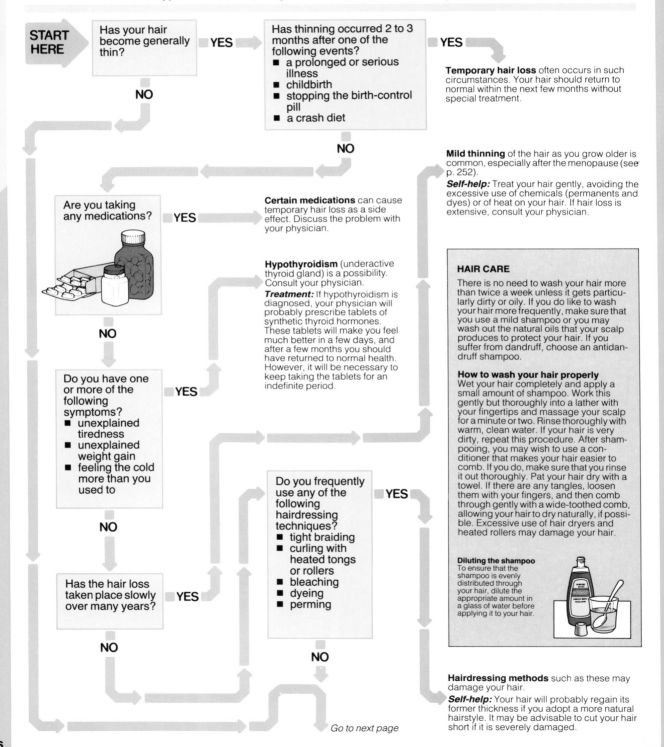

START HERE

Has your hair become generally thin?

YES → **Has thinning occurred 2 to 3 months after one of the following events?**
- a prolonged or serious illness
- childbirth
- stopping the birth-control pill
- a crash diet

YES → **Temporary hair loss** often occurs in such circumstances. Your hair should return to normal within the next few months without special treatment.

NO

Mild thinning of the hair as you grow older is common, especially after the menopause (see p. 252).

Self-help: Treat your hair gently, avoiding the excessive use of chemicals (permanents and dyes) or of heat on your hair. If hair loss is extensive, consult your physician.

Are you taking any medications?

YES → **Certain medications** can cause temporary hair loss as a side effect. Discuss the problem with your physician.

NO

Hypothyroidism (underactive thyroid gland) is a possibility. Consult your physician.

Treatment: If hypothyroidism is diagnosed, your physician will probably prescribe tablets of synthetic thyroid hormones. These tablets will make you feel much better in a few days, and after a few months you should have returned to normal health. However, it will be necessary to keep taking the tablets for an indefinite period.

Do you have one or more of the following symptoms?
- unexplained tiredness
- unexplained weight gain
- feeling the cold more than you used to

YES

NO

Do you frequently use any of the following hairdressing techniques?
- tight braiding
- curling with heated tongs or rollers
- bleaching
- dyeing
- perming

YES

Has the hair loss taken place slowly over many years?

YES

NO

NO

Go to next page

Hairdressing methods such as these may damage your hair.

Self-help: Your hair will probably regain its former thickness if you adopt a more natural hairstyle. It may be advisable to cut your hair short if it is severely damaged.

HAIR CARE

There is no need to wash your hair more than twice a week unless it gets particularly dirty or oily. If you do like to wash your hair more frequently, make sure that you use a mild shampoo or you may wash out the natural oils that your scalp produces to protect your hair. If you suffer from dandruff, choose an antidandruff shampoo.

How to wash your hair properly

Wet your hair completely and apply a small amount of shampoo. Work this gently but thoroughly into a lather with your fingertips and massage your scalp for a minute or two. Rinse thoroughly with warm, clean water. If your hair is very dirty, repeat this procedure. After shampooing, you may wish to use a conditioner that makes your hair easier to comb. If you do, make sure that you rinse it out thoroughly. Pat your hair dry with a towel. If there are any tangles, loosen them with your fingers, and then comb through gently with a wide-toothed comb, allowing your hair to dry naturally, if possible. Excessive use of hair dryers and heated rollers may damage your hair.

Diluting the shampoo
To ensure that the shampoo is evenly distributed through your hair, dilute the appropriate amount in a glass of water before applying it to your hair.

Continued from previous page

Have one or more bald patches suddenly developed?

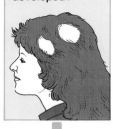

YES

Patchy hair loss may be the result of fungal infection (especially if the scalp is inflamed and itchy) or of alopecia areata (a condition that may be related to emotional stress). Consult your physician.

Treatment: Fungal infection of the scalp is usually treated by an *antifungal* lotion and possibly a course of antifungal tablets. Alopecia areata often clears up without treatment and new hair grows within 6 to 9 months.

NO

Is your scalp flaky and/or itchy?

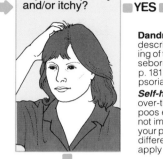

YES

Dandruff is the name used to describe excessive flaking and itching of the scalp. It may be caused by seborrheic dermatitis (see *Eczema*, p. 181) or, less commonly, by psoriasis.

Self-help: Use one of the many over-the-counter *antidandruff* shampoos every 2 to 3 days. If this does not improve the condition, consult your physician, who may prescribe a different shampoo and/or a lotion to apply to your scalp.

NO

Consult your physician if you are unable to make a diagnosis from this chart.

---

75 Nail problems

Fingernails and toenails are made of hard, dead tissue called keratin that protects the sensitive tips of the fingers and toes from damage. Any abnormalities or **diseases affecting the nails may be unsightly and irritating, but they are not harmful to health. Trim your nails regularly.**

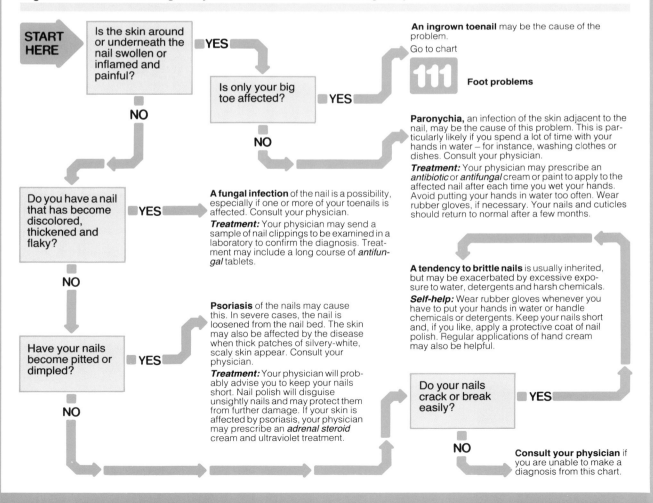

START HERE

Is the skin around or underneath the nail swollen or inflamed and painful?

YES

Is only your big toe affected?

YES

An ingrown toenail may be the cause of the problem.

Go to chart

111

Foot problems

NO

Paronychia, an infection of the skin adjacent to the nail, may be the cause of this problem. This is particularly likely if you spend a lot of time with your hands in water – for instance, washing clothes or dishes. Consult your physician.

Treatment: Your physician may prescribe an *antibiotic* or *antifungal* cream or paint to apply to the affected nail after each time you wet your hands. Avoid putting your hands in water too often. Wear rubber gloves, if necessary. Your nails and cuticles should return to normal after a few months.

NO

Do you have a nail that has become discolored, thickened and flaky?

YES

A fungal infection of the nail is a possibility, especially if one or more of your toenails is affected. Consult your physician.

Treatment: Your physician may send a sample of nail clippings to be examined in a laboratory to confirm the diagnosis. Treatment may include a long course of *antifungal* tablets.

NO

Have your nails become pitted or dimpled?

YES

Psoriasis of the nails may cause this. In severe cases, the nail is loosened from the nail bed. The skin may also be affected by the disease when thick patches of silvery-white, scaly skin appear. Consult your physician.

Treatment: Your physician will probably advise you to keep your nails short. Nail polish will disguise unsightly nails and may protect them from further damage. If your skin is affected by psoriasis, your physician may prescribe an *adrenal steroid* cream and ultraviolet treatment.

NO

A tendency to brittle nails is usually inherited, but may be exacerbated by excessive exposure to water, detergents and harsh chemicals.

Self-help: Wear rubber gloves whenever you have to put your hands in water or handle chemicals or detergents. Keep your nails short and, if you like, apply a protective coat of nail polish. Regular applications of hand cream may also be helpful.

Do your nails crack or break easily?

YES

NO

Consult your physician if you are unable to make a diagnosis from this chart.

76 General skin problems

Many different types of disorders may affect the skin, including infections, inflammation, abnormal cell growth and abnormal skin coloration. Such disorders may be the result of an internal disease, exposure to an irritant or some other external factor. Symptoms may include blemishes, lumps, rashes, change in skin coloring or texture, itching or discomfort. Consult this chart if your symptom is not covered elsewhere in this book.

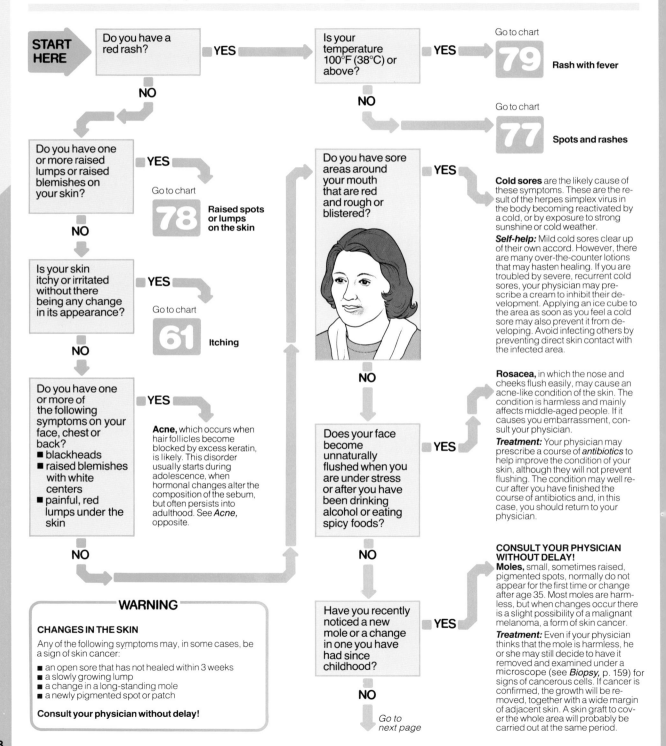

START HERE

Do you have a red rash?

YES → **Is your temperature 100°F (38°C) or above?**

YES → Go to chart **79** **Rash with fever**

NO → Go to chart **77** **Spots and rashes**

NO →

Do you have one or more raised lumps or raised blemishes on your skin?

YES → Go to chart **78** **Raised spots or lumps on the skin**

NO →

Is your skin itchy or irritated without there being any change in its appearance?

YES → Go to chart **61** **Itching**

NO →

Do you have one or more of the following symptoms on your face, chest or back?
- blackheads
- raised blemishes with white centers
- painful, red lumps under the skin

YES → **Acne,** which occurs when hair follicles become blocked by excess keratin, is likely. This disorder usually starts during adolescence, when hormonal changes alter the composition of the sebum, but often persists into adulthood. See *Acne,* opposite.

NO →

Do you have sore areas around your mouth that are red and rough or blistered?

YES → **Cold sores** are the likely cause of these symptoms. These are the result of the herpes simplex virus in the body becoming reactivated by a cold, or by exposure to strong sunshine or cold weather.
Self-help: Mild cold sores clear up of their own accord. However, there are many over-the-counter lotions that may hasten healing. If you are troubled by severe, recurrent cold sores, your physician may prescribe a cream to inhibit their development. Applying an ice cube to the area as soon as you feel a cold sore may also prevent it from developing. Avoid infecting others by preventing direct skin contact with the infected area.

NO →

Does your face become unnaturally flushed when you are under stress or after you have been drinking alcohol or eating spicy foods?

YES → **Rosacea,** in which the nose and cheeks flush easily, may cause an acne-like condition of the skin. The condition is harmless and mainly affects middle-aged people. If it causes you embarrassment, consult your physician.
Treatment: Your physician may prescribe a course of *antibiotics* to help improve the condition of your skin, although they will not prevent flushing. The condition may well recur after you have finished the course of antibiotics and, in this case, you should return to your physician.

NO →

Have you recently noticed a new mole or a change in one you have had since childhood?

YES → **CONSULT YOUR PHYSICIAN WITHOUT DELAY!**
Moles, small, sometimes raised, pigmented spots, normally do not appear for the first time or change after age 35. Most moles are harmless, but when changes occur there is a slight possibility of a malignant melanoma, a form of skin cancer.
Treatment: Even if your physician thinks that the mole is harmless, he or she may still decide to have it removed and examined under a microscope (see *Biopsy,* p. 159) for signs of cancerous cells. If cancer is confirmed, the growth will be removed, together with a wide margin of adjacent skin. A skin graft to cover the whole area will probably be carried out at the same period.

NO → *Go to next page*

WARNING

CHANGES IN THE SKIN

Any of the following symptoms may, in some cases, be a sign of skin cancer:

- an open sore that has not healed within 3 weeks
- a slowly growing lump
- a change in a long-standing mole
- a newly pigmented spot or patch

Consult your physician without delay!

Continued from previous page

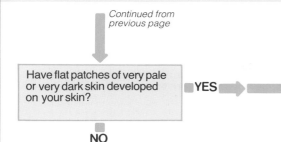

Have flat patches of very pale or very dark skin developed on your skin?

YES →

Are you pregnant?

YES →

Go to chart

139 Skin changes in pregnancy

NO ↓

Uneven skin pigmentation is usually the result of abnormal formation of the cells that produce skin pigment or of an abnormal rate of pigment production. This may sometimes be caused by a fungal infection. Consult your physician.

Treatment: Most disorders of skin pigment are harmless and require no treatment. You can disguise any disfiguring patches with make-up. If your physician suspects a fungal infection, you will be prescribed an *antifungal* cream, which will soon clear up the condition.

NO ↓

Do you have one or more red patches covered with silvery-white, flaky skin?

YES →

Psoriasis, a disorder in which the skin cells grow unusually rapidly and form scales, is a possibility. The most common sites for this to occur are the scalp, elbows and knees, though scaly patches can also appear in the armpits, on the trunk or around the anus. Consult your physician.

Treatment: Your physician will probably prescribe a *steroid* ointment or cream to apply to the affected area. This needs to be done carefully because it may thin the unaffected skin. Alternatively, a combination of ultraviolet light treatment and medication may be recommended, or medication may be prescribed to slow down the rate of cell growth in the skin.

NO ↓

Has a blistery rash appeared on one side of your body in a place in which there has been a burning sensation for a day or two?

YES →

Shingles, a virus infection of the nerves, is a possibility. Consult your physician. This is a matter of urgency if the rash is on your face because it may affect your eyes.

Treatment: Your physician will probably prescribe painkillers and a soothing ointment to put on the skin and, possibly, an antiviral agent. If there is any possibility of damage to the eyes, you will probably be referred to a specialist for treatment.

NO ↓

Do you have one or more open sores on your skin?

YES →

Skin ulcers are usually caused by injury or infection, but may in some cases be encouraged by an underlying disorder such as poor circulation or diabetes.

Self-help: Keep the sore area clean and dry and, if necessary, protect it with an adhesive bandage or light dressing. Consult your physician if the sore has not healed within 3 weeks or if ulcers recur. Tests may be needed to determine the underlying cause of the trouble and determine treatment.

NO ↓

Consult your physician if you are unable to make a diagnosis from this chart.

ACNE

Acne is the name used to describe a group of skin symptoms mainly affecting the face, chest and back, caused by blockage and infection of hair follicles. There are 3 main types of symptoms:

Blackheads
These are tiny black spots caused by excess skin pigment overlying trapped sebum and skin debris in a hair follicle.

Pustules
Pustules are tender, red blemishes that develop raised, white centers. They occur when excess keratin blocks a hair follicle and becomes inflamed (see below).

The development of a pustule

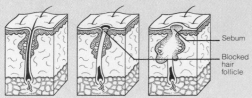

Sebum

Blocked hair follicle

Cysts
These are painful, red, fluid-filled lumps under the skin. They persist for several weeks and are more likely than other types of blemishes to lead to scarring.

Self-help
Mild acne with blackheads and the occasional pustule needs no special treatment other than ensuring that you wash your face thoroughly twice a day. Exposure to sunlight or careful use of an ultraviolet lamp often improves the condition. Avoid squeezing blemishes, as this is likely to increase the risk of infection and scarring. There are many over-the-counter preparations for acne. You may find some of these helpful. But you should avoid using anything too vigorously; this may lead to permanent skin damage.

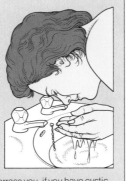

Professional treatment
If your acne is severe enough to embarrass you, if you have cystic blemishes or if there is any sign of scarring, consult your physician. Various treatments may be advised, depending on the type of acne. You may be prescribed a lotion that gently removes the top layer of skin, clearing blocked pores and preventing further blemishes from forming. Or you may be prescribed a long course of low-dose *antibiotics* that counters bacterial activity in the skin. Less commonly, a medication that alters the composition of the sebum may be prescribed. This treatment needs to be monitored carefully because of possible side-effects.

77 Spots and rashes

Groups of inflamed spots or blisters, or larger areas of inflamed skin, are usually caused by infection, irritation or an allergic reaction. Such a rash may come up suddenly or develop over a period of days and may, or may not, cause discomfort or itching. If a rash persists for more than a day, it is wise to consult your physician for diagnosis and treatment. Scratching may extend or enlarge the rash or spread it to other areas.

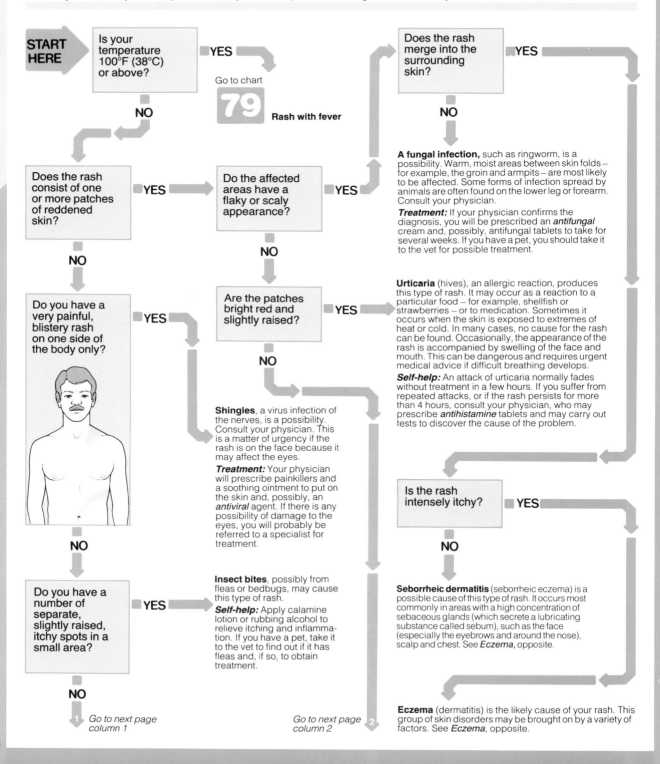

START HERE

Is your temperature 100°F (38°C) or above?

YES → Go to chart **79** Rash with fever

NO

Does the rash consist of one or more patches of reddened skin?

YES → Do the affected areas have a flaky or scaly appearance?

YES → Does the rash merge into the surrounding skin?

YES →

NO

A fungal infection, such as ringworm, is a possibility. Warm, moist areas between skin folds – for example, the groin and armpits – are most likely to be affected. Some forms of infection spread by animals are often found on the lower leg or forearm. Consult your physician.

Treatment: If your physician confirms the diagnosis, you will be prescribed an *antifungal* cream and, possibly, antifungal tablets to take for several weeks. If you have a pet, you should take it to the vet for possible treatment.

NO (from flaky/scaly)

Are the patches bright red and slightly raised?

YES →

Urticaria (hives), an allergic reaction, produces this type of rash. It may occur as a reaction to a particular food – for example, shellfish or strawberries – or to medication. Sometimes it occurs when the skin is exposed to extremes of heat or cold. In many cases, no cause for the rash can be found. Occasionally, the appearance of the rash is accompanied by swelling of the face and mouth. This can be dangerous and requires urgent medical advice if difficult breathing develops.

Self-help: An attack of urticaria normally fades without treatment in a few hours. If you suffer from repeated attacks, or if the rash persists for more than 4 hours, consult your physician, who may prescribe *antihistamine* tablets and may carry out tests to discover the cause of the problem.

NO (from reddened patches)

Do you have a very painful, blistery rash on one side of the body only?

YES →

Shingles, a virus infection of the nerves, is a possibility. Consult your physician. This is a matter of urgency if the rash is on the face because it may affect the eyes.

Treatment: Your physician will prescribe painkillers and a soothing ointment to put on the skin and, possibly, an *antiviral* agent. If there is any possibility of damage to the eyes, you will probably be referred to a specialist for treatment.

NO

Is the rash intensely itchy?

YES →

NO

Seborrheic dermatitis (seborrheic eczema) is a possible cause of this type of rash. It occurs most commonly in areas with a high concentration of sebaceous glands (which secrete a lubricating substance called sebum), such as the face (especially the eyebrows and around the nose), scalp and chest. See *Eczema,* opposite.

Do you have a number of separate, slightly raised, itchy spots in a small area?

YES →

Insect bites, possibly from fleas or bedbugs, may cause this type of rash.

Self-help: Apply calamine lotion or rubbing alcohol to relieve itching and inflammation. If you have a pet, take it to the vet to find out if it has fleas and, if so, to obtain treatment.

NO

1 *Go to next page column 1*

2 *Go to next page column 2*

Eczema (dermatitis) is the likely cause of your rash. This group of skin disorders may be brought on by a variety of factors. See *Eczema,* opposite.

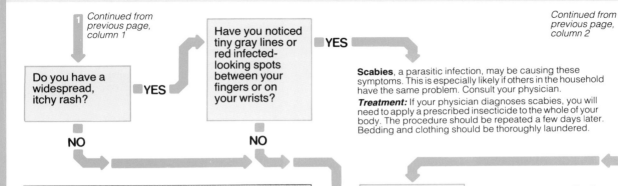

1 Continued from previous page, column 1

2 Continued from previous page, column 2

Do you have a widespread, itchy rash?

YES → **Have you noticed tiny gray lines or red infected-looking spots between your fingers or on your wrists?**

YES →

Scabies, a parasitic infection, may be causing these symptoms. This is especially likely if others in the household have the same problem. Consult your physician.

Treatment: If your physician diagnoses scabies, you will need to apply a prescribed insecticide to the whole of your body. The procedure should be repeated a few days later. Bedding and clothing should be thoroughly laundered.

NO ↓   **NO** ↓

Have you recently started to take any medication?

YES → **Certain medications** may cause rashes as a side effect. Discuss the problem with your physician.

NO ↓

Consult your physician if you are unable to make a diagnosis from this chart.

LYME DISEASE

Lyme disease, a bacterial infection, is transmitted by the bite of a tick that usually lives on deer or dogs, but can bite humans. Most cases of Lyme disease have occurred in northeastern and upper midwestern states, but cases have been reported in almost every state.

At the site of the tick bite, a rash may appear and expand over an area several inches across–although some people do not notice the bite. Symptoms such as fever, headache, lethargy, and muscle pain usually develop, followed by joint inflammation. The symptoms may occur in cycles lasting a week or so. Unless the disease is diagnosed and treated, symptoms may continue for several years, gradually lessening. In some severe cases, complications affecting the heart or nervous system occur; these complications can be fatal.

If you have some of these symptoms, especially if you know you have been bitten by a tick, consult your doctor. Blood tests can confirm your doctor's diagnosis of Lyme disease.

Most cases of Lyme disease can be quickly cleared up with antibiotics. If the disease is advanced, recovery may take longer. Nonsteroidal anti-inflammatory drugs and sometimes corticosteroid drugs may be prescribed.

How can you avoid being bitten by ticks? When you are outside in grassy, wooded, or sandy areas, wear light-colored clothing (so you can spot ticks) with long sleeves and with long pants tucked into your socks. Avoid going barefoot. Insect repellent containing diethyltoluamide (deet) can be helpful. Do not put it on young children's skin–spray their clothing instead. If you spend time outdoors, especially in heavily infested areas, check yourself, your children, and your pets for ticks or tick bites every day.

ECZEMA

Eczema (dermatitis) refers to a group of related conditions in which the skin becomes inflamed and itchy. The main types of eczema are described below.

Infantile (atopic) eczema

This is an allergic condition that usually appears for the first time in early infancy. It tends to get less severe and may clear up completely by early adolescence. Infantile eczema usually affects the wrists, insides of the elbows and backs of the knees but, in severe cases, the whole body may be affected. The usual treatment is to avoid harsh soaps and detergents, to use a special soap substitute and to apply oil after the bath. A rich, moisturizing cream should be applied to the affected areas. If itching is severe, your physician may prescribe medication. Mild *steroid* creams are recommended in some cases and, if the eczema becomes infected, a mixed steroid and *antibiotic* cream or antibiotics by mouth may be necessary. Skin tests may be carried out to identify factors that trigger outbreaks. Going on a special diet may help.

Contact eczema

This type of eczema is caused by a reaction to contact with a substance to which you are allergic. Certain plants, such as poison ivy or poison oak, are common causes. The skin becomes red and itchy and blisters (which break and crust over) may form. Milder forms of contact eczema may be caused by contact with certain metals – for example, nickel used in jewelry or on a watch. The rash will clear up in a week or so if the cause of the trouble is removed.

Irritant eczema

As the name suggests, this type of rash is caused by contact with irritant chemicals – for example, harsh detergents or industrial chemicals in your place of work. The skin becomes dry, red, rough and itchy. The condition usually clears up if you avoid contact with the irritants by protecting your hands with gloves. A moisturizing hand cream should soothe the affected skin, but it is advisable to consult your physician, who may prescribe a mild steroid cream to clear up the rash.

Seborrheic dermatitis

The tendency to develop this type of eczema is probably inherited. Flaky, red, but not especially itchy, patches appear in areas with a high concentration of sebaceous glands (which secrete a lubricating substance called sebum), such as around the nose, eyebrows or on the scalp and chest. Seborrheic dermatitis on the scalp is the most common cause of dandruff. Keep the affected skin clean and dry, but avoid using harsh soaps and detergents. Further treatment is often unnecessary but, if the rash is extensive, consult your physician, who may prescribe a mild cream or ointment.

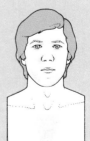

BRUISING

A bruise is a discolored area of skin caused by blood leaking into the dermis (the inner layer of skin) from a blood vessel damaged by injury. A bruise is usually blue, purple or black at first, but gradually fades to yellow before disappearing.

Self-help

If you have a bruise, do not rub or massage the bruised area; this may make matters worse. Applying an ice bag (or an unopened packet of frozen vegetables) immediately after the injury may reduce the extent of bruising. If you have bruised your leg, resting with your feet up may assist healing.

When to consult your physician

Consult your physician in any of the following circumstances:

- If you feel severe pain, or if movement is restricted.
- If bruises appear without injury.
- If you bruise frequently and easily.

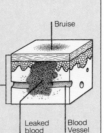

Bruise

Dermis

Leaked blood   **Blood Vessel**

Formation of a bruise
A bruise forms when blood from a damaged blood vessel leaks under the skin (above).

78 Raised spots or lumps on the skin

Consult this chart if you develop any raised lumps, whether they are skin colored or pigmented (brown). In the majority of cases, such lumps are the harmless result of virus infection. Your physician will be willing to give you advice on the problem if skin lumps persist or cause you discomfort or embarrassment.

START HERE

Have you recently noticed a new, dark, mole-like spot on your skin? — YES → **Does it have a caked, crusty appearance?** — YES →

NO ↓ (from first box)

NO ↓ (from second box)

Have you noticed a change in the look of any mole that you have had since childhood? — YES →

A seborrheic keratosis is the most likely diagnosis. This type of keratosis is common and harmless and often appears on the skin in large numbers in later life. Such a keratosis can vary in size from 1 to 3 cm. However, you should show it to your physician so that the diagnosis can be confirmed.

Treatment: Seborrheic keratoses need no treatment, but your physician may decide to have it removed and examined under a microscope (see *Biopsy,* p.159).

CONSULT YOUR PHYSICIAN WITHOUT DELAY!
Moles, small, sometimes raised, pigmented spots, normally do not appear for the first time or change after age 35. Most moles are harmless, but when changes occur, there is a slight possibility of a malignant melanoma, a form of skin cancer.

Treatment: Your physician may be able to reassure you that the mole is harmless. If unsure of the diagnosis, he or she may refer you to a specialist for a *biopsy* (p.159) in order to find out whether or not there is an underlying disorder. If cancerous cells are found, they will be removed together with a wide margin of adjacent skin. A skin graft to cover the whole area will probably be carried out at the same time.

Common warts develop when a virus invades the skin cells and causes them to multiply rapidly. Wart viruses spread by touch or from contact with the skin shed from a wart. When they appear on the feet they are often referred to as plantar warts and can be very painful when pressure is put on them.

Self-help: Most warts disappear naturally in time, but if you find them a nuisance, apply one of the wart remedies that are available over-the-counter in the form of cream or paint. These preparations should be applied very carefully, following the manufacturer's instructions, because they can make surrounding skin sore. Afterward, the dead skin should be removed with a pumice stone. If you have a wart that does not respond to this treatment, ask your physician for advice. He or she may refer you to a skin specialist who may remove the wart by freezing it with liquid nitrogen or carbon dioxide, or by burning it off (diathermy).

Have small, hard, white or pink lumps appeared anywhere on your body that have a roughened, cauliflower-like surface? — YES →

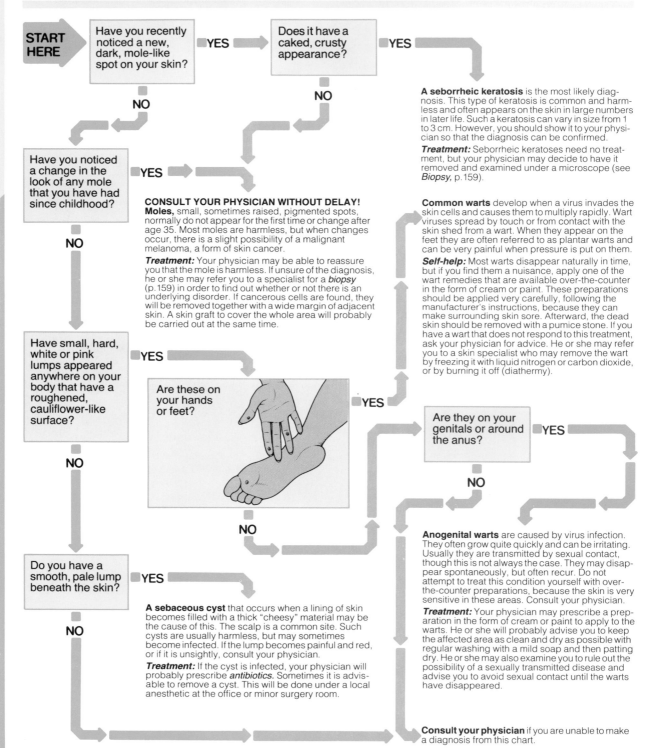

Are these on your hands or feet? — YES →

NO ↓

Are they on your genitals or around the anus? — YES →

NO ↓

Do you have a smooth, pale lump beneath the skin? — YES →

NO ↓

A sebaceous cyst that occurs when a lining of skin becomes filled with a thick "cheesy" material may be the cause of this. The scalp is a common site. Such cysts are usually harmless, but may sometimes become infected. If the lump becomes painful and red, or if it is unsightly, consult your physician.

Treatment: If the cyst is infected, your physician will probably prescribe *antibiotics.* Sometimes it is advisable to remove a cyst. This will be done under a local anesthetic at the office or minor surgery room.

Anogenital warts are caused by virus infection. They often grow quite quickly and can be irritating. Usually they are transmitted by sexual contact, though this is not always the case. They may disappear spontaneously, but often recur. Do not attempt to treat this condition yourself with over-the-counter preparations, because the skin is very sensitive in these areas. Consult your physician.

Treatment: Your physician may prescribe a preparation in the form of cream or paint to apply to the warts. He or she will probably advise you to keep the affected area as clean and dry as possible with regular washing with a mild soap and then patting dry. He or she may also examine you to rule out the possibility of a sexually transmitted disease and advise you to avoid sexual contact until the warts have disappeared.

Consult your physician if you are unable to make a diagnosis from this chart.

79 Rash with fever

Consult this chart if you notice any blemishes or discolored areas of skin and also have a temperature of 100°F (38°C) or above. You may well have one of the infectious diseases that are more common in childhood.

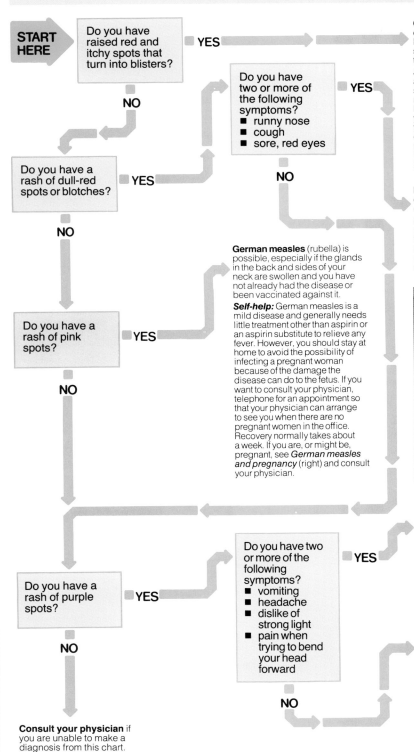

START HERE

Do you have raised red and itchy spots that turn into blisters?

NO ⟶ **Do you have a rash of dull-red spots or blotches?**

YES ⟶ **Do you have two or more of the following symptoms?**
- runny nose
- cough
- sore, red eyes

YES ⟶

NO ⟶ **German measles** (rubella) is possible, especially if the glands in the back and sides of your neck are swollen and you have not already had the disease or been vaccinated against it.

Self-help: German measles is a mild disease and generally needs little treatment other than aspirin or an aspirin substitute to relieve any fever. However, you should stay at home to avoid the possibility of infecting a pregnant woman because of the damage the disease can do to the fetus. If you want to consult your physician, telephone for an appointment so that your physician can arrange to see you when there are no pregnant women in the office. Recovery normally takes about a week. If you are, or might be, pregnant, see *German measles and pregnancy* (right) and consult your physician.

NO ⟶ **Do you have a rash of pink spots?**

YES ⟶

NO ⟶ **Do you have a rash of purple spots?**

YES ⟶ **Do you have two or more of the following symptoms?**
- vomiting
- headache
- dislike of strong light
- pain when trying to bend your head forward

YES ⟶

NO ⟶

NO ⟶ **Consult your physician** if you are unable to make a diagnosis from this chart.

Chickenpox, a childhood infectious disease caused by the herpes varicella-zoster virus, is the likely cause of such symptoms. The rash usually starts on the face and trunk, but later may spread to the limbs.

Self-help: Drink plenty of fluids and take aspirin or an aspirin substitute to relieve any feverish symptoms. Apply calamine lotion to the rash to relieve itching. Try to resist the urge to scratch because scratching leads to scarring. Consult your physician if you are, or might be, pregnant, if your temperature rises above 104°F (40°C), if you develop a severe cough, if your eyes become painful, or if you find it hard not to scratch. You are infectious until all the blisters have formed scabs (after about a week).

Measles (rubeola), a highly contagious viral disease, may be the cause of such symptoms, especially if you did not have measles as a child.

Self-help: There is no specific treatment for measles. Stay at home, drink plenty of fluids and take aspirin or an aspirin substitute to reduce fever. Consult your physician if you are, or might be, pregnant, if you develop a severe headache or earache, or if your cough starts to get worse.

GERMAN MEASLES AND PREGNANCY

The virus responsible for German measles may cross the placenta of a pregnant woman and damage the developing fetus, causing defects such as deafness, blindness and heart problems. The likelihood of damage occurring is strongest if the disease develops in the first 12 weeks of pregnancy. If you are pregnant or trying to become pregnant it is therefore vitally important to avoid contracting this disease.

In most cases you will be given a blood test in early pregnancy to check whether you are immune. If this test shows that you are at risk from the disease, you should be careful to avoid anyone who has the disease or has recently been in contact with it.

CALL YOUR PHYSICIAN NOW!

Meningitis, inflammation of the membranes (due to infection) surrounding the brain or spinal cord, may be the cause of such symptoms.

Treatment: You will probably be required to go to the hospital for a *lumbar puncture* (p. 155). If the infection is found to be bacterial you will be given *antibiotics,* possibly by intravenous drip. If the infection is viral, no specific treatment is necessary, but you will be given painkillers and intravenous fluids. Recovery normally takes 2 to 3 weeks.

CONSULT YOUR PHYSICIAN WITHOUT DELAY!

Purpura, a type of rash caused by blood leaking from blood vessels under the skin, may be produced by an allergic reaction to a food or drug, or by infection. Call your doctor at once if your temperature rises to 104°F (40°C), or if you are suffering from a headache, stiff neck and/or vomiting.

Treatment: You will probably be admitted to the hospital for a blood test (see *Blood analysis,* p. 146) and possibly a *lumbar puncture* (p. 155) to determine the exact nature of the disorder. Further treatment will depend on the results of these tests.

80 Painful or irritated eye

Pain or irritation in or around the eye may be caused by disorders of the eye or surrounding tissues or injury to the eye area. Infection and inflammation are the common causes of eye discomfort. Disorders that threaten sight or that endanger health are uncommon, but should always be ruled out by your physician.

START HERE → **Have you injured your eye?** — YES →

A foreign body in the eye may cause pain, redness and watering. Carry out first aid (opposite). If first aid is not possible, or if it is unsuccessful, seek medical help.

NO ↓

EMERGENCY
GET MEDICAL HELP NOW!

Damage to the eye always requires immediate expert treatment.

Treatment: Carry out first aid (opposite) and get to the emergency room of your local hospital where specialist help will be available, or contact your ophthalmologist.

Is there a foreign body — for example, a piece of dirt — in the eye? — YES →

CALL YOUR PHYSICIAN NOW!
Acute glaucoma (narrow angle glaucoma), a serious disorder in which excess fluid inside the eye causes increased pressure, is a possible cause of the pain, especially if you are over 40.

Treatment: If your physician suspects that you have this disorder, you will probably be referred to an ophthalmologist for treatment. Treatment usually consists of eye drops to enable excess fluid to drain from the eye. In addition, you may be given a drug to prevent fluid retention. Once the pressure has been relieved, an operation to prevent a recurrence is usually carried out.

NO ↓

Is your vision blurred AND/OR do you see halos around lights? — YES →

NO ↓

Is the white of the eye bloodshot? — YES →

NO ↓

Is there a sticky discharge from the eye? — YES →

NO ↓

Does the eyelid seem to be turning inward? — YES →

NO ↓

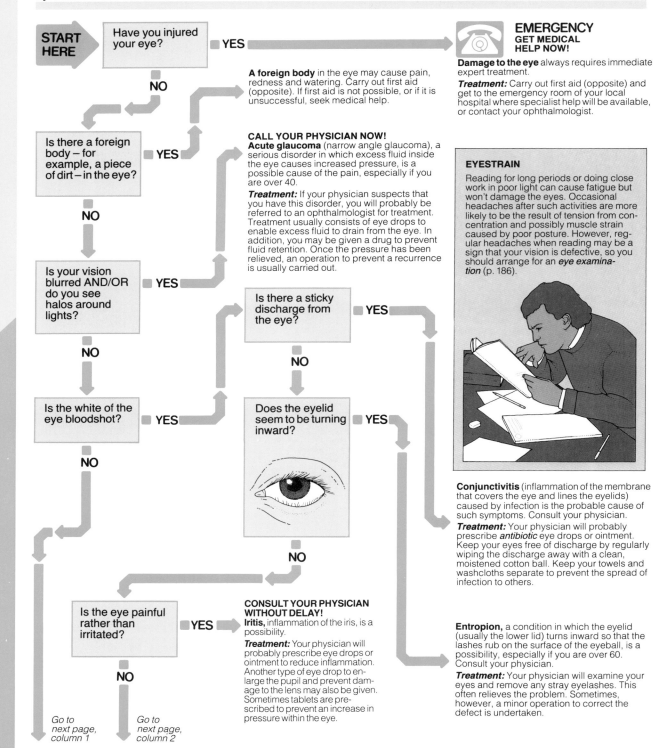

Is the eye painful rather than irritated? — YES →

CONSULT YOUR PHYSICIAN WITHOUT DELAY!
Iritis, inflammation of the iris, is a possibility.

Treatment: Your physician will probably prescribe eye drops or ointment to reduce inflammation. Another type of eye drop to enlarge the pupil and prevent damage to the lens may also be given. Sometimes tablets are prescribed to prevent an increase in pressure within the eye.

NO ↓

Go to next page, column 1

Go to next page, column 2

EYESTRAIN

Reading for long periods or doing close work in poor light can cause fatigue but won't damage the eyes. Occasional headaches after such activities are more likely to be the result of tension from concentration and possibly muscle strain caused by poor posture. However, regular headaches when reading may be a sign that your vision is defective, so you should arrange for an *eye examination* (p. 186).

Conjunctivitis (inflammation of the membrane that covers the eye and lines the eyelids) caused by infection is the probable cause of such symptoms. Consult your physician.

Treatment: Your physician will probably prescribe *antibiotic* eye drops or ointment. Keep your eyes free of discharge by regularly wiping the discharge away with a clean, moistened cotton ball. Keep your towels and washcloths separate to prevent the spread of infection to others.

Entropion, a condition in which the eyelid (usually the lower lid) turns inward so that the lashes rub on the surface of the eyeball, is a possibility, especially if you are over 60. Consult your physician.

Treatment: Your physician will examine your eyes and remove any stray eyelashes. This often relieves the problem. Sometimes, however, a minor operation to correct the defect is undertaken.

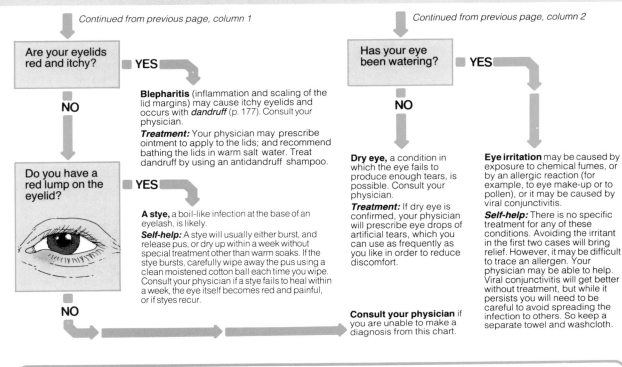

Continued from previous page, column 1

Are your eyelids red and itchy? ■ YES

NO

Blepharitis (inflammation and scaling of the lid margins) may cause itchy eyelids and occurs with *dandruff* (p. 177). Consult your physician.
Treatment: Your physician may prescribe ointment to apply to the lids; and recommend bathing the lids in warm salt water. Treat dandruff by using an antidandruff shampoo.

Do you have a red lump on the eyelid? ■ YES

A stye, a boil-like infection at the base of an eyelash, is likely.
Self-help: A stye will usually either burst, and release pus, or dry up within a week without special treatment other than warm soaks. If the stye bursts, carefully wipe away the pus using a clean moistened cotton ball each time you wipe. Consult your physician if a stye fails to heal within a week, the eye itself becomes red and painful, or if styes recur.

■ **NO**

Continued from previous page, column 2

Has your eye been watering? ■ YES

NO

Dry eye, a condition in which the eye fails to produce enough tears, is possible. Consult your physician.
Treatment: If dry eye is confirmed, your physician will prescribe eye drops of artificial tears, which you can use as frequently as you like in order to reduce discomfort.

Eye irritation may be caused by exposure to chemical fumes, or by an allergic reaction (for example, to eye make-up or to pollen), or it may be caused by viral conjunctivitis.
Self-help: There is no specific treatment for any of these conditions. Avoiding the irritant in the first two cases will bring relief. However, it may be difficult to trace an allergen. Your physician may be able to help. Viral conjunctivitis will get better without treatment, but while it persists you will need to be careful to avoid spreading the infection to others. So keep a separate towel and washcloth.

Consult your physician if you are unable to make a diagnosis from this chart.

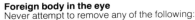

FIRST AID FOR EYE INJURIES

If you suffer an injury to your eye or eyelid, rapid action is essential. Except in the case of a foreign body that has been successfully removed, go to the emergency room of your local hospital or to an ophthalmologist by the fastest means possible, as soon as you have carried out first aid.

Cuts to the eye or eyelid
Cover the eye with a clean pad (such as a folded handkerchief) and hold it lightly in place with a bandage. Apply no pressure. Cover the other eye as well to prevent movement of the eyeball. Seek medical help.

Blows to the eye area
Carry out first aid as for a cut eye (above) but use a cold compress instead of a dry pad over the injured eye.

Corrosive chemicals
If you spill any harsh chemical (for example, bleach or household cleaner) in the eye, immediately flood the eye with large quantities of cold running water. Tilt your head with the injured eye downward so that the water runs from the inside outward. Keep the eyelids apart with your fingers. When all traces of the chemical have been removed, lightly cover the eye with a clean pad and seek medical help.

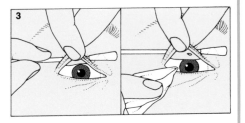

Foreign body in the eye
Never attempt to remove any of the following:

■ an object that is embedded in the eyeball
■ a chip of metal
■ a particle over the colored part of the eye

In any of these cases, cover both eyes as described for cuts to the eye or eyelid (left) and seek medical help. Other foreign bodies – for example, specks of dirt or eyelashes floating on the white of the eye or inside the lids – may be removed as follows:

1 If you can see the particle on the white of the eye or inside the lower lid, pick it off using the moistened corner of a clean handkerchief (below) or sterile cotton-tipped swab.

2 If you cannot see the particle, pull the upper lid down over the lower lid and hold it for a moment (far right). This may dislodge the particle. If the particle remains, it may be on the inside of the upper lid. If you are alone, seek medical help. Another person may be able to remove the foreign body as in step 3.

3 Ask the person to look down. Hold the lashes of the upper lid and pull it down. Place a match or cotton-tipped swab over the upper lid and fold the lid back over it (right). If the particle is now visible, pick it off as described in step 1.

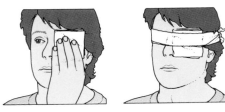
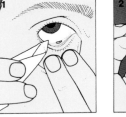
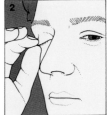

If you do not succeed in removing the foreign body, lightly cover the eye and seek medical help at once.

81 Disturbed or impaired vision

This chart deals with any change in your vision, including blurring, seeing double, seeing flashing lights or floating spots, and loss of part or all of your field of vision. Any such change in vision should be brought to your physician's attention promptly to rule out the possibility of a sight-threatening eye disorder. Successful treatment of many eye disorders may depend on catching the disease in its early stages.

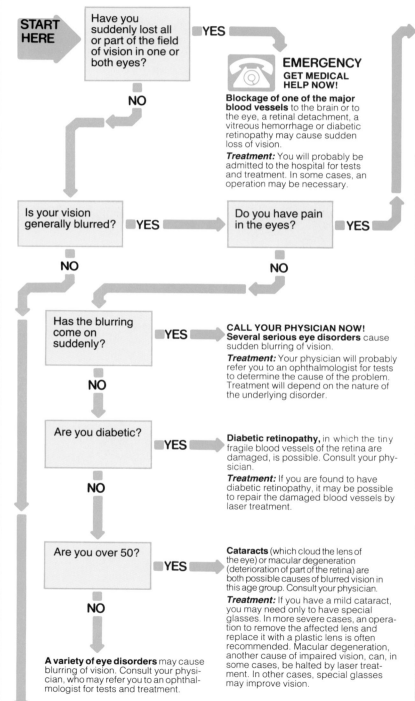

START HERE

Have you suddenly lost all or part of the field of vision in one or both eyes?

YES →

EMERGENCY GET MEDICAL HELP NOW!

Blockage of one of the major blood vessels to the brain or to the eye, a retinal detachment, a vitreous hemorrhage or diabetic retinopathy may cause sudden loss of vision.

Treatment: You will probably be admitted to the hospital for tests and treatment. In some cases, an operation may be necessary.

NO ↓

Is your vision generally blurred? — YES → **Do you have pain in the eyes?** — YES →

CALL YOUR PHYSICIAN NOW!
Acute glaucoma (narrow angle glaucoma) is a possibility, especially if you are over 40. This is a serious disorder in which obstruction to the normal draining mechanism causes a buildup of fluid, and a consequent increase of pressure in the eye.

Treatment: If your physician suspects this disorder, you will probably be referred to an ophthalmologist for treatment. Treatment usually consists of drugs to help lower the pressure within the eye and to relieve pain. You will also probably be given eye drops to help fluid drain from the eye. Later on you may need to have an operation to prevent a recurrence of the problem.

NO ↓ (blurred)   NO ↓ (pain)

Has the blurring come on suddenly? — YES →

CALL YOUR PHYSICIAN NOW!
Several serious eye disorders cause sudden blurring of vision.

Treatment: Your physician will probably refer you to an ophthalmologist for tests to determine the cause of the problem. Treatment will depend on the nature of the underlying disorder.

NO ↓

Are you diabetic? — YES →

Diabetic retinopathy, in which the tiny fragile blood vessels of the retina are damaged, is possible. Consult your physician.

Treatment: If you are found to have diabetic retinopathy, it may be possible to repair the damaged blood vessels by laser treatment.

NO ↓

Are you over 50? — YES →

Cataracts (which cloud the lens of the eye) or **macular degeneration** (deterioration of part of the retina) are both possible causes of blurred vision in this age group. Consult your physician.

Treatment: If you have a mild cataract, you may need only to have special glasses. In more severe cases, an operation to remove the affected lens and replace it with a plastic lens is often recommended. Macular degeneration, another cause of impaired vision, can, in some cases, be halted by laser treatment. In other cases, special glasses may improve vision.

NO ↓

A variety of eye disorders may cause blurring of vision. Consult your physician, who may refer you to an ophthalmologist for tests and treatment.

Go to next page

EYE TESTING

After age 40 you should have your eyes tested routinely every year (or less often if the ophthalmologist recommends it), or at any age if you have any visual problem. The ophthalmologist will test the sharpness of your vision by asking you to read letters on a Snellen chart (named after its inventor). The result of the test is given as two figures. So, for example, the result 20/40 means that the lowest row of letters that you were able to read at a distance of 20 feet is one that a person with normal vision would read at 40 feet.

The ophthalmologist also looks at each eye through an instrument called an ophthalmoscope (below) to check that the back of the eye looks normal and make sure that there are no signs suggestive of a general disorder, such as high blood pressure or diabetes. Also, he or she will test the balance of the muscles that control the movements of the eyes to detect any eye muscle disorder.

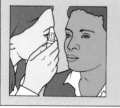

Eye examination
The ophthalmologist looks at each eye through an instrument called an ophthalmoscope (left). With this, he or she can check that the back of the eye looks normal and that there are no signs of an underlying condition.

COLOR BLINDNESS

Color blindness is a term used to describe the hereditary inability to distinguish between certain colors. All the colors we see are thought to be made up of combinations of red, green and blue – the basic colors in the light rays that enter our eyes. Literal color blindness in which everything is seen in shades of gray is rare. The most common defect, which primarily affects men, is an inability to distinguish between red and green. Most people learn to live with this minor disability without problems. However, perfect color vision is required for certain jobs – for example, that of an airline pilot – and anyone applying for such a job will be required to have a full eye examination, including tests for color vision.

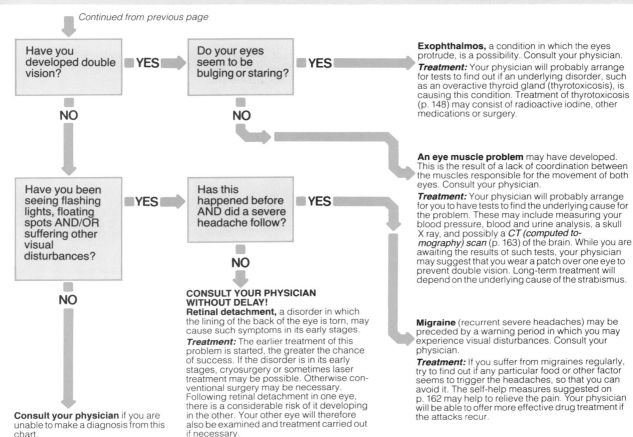

Continued from previous page

Have you developed double vision?

YES → **Do your eyes seem to be bulging or staring?**

YES → **Exophthalmos,** a condition in which the eyes protrude, is a possibility. Consult your physician.

Treatment: Your physician will probably arrange for tests to find out if an underlying disorder, such as an overactive thyroid gland (thyrotoxicosis), is causing this condition. Treatment of thyrotoxicosis (p. 148) may consist of radioactive iodine, other medications or surgery.

NO (under first box)

NO (under "Do your eyes seem to be bulging or staring?")

An eye muscle problem may have developed. This is the result of a lack of coordination between the muscles responsible for the movement of both eyes. Consult your physician.

Treatment: Your physician will probably arrange for you to have tests to find the underlying cause for the problem. These may include measuring your blood pressure, blood and urine analysis, a skull X ray, and possibly a *CT (computed tomography) scan* (p. 163) of the brain. While you are awaiting the results of such tests, your physician may suggest that you wear a patch over one eye to prevent double vision. Long-term treatment will depend on the underlying cause of the strabismus.

Have you been seeing flashing lights, floating spots AND/OR suffering other visual disturbances?

YES → **Has this happened before AND did a severe headache follow?**

YES → **Migraine** (recurrent severe headaches) may be preceded by a warning period in which you may experience visual disturbances. Consult your physician.

Treatment: If you suffer from migraines regularly, try to find out if any particular food or other factor seems to trigger the headaches, so that you can avoid it. The self-help measures suggested on p. 162 may help to relieve the pain. Your physician will be able to offer more effective drug treatment if the attacks recur.

NO (under flashing lights box)

NO (under "Has this happened before...")

CONSULT YOUR PHYSICIAN WITHOUT DELAY!
Retinal detachment, a disorder in which the lining of the back of the eye is torn, may cause such symptoms in its early stages.

Treatment: The earlier treatment of this problem is started, the greater the chance of success. If the disorder is in its early stages, cryosurgery or sometimes laser treatment may be possible. Otherwise conventional surgery may be necessary. Following retinal detachment in one eye, there is a considerable risk of it developing in the other. Your other eye will therefore also be examined and treatment carried out if necessary.

Consult your physician if you are unable to make a diagnosis from this chart.

THE STRUCTURE OF THE EYE

The eye is a complex and delicate structure. The eyeball itself consists of 3 layers:

The sclera, the tough outer layer, is visible as the white of the eye. It is protected at the front by the conjunctiva, a clear membrane that also lines the inner surface of the eyelids. The colored part of the eye, the iris, is covered by the cornea.

The choroid layer beneath the sclera is rich in blood vessels that supply the retina (the light-sensitive inner lining of the eyeball) with oxygen. At the front of the eye, the choroid layer thickens to form the ciliary body, a circle of muscles that supports and controls the lens. In front of the ciliary body lies the iris, which contains muscular fibers that control the amount of light that passes through the lens. The area between the iris and the cornea is filled with watery fluid known as the aqueous humor.

The retina is the innermost layer of the eyeball. This contains the light-sensitive nerve cells that pick up images and transmit the information through the optic nerve to the brain. The inner part of the eyeball is filled with a thick, jelly-like substance called the vitreous humor.

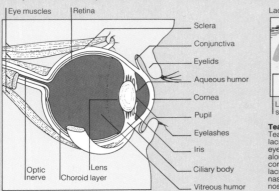

Eye muscles · Retina · Sclera · Conjunctiva · Eyelids · Aqueous humor · Cornea · Pupil · Eyelashes · Iris · Ciliary body · Vitreous humor · Optic nerve · Lens · Choroid layer

Lacrimal gland · Tear duct · Lacrimal sac · Nasolacrimal duct

Tear glands and ducts
Tears are produced in the lacrimal glands above each eyeball and drain away along tear ducts in the inner corners of the lids, into the lacrimal sac, and via the nasolacrimal duct into the nose.

CONTACT LENSES

In recent years, contact lenses have become a popular alternative to eyeglasses as a means of correcting defects in vision such as nearsightedness or farsightedness. There are two main types of lenses: the rigid lens, which is made of hard-wearing plastic and may be impermeable or gas-permeable, and the soft lens, which is often more comfortable but is more easily damaged and not so long-lasting. Your ophthalmologist will help you decide which type of lens is most suitable.

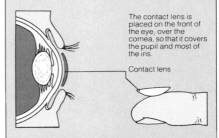

The contact lens is placed on the front of the eye, over the cornea, so that it covers the pupil and most of the iris.

Contact lens

Care of contact lenses
All types of contact lenses need regular and careful cleaning to remove dirt and prevent the buildup of protein deposits on the lens. If this is not done there is a danger of infection and permanent damage to the eye. Always use the special cleaning and soaking solutions recommended for your type of lens, and follow your ophthalmologist's detailed advice on the care of your lenses precisely.

82 Earache

Earache may vary from a dull, throbbing sensation to a sharp, stabbing pain that can be most distressing. It is a common symptom in childhood, but occurs much less frequently in adults. Pain in the ear is usually caused by infection and normally requires medical attention and antibiotic treatment.

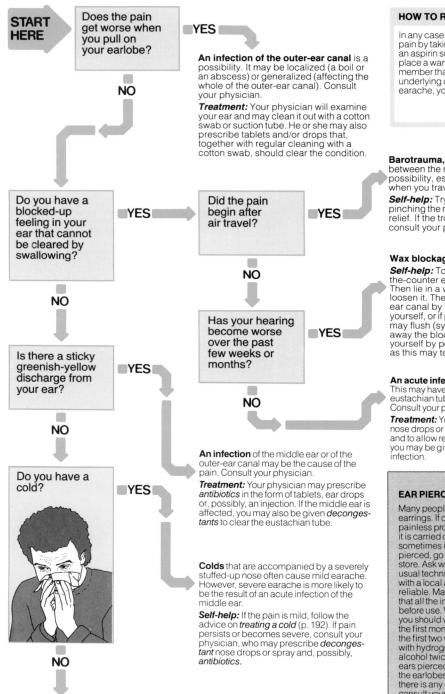

START HERE

Does the pain get worse when you pull on your earlobe?

YES → An infection of the outer-ear canal is a possibility. It may be localized (a boil or an abscess) or generalized (affecting the whole of the outer-ear canal). Consult your physician.

Treatment: Your physician will examine your ear and may clean it out with a cotton swab or suction tube. He or she may also prescribe tablets and/or drops that, together with regular cleaning with a cotton swab, should clear the condition.

NO ↓

Do you have a blocked-up feeling in your ear that cannot be cleared by swallowing?

YES → **Did the pain begin after air travel?**

YES → Barotrauma, in which the air-pressure balance between the middle and outer ears is disrupted, is a possibility, especially if you had a cold or a stuffy nose when you traveled.

Self-help: Try blowing through your nose while pinching the nostrils closed. In many cases, this brings relief. If the trouble persists for more than 24 hours, consult your physician.

NO ↓

Has your hearing become worse over the past few weeks or months?

YES → Wax blockage may be causing the pain.

Self-help: To remove wax yourself, soften it with over-the-counter ear drops or warm oil for several days. Then lie in a warm bath with your ears submerged to loosen it. The wax should work its way out of the outer-ear canal by itself. If you cannot remove the wax yourself, or if pain persists, consult your physician, who may flush (syringe) the ear with warm water to wash away the blockage. Never attempt to lever the wax out yourself by poking a pointed instrument into your ear, as this may tear a hole in the eardrum or canal skin.

NO ↓

An acute infection of the middle ear is a possibility. This may have occurred as a result of blockage of the eustachian tube (see *The structure of the ear*, opposite). Consult your physician.

Treatment: Your physician may prescribe *decongestant* nose drops or spray to help unblock the eustachian tube and to allow restoration of normal ear pressure. In addition, you may be given *antibiotics* to clear up a bacterial infection.

NO ↓

Is there a sticky greenish-yellow discharge from your ear?

YES → An infection of the middle ear or of the outer-ear canal may be the cause of the pain. Consult your physician.

Treatment: Your physician may prescribe *antibiotics* in the form of tablets, ear drops or, possibly, an injection. If the middle ear is affected, you may also be given *decongestants* to clear the eustachian tube.

NO ↓

Do you have a cold?

YES → Colds that are accompanied by a severely stuffed-up nose often cause mild earache. However, severe earache is more likely to be the result of an acute infection of the middle ear.

Self-help: If the pain is mild, follow the advice on *treating a cold* (p. 192). If pain persists or becomes severe, consult your physician, who may prescribe *decongestant* nose drops or spray and, possibly, *antibiotics*.

NO ↓

Consult your physician if you are unable to make a diagnosis from this chart.

HOW TO RELIEVE AN EARACHE

In any case of earache, you will be able to relieve the pain by taking the recommended dose of aspirin or an aspirin substitute. It may also be comforting to place a warm heating pad against the ear. But remember that these measures alone will not cure the underlying disorder. With persistent cases of earache, you should always consult your physician.

EAR PIERCING

Many people have holes pierced in their earlobes for earrings. If done properly, this is a perfectly safe and painless procedure, but unfortunately, in many cases it is carried out inexpertly, leading to discomfort and sometimes infection. If you want to have your ears pierced, go to a reputable jeweler or department store. Ask what method of ear piercing they use. The usual technique is to use a special ear punch along with a local anesthetic. Other methods may not be reliable. Make sure that the conditions look clean and that all the instruments and earrings are sterilized before use. When you have had your ears pierced, you should wear only earrings of high-carat gold for the first month and these should not be removed for the first two weeks. You will need to bathe the earlobe with hydrogen peroxide or isopropyl (rubbing) alcohol twice a day during this time. Do not have your ears pierced if you have any skin infection affecting the earlobes. If either earlobe becomes inflamed or if there is any pus after having your ears pierced, consult your physician.

83 Noises in the ear

If you sometimes hear noises inside your ears, such as buzzing, ringing or hissing, you are probably suffering from a symptom known as tinnitus. This symptom can indicate a variety of ear disorders.

START HERE

Did the noises start during or after air travel? — **YES** →

Barotrauma, in which the air-pressure balance between the middle and outer ears is disrupted, is a possibility, especially if you had a cold or a blocked nose when you traveled.

Self-help: Try blowing through your nose while pinching the nostrils closed. In many cases, this restores hearing to normal. If the trouble persists for more than 24 hours, consult your physician.

NO ↓

Have you noticed any loss of hearing? — **YES** →

Deafness often occurs together with noises in the ear.

Go to chart

84 **Deafness**

NO ↓

Are you taking, or have you recently taken, any prescribed or over-the-counter medications? — **YES** →

Certain drugs can cause noises in the ear as a side effect. Discuss the problem with your physician.

FIRST AID FOR AN INSECT IN THE EAR

If an insect has become trapped in your ear, you can safely try to remove it by tilting your head so that the affected side is uppermost and then pouring warm olive oil, mineral oil or baby oil into the ear (it is easiest if someone helps you do this). After 15 to 20 minutes, the insect should then float out. Alternatively, you can simply lie back in a bath with your ears submerged. If these measures do not succeed in removing the insect, consult your physician.

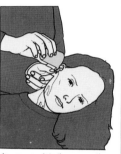

As you pour into the ear, gently pull the ear up and back

An insect, or other foreign body, may have become trapped in your outer-ear canal.

Self-help: Carry out the first-aid suggestions described above. If these are not effective, consult your physician. Never attempt to remove anything by inserting an object into the ear.

NO ↓

Do you have a tickling sensation in the ear? — **YES** →

NO ↓

Consult your physician if you are unable to make a diagnosis from this chart, especially if associated with hearing loss, dizziness, headache or ear pressure.

THE STRUCTURE OF THE EAR

The ear is made up of three main parts:

The outer ear includes the external part of the ear, the pinna, which collects and funnels sound waves along the outer-ear canal to the eardrum, which then vibrates.

The middle ear contains the eardrum and three small bones (hammer, anvil and stirrup) that transmit the vibrations of the eardrum to the inner ear. Air pressure in the middle ear is kept normal by means of the eustachian tube, which links the middle-ear cavity to the back of the throat.

The inner ear is filled with fluid and contains the cochlea, which converts the vibrations from the middle ear into nerve impulses. These are passed to the brain by the auditory nerve. The inner ear also contains the semicircular canals which control the body's balance.

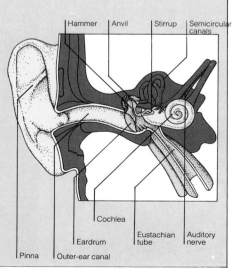

Hammer | Anvil | Stirrup | Semicircular canals

Cochlea

Eustachian tube | Auditory nerve

Eardrum

Pinna | Outer-ear canal

84 Deafness

Deafness – decreased ability to hear some or all sounds –
may come on gradually over a period of months or
years, or may occur suddenly over a matter of days or

hours. One or both ears may be affected. In most cases,
deafness is the result of infection or wax blockage and
can be treated.

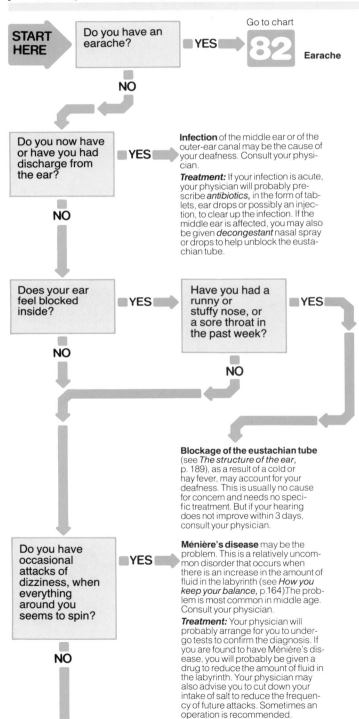

START HERE

Do you have an earache?

YES → **Go to chart 82** Earache

NO

Do you now have or have you had discharge from the ear?

YES → **Infection** of the middle ear or of the outer-ear canal may be the cause of your deafness. Consult your physician.

Treatment: If your infection is acute, your physician will probably prescribe *antibiotics,* in the form of tablets, ear drops or possibly an injection, to clear up the infection. If the middle ear is affected, you may also be given *decongestant* nasal spray or drops to help unblock the eustachian tube.

NO

Does your ear feel blocked inside?

YES → **Have you had a runny or stuffy nose, or a sore throat in the past week?**

YES →

NO

NO

Blockage of the eustachian tube (see *The structure of the ear,* p. 189), as a result of a cold or hay fever, may account for your deafness. This is usually no cause for concern and needs no specific treatment. But if your hearing does not improve within 3 days, consult your physician.

Do you have occasional attacks of dizziness, when everything around you seems to spin?

YES → **Ménière's disease** may be the problem. This is a relatively uncommon disorder that occurs when there is an increase in the amount of fluid in the labyrinth (see *How you keep your balance,* p 164)The problem is most common in middle age. Consult your physician.

Treatment: Your physician will probably arrange for you to undergo tests to confirm the diagnosis. If you are found to have Ménière's disease, you will probably be given a drug to reduce the amount of fluid in the labyrinth. Your physician may also advise you to cut down your intake of salt to reduce the frequency of future attacks. Sometimes an operation is recommended.

NO

Go to next page

HEARING TESTS

If, after examining you, your physician suspects that your hearing is impaired, he or she may refer you for specialized hearing tests known as audiometry and acoustic impedance testing.

Audiometry
The first part of this test measures your ability to hear sounds conducted through the air. You are asked to listen through headphones, one ear at a time, to different pitches of sound. Each sound is played first at an inaudible level, then the volume is gradually increased until you signal that you can hear it.
  The second part of the test measures your ability to hear the same sounds conducted through the bones in your head. For this test you wear a special headset that vibrates against your skull, usually behind the ear.
  The third part of the test measures your ability to understand and repeat certain words.
  The results of the tests are recorded on an audiogram and show what sounds you have difficulty hearing.

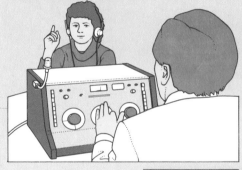

In the first part of the test, your ability to hear sound through headphones is measured (above). In the second part of the test, you wear a special headset behind your ears that transmits vibrations through the bones in your skull (right).

Acoustic impedance testing
Acoustic impedance testing is used to assess the movement of the eardrum, which may be impaired as a result of a disorder of the middle ear. A special probe containing a sound transmitter and receiver is inserted into the outer-ear canal. Air is pumped through the probe and the ability of the eardrum to reflect sound emitted by the sound transmitter at different air pressure levels is measured. From the results it is possible to determine the ease with which sound is transmitted through the eardrum and into the inner ear.

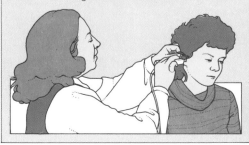

Continued from previous page

Do you regularly spend time listening to loud music, for example, at rock concerts or discos, or through headphones; are you often exposed to loud noise at work; or are you exposed to loud noise through hobbies involving power tools or firearms?

YES →

Repeated exposure to loud noise has probably caused your hearing loss. Even noise levels that do not cause discomfort can result in permanent damage to your hearing. Headphones can be particularly dangerous, since it is easy to have the volume too high (to overcome external noises such as traffic) without realizing it.

Self-help: Take appropriate steps to avoid noise exposure. Keep well away from the speakers at rock concerts and discos, and reduce the volume on your headphones so that others in the same room cannot hear the music. If you work in noisy surroundings (in a factory, for example), your employer should supply you with ear protectors, or you can buy your own earplugs. You should consult your physician, who may arrange for you to have special hearing tests and, if necessary, recommend a hearing aid.

NO ↓

Have you recently taken any prescribed or over-the-counter medications?

YES →

Certain drugs can cause deafness as a side effect. Discuss the problem with your physician.

NO ↓

Has your hearing been getting worse over a period of several weeks or more?

YES →

Have other members of your family suffered from gradual hearing loss?

YES →

NO ↓

Wax blockage may be the cause of your deafness.

Self-help: To remove wax yourself, soften it with over-the-counter ear drops or warm oil for several days. Then lie in a warm bath with your ears submerged to loosen the wax, which should work its way out of the outer ear by itself. If you cannot remove the wax this way, do not attempt to lever it out by poking a pointed instrument into your ear. Consult your physician, who will flush (syringe) the ear with warm water to wash away the blockage.

NO ↓

Consult your physician if you are unable to make a diagnosis from this chart.

Are you over 50 years old?

YES →

NO ↓

Otosclerosis, a disorder that affects the working of the bones in the middle ear, may be the problem. This type of deafness usually affects young adults and is especially common in women. The disorder may get worse during pregnancy (see *Deafness and pregnancy,* below left). Consult your physician.

Treatment: If your physician suspects otosclerosis, he or she will probably arrange for you to undergo *hearing tests* (opposite). If you have serious loss of hearing in one or both ears, a *stapedectomy* (above) may be recommended.

Presbycusis, gradual loss of hearing as you get older, is common, especially if other members of your family have become deaf in old age. Consult your physician.

Treatment: Your physician may refer you for *hearing tests* (opposite). If these confirm the diagnosis, you will probably be offered a hearing aid.

STAPEDECTOMY

Stapedectomy is an operation on the stirrup bone in the middle ear that is often carried out in severe cases of otosclerosis. Usually the operation produces a marked improvement in hearing but, unfortunately, in a small proportion of cases it results in complete deafness in that ear.

The operation

During the operation, the eardrum is moved aside and the stirrup *(stapes),* one of the three tiny bones in the middle ear that is immobilized by the disease, is replaced by a metal or plastic substitute. This improves the conduction of sound through the middle ear.

Stapedectomy usually involves a hospital stay of 2 to 3 days and convalescence at home for another week or so. You may feel dizzy for a few days following the operation.

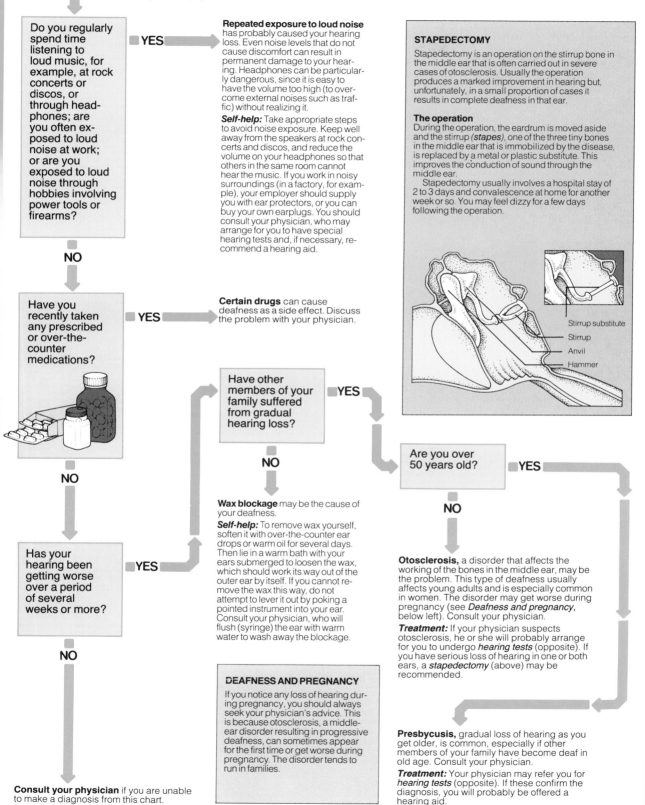

Stirrup substitute
Stirrup
Anvil
Hammer

DEAFNESS AND PREGNANCY

If you notice any loss of hearing during pregnancy, you should always seek your physician's advice. This is because otosclerosis, a middle-ear disorder resulting in progressive deafness, can sometimes appear for the first time or get worse during pregnancy. The disorder tends to run in families.

85 Runny nose

Blockage of the nose by a thick or watery discharge is probably one of the most familiar symptoms. It is nearly always caused by irritation of the mucous membrane lining of the nose. This is usually the result of infection, but may sometimes occur as an allergic reaction. A runny nose rarely indicates a serious disorder.

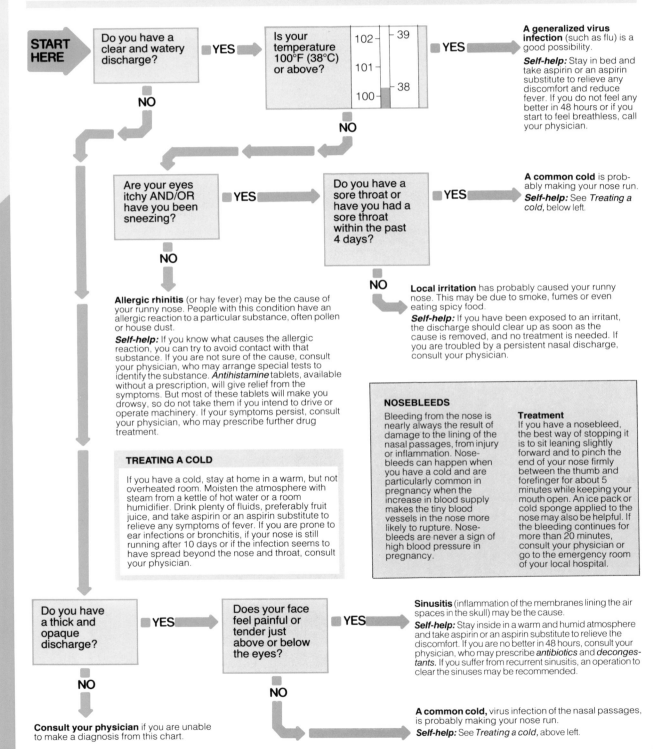

START HERE

Do you have a clear and watery discharge? YES → **Is your temperature 100°F (38°C) or above?** YES → **A generalized virus infection** (such as flu) is a good possibility.

Self-help: Stay in bed and take aspirin or an aspirin substitute to relieve any discomfort and reduce fever. If you do not feel any better in 48 hours or if you start to feel breathless, call your physician.

102 — 39
101
100 — 38

NO (from discharge) / NO (from temperature)

Are your eyes itchy AND/OR have you been sneezing? YES → **Do you have a sore throat or have you had a sore throat within the past 4 days?** YES → **A common cold** is probably making your nose run.
Self-help: See *Treating a cold,* below left.

NO (from eyes/sneezing)

NO (from sore throat) → **Local irritation** has probably caused your runny nose. This may be due to smoke, fumes or even eating spicy food.
Self-help: If you have been exposed to an irritant, the discharge should clear up as soon as the cause is removed, and no treatment is needed. If you are troubled by a persistent nasal discharge, consult your physician.

Allergic rhinitis (or hay fever) may be the cause of your runny nose. People with this condition have an allergic reaction to a particular substance, often pollen or house dust.

Self-help: If you know what causes the allergic reaction, you can try to avoid contact with that substance. If you are not sure of the cause, consult your physician, who may arrange special tests to identify the substance. *Antihistamine* tablets, available without a prescription, will give relief from the symptoms. But most of these tablets will make you drowsy, so do not take them if you intend to drive or operate machinery. If your symptoms persist, consult your physician, who may prescribe further drug treatment.

TREATING A COLD

If you have a cold, stay at home in a warm, but not overheated room. Moisten the atmosphere with steam from a kettle of hot water or a room humidifier. Drink plenty of fluids, preferably fruit juice, and take aspirin or an aspirin substitute to relieve any symptoms of fever. If you are prone to ear infections or bronchitis, if your nose is still running after 10 days or if the infection seems to have spread beyond the nose and throat, consult your physician.

NOSEBLEEDS

Bleeding from the nose is nearly always the result of damage to the lining of the nasal passages, from injury or inflammation. Nosebleeds can happen when you have a cold and are particularly common in pregnancy when the increase in blood supply makes the tiny blood vessels in the nose more likely to rupture. Nosebleeds are never a sign of high blood pressure in pregnancy.

Treatment
If you have a nosebleed, the best way of stopping it is to sit leaning slightly forward and to pinch the end of your nose firmly between the thumb and forefinger for about 5 minutes while keeping your mouth open. An ice pack or cold sponge applied to the nose may also be helpful. If the bleeding continues for more than 20 minutes, consult your physician or go to the emergency room of your local hospital.

Do you have a thick and opaque discharge? YES → **Does your face feel painful or tender just above or below the eyes?** YES → **Sinusitis** (inflammation of the membranes lining the air spaces in the skull) may be the cause.

Self-help: Stay inside in a warm and humid atmosphere and take aspirin or an aspirin substitute to relieve the discomfort. If you are no better in 48 hours, consult your physician, who may prescribe *antibiotics* and *decongestants.* If you suffer from recurrent sinusitis, an operation to clear the sinuses may be recommended.

NO (from thick discharge)

NO (from face pain) → **A common cold,** virus infection of the nasal passages, is probably making your nose run.
Self-help: See *Treating a cold,* above left.

Consult your physician if you are unable to make a diagnosis from this chart.

86 Sore throat

Most people suffer from a painful, rough or raw feeling in the throat from time to time. This is usually the result of a minor infection or local irritation, and almost always disappears within a few days without medical treatment.

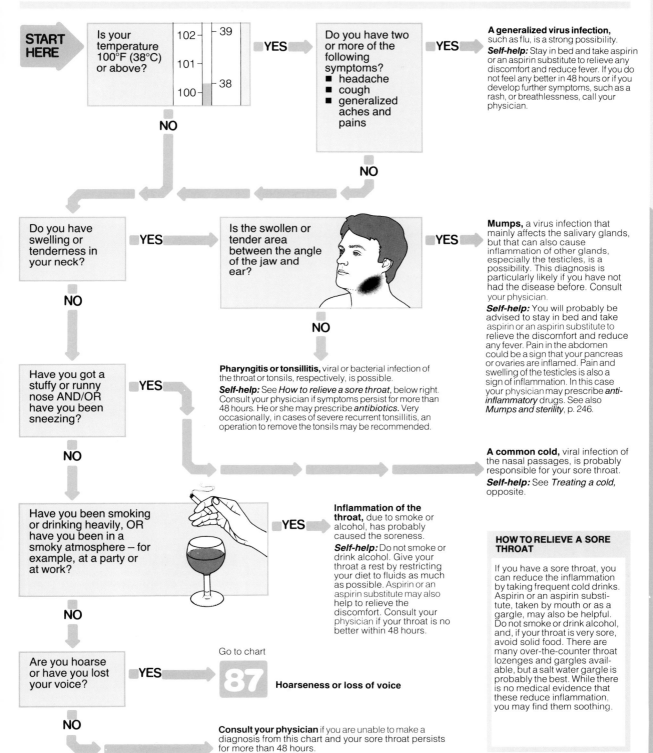

START HERE

Is your temperature 100°F (38°C) or above?

102 — 39
101 —
100 — 38

YES → Do you have two or more of the following symptoms?
■ headache
■ cough
■ generalized aches and pains

YES → **A generalized virus infection,** such as flu, is a strong possibility.
Self-help: Stay in bed and take aspirin or an aspirin substitute to relieve any discomfort and reduce fever. If you do not feel any better in 48 hours or if you develop further symptoms, such as a rash, or breathlessness, call your physician.

NO (temperature)

NO (symptoms)

Do you have swelling or tenderness in your neck?

YES → Is the swollen or tender area between the angle of the jaw and ear?

YES → **Mumps,** a virus infection that mainly affects the salivary glands, but that can also cause inflammation of other glands, especially the testicles, is a possibility. This diagnosis is particularly likely if you have not had the disease before. Consult your physician.
Self-help: You will probably be advised to stay in bed and take aspirin or an aspirin substitute to relieve the discomfort and reduce any fever. Pain in the abdomen could be a sign that your pancreas or ovaries are inflamed. Pain and swelling of the testicles is also a sign of inflammation. In this case your physician may prescribe *anti-inflammatory* drugs. See also *Mumps and sterility*, p. 246.

NO (neck)

NO (jaw/ear)

Have you got a stuffy or runny nose AND/OR have you been sneezing?

YES → **Pharyngitis or tonsillitis,** viral or bacterial infection of the throat or tonsils, respectively, is possible.
Self-help: See *How to relieve a sore throat,* below right. Consult your physician if symptoms persist for more than 48 hours. He or she may prescribe *antibiotics.* Very occasionally, in cases of severe recurrent tonsillitis, an operation to remove the tonsils may be recommended.

A common cold, viral infection of the nasal passages, is probably responsible for your sore throat.
Self-help: See *Treating a cold,* opposite.

NO (nose)

Have you been smoking or drinking heavily, OR have you been in a smoky atmosphere – for example, at a party or at work?

YES → **Inflammation of the throat,** due to smoke or alcohol, has probably caused the soreness.
Self-help: Do not smoke or drink alcohol. Give your throat a rest by restricting your diet to fluids as much as possible. Aspirin or an aspirin substitute may also help to relieve the discomfort. Consult your physician if your throat is no better within 48 hours.

NO (smoking)

Are you hoarse or have you lost your voice?

YES → Go to chart **87** Hoarseness or loss of voice

NO

Consult your physician if you are unable to make a diagnosis from this chart and your sore throat persists for more than 48 hours.

HOW TO RELIEVE A SORE THROAT

If you have a sore throat, you can reduce the inflammation by taking frequent cold drinks. Aspirin or an aspirin substitute, taken by mouth or as a gargle, may also be helpful. Do not smoke or drink alcohol, and, if your throat is very sore, avoid solid food. There are many over-the-counter throat lozenges and gargles available, but a salt water gargle is probably the best. While there is no medical evidence that these reduce inflammation, you may find them soothing.

87 Hoarseness or loss of voice

Hoarseness, huskiness or loss of voice is almost always caused by laryngitis – inflammation and swelling of the vocal cords that interferes with their ability to vibrate normally to produce sounds. There can be a variety of underlying causes for this inflammation, including infections or irritations, most of which are minor and easily treated at home. However, persistent or recurrent hoarseness or loss of voice may have a more serious cause and should always be brought to your physician's attention without delay.

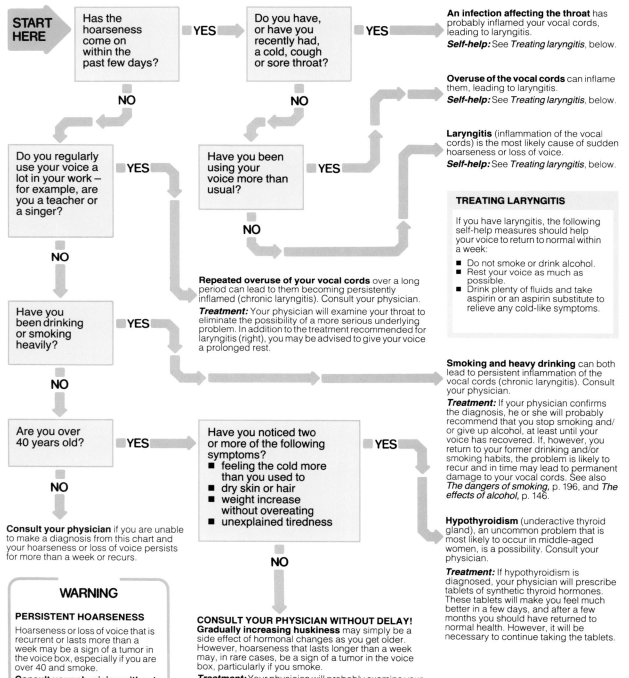

START HERE

Has the hoarseness come on within the past few days? — **YES** → Do you have, or have you recently had, a cold, cough or sore throat? — **YES** →

An infection affecting the throat has probably inflamed your vocal cords, leading to laryngitis.
Self-help: See *Treating laryngitis*, below.

NO ↓ (from first question)

NO ↓ (from cold/cough question)

Do you regularly use your voice a lot in your work – for example, are you a teacher or a singer? — **YES** →

Have you been using your voice more than usual? — **YES** →

Overuse of the vocal cords can inflame them, leading to laryngitis.
Self-help: See *Treating laryngitis*, below.

NO ↓ (Have you been using your voice)

Laryngitis (inflammation of the vocal cords) is the most likely cause of sudden hoarseness or loss of voice.
Self-help: See *Treating laryngitis*, below.

NO ↓ (Do you regularly use your voice)

Have you been drinking or smoking heavily? — **YES** →

Repeated overuse of your vocal cords over a long period can lead to them becoming persistently inflamed (chronic laryngitis). Consult your physician.

Treatment: Your physician will examine your throat to eliminate the possibility of a more serious underlying problem. In addition to the treatment recommended for laryngitis (right), you may be advised to give your voice a prolonged rest.

NO ↓

Are you over 40 years old? — **YES** →

Have you noticed two or more of the following symptoms?
■ feeling the cold more than you used to
■ dry skin or hair
■ weight increase without overeating
■ unexplained tiredness
— **YES** →

NO ↓

Consult your physician if you are unable to make a diagnosis from this chart and your hoarseness or loss of voice persists for more than a week or recurs.

NO ↓ (symptoms)

TREATING LARYNGITIS

If you have laryngitis, the following self-help measures should help your voice to return to normal within a week:

■ Do not smoke or drink alcohol.
■ Rest your voice as much as possible.
■ Drink plenty of fluids and take aspirin or an aspirin substitute to relieve any cold-like symptoms.

Smoking and heavy drinking can both lead to persistent inflammation of the vocal cords (chronic laryngitis). Consult your physician.

Treatment: If your physician confirms the diagnosis, he or she will probably recommend that you stop smoking and/or give up alcohol, at least until your voice has recovered. If, however, you return to your former drinking and/or smoking habits, the problem is likely to recur and in time may lead to permanent damage to your vocal cords. See also *The dangers of smoking,* p. 196, and *The effects of alcohol,* p. 146.

Hypothyroidism (underactive thyroid gland), an uncommon problem that is most likely to occur in middle-aged women, is a possibility. Consult your physician.

Treatment: If hypothyroidism is diagnosed, your physician will prescribe tablets of synthetic thyroid hormones. These tablets will make you feel much better in a few days, and after a few months you should have returned to normal health. However, it will be necessary to continue taking the tablets.

WARNING

PERSISTENT HOARSENESS

Hoarseness or loss of voice that is recurrent or lasts more than a week may be a sign of a tumor in the voice box, especially if you are over 40 and smoke.

Consult your physician without delay!

CONSULT YOUR PHYSICIAN WITHOUT DELAY!
Gradually increasing huskiness may simply be a side effect of hormonal changes as you get older. However, hoarseness that lasts longer than a week may, in rare cases, be a sign of a tumor in the voice box, particularly if you smoke.

Treatment: Your physician will probably examine your throat and may arrange for you to have a *biopsy* (p. 159) of the voice box. Many growths can be removed surgically.

88 Wheezing

Wheezing sometimes occurs when breathing out if you have a chest cold, and this is no cause for concern as long as breathing is otherwise normal. Such wheezing can usually be heard only through a stethoscope, but it may become more apparent to you when you exhale violently (during exercise, for example). Loud wheezing, especially if you also feel breathless or if breathing is painful, may be a sign of a number of more serious conditions, including congestive heart failure, asthma and bronchitis, which require medical attention.

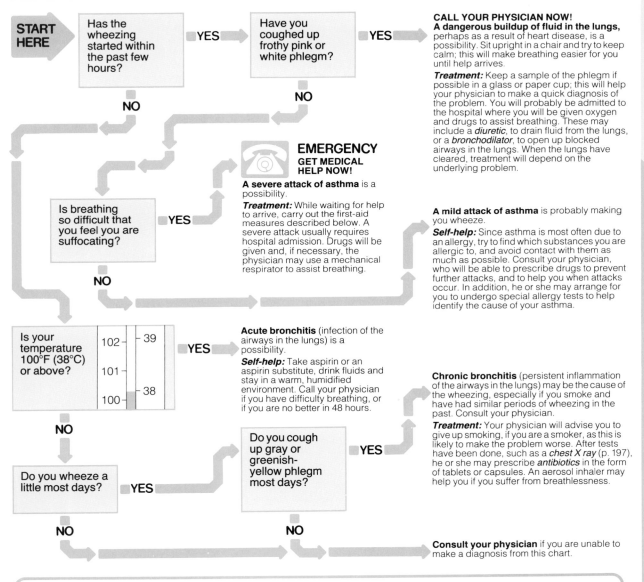

START HERE

Has the wheezing started within the past few hours? — **YES** → **Have you coughed up frothy pink or white phlegm?** — **YES** →

CALL YOUR PHYSICIAN NOW!
A dangerous buildup of fluid in the lungs, perhaps as a result of heart disease, is a possibility. Sit upright in a chair and try to keep calm; this will make breathing easier for you until help arrives.

Treatment: Keep a sample of the phlegm if possible in a glass or paper cup; this will help your physician to make a quick diagnosis of the problem. You will probably be admitted to the hospital where you will be given oxygen and drugs to assist breathing. These may include a *diuretic*, to drain fluid from the lungs, or a *bronchodilator*, to open up blocked airways in the lungs. When the lungs have cleared, treatment will depend on the underlying problem.

NO ↓   **NO** ↓

EMERGENCY GET MEDICAL HELP NOW!
A severe attack of asthma is a possibility.

Treatment: While waiting for help to arrive, carry out the first-aid measures described below. A severe attack usually requires hospital admission. Drugs will be given and, if necessary, the physician may use a mechanical respirator to assist breathing.

Is breathing so difficult that you feel you are suffocating? — **YES** ↑

A mild attack of asthma is probably making you wheeze.

Self-help: Since asthma is most often due to an allergy, try to find which substances you are allergic to, and avoid contact with them as much as possible. Consult your physician, who will be able to prescribe drugs to prevent further attacks, and to help you when attacks occur. In addition, he or she may arrange for you to undergo special allergy tests to help identify the cause of your asthma.

NO ↓

Is your temperature 100°F (38°C) or above?

102 –	– 39
101 –	
100 –	– 38

— **YES** →

Acute bronchitis (infection of the airways in the lungs) is a possibility.

Self-help: Take aspirin or an aspirin substitute, drink fluids and stay in a warm, humidified environment. Call your physician if you have difficulty breathing, or if you are no better in 48 hours.

Chronic bronchitis (persistent inflammation of the airways in the lungs) may be the cause of the wheezing, especially if you smoke and have had similar periods of wheezing in the past. Consult your physician.

Treatment: Your physician will advise you to give up smoking, if you are a smoker, as this is likely to make the problem worse. After tests have been done, such as a *chest X ray* (p. 197), he or she may prescribe *antibiotics* in the form of tablets or capsules. An aerosol inhaler may help you if you suffer from breathlessness.

NO ↓

Do you wheeze a little most days? — **YES** → **Do you cough up gray or greenish-yellow phlegm most days?** — **YES** ↑

NO ↓   **NO** ↓

Consult your physician if you are unable to make a diagnosis from this chart.

FIRST AID FOR ASTHMA

A severe attack of asthma, in which the person is fighting for breath and/or becomes pale and clammy with a blue tinge to the tongue or lips, is an emergency and admission to the hospital is essential. Call an ambulance or go to the emergency room of your local hospital immediately. Most people with asthma already have drugs or an inhaling apparatus, both of which should be administered. If one dose of inhalant does not quickly relieve the wheezing, it should be repeated only once.

In all cases, help the asthmatic to find the most comfortable position while you are waiting for medical help. The best position is sitting up, leaning forward on the back of a chair, and taking some of the weight on the arms (right). Plenty of fresh air will also help. A sudden severe attack of asthma can be very frightening for the family as well as the asthmatic. However, anxiety can make the attack worse, so only one other person should remain with the asthmatic and this person should be calm until help is provided.

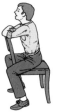

89 Coughing

A cough may produce phlegm or be "dry." It is the body's response to any foreign body, congestion or irritation in the lungs or the throat (for instance, as a result of a cold, smoking or an allergy). Sometimes, however, coughing signals a more serious disorder in the respiratory tract and requires medical attention.

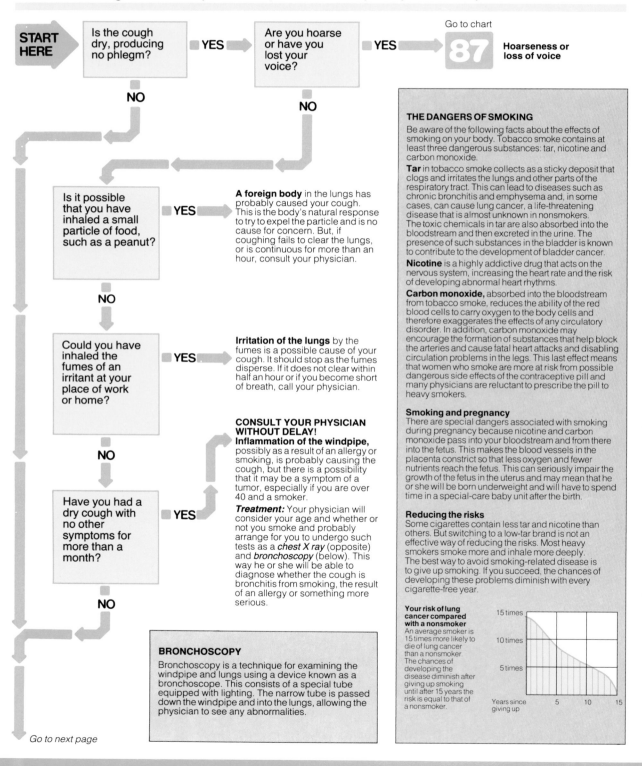

START HERE

Is the cough dry, producing no phlegm?

YES → **Are you hoarse or have you lost your voice?**

YES → Go to chart **87** Hoarseness or loss of voice

NO ↓ (cough box) / NO ↓ (hoarse box)

Is it possible that you have inhaled a small particle of food, such as a peanut?

YES → **A foreign body** in the lungs has probably caused your cough. This is the body's natural response to try to expel the particle and is no cause for concern. But, if coughing fails to clear the lungs, or is continuous for more than an hour, consult your physician.

NO ↓

Could you have inhaled the fumes of an irritant at your place of work or home?

YES → **Irritation of the lungs** by the fumes is a possible cause of your cough. It should stop as the fumes disperse. If it does not clear within half an hour or if you become short of breath, call your physician.

NO ↓

Have you had a dry cough with no other symptoms for more than a month?

YES → **CONSULT YOUR PHYSICIAN WITHOUT DELAY!**
Inflammation of the windpipe, possibly as a result of an allergy or smoking, is probably causing the cough, but there is a possibility that it may be a symptom of a tumor, especially if you are over 40 and a smoker.

Treatment: Your physician will consider your age and whether or not you smoke and probably arrange for you to undergo such tests as a *chest X ray* (opposite) and *bronchoscopy* (below). This way he or she will be able to diagnose whether the cough is bronchitis from smoking, the result of an allergy or something more serious.

NO ↓

BRONCHOSCOPY

Bronchoscopy is a technique for examining the windpipe and lungs using a device known as a bronchoscope. This consists of a special tube equipped with lighting. The narrow tube is passed down the windpipe and into the lungs, allowing the physician to see any abnormalities.

Go to next page

THE DANGERS OF SMOKING

Be aware of the following facts about the effects of smoking on your body. Tobacco smoke contains at least three dangerous substances: tar, nicotine and carbon monoxide.

Tar in tobacco smoke collects as a sticky deposit that clogs and irritates the lungs and other parts of the respiratory tract. This can lead to diseases such as chronic bronchitis and emphysema and, in some cases, can cause lung cancer, a life-threatening disease that is almost unknown in nonsmokers. The toxic chemicals in tar are also absorbed into the bloodstream and then excreted in the urine. The presence of such substances in the bladder is known to contribute to the development of bladder cancer.

Nicotine is a highly addictive drug that acts on the nervous system, increasing the heart rate and the risk of developing abnormal heart rhythms.

Carbon monoxide, absorbed into the bloodstream from tobacco smoke, reduces the ability of the red blood cells to carry oxygen to the body cells and therefore exaggerates the effects of any circulatory disorder. In addition, carbon monoxide may encourage the formation of substances that help block the arteries and cause fatal heart attacks and disabling circulation problems in the legs. This last effect means that women who smoke are more at risk from possible dangerous side effects of the contraceptive pill and many physicians are reluctant to prescribe the pill to heavy smokers.

Smoking and pregnancy
There are special dangers associated with smoking during pregnancy because nicotine and carbon monoxide pass into your bloodstream and from there into the fetus. This makes the blood vessels in the placenta constrict so that less oxygen and fewer nutrients reach the fetus. This can seriously impair the growth of the fetus in the uterus and may mean that he or she will be born underweight and will have to spend time in a special-care baby unit after the birth.

Reducing the risks
Some cigarettes contain less tar and nicotine than others. But switching to a low-tar brand is not an effective way of reducing the risks. Most heavy smokers smoke more and inhale more deeply. The best way to avoid smoking-related disease is to give up smoking. If you succeed, the chances of developing these problems diminish with every cigarette-free year.

Your risk of lung cancer compared with a nonsmoker
An average smoker is 15 times more likely to die of lung cancer than a nonsmoker. The chances of developing the disease diminish after giving up smoking until after 15 years the risk is equal to that of a nonsmoker.

15 times
10 times
5 times

Years since giving up   5   10   15

Continued from previous page

Has the cough started within the past week? → **YES** → **Is your temperature 100°F (38°C) or above?**

102 — 39
101 —
100 — 38

YES → **Are you short of breath?** → **YES**

NO (from temperature) ↓

NO (from cough started) ↓

NO (from short of breath) ↓

Do you have a runny nose AND/OR a sore throat? → **YES** → **A common cold,** a viral infection of the nasal passages, has probably caused these symptoms.

Self-help: For advice on the treatment of colds, see p. 192.

NO ↓

Acute bronchitis (infection of the airways in the lungs) is a possibility.

Self-help: Take aspirin or an aspirin substitute and cough medicine following the instructions on the labels. Stay in a humid environment but it is not necessary to go to bed. Call your physician if you have difficulty in breathing, or if you are no better in 48 hours.

Are you short of breath, even when you have not been exercising? → **YES** → Go to chart

90 **Difficulty breathing**

NO ↓

CALL YOUR PHYSICIAN NOW!
Pneumonia is a possibility. This is an infection of the lungs that can be dangerous, especially for the elderly and those in poor health.

Treatment: Your physician will probably recommend that you take aspirin or an aspirin substitute to reduce your fever and relieve any discomfort. He or she may prescribe *antibiotics* and, in a severe case, may advise admission to a hospital.

Do you cough up thick, gray or greenish-yellow phlegm most days? → **YES**

Chronic bronchitis, persistent inflammation of the airways to the lungs, may be the cause of a cough, especially if you smoke and have had similar periods of persistent coughing in the past. Consult your physician.

Treatment: Your physician may prescribe *antibiotics* in the form of tablets or capsules. An aerosol inhaler may help you if you are suffering from shortness of breath. However, the problem is likely to get worse over the years unless you stop smoking.

NO ↓

CONSULT YOUR PHYSICIAN WITHOUT DELAY!
A serious lung disorder, such as tuberculosis or lung cancer, may cause persistent coughing although a simpler explanation, such as an allergy or chronic bronchitis, is more likely.

Treatment: Your physician will probably arrange for tests to find out which underlying disorder is causing the symptoms. You may be asked to give blood and phlegm samples for analysis. A *chest X ray* (below) and *bronchoscopy* (opposite) may also be necessary.

Have you had your cough for several weeks or months AND has it been getting more severe? → **YES**

CHEST X RAY

A chest X ray is an effective way of examining the lungs and is used by chest specialists as their main diagnostic test. It will show up infections, tumors, other lung disorders, fluid or air in the chest cavity and damage to the rib cage.

This chest X ray shows a condition called pericardial effusion, in which fluid collects around the heart.

NO ↓

Consult your physician if you are unable to make a diagnosis from this chart.

COUGHING UP BLOOD

Phlegm that is colored or streaked bright red or rusty brown may contain blood. Although coughing up blood may simply mean that you have ruptured a small blood vessel in the lung, it may also indicate congestion of the lungs, an infection such as pneumonia or tuberculosis, or a tumor. If you feel quite well and cough up blood on a single occasion, you need not feel alarmed; but coughing up blood more than once, or if you have any of the additional symptoms described, may indicate one of the following serious problems and you should seek medical advice without delay.

A chest infection, such as pneumonia – if your temperature is above 102°F (39°C).

A blood clot in the lung – which is most likely if you have recently had an operation or been confined to bed by an injury or illness. This is an EMERGENCY.

Lung cancer or tuberculosis – especially if you have had a cough for many weeks or months.

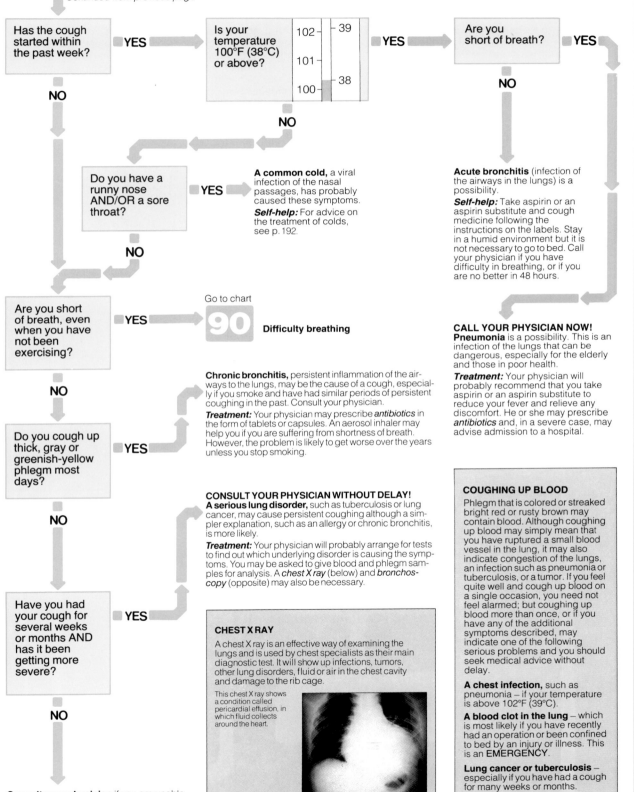

90 Difficulty breathing

If you have the feeling that you cannot get enough air or are breathless to the extent that you are breathing rapidly or "puffing," either at rest or after gentle exercise, this suggests the possibility of a problem affecting the heart or the respiratory system. The sudden onset of difficult breathing while eating is more likely to be caused by choking, and you should immediately carry out first aid as described in the box opposite. Because of the possibility of a disorder that may threaten the supply of oxygen to the body, it is important to seek medical advice promptly if you notice any of the symptoms mentioned in this diagnostic chart.

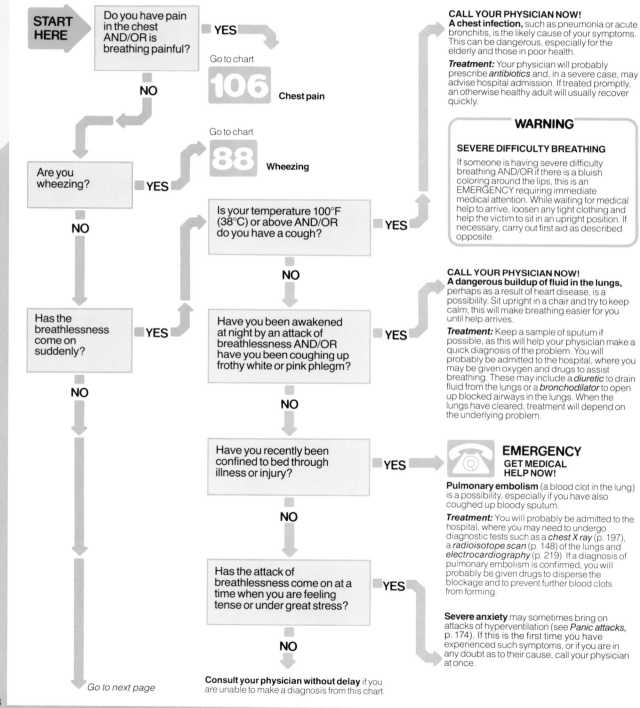

START HERE

Do you have pain in the chest AND/OR is breathing painful? — **YES** → Go to chart **106** Chest pain

NO

Are you wheezing? — **YES** → Go to chart **88** Wheezing

NO

Has the breathlessness come on suddenly? — **YES** →

NO

Is your temperature 100°F (38°C) or above AND/OR do you have a cough? — **YES** →

NO

Have you been awakened at night by an attack of breathlessness AND/OR have you been coughing up frothy white or pink phlegm? — **YES** →

NO

Have you recently been confined to bed through illness or injury? — **YES** →

NO

Has the attack of breathlessness come on at a time when you are feeling tense or under great stress? — **YES** →

NO

Go to next page

Consult your physician without delay if you are unable to make a diagnosis from this chart.

CALL YOUR PHYSICIAN NOW!
A chest infection, such as pneumonia or acute bronchitis, is the likely cause of your symptoms. This can be dangerous, especially for the elderly and those in poor health.

Treatment: Your physician will probably prescribe *antibiotics* and, in a severe case, may advise hospital admission. If treated promptly, an otherwise healthy adult will usually recover quickly.

WARNING

SEVERE DIFFICULTY BREATHING

If someone is having severe difficulty breathing AND/OR if there is a bluish coloring around the lips, this is an EMERGENCY requiring immediate medical attention. While waiting for medical help to arrive, loosen any tight clothing and help the victim to sit in an upright position. If necessary, carry out first aid as described opposite.

CALL YOUR PHYSICIAN NOW!
A dangerous buildup of fluid in the lungs, perhaps as a result of heart disease, is a possibility. Sit upright in a chair and try to keep calm; this will make breathing easier for you until help arrives.

Treatment: Keep a sample of sputum if possible, as this will help your physician make a quick diagnosis of the problem. You will probably be admitted to the hospital, where you may be given oxygen and drugs to assist breathing. These may include a *diuretic* to drain fluid from the lungs or a *bronchodilator* to open up blocked airways in the lungs. When the lungs have cleared, treatment will depend on the underlying problem.

EMERGENCY
GET MEDICAL HELP NOW!

Pulmonary embolism (a blood clot in the lung) is a possibility, especially if you have also coughed up bloody sputum.

Treatment: You will probably be admitted to the hospital, where you may need to undergo diagnostic tests such as a *chest X ray* (p. 197), a *radioisotope scan* (p. 148) of the lungs and *electrocardiography* (p. 219). If a diagnosis of pulmonary embolism is confirmed, you will probably be given drugs to disperse the blockage and to prevent further blood clots from forming.

Severe anxiety may sometimes bring on attacks of hyperventilation (see *Panic attacks,* p. 174). If this is the first time you have experienced such symptoms, or if you are in any doubt as to their cause, call your physician at once.

Continued from previous page

Do you cough up thick, gray or greenish-yellow phlegm most days?

YES → **Do you, or have you, worked in a dusty atmosphere – for example in a mine or quarry?**

YES →

NO ↓

NO ↓

Chronic bronchitis (persistent inflammation of the airways in the lungs) may be the cause of your breathing difficulty, especially if you smoke and have had similar periods of coughing in the past winter. If your work involves regular exposure to mineral dusts, an industrial lung disease such as pneumoconiosis is also possible. Consult your physician.
Treatment: Your physician will advise you to give up smoking, if you are a smoker, as this is likely to make the problem worse. Following tests such as a *chest X-ray* (p.197), he or she may prescribe *antibiotics* in the form of tablets or capsules. An aerosol inhaler may help to relieve breathlessness.

Does your work involve regular contact with grain or other crops AND/OR caged birds or animals?

YES →

NO ↓

Pneumoconiosis, a reaction to coal-dust in the lungs or another dust disease, is a possibility. Consult your physician.
Treatment: A *chest X-ray* (p.197) will indicate how seriously your lungs have been affected. Your physician may advise you to change your job and, if you are a smoker, to give up smoking.

Farmer's lung, an allergic reaction to fungus in moldy grain or hay or a similar sort of allergy to bird or animal droppings, can cause breathless attacks, often with coughing. Consult your physician.
Treatment: Your physician will probably arrange for you to have diagnostic tests including a *chest X-ray* (p.197) and skin tests for allergic sensitivity. If the diagnosis is confirmed, you will probably be advised to avoid further exposure to the substance causing the reaction by changing your job or by wearing a protective mask at work. You may also be given drugs to reduce inflammation of the lung.

Are you pregnant?

YES → Go to chart

143 **Shortness of breath in pregnancy**

NO ↓

Consult your physician without further delay if you are unable to make a diagnosis from this chart.

FIRST AID FOR CHOKING

If severe breathing difficulties occur and the victim is unable to cough up the object, such as a piece of food, use the Heimlich maneuver to dislodge it. Call for emergency help.

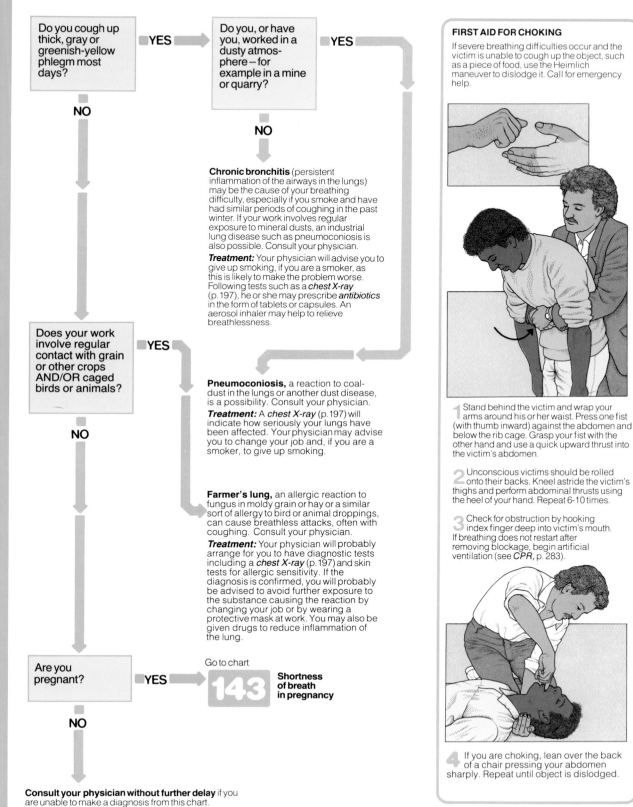

1 Stand behind the victim and wrap your arms around his or her waist. Press one fist (with thumb inward) against the abdomen and below the rib cage. Grasp your fist with the other hand and use a quick upward thrust into the victim's abdomen.

2 Unconscious victims should be rolled onto their backs. Kneel astride the victim's thighs and perform abdominal thrusts using the heel of your hand. Repeat 6-10 times.

3 Check for obstruction by hooking index finger deep into victim's mouth. If breathing does not restart after removing blockage, begin artificial ventilation (see *CPR,* p. 283).

4 If you are choking, lean over the back of a chair pressing your abdomen sharply. Repeat until object is dislodged.

91 Toothache

Teeth are just as much living structures as any other part of the body, despite their tough appearance. They are constantly under threat from our diet because of the high level of sugar we consume. Bacteria act on sugar to produce acids that attack enamel, the tooth's protective layer. When this happens, bacterial destruction (decay) spreads down the root canal to the nerve, causing inflammation and pain. Any pain in one tooth or from teeth and gums in general, whether it is a dull throb or a sharp twinge, should be brought to your dentist's attention.

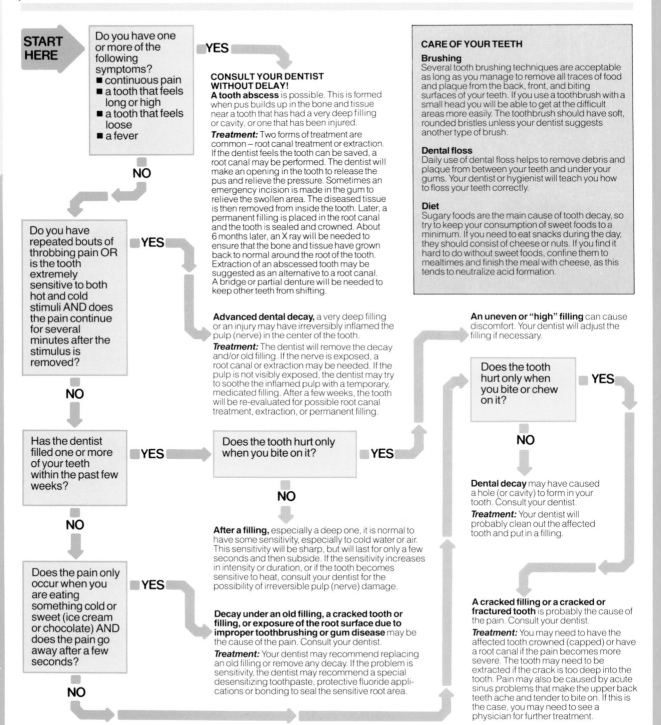

START HERE

Do you have one or more of the following symptoms?
- continuous pain
- a tooth that feels long or high
- a tooth that feels loose
- a fever

YES

CONSULT YOUR DENTIST WITHOUT DELAY!
A tooth abscess is possible. This is formed when pus builds up in the bone and tissue near a tooth that has had a very deep filling or cavity, or one that has been injured.
Treatment: Two forms of treatment are common – root canal treatment or extraction. If the dentist feels the tooth can be saved, a root canal may be performed. The dentist will make an opening in the tooth to release the pus and relieve the pressure. Sometimes an emergency incision is made in the gum to relieve the swollen area. The diseased tissue is then removed from inside the tooth. Later, a permanent filling is placed in the root canal and the tooth is sealed and crowned. About 6 months later, an X ray will be needed to ensure that the bone and tissue have grown back to normal around the root of the tooth. Extraction of an abscessed tooth may be suggested as an alternative to a root canal. A bridge or partial denture will be needed to keep other teeth from shifting.

NO

Do you have repeated bouts of throbbing pain OR is the tooth extremely sensitive to both hot and cold stimuli AND does the pain continue for several minutes after the stimulus is removed?

YES

Advanced dental decay, a very deep filling or an injury may have irreversibly inflamed the pulp (nerve) in the center of the tooth.
Treatment: The dentist will remove the decay and/or old filling. If the nerve is exposed, a root canal or extraction may be needed. If the pulp is not visibly exposed, the dentist may try to soothe the inflamed pulp with a temporary, medicated filling. After a few weeks, the tooth will be re-evaluated for possible root canal treatment, extraction, or permanent filling.

NO

Has the dentist filled one or more of your teeth within the past few weeks?

YES

Does the tooth hurt only when you bite on it?

YES

NO

After a filling, especially a deep one, it is normal to have some sensitivity, especially to cold water or air. This sensitivity will be sharp, but will last for only a few seconds and then subside. If the sensitivity increases in intensity or duration, or if the tooth becomes sensitive to heat, consult your dentist for the possibility of irreversible pulp (nerve) damage.

NO

Does the pain only occur when you are eating something cold or sweet (ice cream or chocolate) AND does the pain go away after a few seconds?

YES

Decay under an old filling, a cracked tooth or filling, or exposure of the root surface due to improper toothbrushing or gum disease may be the cause of the pain. Consult your dentist.
Treatment: Your dentist may recommend replacing an old filling or remove any decay. If the problem is sensitivity, the dentist may recommend a special desensitizing toothpaste, protective fluoride applications or bonding to seal the sensitive root area.

NO

An uneven or "high" filling can cause discomfort. Your dentist will adjust the filling if necessary.

Does the tooth hurt only when you bite or chew on it?

YES

NO

Dental decay may have caused a hole (or cavity) to form in your tooth. Consult your dentist.
Treatment: Your dentist will probably clean out the affected tooth and put in a filling.

A cracked filling or a cracked or fractured tooth is probably the cause of the pain. Consult your dentist.
Treatment: You may need to have the affected tooth crowned (capped) or have a root canal if the pain becomes more severe. The tooth may need to be extracted if the crack is too deep into the tooth. Pain may also be caused by acute sinus problems that make the upper back teeth ache and tender to bite on. If this is the case, you may need to see a physician for further treatment.

CARE OF YOUR TEETH

Brushing
Several tooth brushing techniques are acceptable as long as you manage to remove all traces of food and plaque from the back, front, and biting surfaces of your teeth. If you use a toothbrush with a small head you will be able to get at the difficult areas more easily. The toothbrush should have soft, rounded bristles unless your dentist suggests another type of brush.

Dental floss
Daily use of dental floss helps to remove debris and plaque from between your teeth and under your gums. Your dentist or hygienist will teach you how to floss your teeth correctly.

Diet
Sugary foods are the main cause of tooth decay, so try to keep your consumption of sweet foods to a minimum. If you need to eat snacks during the day, they should consist of cheese or nuts. If you find it hard to do without sweet foods, confine them to mealtimes and finish the meal with cheese, as this tends to neutralize acid formation.

92 Difficulty swallowing

Difficulty swallowing is most often the result of an infection causing soreness, swelling and excess mucus at the back of the throat. Difficulty or pain when swallowing that is not related to a sore throat may be a sign of a more serious disorder affecting the esophagus and should be brought to your physician's attention.

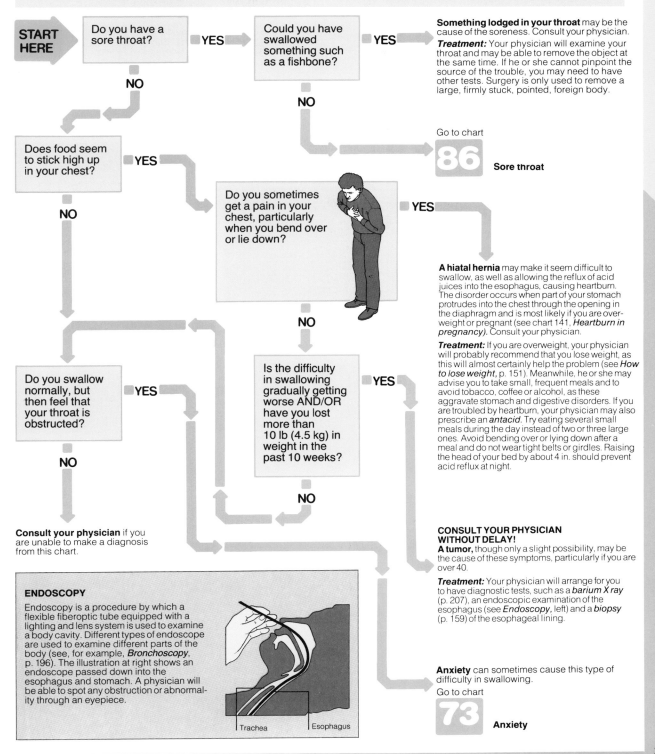

START HERE

Do you have a sore throat?
YES → **Could you have swallowed something such as a fishbone?**
YES → **Something lodged in your throat** may be the cause of the soreness. Consult your physician.

Treatment: Your physician will examine your throat and may be able to remove the object at the same time. If he or she cannot pinpoint the source of the trouble, you may need to have other tests. Surgery is only used to remove a large, firmly stuck, pointed, foreign body.

Do you have a sore throat? **NO**

Could you have swallowed something such as a fishbone? **NO**

Go to chart **86** **Sore throat**

Does food seem to stick high up in your chest?
YES → **Do you sometimes get a pain in your chest, particularly when you bend over or lie down?**
YES →

Does food seem to stick high up in your chest? **NO**

A hiatal hernia may make it seem difficult to swallow, as well as allowing the reflux of acid juices into the esophagus, causing heartburn. The disorder occurs when part of your stomach protrudes into the chest through the opening in the diaphragm and is most likely if you are overweight or pregnant (see chart 141, *Heartburn in pregnancy*). Consult your physician.

Treatment: If you are overweight, your physician will probably recommend that you lose weight, as this will almost certainly help the problem (see *How to lose weight*, p. 151). Meanwhile, he or she may advise you to take small, frequent meals and to avoid tobacco, coffee or alcohol, as these aggravate stomach and digestive disorders. If you are troubled by heartburn, your physician may also prescribe an *antacid*. Try eating several small meals during the day instead of two or three large ones. Avoid bending over or lying down after a meal and do not wear tight belts or girdles. Raising the head of your bed by about 4 in. should prevent acid reflux at night.

Do you sometimes get a pain in your chest...? **NO**

Do you swallow normally, but then feel that your throat is obstructed?
YES →

Is the difficulty in swallowing gradually getting worse AND/OR have you lost more than 10 lb (4.5 kg) in weight in the past 10 weeks?
YES →

Do you swallow normally...? **NO**

Is the difficulty in swallowing...? **NO**

Consult your physician if you are unable to make a diagnosis from this chart.

CONSULT YOUR PHYSICIAN WITHOUT DELAY!
A tumor, though only a slight possibility, may be the cause of these symptoms, particularly if you are over 40.

Treatment: Your physician will arrange for you to have diagnostic tests, such as a *barium X ray* (p. 207), an endoscopic examination of the esophagus (see *Endoscopy,* left) and a *biopsy* (p. 159) of the esophageal lining.

ENDOSCOPY

Endoscopy is a procedure by which a flexible fiberoptic tube equipped with a lighting and lens system is used to examine a body cavity. Different types of endoscope are used to examine different parts of the body (see, for example, *Bronchoscopy*, p. 196). The illustration at right shows an endoscope passed down into the esophagus and stomach. A physician will be able to spot any obstruction or abnormality through an eyepiece.

Trachea   Esophagus

Anxiety can sometimes cause this type of difficulty in swallowing.
Go to chart **73** **Anxiety**

93 Sore mouth or tongue

Most painful areas on the lips or tongue or around the teeth are symptoms of minor conditions. You will be able to tell the mild from the serious by the length of time they take to heal. Any condition lasting longer than 3 weeks should be seen by your physician or dentist. It is important to keep the delicate mucous membrane that lines the mouth healthy by maintaining good oral hygiene at all times (see Care of your teeth, p.200).

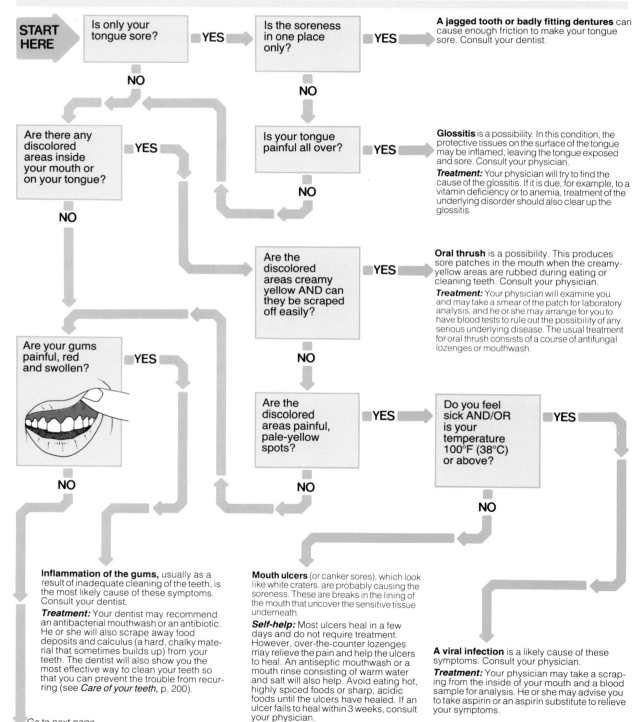

START HERE

Is only your tongue sore?

→ YES → **Is the soreness in one place only?** → YES → **A jagged tooth or badly fitting dentures** can cause enough friction to make your tongue sore. Consult your dentist.

NO ↓ (from "Is only your tongue sore?")

NO ↓ (from "Is the soreness in one place only?")

Are there any discolored areas inside your mouth or on your tongue? → YES →

Is your tongue painful all over? → YES → **Glossitis** is a possibility. In this condition, the protective tissues on the surface of the tongue may be inflamed, leaving the tongue exposed and sore. Consult your physician.

Treatment: Your physician will try to find the cause of the glossitis. If it is due, for example, to a vitamin deficiency or to anemia, treatment of the underlying disorder should also clear up the glossitis.

NO ↓ (from "Is your tongue painful all over?")

Are the discolored areas creamy yellow AND can they be scraped off easily? → YES → **Oral thrush** is a possibility. This produces sore patches in the mouth when the creamy-yellow areas are rubbed during eating or cleaning teeth. Consult your physician.

Treatment: Your physician will examine you and may take a smear of the patch for laboratory analysis, and he or she may arrange for you to have blood tests to rule out the possibility of any serious underlying disease. The usual treatment for oral thrush consists of a course of antifungal lozenges or mouthwash.

NO ↓

Are your gums painful, red and swollen? → YES →

Are the discolored areas painful, pale-yellow spots? → YES → **Do you feel sick AND/OR is your temperature 100°F (38°C) or above?** → YES →

NO ↓ (gums)

NO ↓ (discolored areas painful)

NO ↓ (feel sick)

Inflammation of the gums, usually as a result of inadequate cleaning of the teeth, is the most likely cause of these symptoms. Consult your dentist.

Treatment: Your dentist may recommend an antibacterial mouthwash or an antibiotic. He or she will also scrape away food deposits and calculus (a hard, chalky material that sometimes builds up) from your teeth. The dentist will also show you the most effective way to clean your teeth so that you can prevent the trouble from recurring (see *Care of your teeth,* p. 200).

Mouth ulcers (or canker sores), which look like white craters, are probably causing the soreness. These are breaks in the lining of the mouth that uncover the sensitive tissue underneath.

Self-help: Most ulcers heal in a few days and do not require treatment. However, over-the-counter lozenges may relieve the pain and help the ulcers to heal. An antiseptic mouthwash or a mouth rinse consisting of warm water and salt will also help. Avoid eating hot, highly spiced foods or sharp, acidic foods until the ulcers have healed. If an ulcer fails to heal within 3 weeks, consult your physician.

A viral infection is a likely cause of these symptoms. Consult your physician.

Treatment: Your physician may take a scraping from the inside of your mouth and a blood sample for analysis. He or she may advise you to take aspirin or an aspirin substitute to relieve your symptoms.

Go to next page

Continued from previous page

Do you have sore places on or around the lips?

→ **YES** → **Did the sores start as painful blisters?** → **YES** →

Cold sores are the likely cause of these symptoms. They are the result of a virus in the body becoming reactivated by a cold, or exposure to strong sunshine or cold weather.

Self-help: Mild cases of cold sores clear up on their own. However, there are many over-the-counter preparations that may relieve symptoms. If you are troubled by severe, recurrent cold sores, your physician may prescribe a cream for you to apply when a sore is in its early stages to inhibit its development.

NO ↓ ... **NO** ↓

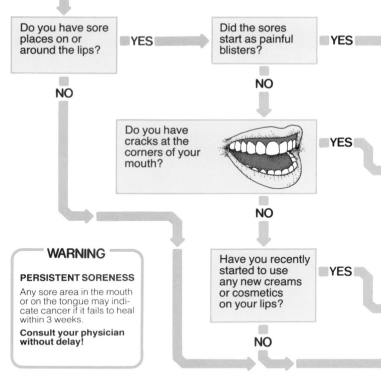

Do you have cracks at the corners of your mouth? → **YES** →

Ill-fitting dentures may be the cause of such soreness. Occasionally, however, cracking at the corners of the mouth may also be a sign of a vitamin deficiency. If you wear dentures, consult your dentist. Otherwise, consult your physician.

Treatment: If dentures are the problem, your dentist may adjust your old baseplate or supply a new set. He or she may also prescribe lozenges to relieve the soreness. If there is a possibility of a vitamin deficiency, your physician will ask you about your diet and examine you to eliminate the possibility of an underlying disease. He or she may prescribe vitamin supplements.

NO ↓

Have you recently started to use any new creams or cosmetics on your lips? → **YES** →

An allergic reaction to one of the ingredients is a possibility (see also *Eczema,* p. 181).
Self-help: Avoid contact with the substance that causes the reaction. If the soreness continues, consult your physician, who may prescribe a salve.

NO ↓

Consult your physician if you are unable to make a diagnosis from this chart.

WARNING

PERSISTENT SORENESS

Any sore area in the mouth or on the tongue may indicate cancer if it fails to heal within 3 weeks.

Consult your physician without delay!

BAD BREATH

You are unlikely to notice that you have bad breath unless it is pointed out to you by a friend. The following are the most common causes of bad breath and are easily remedied:

Sore mouth
Infection or ulceration of the mouth, gums or tongue may cause bad breath. Rinsing out your mouth with an antiseptic mouthwash usually clears up the problem within a few days. If the problem persists, consult your physician.

Inadequately cleaned teeth or dentures
If you do not clean your teeth (or dentures, if you wear them) thoroughly at least twice a day, this may be the cause of your bad breath. Decaying food particles lodge between the teeth or stick to the dentures (see *Care of your teeth*, p. 200, and *Caring for your dentures*, right).

Garlic, onions and alcohol
These contain volatile substances that, when absorbed into the bloodstream and then released into the lungs, may cause bad breath. Your breath should return to normal within 24 hours after consuming these foods.

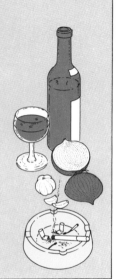

Smoking
Smoking always causes a form of bad breath (see also *The dangers of smoking*, p. 196).

If your bad breath continues for some time, it may be a symptom of something more serious such as a mouth infection or a lung disease. Consult your physician.

CARING FOR YOUR DENTURES

Always remove your dentures at night and keep them in a glass of water containing a cleansing agent so that they do not dry out and warp. This will also give the gum tissues a regular rest period. Brush your dentures thoroughly every day. Your dentist will show you the best way to do this. It is also important to remember to clean any remaining natural teeth thoroughly, especially where teeth and gums meet. Partial dentures may feel a little tight when inserted in the morning, but this is normal and the feeling disappears in a few minutes. The useful life of dentures varies greatly – from 6 months to 5 years or more – depending on how well your gums and jaws keep their shape. If you have a full set of dentures, you should visit the dentist every 2 years. If you still have some natural teeth, you should go for a check-up every 6 months.

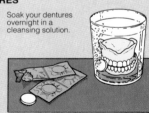
Soak your dentures overnight in a cleansing solution.

Brush your dentures daily on both sides to remove all food deposits. Rinse throughly before replacing them in your mouth.

Brush any remaining natural teeth carefully twice a day.

94 Vomiting

Vomiting occurs when the muscles around the stomach suddenly contract and "throw up" the stomach contents. This is usually the result of irritation of the stomach from infection or overindulgence in rich food or alcohol, but may also occur as a result of disturbance elsewhere in the digestive tract. Occasionally, a dis-order affecting the nerve signals from the brain, or from the balance mechanism in the inner ear (p. 40), can also produce vomiting. Most cases of vomiting can be treated at home, but vomiting that is accompanied by severe abdominal pain, or by severe headache or eye pain, requires urgent medical attention.

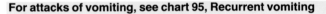

For attacks of vomiting, see chart 95, Recurrent vomiting

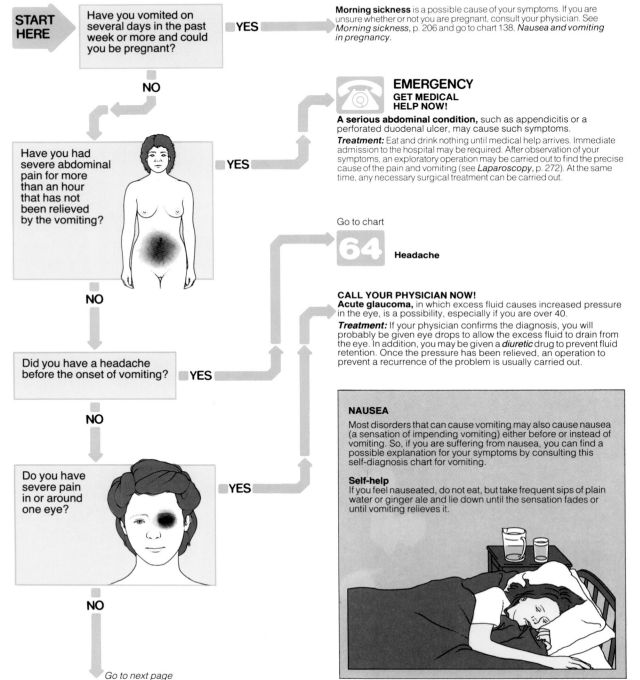

START HERE

Have you vomited on several days in the past week or more and could you be pregnant?

YES → **Morning sickness** is a possible cause of your symptoms. If you are unsure whether or not you are pregnant, consult your physician. See *Morning sickness*, p. 206 and go to chart 138, *Nausea and vomiting in pregnancy*.

NO

Have you had severe abdominal pain for more than an hour that has not been relieved by the vomiting?

YES → **EMERGENCY**
GET MEDICAL HELP NOW!

A serious abdominal condition, such as appendicitis or a perforated duodenal ulcer, may cause such symptoms.

Treatment: Eat and drink nothing until medical help arrives. Immediate admission to the hospital may be required. After observation of your symptoms, an exploratory operation may be carried out to find the precise cause of the pain and vomiting (see *Laparoscopy*, p. 272). At the same time, any necessary surgical treatment can be carried out.

NO

Did you have a headache before the onset of vomiting?

YES → Go to chart

64 **Headache**

NO

Do you have severe pain in or around one eye?

YES → **CALL YOUR PHYSICIAN NOW!**
Acute glaucoma, in which excess fluid causes increased pressure in the eye, is a possibility, especially if you are over 40.

Treatment: If your physician confirms the diagnosis, you will probably be given eye drops to allow the excess fluid to drain from the eye. In addition, you may be given a *diuretic* drug to prevent fluid retention. Once the pressure has been relieved, an operation to prevent a recurrence of the problem is usually carried out.

NO

Go to next page

NAUSEA

Most disorders that can cause vomiting may also cause nausea (a sensation of impending vomiting) either before or instead of vomiting. So, if you are suffering from nausea, you can find a possible explanation for your symptoms by consulting this self-diagnosis chart for vomiting.

Self-help
If you feel nauseated, do not eat, but take frequent sips of plain water or ginger ale and lie down until the sensation fades or until vomiting relieves it.

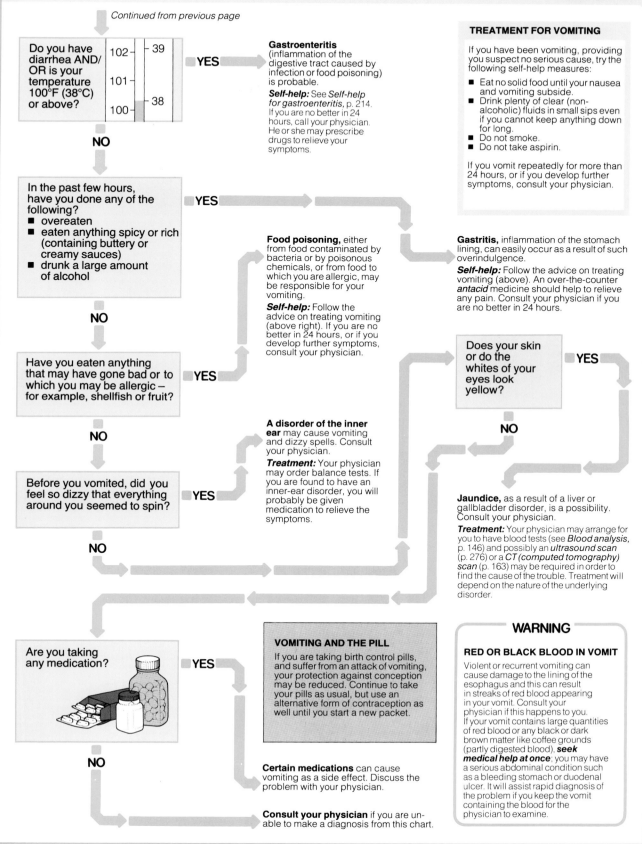

Continued from previous page

Do you have diarrhea AND/OR is your temperature 100°F (38°C) or above?

102 –	– 39
101 –	
100 –	– 38

YES →

Gastroenteritis (inflammation of the digestive tract caused by infection or food poisoning) is probable.
Self-help: See *Self-help for gastroenteritis,* p. 214. If you are no better in 24 hours, call your physician. He or she may prescribe drugs to relieve your symptoms.

NO ↓

In the past few hours, have you done any of the following?
- overeaten
- eaten anything spicy or rich (containing buttery or creamy sauces)
- drunk a large amount of alcohol

YES →

Food poisoning, either from food contaminated by bacteria or by poisonous chemicals, or from food to which you are allergic, may be responsible for your vomiting.
Self-help: Follow the advice on treating vomiting (above right). If you are no better in 24 hours, or if you develop further symptoms, consult your physician.

NO ↓

Have you eaten anything that may have gone bad or to which you may be allergic — for example, shellfish or fruit?

YES →

NO ↓

Before you vomited, did you feel so dizzy that everything around you seemed to spin?

YES →

A disorder of the inner ear may cause vomiting and dizzy spells. Consult your physician.
Treatment: Your physician may order balance tests. If you are found to have an inner-ear disorder, you will probably be given medication to relieve the symptoms.

NO ↓

Are you taking any medication?

YES →

NO ↓

Does your skin or do the whites of your eyes look yellow?

YES →

NO ↓

Gastritis, inflammation of the stomach lining, can easily occur as a result of such overindulgence.
Self-help: Follow the advice on treating vomiting (above). An over-the-counter *antacid* medicine should help to relieve any pain. Consult your physician if you are no better in 24 hours.

Jaundice, as a result of a liver or gallbladder disorder, is a possibility. Consult your physician.
Treatment: Your physician may arrange for you to have blood tests (see *Blood analysis,* p. 146) and possibly an *ultrasound scan* (p. 276) or a *CT (computed tomography) scan* (p. 163) may be required in order to find the cause of the trouble. Treatment will depend on the nature of the underlying disorder.

TREATMENT FOR VOMITING

If you have been vomiting, providing you suspect no serious cause, try the following self-help measures:

- Eat no solid food until your nausea and vomiting subside.
- Drink plenty of clear (non-alcoholic) fluids in small sips even if you cannot keep anything down for long.
- Do not smoke.
- Do not take aspirin.

If you vomit repeatedly for more than 24 hours, or if you develop further symptoms, consult your physician.

VOMITING AND THE PILL

If you are taking birth control pills, and suffer from an attack of vomiting, your protection against conception may be reduced. Continue to take your pills as usual, but use an alternative form of contraception as well until you start a new packet.

Certain medications can cause vomiting as a side effect. Discuss the problem with your physician.

Consult your physician if you are unable to make a diagnosis from this chart.

WARNING

RED OR BLACK BLOOD IN VOMIT

Violent or recurrent vomiting can cause damage to the lining of the esophagus and this can result in streaks of red blood appearing in your vomit. Consult your physician if this happens to you. If your vomit contains large quantities of red blood or any black or dark brown matter like coffee grounds (partly digested blood), **seek medical help at once**; you may have a serious abdominal condition such as a bleeding stomach or duodenal ulcer. It will assist rapid diagnosis of the problem if you keep the vomit containing the blood for the physician to examine.

95 Recurrent vomiting

Consult this chart if you have vomited (or felt nauseated) for several days in the past week. Apart from the nausea and vomiting of early pregnancy, most cases of recurrent vomiting are caused by persistent inflammation of the stomach lining or ulceration. However, it is important to seek medical advice so that you can obtain effective treatment and to eliminate the slight possibility of a more serious underlying disorder.

For isolated attacks of vomiting, see chart 94, Vomiting

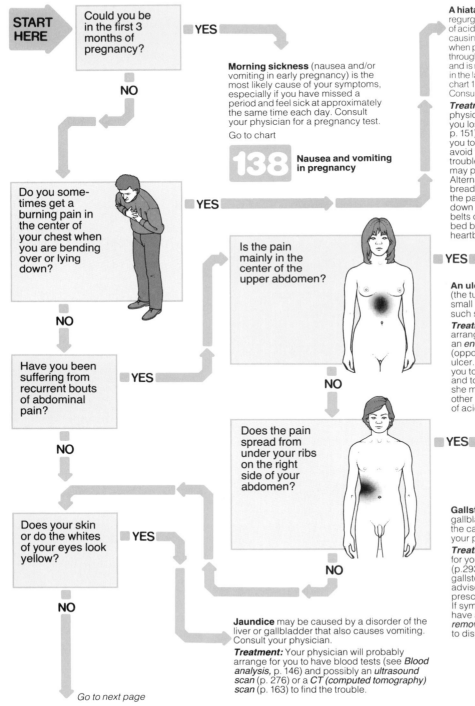

START HERE

Could you be in the first 3 months of pregnancy?

YES

Morning sickness (nausea and/or vomiting in early pregnancy) is the most likely cause of your symptoms, especially if you have missed a period and feel sick at approximately the same time each day. Consult your physician for a pregnancy test.

Go to chart

138 **Nausea and vomiting in pregnancy**

NO

Do you sometimes get a burning pain in the center of your chest when you are bending over or lying down?

YES

A hiatal hernia with reflux causes regurgitation of food and leakage of acid juices into the esophagus, causing heartburn. The disorder occurs when part of the stomach protrudes through the opening in the diaphragm and is most likely if you are overweight or in the last months of pregnancy (see chart 141, *Heartburn in pregnancy*). Consult your physician.

Treatment: If you are overweight, your physician will probably recommend that you lose weight (see *How to lose weight*, p. 151). Meanwhile, he or she may advise you to take small, frequent meals and to avoid tobacco and alcohol. If you are troubled by heartburn, your physician may prescribe an *antacid* medication. Alternatively you might try eating a little bread or drinking a glass of milk to relieve the pain. Avoid bending over or lying down after meals and do not wear tight belts or girdles. Raising the head of your bed by about 4 in. should prevent heartburn.

NO

Is the pain mainly in the center of the upper abdomen?

YES

An ulcer in the stomach or duodenum (the tube connecting the stomach to the small intestine) is a common cause of such symptoms. Consult your physician.

Treatment: Your physician will probably arrange for you to undergo tests such as an *endoscopy* (p. 201) or a *barium X ray* (opposite) to locate the exact site of the ulcer. Your physician is likely to advise you to rest, to avoid tobacco and alcohol and to eat small, frequent meals. He or she may also prescribe an *antacid* or other medications to reduce the amount of acid produced in your stomach.

NO

Have you been suffering from recurrent bouts of abdominal pain?

YES

Does the pain spread from under your ribs on the right side of your abdomen?

YES

Gallstones in the tube connecting the gallbladder to the digestive tract may be the cause of such symptoms. Consult your physician.

Treatment: Your physician may arrange for you to undergo *cholecystography* (p.293) or an *ultrasound scan* (p. 276). If gallstones are diagnosed, you will be advised to avoid fatty foods and may be prescribed muscle relaxants for the pain. If symptoms persist, you may need to have an operation (see *Gallbladder removal*, opposite). In some cases, drugs to dissolve the stones may be given.

NO

NO

Does your skin or do the whites of your eyes look yellow?

YES

Jaundice may be caused by a disorder of the liver or gallbladder that also causes vomiting. Consult your physician.

Treatment: Your physician will probably arrange for you to have blood tests (see *Blood analysis,* p. 146) and possibly an *ultrasound scan* (p. 276) or a *CT (computed tomography) scan* (p. 163) to find the trouble.

NO

Go to next page

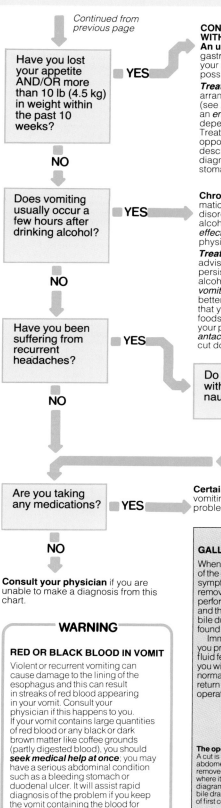

Continued from previous page

Have you lost your appetite AND/OR more than 10 lb (4.5 kg) in weight within the past 10 weeks? — **YES** →

CONSULT YOUR PHYSICIAN WITHOUT DELAY!
An ulcer in the stomach or duodenum or gastritis are the most likely causes of your symptoms, but there is a slight possibility of stomach cancer.

Treatment: Your physician will probably arrange for you to have a barium meal (see *Barium X rays*, right) and possibly an *endoscopy* (p. 201). Treatment will depend on the underlying disorder. Treatments for an ulcer are described opposite and treatments for gastritis are described below. If stomach cancer is diagnosed, the affected part of the stomach may be removed.

NO ↓

Does vomiting usually occur a few hours after drinking alcohol? — **YES** →

Chronic gastritis (persistent inflammation of the lining of the stomach), a disorder that is aggravated by drinking alcohol, is a possibility (see also *The effects of alcohol,* p. 146). Consult your physician.

Treatment: Your physician will probably advise you to eat nothing while vomiting persists and to drink plenty of clear (non-alcoholic) fluids (see *Treatment for vomiting,* p. 205). As you start to feel better, he or she will probably suggest that you gradually introduce some bland foods. If you suffer from abdominal pain, your physician will probably prescribe an *antacid.* And he or she may advise you to cut down on your regular alcohol intake.

NO ↓

Have you been suffering from recurrent headaches? — **YES** →

Do you vomit without preceding nausea? — **YES** →

NO ↓

NO ↓

Are you taking any medications? — **YES** →

Certain drugs can cause nausea and vomiting as a side effect. Discuss the problem with your physician.

NO ↓

Consult your physician if you are unable to make a diagnosis from this chart.

BARIUM X RAYS

Barium sulfate is a metallic compound that is visible on X-ray pictures and is used to show up areas of the digestive tract under investigation. If you need to have an X ray of the esophagus, stomach or small intestine, you will probably be given barium in the form of a drink (a barium swallow or meal). X rays will then be taken when the liquid reaches the relevant part of the digestive tract (after about 10 minutes for the esophagus, after 2 to 3 hours for the small intestine). If the large intestine (colon and rectum) is being examined, barium will be given in the form of an enema and the X rays will be taken immediately. Normally, you will be told to eat nothing after midnight on the day before your barium meal or enema. If you are having an enema, you may also be given a laxative to clear the bowel.

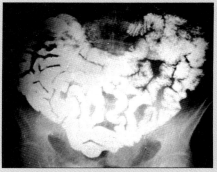

A barium X ray of normal intestines

CONSULT YOUR PHYSICIAN WITHOUT DELAY!
Pressure on the brain as a result of bleeding or a tumor is possible.

Treatment: Your physician will probably arrange for tests such as a *CT (computed tomography)* scan (p. 163) and a *radioisotope scan* (p. 148) of the brain tissues. Treatment usually consists of either surgery or drugs to reduce the pressure and relieve symptoms.

WARNING

RED OR BLACK BLOOD IN VOMIT

Violent or recurrent vomiting can cause damage to the lining of the esophagus and this can result in streaks of red blood appearing in your vomit. Consult your physician if this happens to you. If your vomit contains large quantities of red blood or any black or dark brown matter like coffee grounds (partly digested blood), you should **seek medical help at once**; you may have a serious abdominal condition such as a bleeding stomach or duodenal ulcer. It will assist rapid diagnosis of the problem if you keep the vomit containing the blood for the physician to examine.

GALLBLADDER REMOVAL

When gallstones or another disorder of the gallbladder cause serious symptoms, the gallbladder is often removed surgically. The operation is performed under general anesthetic, and the surgeon will also explore the bile duct and remove any stones found there.

Immediately after the operation, you probably will have intravenous fluid feedings, but after a few days you will be able to eat and drink normally. You should be able to return home about 7 days after the operation.

The operation
A cut is made in the right side of the abdomen (right). The gallbladder is then removed by cutting the cystic duct near where it joins the bile duct as shown in the diagram (above right). After the operation, bile drains straight into the intestine instead of first collecting in the gallbladder.

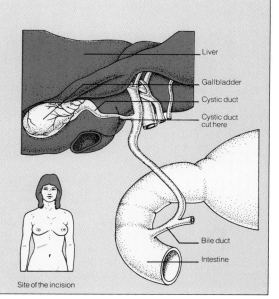

Liver
Gallbladder
Cystic duct
Cystic duct cut here
Bile duct
Intestine

Site of the incision

96 Abdominal pain

Pain between the bottom of the ribcage and the groin can be a sign of a wide number of different disorders of the digestive tract, urinary tract or reproductive organs.

Most cases of abdominal pain are due to minor digestive upsets, but severe and persistent pain should always receive prompt medical attention.

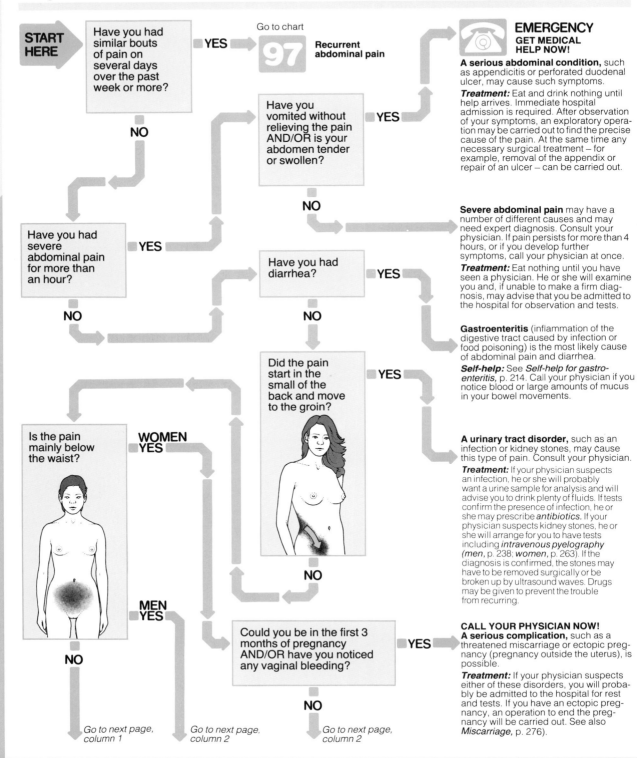

START HERE

Have you had similar bouts of pain on several days over the past week or more?

YES → Go to chart **97** Recurrent abdominal pain

NO

Have you had severe abdominal pain for more than an hour?

YES

NO

Have you vomited without relieving the pain AND/OR is your abdomen tender or swollen?

YES

NO

Have you had diarrhea?

YES

NO

Did the pain start in the small of the back and move to the groin?

YES

NO

Is the pain mainly below the waist?

WOMEN YES

MEN YES

NO

Could you be in the first 3 months of pregnancy AND/OR have you noticed any vaginal bleeding?

YES

NO

EMERGENCY
GET MEDICAL HELP NOW!

A serious abdominal condition, such as appendicitis or perforated duodenal ulcer, may cause such symptoms.
Treatment: Eat and drink nothing until help arrives. Immediate hospital admission is required. After observation of your symptoms, an exploratory operation may be carried out to find the precise cause of the pain. At the same time any necessary surgical treatment – for example, removal of the appendix or repair of an ulcer – can be carried out.

Severe abdominal pain may have a number of different causes and may need expert diagnosis. Consult your physician. If pain persists for more than 4 hours, or if you develop further symptoms, call your physician at once.
Treatment: Eat nothing until you have seen a physician. He or she will examine you and, if unable to make a firm diagnosis, may advise that you be admitted to the hospital for observation and tests.

Gastroenteritis (inflammation of the digestive tract caused by infection or food poisoning) is the most likely cause of abdominal pain and diarrhea.
Self-help: See *Self-help for gastro-enteritis*, p. 214. Call your physician if you notice blood or large amounts of mucus in your bowel movements.

A urinary tract disorder, such as an infection or kidney stones, may cause this type of pain. Consult your physician.
Treatment: If your physician suspects an infection, he or she will probably want a urine sample for analysis and will advise you to drink plenty of fluids. If tests confirm the presence of infection, he or she may prescribe *antibiotics*. If your physician suspects kidney stones, he or she will arrange for you to have tests including *intravenous pyelography (men*, p. 238; *women*, p. 263). If the diagnosis is confirmed, the stones may have to be removed surgically or be broken up by ultrasound waves. Drugs may be given to prevent the trouble from recurring.

CALL YOUR PHYSICIAN NOW!
A serious complication, such as a threatened miscarriage or ectopic pregnancy (pregnancy outside the uterus), is possible.
Treatment: If your physician suspects either of these disorders, you will probably be admitted to the hospital for rest and tests. If you have an ectopic pregnancy, an operation to end the pregnancy will be carried out. See also *Miscarriage*, p. 276).

Go to next page, column 1

Go to next page, column 2

Go to next page, column 2

Continued from previous page column 1

Continued from previous page column 2

Do you have intermittent cramping pains?

YES → **Are you having a period?** → **YES** → Go to chart

127 Painful periods

NO

Disturbance of the intestines as a result of a recent change in diet or anxiety is likely. Consult your physician if pain persists for more than 4 hours or becomes severe.

MEN NO **WOMEN NO**

A urinary-tract infection is likely.

Go to chart

Do you have a fever, and pain on one side, with or without vaginal discharge? → **YES**

Infection of the fallopian tubes (sometimes known as salpingitis) is possible. Consult your physician.

Treatment: Your physician will probably do a *vaginal examination* (p. 258) and may take a sample of any discharge for analysis. He or she is likely to prescribe aspirin or an aspirin substitute for the pain and *antibiotics* to counter infection. In severe cases, hospital admission may be necessary.

117 Men   ## 132 Women   Painful urination

or to chart

133 Abnormally frequent urination

NO

WARNING

SEVERE ABDOMINAL PAIN

Severe and continuous abdominal pain requires urgent medical attention in the following cases:

- if it persists for more than 4 hours
- if it is accompanied but unrelieved by vomiting
- if the abdomen is swollen and tender
- if it is accompanied by faintness, drowsiness or confusion

Do you have a burning pain when you urinate AND/OR are you urinating more frequently than usual? → **YES**

Is the pain spreading from below the ribs on the right? → **YES**

Waiting for medical attention
While waiting for medical help to arrive do not eat or drink anything, in case you need to undergo surgery immediately. Do not take aspirin to relieve the pain or drink alcohol; these can further inflame an irritated stomach and in some circumstances can cause dangerous internal bleeding.

NO

Consult your physician if you are unable to make a diagnosis from this chart.

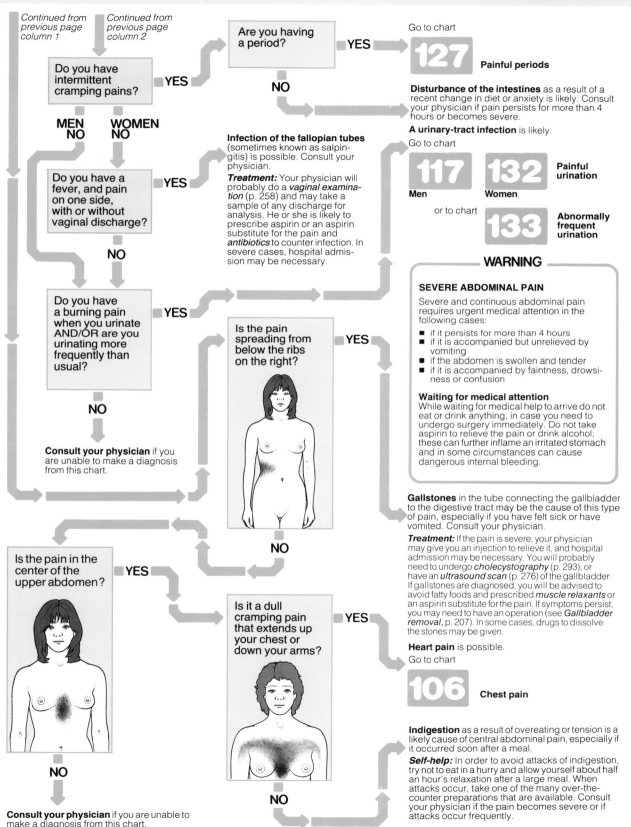

Gallstones in the tube connecting the gallbladder to the digestive tract may be the cause of this type of pain, especially if you have felt sick or have vomited. Consult your physician.

Treatment: If the pain is severe, your physician may give you an injection to relieve it, and hospital admission may be necessary. You will probably need to undergo *cholecystography* (p. 293), or have an *ultrasound scan* (p. 276) of the gallbladder. If gallstones are diagnosed, you will be advised to avoid fatty foods and prescribed *muscle relaxants* or an aspirin substitute for the pain. If symptoms persist, you may need to have an operation (see *Gallbladder removal*, p. 207). In some cases, drugs to dissolve the stones may be given.

NO

Is the pain in the center of the upper abdomen? → **YES**

Is it a dull cramping pain that extends up your chest or down your arms? → **YES**

Heart pain is possible.

Go to chart

106 Chest pain

NO

Indigestion as a result of overeating or tension is a likely cause of central abdominal pain, especially if it occurred soon after a meal.

Self-help: In order to avoid attacks of indigestion, try not to eat in a hurry and allow yourself about half an hour's relaxation after a large meal. When attacks occur, take one of the many over-the-counter preparations that are available. Consult your physician if the pain becomes severe or if attacks occur frequently.

NO

Consult your physician if you are unable to make a diagnosis from this chart.

97 Recurrent abdominal pain

Consult this chart if you have pain in the abdomen (between the bottom of the ribcage and the groin) of a similar type on several days in the course of a week or more. Most cases of recurrent abdominal pain are the result of long-standing digestive problems, and can be remedied by drugs from your physician, possibly combined with a change in eating habits. However, early diagnosis is always necessary to eliminate the slight possibility of serious underlying disease of the stomach, bowel or reproductive organs.

For isolated attacks of abdominal pain, see chart 96, Abdominal pain.

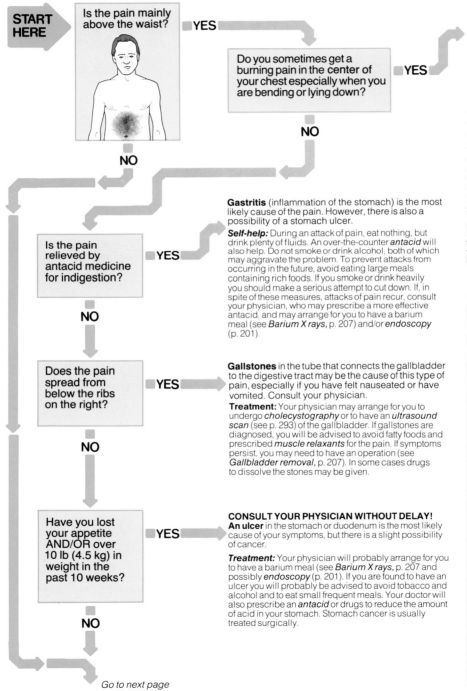

START HERE

Is the pain mainly above the waist? **YES**

Do you sometimes get a burning pain in the center of your chest especially when you are bending or lying down? **YES**

NO

NO

Is the pain relieved by antacid medicine for indigestion? **YES**

NO

Does the pain spread from below the ribs on the right? **YES**

NO

Have you lost your appetite AND/OR over 10 lb (4.5 kg) in weight in the past 10 weeks? **YES**

NO

Go to next page

A hiatal hernia with backup of acid juices (acid reflux) into the esophagus may be causing heartburn. This disorder can occur when part of the stomach protrudes through the opening in the diaphragm and is most likely if you are overweight or pregnant (see chart 141, *Heartburn in pregnancy).* Consult your physician.

Treatment: If you are overweight, your physician will probably recommend that you lose weight, as this will almost certainly help the problem (see *How to lose weight,* p. 151). Meanwhile, he or she may also advise you to take small, frequent meals and to avoid tobacco, coffee or alcohol, as these may aggravate stomach and digestive disorders. If you are troubled by heartburn, your physician may also prescribe an *antacid* medication. Alternatively, you might try eating a little bread or drinking a glass of milk to relieve the pain. Avoid bending over or lying down after meals and do not wear tight belts or girdles. Raising the head of your bed by about 4 in. should prevent heartburn at night.

Gastritis (inflammation of the stomach) is the most likely cause of the pain. However, there is also a possibility of a stomach ulcer.

Self-help: During an attack of pain, eat nothing, but drink plenty of fluids. An over-the-counter *antacid* will also help. Do not smoke or drink alcohol, both of which may aggravate the problem. To prevent attacks from occurring in the future, avoid eating large meals containing rich foods. If you smoke or drink heavily you should make a serious attempt to cut down. If, in spite of these measures, attacks of pain recur, consult your physician, who may prescribe a more effective antacid, and may arrange for you to have a barium meal (see *Barium X rays,* p. 207) and/or *endoscopy* (p. 201).

Gallstones in the tube that connects the gallbladder to the digestive tract may be the cause of this type of pain, especially if you have felt nauseated or have vomited. Consult your physician.

Treatment: Your physician may arrange for you to undergo *cholecystography* or to have an *ultrasound scan* (see p. 293) of the gallbladder. If gallstones are diagnosed, you will be advised to avoid fatty foods and prescribed *muscle relaxants* for the pain. If symptoms persist, you may need to have an operation (see *Gallbladder removal,* p. 207). In some cases drugs to dissolve the stones may be given.

CONSULT YOUR PHYSICIAN WITHOUT DELAY!
An ulcer in the stomach or duodenum is the most likely cause of your symptoms, but there is a slight possibility of cancer.

Treatment: Your physician will probably arrange for you to have a barium meal (see *Barium X rays,* p. 207 and possibly *endoscopy* (p. 201). If you are found to have an ulcer you will probably be advised to avoid tobacco and alcohol and to eat small frequent meals. Your doctor will also prescribe an *antacid* or drugs to reduce the amount of acid in your stomach. Stomach cancer is usually treated surgically.

IRRITABLE COLON

Many people who suffer from recurrent cramping pains in the lower abdomen with or without intermittent diarrhea and/or constipation have no serious underlying disorder and are diagnosed as having an irritable colon (or irritable bowel syndrome).

It is thought that the disorder is caused by abnormally strong and irregular muscle contractions in the bowel. This may be due to sensitivity to the passage of matter through the intestines, but it may also be linked to psychological stress (see *What is stress?,* p. 175). A large proportion of those with this complaint are anxious, and attacks seem to be made worse by worry. Most sufferers learn to live with the problem without specific treatment. A high-fiber diet (p. 215) often relieves the symptoms. Those who suffer from severe pain may be prescribed *antispasmodic* drugs.

Continued from previous page

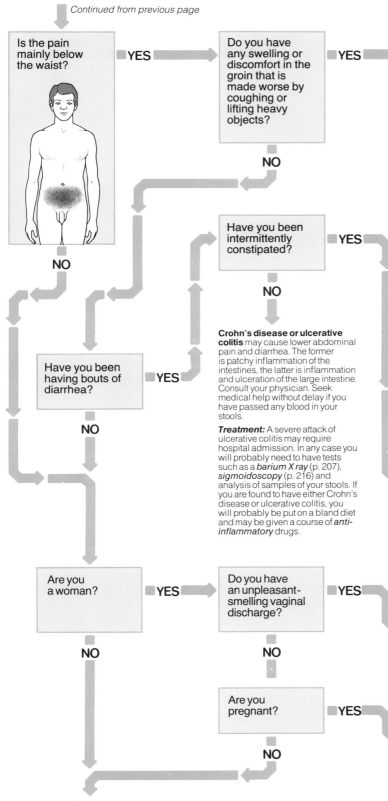

Is the pain mainly below the waist?

YES →

Do you have any swelling or discomfort in the groin that is made worse by coughing or lifting heavy objects?

YES →

A hernia (see *What is a hernia?*, below) may be the cause of such pain. Consult your physician.

Treatment: Your physician will examine you to confirm the diagnosis. If you have a hernia, it may be necessary for you to have a minor operation to repair the abdominal wall.

NO (pain below waist)

NO (groin swelling)

Have you been intermittently constipated?

YES →

NO

Crohn's disease or ulcerative colitis may cause lower abdominal pain and diarrhea. The former is patchy inflammation of the intestines, the latter is inflammation and ulceration of the large intestine. Consult your physician. Seek medical help without delay if you have passed any blood in your stools.

Treatment: A severe attack of ulcerative colitis may require hospital admission. In any case you will probably need to have tests such as a *barium X ray* (p. 207), *sigmoidoscopy* (p. 216) and analysis of samples of your stools. If you are found to have either Crohn's disease or ulcerative colitis, you will probably be put on a bland diet and may be given a course of *anti-inflammatory* drugs.

Have you been having bouts of diarrhea?

YES →

NO

Are you a woman?

YES →

Do you have an unpleasant-smelling vaginal discharge?

YES →

NO

NO

Are you pregnant?

YES →

NO

Consult your physician if you are unable to make a diagnosis from this chart.

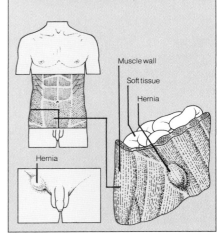

WHAT IS A HERNIA?

A hernia occurs when soft tissue in the abdomen bulges through a weak area in the abdominal wall. Hernias may occur in various places. In men, one of the most common sites is the groin, where the abdominal organs either push aside the weak muscles of the groin or protrude down the inguinal canal (the tube down which the testicles descend before birth).

Muscle wall

Soft tissue

Hernia

Hernia

CONSULT YOUR PHYSICIAN WITHOUT DELAY!
Irritable colon (see opposite) or *diverticular disease* (in which swellings develop on the walls of the large intestine) may be the cause of your symptoms. However, the slight possibility of bowel cancer also needs to be ruled out.

Treatment: To make an exact diagnosis, your physician may need to arrange tests such as a barium enema (see *Barium X rays*, p. 207) and *endoscopy* (p. 201). The long-term treatment for both irritable colon and diverticular disease is based on a high-fiber diet (p. 215). Your physician may also prescribe drugs to relieve your symptoms.

Infection of the fallopian tubes (sometimes known as salpingitis) is possible. Consult your physician.

Treatment: Your physician will probably do a *vaginal examination* (p. 258) and take a sample of the discharge from your vagina for analysis. You may also need to have a *D and C* (p. 254) and/or *laparoscopy* (p. 272). If the diagnosis is confirmed, your physician is likely to prescribe aspirin or an aspirin substitute for the pain and *antibiotics* to counter infection. In severe cases, admission to the hospital may be necessary.

Periodic tightening of the smooth muscles of the uterus, known as Braxton Hicks contractions, occurs throughout pregnancy. These make your abdomen feel hard and tense for about 30 seconds, but should not cause actual pain. Call your physician if contractions are accompanied by vaginal bleeding, or if they are painful. In late pregnancy, an increase in the frequency and strength of these contractions may signal the start of labor (see chart 145, *Am I in labor?*).

98 Swollen abdomen

A generalized swelling over the whole abdomen (the area between the bottom of the rib cage and the groin) suggests a condition affecting the digestive or repro-ductive organs. If your abdomen is painful as well as swollen, this is an emergency and you should seek medical advice immediately.

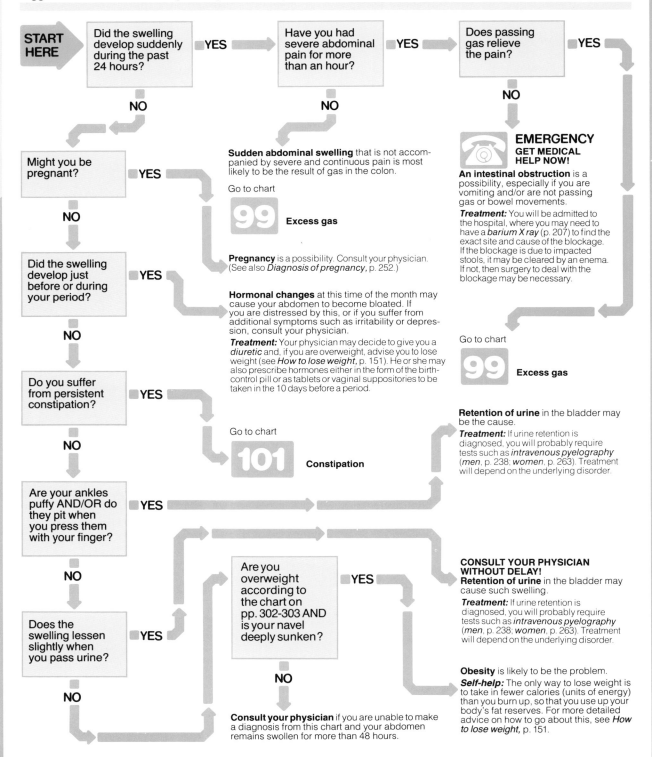

START HERE

Did the swelling develop suddenly during the past 24 hours?
YES → **Have you had severe abdominal pain for more than an hour?**
YES → **Does passing gas relieve the pain?**
YES →

NO

NO

NO → **EMERGENCY GET MEDICAL HELP NOW!**

Might you be pregnant?
YES →

NO

Sudden abdominal swelling that is not accompanied by severe and continuous pain is most likely to be the result of gas in the colon.

Go to chart

99 Excess gas

Did the swelling develop just before or during your period?
YES →

NO

Pregnancy is a possibility. Consult your physician. (See also *Diagnosis of pregnancy*, p. 252.)

Hormonal changes at this time of the month may cause your abdomen to become bloated. If you are distressed by this, or if you suffer from additional symptoms such as irritability or depression, consult your physician.

Treatment: Your physician may decide to give you a *diuretic* and, if you are overweight, advise you to lose weight (see *How to lose weight*, p. 151). He or she may also prescribe hormones either in the form of the birth-control pill or as tablets or vaginal suppositories to be taken in the 10 days before a period.

An intestinal obstruction is a possibility, especially if you are vomiting and/or are not passing gas or bowel movements.

Treatment: You will be admitted to the hospital, where you may need to have a *barium X ray* (p. 207) to find the exact site and cause of the blockage. If the blockage is due to impacted stools, it may be cleared by an enema. If not, then surgery to deal with the blockage may be necessary.

Go to chart

99 Excess gas

Do you suffer from persistent constipation?
YES →

NO

Go to chart

101 Constipation

Retention of urine in the bladder may be the cause.

Treatment: If urine retention is diagnosed, you will probably require tests such as *intravenous pyelography* (*men*, p. 238; *women*, p. 263). Treatment will depend on the underlying disorder.

Are your ankles puffy AND/OR do they pit when you press them with your finger?
YES →

NO

Are you overweight according to the chart on pp. 302-303 AND is your navel deeply sunken?
YES →

NO

Does the swelling lessen slightly when you pass urine?
YES →

NO

CONSULT YOUR PHYSICIAN WITHOUT DELAY!
Retention of urine in the bladder may cause such swelling.

Treatment: If urine retention is diagnosed, you will probably require tests such as *intravenous pyelography* (*men*, p. 238; *women*, p. 263). Treatment will depend on the underlying disorder.

Obesity is likely to be the problem.
Self-help: The only way to lose weight is to take in fewer calories (units of energy) than you burn up, so that you use up your body's fat reserves. For more detailed advice on how to go about this, see *How to lose weight*, p. 151.

Consult your physician if you are unable to make a diagnosis from this chart and your abdomen remains swollen for more than 48 hours.

99 Excess gas

Excess gas in the digestive system may cause an uncomfortable, distended feeling in the abdomen and may produce rumbling noises in the intestines. Expulsion of gas, either through the mouth or the anus, generally relieves these symptoms temporarily. Although it may be embarrassing, passing gas is rarely a sign of an underlying disease. In most cases, gas is caused by swallowing air or by certain foods not being properly digested, leaving a residue that ferments, producing gas in the intestines. Different foods affect different people – though onions, cabbage and beans are common causes of gas.

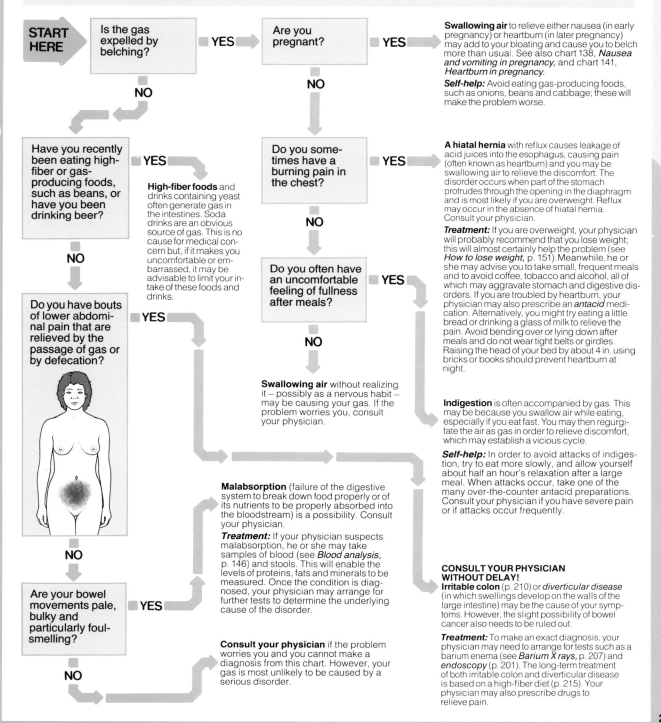

START HERE

Is the gas expelled by belching?
- **YES** →
- **NO** ↓

Are you pregnant?
- **YES** →
- **NO** ↓

Swallowing air to relieve either nausea (in early pregnancy) or heartburn (in later pregnancy) may add to your bloating and cause you to belch more than usual. See also chart 138, *Nausea and vomiting in pregnancy*, and chart 141, *Heartburn in pregnancy*.

Self-help: Avoid eating gas-producing foods, such as onions, beans and cabbage; these will make the problem worse.

Have you recently been eating high-fiber or gas-producing foods, such as beans, or have you been drinking beer?
- **YES** →
- **NO** ↓

High-fiber foods and drinks containing yeast often generate gas in the intestines. Soda drinks are an obvious source of gas. This is no cause for medical concern but, if it makes you uncomfortable or embarrassed, it may be advisable to limit your intake of these foods and drinks.

Do you sometimes have a burning pain in the chest?
- **YES** →
- **NO** ↓

A hiatal hernia with reflux causes leakage of acid juices into the esophagus, causing pain (often known as heartburn) and you may be swallowing air to relieve the discomfort. The disorder occurs when part of the stomach protrudes through the opening in the diaphragm and is most likely if you are overweight. Reflux may occur in the absence of hiatal hernia. Consult your physician.

Treatment: If you are overweight, your physician will probably recommend that you lose weight; this will almost certainly help the problem (see *How to lose weight,* p. 151). Meanwhile, he or she may advise you to take small, frequent meals and to avoid coffee, tobacco and alcohol, all of which may aggravate stomach and digestive disorders. If you are troubled by heartburn, your physician may also prescribe an *antacid* medication. Alternatively, you might try eating a little bread or drinking a glass of milk to relieve the pain. Avoid bending over or lying down after meals and do not wear tight belts or girdles. Raising the head of your bed by about 4 in. using bricks or books should prevent heartburn at night.

Do you have bouts of lower abdominal pain that are relieved by the passage of gas or by defecation?
- **YES** →
- **NO** ↓

Do you often have an uncomfortable feeling of fullness after meals?
- **YES** →
- **NO** ↓

Swallowing air without realizing it – possibly as a nervous habit – may be causing your gas. If the problem worries you, consult your physician.

Indigestion is often accompanied by gas. This may be because you swallow air while eating, especially if you eat fast. You may then regurgitate the air as gas in order to relieve discomfort, which may establish a vicious cycle.

Self-help: In order to avoid attacks of indigestion, try to eat more slowly, and allow yourself about half an hour's relaxation after a large meal. When attacks occur, take one of the many over-the-counter antacid preparations. Consult your physician if you have severe pain or if attacks occur frequently.

Malabsorption (failure of the digestive system to break down food properly or of its nutrients to be properly absorbed into the bloodstream) is a possibility. Consult your physician.

Treatment: If your physician suspects malabsorption, he or she may take samples of blood (see *Blood analysis*, p. 146) and stools. This will enable the levels of proteins, fats and minerals to be measured. Once the condition is diagnosed, your physician may arrange for further tests to determine the underlying cause of the disorder.

Are your bowel movements pale, bulky and particularly foul-smelling?
- **YES** →
- **NO** ↓

CONSULT YOUR PHYSICIAN WITHOUT DELAY!
Irritable colon (p. 210) or *diverticular disease* (in which swellings develop on the walls of the large intestine) may be the cause of your symptoms. However, the slight possibility of bowel cancer also needs to be ruled out.

Treatment: To make an exact diagnosis, your physician may need to arrange for tests such as a barium enema (see *Barium X rays*, p. 207) and *endoscopy* (p. 201). The long-term treatment of both irritable colon and diverticular disease is based on a high-fiber diet (p. 215). Your physician may also prescribe drugs to relieve pain.

Consult your physician if the problem worries you and you cannot make a diagnosis from this chart. However, your gas is most unlikely to be caused by a serious disorder.

213

100 Diarrhea

Diarrhea is the passing of unusually loose and frequent bowel movements. It is rarely a dangerous symptom, but it may cause discomfort and is often accompanied or preceded by cramping pains in the lower abdomen. In this country, most attacks of diarrhea are the result of infection and last no more than 48 hours. No special treatment is usually needed other than ensuring that you drink enough fluids. However, if diarrhea persists or recurs, it should be reported to your physician. Remember, if you are taking a birth-control pill and have diarrhea for more than 24 hours, your protection against pregnancy may be reduced and you should use another means of contraception for the remainder of your cycle (see chart 136, Choosing a contraceptive method).

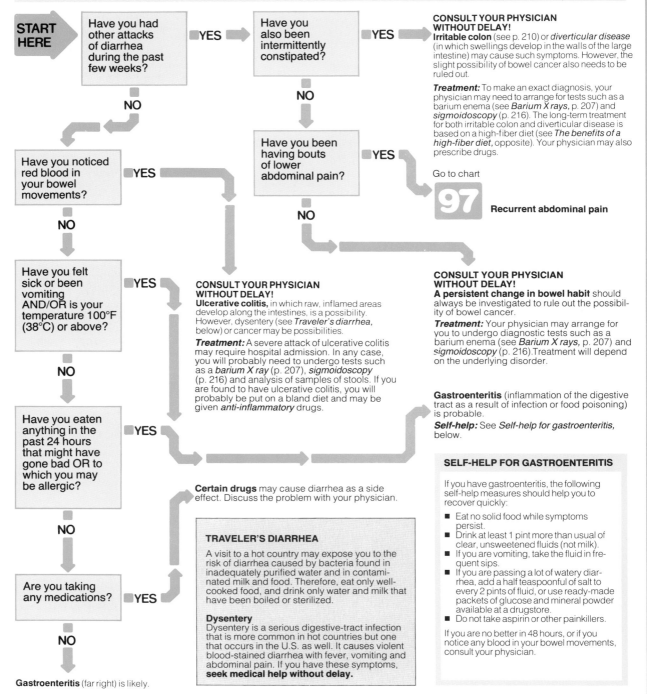

START HERE

Have you had other attacks of diarrhea during the past few weeks?

→ **YES** → **Have you also been intermittently constipated?** → **YES** →

NO ↓

Have you noticed red blood in your bowel movements? → **YES** →

NO ↓

Have you felt sick or been vomiting AND/OR is your temperature 100°F (38°C) or above? → **YES** →

NO ↓

Have you eaten anything in the past 24 hours that might have gone bad OR to which you may be allergic? → **YES** →

NO ↓

Are you taking any medications? → **YES** →

NO ↓

Gastroenteritis (far right) is likely.

Have you been having bouts of lower abdominal pain? → **YES** →

NO ↓

CONSULT YOUR PHYSICIAN WITHOUT DELAY!
Irritable colon (see p. 210) or *diverticular disease* (in which swellings develop in the walls of the large intestine) may cause such symptoms. However, the slight possibility of bowel cancer also needs to be ruled out.

Treatment: To make an exact diagnosis, your physician may need to arrange for tests such as a barium enema (see *Barium X rays,* p. 207) and *sigmoidoscopy* (p. 216). The long-term treatment for both irritable colon and diverticular disease is based on a high-fiber diet (see *The benefits of a high-fiber diet,* opposite). Your physician may also prescribe drugs.

Go to chart

97 Recurrent abdominal pain

CONSULT YOUR PHYSICIAN WITHOUT DELAY!
Ulcerative colitis, in which raw, inflamed areas develop along the intestines, is a possibility. However, dysentery (see *Traveler's diarrhea,* below) or cancer may be possibilities.

Treatment: A severe attack of ulcerative colitis may require hospital admission. In any case, you will probably need to undergo tests such as a barium X ray (p. 207), *sigmoidoscopy* (p. 216) and analysis of samples of stools. If you are found to have ulcerative colitis, you will probably be put on a bland diet and may be given *anti-inflammatory* drugs.

CONSULT YOUR PHYSICIAN WITHOUT DELAY!
A persistent change in bowel habit should always be investigated to rule out the possibility of bowel cancer.

Treatment: Your physician may arrange for you to undergo diagnostic tests such as a barium enema (see *Barium X rays,* p. 207) and *sigmoidoscopy* (p. 216).Treatment will depend on the underlying disorder.

Gastroenteritis (inflammation of the digestive tract as a result of infection or food poisoning) is probable.

Self-help: See *Self-help for gastroenteritis,* below.

Certain drugs may cause diarrhea as a side effect. Discuss the problem with your physician.

TRAVELER'S DIARRHEA

A visit to a hot country may expose you to the risk of diarrhea caused by bacteria found in inadequately purified water and in contaminated milk and food. Therefore, eat only well-cooked food, and drink only water and milk that have been boiled or sterilized.

Dysentery
Dysentery is a serious digestive-tract infection that is more common in hot countries but one that occurs in the U.S. as well. It causes violent blood-stained diarrhea with fever, vomiting and abdominal pain. If you have these symptoms, **seek medical help without delay.**

SELF-HELP FOR GASTROENTERITIS

If you have gastroenteritis, the following self-help measures should help you to recover quickly:

- Eat no solid food while symptoms persist.
- Drink at least 1 pint more than usual of clear, unsweetened fluids (not milk).
- If you are vomiting, take the fluid in frequent sips.
- If you are passing a lot of watery diarrhea, add a half teaspoonful of salt to every 2 pints of fluid, or use ready-made packets of glucose and mineral powder available at a drugstore.
- Do not take aspirin or other painkillers.

If you are no better in 48 hours, or if you notice any blood in your bowel movements, consult your physician.

101 Constipation

Normal bowel habits vary from person to person – many people have one or more bowel movements a day, but a few have four or five a day. Constipation occurs only when the stools are dry, hard and painful or difficult to pass. This is more likely to occur when stools are passed more infrequently than you are used to.

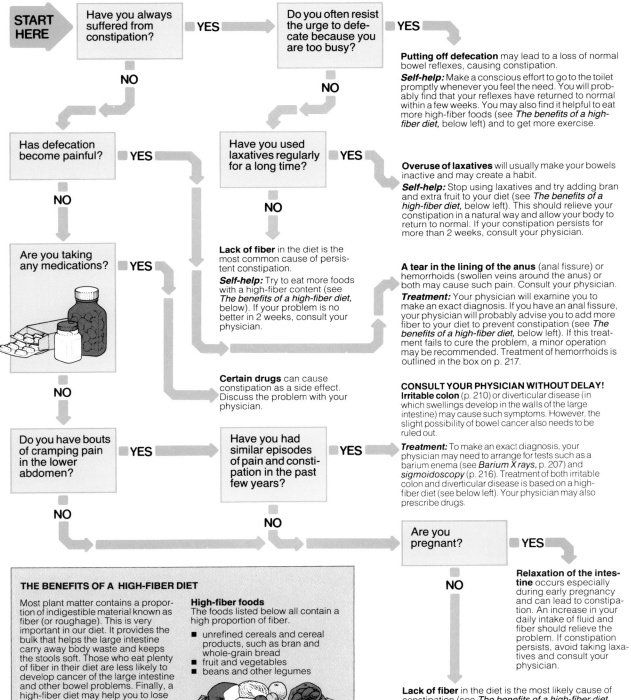

START HERE

Have you always suffered from constipation?

YES → **Do you often resist the urge to defecate because you are too busy?** → **YES**

Putting off defecation may lead to a loss of normal bowel reflexes, causing constipation.
Self-help: Make a conscious effort to go to the toilet promptly whenever you feel the need. You will probably find that your reflexes have returned to normal within a few weeks. You may also find it helpful to eat more high-fiber foods (see *The benefits of a high-fiber diet,* below left) and to get more exercise.

NO ↓   **NO** ↓

Has defecation become painful? **YES** →

Have you used laxatives regularly for a long time? **YES** →

Overuse of laxatives will usually make your bowels inactive and may create a habit.
Self-help: Stop using laxatives and try adding bran and extra fruit to your diet (see *The benefits of a high-fiber diet,* below left). This should relieve your constipation in a natural way and allow your body to return to normal. If your constipation persists for more than 2 weeks, consult your physician.

NO ↓   **NO** ↓

Lack of fiber in the diet is the most common cause of persistent constipation.
Self-help: Try to eat more foods with a high-fiber content (see *The benefits of a high-fiber diet,* below). If your problem is no better in 2 weeks, consult your physician.

Are you taking any medications? **YES** →

A tear in the lining of the anus (anal fissure) or hemorrhoids (swollen veins around the anus) or both may cause such pain. Consult your physician.
Treatment: Your physician will examine you to make an exact diagnosis. If you have an anal fissure, your physician will probably advise you to add more fiber to your diet to prevent constipation (see *The benefits of a high-fiber diet,* below left). If this treatment fails to cure the problem, a minor operation may be recommended. Treatment of hemorrhoids is outlined in the box on p. 217.

Certain drugs can cause constipation as a side effect. Discuss the problem with your physician.

CONSULT YOUR PHYSICIAN WITHOUT DELAY!
Irritable colon (p. 210) or diverticular disease (in which swellings develop in the walls of the large intestine) may cause such symptoms. However, the slight possibility of bowel cancer also needs to be ruled out.

NO ↓

Do you have bouts of cramping pain in the lower abdomen? **YES** →

Have you had similar episodes of pain and constipation in the past few years? **YES** →

Treatment: To make an exact diagnosis, your physician may need to arrange for tests such as a barium enema (see *Barium X rays,* p. 207) and *sigmoidoscopy* (p. 216). Treatment of both irritable colon and diverticular disease is based on a high-fiber diet (see below left). Your physician may also prescribe drugs.

NO ↓   **NO** ↓

Are you pregnant? **YES** →

Relaxation of the intestine occurs especially during early pregnancy and can lead to constipation. An increase in your daily intake of fluid and fiber should relieve the problem. If constipation persists, avoid taking laxatives and consult your physician.

NO ↓

Lack of fiber in the diet is the most likely cause of constipation (see *The benefits of a high-fiber diet,* left). If your bowel habits have not returned to normal within 2 weeks, consult your physician.

THE BENEFITS OF A HIGH-FIBER DIET

Most plant matter contains a proportion of indigestible material known as fiber (or roughage). This is very important in our diet. It provides the bulk that helps the large intestine carry away body waste and keeps the stools soft. Those who eat plenty of fiber in their diet are less likely to develop cancer of the large intestine and other bowel problems. Finally, a high-fiber diet may help you to lose weight, because fiber fills you up without providing extra calories.

High-fiber foods
The foods listed below all contain a high proportion of fiber.

- unrefined cereals and cereal products, such as bran and whole-grain bread
- fruit and vegetables
- beans and other legumes

102 Abnormal-looking bowel movements

Most minor changes in the color, shape and consistency of your bowel movements are due to a recent change in diet. But if the stools are black or significantly lighter than usual, or if they are streaked with blood, this may indicate something more serious and you should consult your physician.

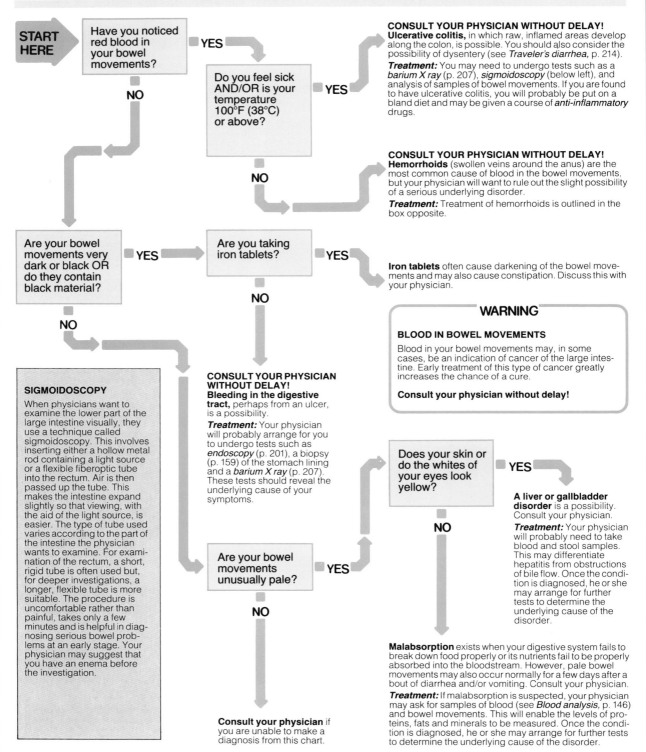

START HERE

Have you noticed red blood in your bowel movements?

YES → **Do you feel sick AND/OR is your temperature 100°F (38°C) or above?**

YES → **CONSULT YOUR PHYSICIAN WITHOUT DELAY!**
Ulcerative colitis, in which raw, inflamed areas develop along the colon, is possible. You should also consider the possibility of dysentery (see *Traveler's diarrhea*, p. 214).
Treatment: You may need to undergo tests such as a *barium X ray* (p. 207), *sigmoidoscopy* (below left), and analysis of samples of bowel movements. If you are found to have ulcerative colitis, you will probably be put on a bland diet and may be given a course of *anti-inflammatory* drugs.

NO → **CONSULT YOUR PHYSICIAN WITHOUT DELAY!**
Hemorrhoids (swollen veins around the anus) are the most common cause of blood in the bowel movements, but your physician will want to rule out the slight possibility of a serious underlying disorder.
Treatment: Treatment of hemorrhoids is outlined in the box opposite.

NO → **Are your bowel movements very dark or black OR do they contain black material?**

YES → **Are you taking iron tablets?**

YES → **Iron tablets** often cause darkening of the bowel movements and may also cause constipation. Discuss this with your physician.

NO →

WARNING

BLOOD IN BOWEL MOVEMENTS

Blood in your bowel movements may, in some cases, be an indication of cancer of the large intestine. Early treatment of this type of cancer greatly increases the chance of a cure.

Consult your physician without delay!

NO →

SIGMOIDOSCOPY

When physicians want to examine the lower part of the large intestine visually, they use a technique called sigmoidoscopy. This involves inserting either a hollow metal rod containing a light source or a flexible fiberoptic tube into the rectum. Air is then passed up the tube. This makes the intestine expand slightly so that viewing, with the aid of the light source, is easier. The type of tube used varies according to the part of the intestine the physician wants to examine. For examination of the rectum, a short, rigid tube is often used but, for deeper investigations, a longer, flexible tube is more suitable. The procedure is uncomfortable rather than painful, takes only a few minutes and is helpful in diagnosing serious bowel problems at an early stage. Your physician may suggest that you have an enema before the investigation.

CONSULT YOUR PHYSICIAN WITHOUT DELAY!
Bleeding in the digestive tract, perhaps from an ulcer, is a possibility.
Treatment: Your physician will probably arrange for you to undergo tests such as *endoscopy* (p. 201), a biopsy (p. 159) of the stomach lining and a *barium X ray* (p. 207). These tests should reveal the underlying cause of your symptoms.

Are your bowel movements unusually pale?

YES →

Does your skin or do the whites of your eyes look yellow?

YES → **A liver or gallbladder disorder** is a possibility. Consult your physician.
Treatment: Your physician will probably need to take blood and stool samples. This may differentiate hepatitis from obstructions of bile flow. Once the condition is diagnosed, he or she may arrange for further tests to determine the underlying cause of the disorder.

NO →

Malabsorption exists when your digestive system fails to break down food properly or its nutrients fail to be properly absorbed into the bloodstream. However, pale bowel movements may also occur normally for a few days after a bout of diarrhea and/or vomiting. Consult your physician.
Treatment: If malabsorption is suspected, your physician may ask for samples of blood (see *Blood analysis,* p. 146) and bowel movements. This will enable the levels of proteins, fats and minerals to be measured. Once the condition is diagnosed, he or she may arrange for further tests to determine the underlying cause of the disorder.

NO →

Consult your physician if you are unable to make a diagnosis from this chart.

103 Anal problems

The anus is a short tube that leads from the last part of the digestive tract (rectum) to the outside. The anus is closed by a ring of muscles (or sphincter). The most common disorder affecting this area is swelling of the veins around the anus (hemorroids). This is often related to painful constipation.

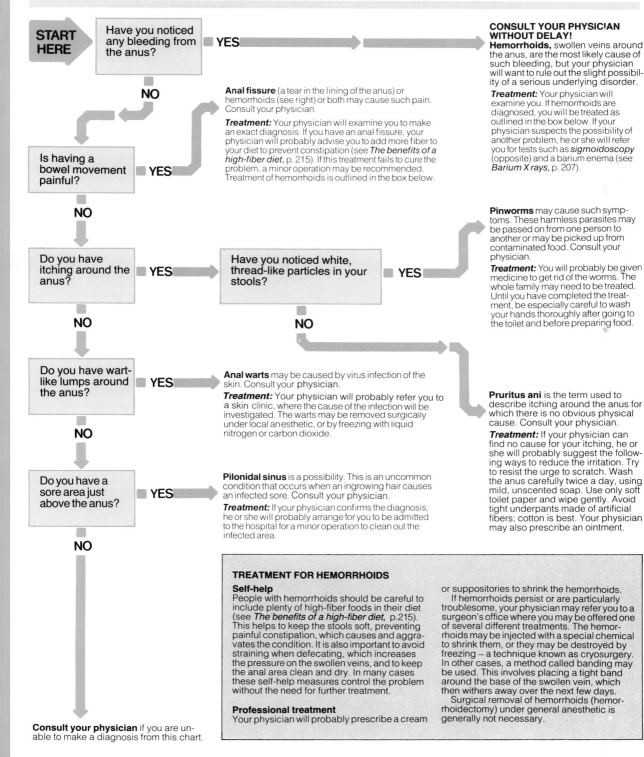

START HERE

Have you noticed any bleeding from the anus? — **YES** →

CONSULT YOUR PHYSICIAN WITHOUT DELAY!
Hemorrhoids, swollen veins around the anus, are the most likely cause of such bleeding, but your physician will want to rule out the slight possibility of a serious underlying disorder.

Treatment: Your physician will examine you. If hemorrhoids are diagnosed, you will be treated as outlined in the box below. If your physician suspects the possibility of another problem, he or she will refer you for tests such as *sigmoidoscopy* (opposite) and a barium enema (see *Barium X rays,* p. 207).

NO ↓

Is having a bowel movement painful? — **YES** →

Anal fissure (a tear in the lining of the anus) or hemorrhoids (see right) or both may cause such pain. Consult your physician.

Treatment: Your physician will examine you to make an exact diagnosis. If you have an anal fissure, your physician will probably advise you to add more fiber to your diet to prevent constipation (see *The benefits of a high-fiber diet,* p. 215). If this treatment fails to cure the problem, a minor operation may be recommended. Treatment of hemorrhoids is outlined in the box below.

NO ↓

Do you have itching around the anus? — **YES** → **Have you noticed white, thread-like particles in your stools?** — **YES** →

Pinworms may cause such symptoms. These harmless parasites may be passed on from one person to another or may be picked up from contaminated food. Consult your physician.

Treatment: You will probably be given medicine to get rid of the worms. The whole family may need to be treated. Until you have completed the treatment, be especially careful to wash your hands thoroughly after going to the toilet and before preparing food.

NO ↓ (from stools question)

NO ↓

Do you have wart-like lumps around the anus? — **YES** →

Anal warts may be caused by virus infection of the skin. Consult your physician.

Treatment: Your physician will probably refer you to a skin clinic, where the cause of the infection will be investigated. The warts may be removed surgically under local anesthetic, or by freezing with liquid nitrogen or carbon dioxide.

Pruritus ani is the term used to describe itching around the anus for which there is no obvious physical cause. Consult your physician.

Treatment: If your physician can find no cause for your itching, he or she will probably suggest the following ways to reduce the irritation. Try to resist the urge to scratch. Wash the anus carefully twice a day, using mild, unscented soap. Use only soft toilet paper and wipe gently. Avoid tight underpants made of artificial fibers; cotton is best. Your physician may also prescribe an ointment.

NO ↓

Do you have a sore area just above the anus? — **YES** →

Pilonidal sinus is a possibility. This is an uncommon condition that occurs when an ingrowing hair causes an infected sore. Consult your physician.

Treatment: If your physician confirms the diagnosis, he or she will probably arrange for you to be admitted to the hospital for a minor operation to clean out the infected area.

NO ↓

Consult your physician if you are unable to make a diagnosis from this chart.

TREATMENT FOR HEMORRHOIDS

Self-help
People with hemorrhoids should be careful to include plenty of high-fiber foods in their diet (see *The benefits of a high-fiber diet,* p.215). This helps to keep the stools soft, preventing painful constipation, which causes and aggravates the condition. It is also important to avoid straining when defecating, which increases the pressure on the swollen veins, and to keep the anal area clean and dry. In many cases these self-help measures control the problem without the need for further treatment.

Professional treatment
Your physician will probably prescribe a cream or suppositories to shrink the hemorrhoids.

If hemorrhoids persist or are particularly troublesome, your physician may refer you to a surgeon's office where you may be offered one of several different treatments. The hemorrhoids may be injected with a special chemical to shrink them, or they may be destroyed by freezing – a technique known as cryosurgery. In other cases, a method called banding may be used. This involves placing a tight band around the base of the swollen vein, which then withers away over the next few days.

Surgical removal of hemorrhoids (hemorrhoidectomy) under general anesthetic is generally not necessary.

104 General urinary problems

Consult this chart if you notice a change in your urinary habits – for instance, a change in the number of times you need to pass urine daily – or if you have difficulty in starting or controlling the flow of urine.

START HERE

Is urination painful?

YES → **Go to chart** **117** Men **132** Women **Painful urination**

NO ↓

Are you passing abnormally large amounts of urine?

YES →

Have you noticed one or more of the following symptoms?
- unexplained tiredness
- increased thirst
- unexplained weight loss

YES →

Diabetes mellitus is a possibility. This disorder is caused by insufficient production of the hormone insulin. Consult your physician.

Treatment: If tests on blood (see *Blood analysis*, p. 146) and urine confirm the diagnosis, you may need treatment with drugs or with regular injections of insulin. Your physician will also advise you on diet.

NO ↓

CONSULT YOUR PHYSICIAN WITHOUT DELAY!
A kidney or hormonal disorder may cause increased urination.

Treatment: Your physician will examine you and take specimens of blood and urine for analysis (see *Blood analysis*, p. 146). He or she may also arrange for you to have a special X ray of the kidneys (see *Intravenous pyelography, men*, p. 238; *women*, p. 263). Further treatment will depend on the results of these tests.

NO ↓

When you want to pass urine, do you have to wait a few moments before the flow starts?

YES →

NO ↓

Do you often need to pass small amounts of urine, AND/OR is your urinary stream weak?

YES →

Narrowing of the urethra, occurring more frequently in women (see chart 131), or enlargement of the prostate gland especially in men over 50 is a possibility (see *Enlargement of the prostate gland*, below).
Treatment: You will be probably be referred to the hospital for tests. If you are found to have a narrowed urethra, a simple operation to enlarge the outlet will be carried out. If you are a man and tests reveal that there is a serious obstruction to the flow of urine, an operation may be recommended (see *Prostatectomy*, right).

NO ↓

Consult your doctor if you are unable to make a diagnosis from this chart.

WARNING

INABILITY TO PASS URINE

If you find that you are unable to urinate even though you feel the urge, you may have a blocked urethra. This requires urgent medical attention to prevent damage to the bladder and kidneys. While waiting for medical help to arrive, try taking a warm bath; this may enable you to pass some urine.

SUDDEN LOSS OF BLADDER CONTROL
Sudden inability to control urination may be a sign of damage to the spinal cord or nervous system, especially if you have recently had a back injury or if you have experienced weakness in your legs.

Seek medical help at once!

PROSTATECTOMY

When the prostate gland becomes so enlarged that it seriously interferes with the flow of urine, an operation to remove part or all of the gland is usually necessary. This is known as prostatectomy. There are two main alternative types of operation available. The choice of method depends on the details of the case. Both methods successfully relieve urinary symptoms of an enlarged prostate, but occasionally impotence or sterility may result. Your physician will discuss these risks with you. Both methods require a general anesthetic.

Traditional surgery
In a traditional prostatectomy, access to the gland is gained through an incision in the lower abdomen. The surgeon can then remove tissue from the gland as necessary.

Transurethral resection of the prostate (TURP)
In this form of prostatectomy, a tube is passed up the urethra from the penis to the prostate. This tube is fitted with a lens system and a cutting tool so that the surgeon can see the gland and cut away as much tissue as necessary.

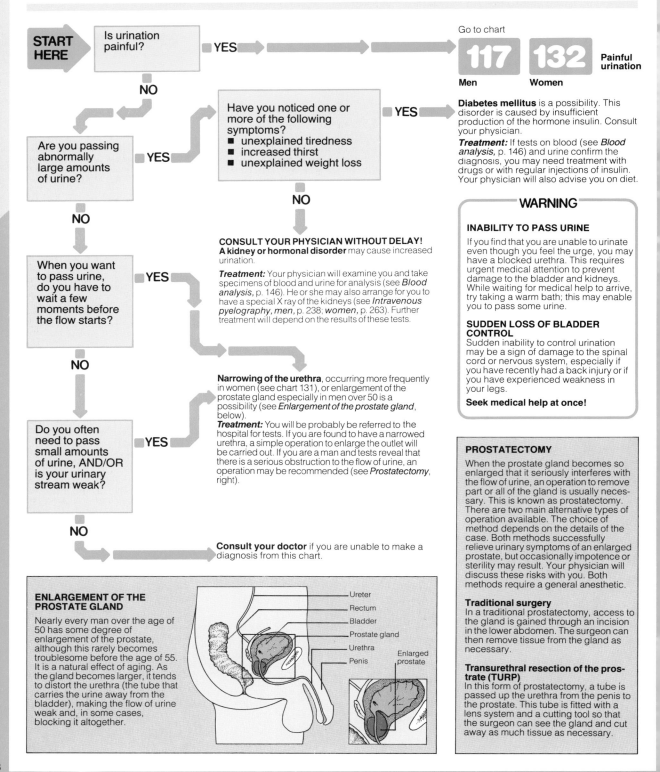

ENLARGEMENT OF THE PROSTATE GLAND

Nearly every man over the age of 50 has some degree of enlargement of the prostate, although this rarely becomes troublesome before the age of 55. It is a natural effect of aging. As the gland becomes larger, it tends to distort the urethra (the tube that carries the urine away from the bladder), making the flow of urine weak and, in some cases, blocking it altogether.

Ureter
Rectum
Bladder
Prostate gland
Urethra
Penis
Enlarged prostate

105 Palpitations

Palpitations is a term used to describe unusually rapid, strong, or irregular beating of the heart. It is normal for the heart rate to speed up during strenuous exercise and you may feel your heart "thumping" for some minutes after. This is no cause for concern. Consult this chart if you have palpitations unconnected with physical exertion. In most cases such palpitations are caused by nicotine and caffeine, or by anxiety. But in a small proportion of cases they are a symptom of an underlying illness. Palpitations that recur on several days or that are connected with pain or breathlessness should always be brought to your physician's attention.

START HERE

Before the onset of palpitations had you been drinking more tea or coffee than usual?
YES → **Caffeine** in large doses can cause the heart rate to speed up or become irregular. See *Caffeine*, below.

NO ↓

Are you feeling tense or worried?
YES →

Have you been smoking more than usual?
YES →

NO ↓

Have you recently lost weight in spite of eating more than usual?
YES →

NO ↓

Have you been feeling breathless, weak, or tired recently?
YES →

NO ↓

Do you feel sick AND/OR do you have a history of heart disease?
YES → **CONSULT YOUR PHYSICIAN WITHOUT DELAY!**

NO ↓

Consult your physician if you are unable to make a diagnosis from this chart.

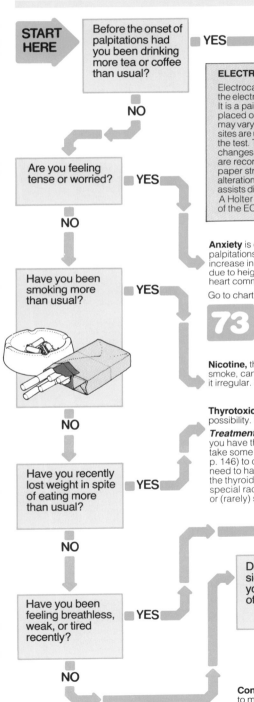

ELECTROCARDIOGRAPHY

Electrocardiography is a technique used to record the electrical impulses that control the heart's activity. It is a painless procedure in which electrodes are placed on the surface of the body. The exact sites may vary, and often several different combinations of sites are used. You may be asked to exercise during the test. The electrodes pick up the electrical changes in the heart with each beat and the results are recorded as an electrocardiogram (ECG) on a paper strip or on a screen. An ECG shows up any alteration in the normal pattern of heart activity and assists diagnosis of a wide variety of heart disorders. A Holter monitor is a portable 24-hour recording of the ECG that may detect rhythm changes.

Anxiety is one of the most common causes of palpitations. This may be partly because of a real increase in heart rate at times of stress, but may also be due to heightened awareness of the normal action of the heart common in people suffering from anxiety.

Go to chart

73 Anxiety

Nicotine, the addictive substance in tobacco smoke, can speed up the heartbeat rate or make it irregular. See *The dangers of smoking*, p. 196.

Thyrotoxicosis (overactive thyroid gland) is a possibility. Consult your physician.

Treatment: If your physician suspects that you have this disorder, he or she will probably take some blood for tests (see *Blood analysis*, p. 146) to confirm the diagnosis. You may also need to have a *radioisotope scan* (p. 148) of the thyroid gland. Treatment may consist of special radioactive iodine, other medications or (rarely) surgery.

CAFFEINE

Caffeine is a substance present in tea, coffee and some soft drinks, notably cola. It stimulates the nervous system, making you feel more energetic and also speeds up the production of urine. Small amounts of caffeine do no harm, but in large doses it may produce symptoms such as palpitations, trembling, and sleeplessness. The table below shows the average amount of caffeine in coffee, tea and cola. It is advisable to keep your total consumption of caffeine below 800 mg a day.

Caffeine content of common drinks

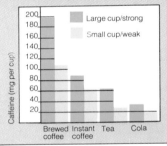

Legend: Large cup/strong · Small cup/weak. Y axis: Caffeine (mg per cup). X axis: Brewed coffee, Instant coffee, Tea, Cola.

Anemia, a disorder in which there are too few red blood cells, is a possibility. Consult your physician.

Treatment: Your physician will probably take a sample of blood for analysis (see *Blood analysis*, p. 146). If you are found to have anemia due to iron deficiency, your physician may give you iron in the form of tablets or injections. In addition, your physician may advise you about a diet. Other causes of anemia are less common and require further tests before treatment can be given.

CONSULT YOUR PHYSICIAN WITHOUT DELAY!
A serious disorder of heart rate or rhythm, as a result of abnormal electrical impulses in the heart, is possible.

Treatment: If your physician suspects such a disorder, he or she will arrange for you to undergo *electrocardiography* (above left), a Holter monitor and a *chest X ray* (p. 197). If your heart rhythms are found to be abnormal, you will probably be given *beta-blocker drugs* to regulate the heart's activity.

106 Chest pain

Pain in the chest (anywhere between the neck and the bottom of the rib cage) may be dull and persistent, sharp and stabbing, or crushing. Although it may be alarming, most chest pain does not have a serious cause. However, severe, crushing central chest pain, or pain that is associated with breathlessness or irregular heartbeat, may be a sign of a serious disorder of the heart or lungs and may warrant emergency treatment.

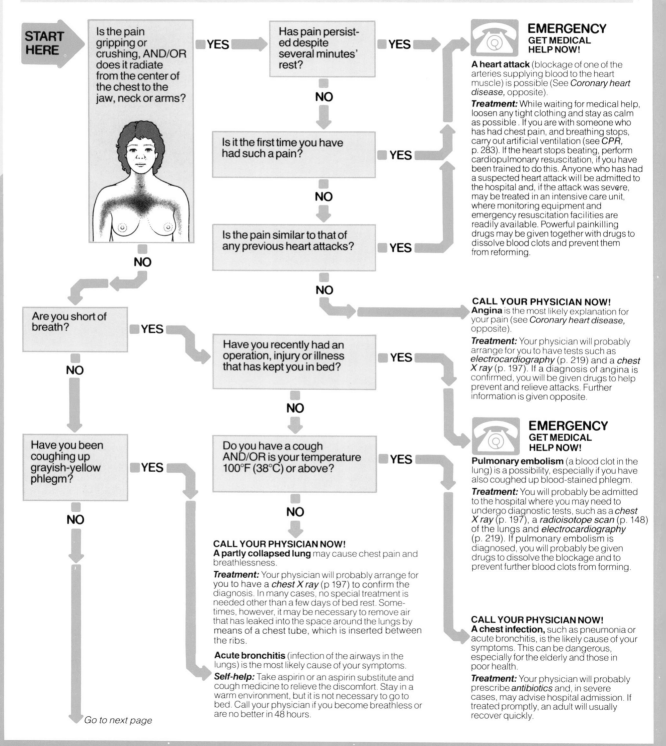

START HERE

Is the pain gripping or crushing, AND/OR does it radiate from the center of the chest to the jaw, neck or arms?

YES → Has pain persisted despite several minutes' rest?

YES → **EMERGENCY GET MEDICAL HELP NOW!**

A heart attack (blockage of one of the arteries supplying blood to the heart muscle) is possible (See *Coronary heart disease,* opposite).

Treatment: While waiting for medical help, loosen any tight clothing and stay as calm as possible . If you are with someone who has had chest pain, and breathing stops, carry out artificial ventilation (see *CPR,* p. 283). If the heart stops beating, perform cardiopulmonary resuscitation, if you have been trained to do this. Anyone who has had a suspected heart attack will be admitted to the hospital and, if the attack was severe, may be treated in an intensive care unit, where monitoring equipment and emergency resuscitation facilities are readily available. Powerful painkilling drugs may be given together with drugs to dissolve blood clots and prevent them from reforming.

NO ↓

Is it the first time you have had such a pain?

YES →

NO ↓

Is the pain similar to that of any previous heart attacks?

YES →

NO ↓

CALL YOUR PHYSICIAN NOW!
Angina is the most likely explanation for your pain (see *Coronary heart disease,* opposite).

Treatment: Your physician will probably arrange for you to have tests such as *electrocardiography* (p. 219) and a *chest X ray* (p. 197). If a diagnosis of angina is confirmed, you will be given drugs to help prevent and relieve attacks. Further information is given opposite.

NO (from first box) ↓

Are you short of breath?

YES → Have you recently had an operation, injury or illness that has kept you in bed?

YES → **EMERGENCY GET MEDICAL HELP NOW!**

Pulmonary embolism (a blood clot in the lung) is a possibility, especially if you have also coughed up blood-stained phlegm.

Treatment: You will probably be admitted to the hospital where you may need to undergo diagnostic tests, such as a *chest X ray* (p. 197), a *radioisotope scan* (p. 148) of the lungs and *electrocardiography* (p. 219). If pulmonary embolism is diagnosed, you will probably be given drugs to dissolve the blockage and to prevent further blood clots from forming.

NO ↓

Have you been coughing up grayish-yellow phlegm?

YES → Do you have a cough AND/OR is your temperature 100°F (38°C) or above?

YES → **CALL YOUR PHYSICIAN NOW!**
A chest infection, such as pneumonia or acute bronchitis, is the likely cause of your symptoms. This can be dangerous, especially for the elderly and those in poor health.

Treatment: Your physician will probably prescribe *antibiotics* and, in severe cases, may advise hospital admission. If treated promptly, an adult will usually recover quickly.

NO ↓

CALL YOUR PHYSICIAN NOW!
A partly collapsed lung may cause chest pain and breathlessness.

Treatment: Your physician will probably arrange for you to have a *chest X ray* (p 197) to confirm the diagnosis. In many cases, no special treatment is needed other than a few days of bed rest. Sometimes, however, it may be necessary to remove air that has leaked into the space around the lungs by means of a chest tube, which is inserted between the ribs.

Acute bronchitis (infection of the airways in the lungs) is the most likely cause of your symptoms.

Self-help: Take aspirin or an aspirin substitute and cough medicine to relieve the discomfort. Stay in a warm environment, but it is not necessary to go to bed. Call your physician if you become breathless or are no better in 48 hours.

Go to next page

Continued from previous page

Is there a burning pain in the center of the chest that gets worse when you bend over or lie down?

YES → **A hiatal hernia** may accompany leakage of acid juices (reflux) into the esophagus, causing pain. The disorder occurs when part of the stomach protudes through the opening in the diaphragm and is more likely if you are overweight or in the last months of pregnancy (see chart 141, *Heartburn in pregnancy*). However, reflux may occur in the absence of hiatal hernia. Consult your physician.
Treatment: See *Hiatal hernia*, p.210.

NO ↓

Do you have a pain in the middle of the chest that came on soon after eating?

YES → **Indigestion** is the most likely explanation for such pain. This may occur as a result of overeating or tension.
Self-help: In order to avoid attacks of indigestion, try not to eat in a hurry and allow yourself about half an hour's relaxation after a large meal. When attacks occur, take one of the many over-the-counter preparations that are available. Consult your physician if pain becomes severe, or if attacks occur frequently.

NO ↓

Is the pain on one side only?

YES →

NO ↓

Consult your physician without delay if you are unable to make a diagnosis from this chart.

Have you recently had a chest injury or a severe cough?

YES →

NO ↓

Is the painful region tender to the touch?

YES → **A pulled muscle** or injury to the ligaments and cartilages of the rib cage are the most likely causes of your pain.
Self-help: Try not to strain the muscle further while you are feeling pain. A painkiller, such as aspirin or an aspirin substitute, will give relief, but, if pain persists for more than 48 hours, consult your physician, who may arrange for you to have a *chest X ray* (p. 197) to rule out the possibility of a broken rib.

NO ↓

Do you have a burning pain in the skin that is unaffected by breathing?

YES → **Shingles,** a virus infection of the nerves, is a possibility. The appearance of a blistery rash along the site of the pain a few days after the onset of pain will confirm the diagnosis. Consult your physician.
Treatment: Your physician will probably prescribe a painkiller and a soothing ointment to put on the skin. He or she may also prescribe an *antiviral* agent to hasten healing.

NO ↓

Consult your physician without delay if you are unable to make a diagnosis from this chart.

CORONARY HEART DISEASE

Coronary heart disease occurs when fatty deposits, or plaques, called atheromas, build up on the inside walls of the arteries that supply oxygenated blood to the heart muscle. This causes the arteries to become narrowed and disturbs the flow of blood.

Coronary heart disease may cause chest pain (angina). This can occur after exertion or emotional stress, when the increased oxygen needs of the heart cannot be supplied through the narrowed coronary arteries. However, many people with coronary heart disease have no symptoms. Often their first indication of the disease is when they experience a heart attack, which occurs when a blood clot or buildup of atheroma blocks a coronary artery, cutting off the blood supply to part of the heart muscle. This can be fatal; even if it is not, it usually results in some permanent damage to the heart muscle.

What is the treatment?
If you are found to have coronary heart disease, you will probably be advised to change any aspects of your life-style that seem to be contributing to the disease (see *Preventing coronary heart disease,* right). You will probably be given medication to reduce the likelihood of angina attacks and others to take if attacks do occur. If you are found to have high blood pressure, this may also need drug treatment.

Coronary artery bypass graft (CABG) surgery
If your coronary arteries are found to be dangerously narrowed, you may be advised to have an operation in which the diseased sections of the coronary arteries are bypassed using healthy veins from the leg or an artery in the chest wall. This is a major operation, but the prospects for an active life and relief of chest pain are good.

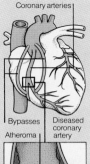
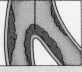

Coronary arteries

Bypasses | Diseased coronary artery

Atheroma

If surgery is necessary, the diseased sections of the coronary arteries containing atheromas are bypassed, usually with multiple bypass sections.

Preventing coronary heart disease
There are many factors that are known to increase the risk of developing coronary heart disease – notably, the tendency for the disease to run in families. But anyone who has a family history of heart disease can reduce the risk of developing serious problems by avoiding the factors listed below.

■ **Smoking** Smokers are at least twice as likely to die of a heart attack than nonsmokers. This is because substances in tobacco smoke increase the level of atheroma-forming fats in the bloodstream.

■ **Obesity** Overweight people tend to eat higher-than-average amounts of fat, increasing the risk of atheroma buildup. Carrying too much weight places an increased strain on the heart, making it less able to withstand any restriction of its blood supply.

■ **Too much fat in the diet** The tendency for atheromas to form in the arteries seems to be related to the level of certain types of fat in the bloodstream, which in turn is related partly to heredity, and partly to the amount of fat in the diet. Cutting down on all types of fat should help to reduce your risk of developing coronary heart disease.

■ **Lack of exercise** Regular strenuous exercise increases the efficiency of the heart, so that it needs less oxygen to function well. If you gradually increase your physical fitness, your heart will be under less strain should its blood supply be reduced by coronary heart disease.

107 Back pain

Your backbone (or spine) extends from the base of your skull to the buttocks. It consists of the spinal column, which is made up of more than 30 separate bones called vertebrae stacked on top of one another. In between each pair of vertebrae is an elastic disc. The vertebrae and discs are held together by ligaments. Along the length of the spinal column is a space containing the spinal cord and the nerves that run from it to the rest of

the body. Most people suffer from mild back pain from time to time, the exact cause of which may be difficult to diagnose. It is usually a sign that you have damaged one or more joints, ligaments or discs by overstretching or twisting your back into an awkward position. Severe pain, however, may be the result of pressure on the nerves from malalignment of the bones or discs in the back. Consult your physician.

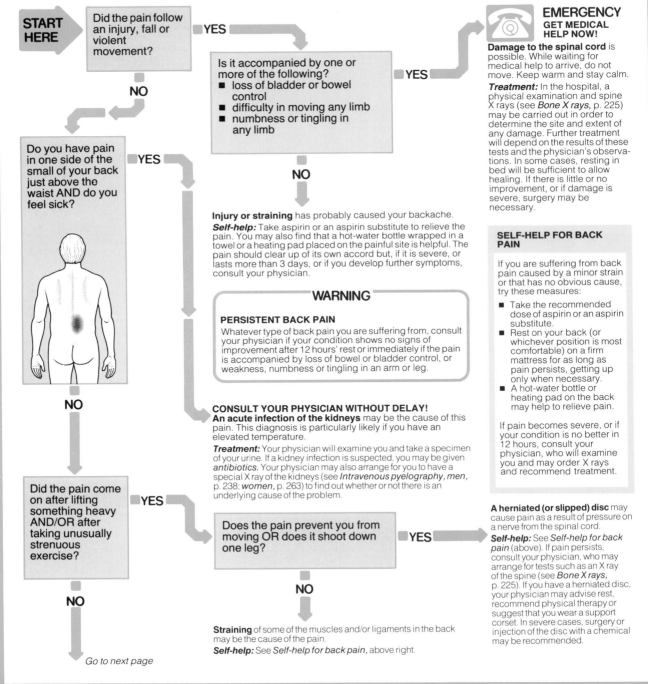

START HERE

Did the pain follow an injury, fall or violent movement?

YES →

NO

Do you have pain in one side of the small of your back just above the waist AND do you feel sick?

YES

NO

Is it accompanied by one or more of the following?
- loss of bladder or bowel control
- difficulty in moving any limb
- numbness or tingling in any limb

YES →

NO

EMERGENCY
GET MEDICAL HELP NOW!

Damage to the spinal cord is possible. While waiting for medical help to arrive, do not move. Keep warm and stay calm.

Treatment: In the hospital, a physical examination and spine X rays (see *Bone X rays,* p. 225) may be carried out in order to determine the site and extent of any damage. Further treatment will depend on the results of these tests and the physician's observations. In some cases, resting in bed will be sufficient to allow healing. If there is little or no improvement, or if damage is severe, surgery may be necessary.

Injury or straining has probably caused your backache.
Self-help: Take aspirin or an aspirin substitute to relieve the pain. You may also find that a hot-water bottle wrapped in a towel or a heating pad placed on the painful site is helpful. The pain should clear up of its own accord but, if it is severe, or lasts more than 3 days, or if you develop further symptoms, consult your physician.

WARNING

PERSISTENT BACK PAIN

Whatever type of back pain you are suffering from, consult your physician if your condition shows no signs of improvement after 12 hours' rest or immediately if the pain is accompanied by loss of bowel or bladder control, or weakness, numbness or tingling in an arm or leg.

CONSULT YOUR PHYSICIAN WITHOUT DELAY!
An acute infection of the kidneys may be the cause of this pain. This diagnosis is particularly likely if you have an elevated temperature.
Treatment: Your physician will examine you and take a specimen of your urine. If a kidney infection is suspected, you may be given *antibiotics.* Your physician may also arrange for you to have a special X ray of the kidneys (see *Intravenous pyelography, men,* p. 238; *women,* p. 263) to find out whether or not there is an underlying cause of the problem.

Did the pain come on after lifting something heavy AND/OR after taking unusually strenuous exercise?

YES

NO

Does the pain prevent you from moving OR does it shoot down one leg?

YES →

NO

Straining of some of the muscles and/or ligaments in the back may be the cause of the pain.
Self-help: See *Self-help for back pain,* above right.

Go to next page

SELF-HELP FOR BACK PAIN

If you are suffering from back pain caused by a minor strain or that has no obvious cause, try these measures:

- Take the recommended dose of aspirin or an aspirin substitute.
- Rest on your back (or whichever position is most comfortable) on a firm mattress for as long as pain persists, getting up only when necessary.
- A hot-water bottle or heating pad on the back may help to relieve pain.

If pain becomes severe, or if your condition is no better in 12 hours, consult your physician, who will examine you and may order X rays and recommend treatment.

A herniated (or slipped) disc may cause pain as a result of pressure on a nerve from the spinal cord.
Self-help: See *Self-help for back pain* (above). If pain persists, consult your physician, who may arrange for tests such as an X ray of the spine (see *Bone X rays,* p. 225). If you have a herniated disc, your physician may advise rest, recommend physical therapy or suggest that you wear a support corset. In severe cases, surgery or injection of the disc with a chemical may be recommended.

Continued from previous page

Has your back gradually become stiff as well as painful over a period of months or years? — **YES** → **Are you over 45?** — **YES** → **Is the pain mainly between the shoulder blades?** — **YES** →

NO (from "Has your back gradually become stiff...")

NO (from "Are you over 45?")

Ankylosing spondylitis (inflammation of the joints between the vertebrae so that the spinal column gradually becomes hard and inflexible) may be the cause of this, especially if you are between 20 and 40. Consult your physician.

Treatment: Your physician will examine you and arrange for you to have a blood test (see *Blood analysis,* p. 146) and an X ray of your back and pelvic area (see *Bone X rays,* p. 225). If you are found to have ankylosing spondylitis, you will probably be given *anti-inflammatory* drugs. You will also be referred to a physiotherapist, who will teach you exercises that will help to keep your back mobile. Such mobility exercises are an essential part of the treatment for this disorder and can be supplemented by other physical activities such as swimming.

NO (from "Is the pain mainly between the shoulder blades?")

Lumbar osteoarthritis, a form of arthritis, is a possible diagnosis. This normally occurs as a result of wear and tear on the spine as you grow older. Consult your doctor.

Treatment: Your doctor will examine you and possibly arrange for you to have an X ray (see *Bone X rays,* p. 225) and possibly a blood test (see *Blood analysis,* p. 146) to check that no other disorder is responsible for these symptoms. If the diagnosis is confirmed, you will probably be prescribed painkillers and advised to exercise to strengthen the muscles in your back. You may be advised to wear a specially fitted support corset. If you are overweight, your doctor will probably advise you to go on a weight-reducing diet (see *How to lose weight,* p. 151).

Did the pain come on suddenly after an extended stay in bed or confinement to a wheelchair, OR are you over 60? — **YES** →

NO

CONSULT YOUR PHYSICIAN WITHOUT DELAY!
Sudden compression of a bone in the spine as a result of thinning of the bones (osteoporosis) is possible.

Treatment: Your doctor will examine you and arrange for you to have an X ray of the spine (see *Bone X rays,* p. 225) to confirm the diagnosis and to help him or her to determine the treatment that should follow. Your doctor will also probably advise you to eat a diet rich in calcium to keep your bones healthy. If you are in pain, he or she will prescribe painkillers and you may be prescribed other drugs to try to slow down the thinning process.

Cervical osteoarthritis, arthritis of the bones in the neck as a result of wear and tear, may be the cause of this pain. Consult your physician.

Treatment: Your physician will examine you and may arrange for you to have an X ray of the bones in your neck (see *Bone X rays,* p. 225). If he or she thinks that the symptoms are due to this disorder, you may be given a supportive collar to wear to reduce neck mobility. Aspirin or an aspirin substitute can be taken to relieve the discomfort. If these measures fail to help, your physician may send you to a physiotherapist for further treatment.

Go to chart
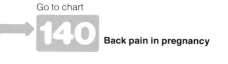
140 **Back pain in pregnancy**

Are you pregnant? — **YES** →

NO

Consult your physician if you are unable to make a diagnosis from this chart and if your back pain has not been relieved within 24 hours.

PREVENTING BACKACHE

There are several practical ways in which you can minimize the amount of strain on your back to help prevent backaches. Feeling comfortable in any movement or position is a general guide to whether or not you are putting strain on your back. Below are some precautions you can take.

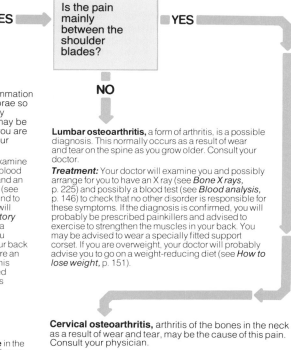

Sitting correctly
When sitting for any length of time, try to keep your back straight and avoid slumping. Choose a chair that has a firm, upright back that will support the length of your spine. You should be able to rest your feet flat on the floor with your knees bent at a right angle.

Posture
The correct way to stand to avoid placing unnecessary strain on your back is with your head, trunk and legs aligned.

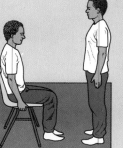

Sleeping
Sleep on a firm mattress or put a board under your existing mattress. Use a single, flat pillow to support your head. These measures will support your back and prevent your spine from sagging into an unhealthy bend.

Lifting
When lifting a heavy object, get as close to it as possible. Keep your back straight and bend your knees so that your leg muscles, not the weaker back muscles, take the strain.

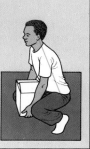

108 Painful or stiff neck

A stiff or painful neck is most often the result of a muscle stiffness brought on by sitting in a cold draft, sleeping in an uncomfortable position or doing some form of exercise or activity to which you are not accustomed.

This type of problem should resolve itself within a day or so. If pain and/or stiffness persist, ask your physician for advice. Occasionally, a stiff or painful neck may be a sign of a disorder that requires medical treatment.

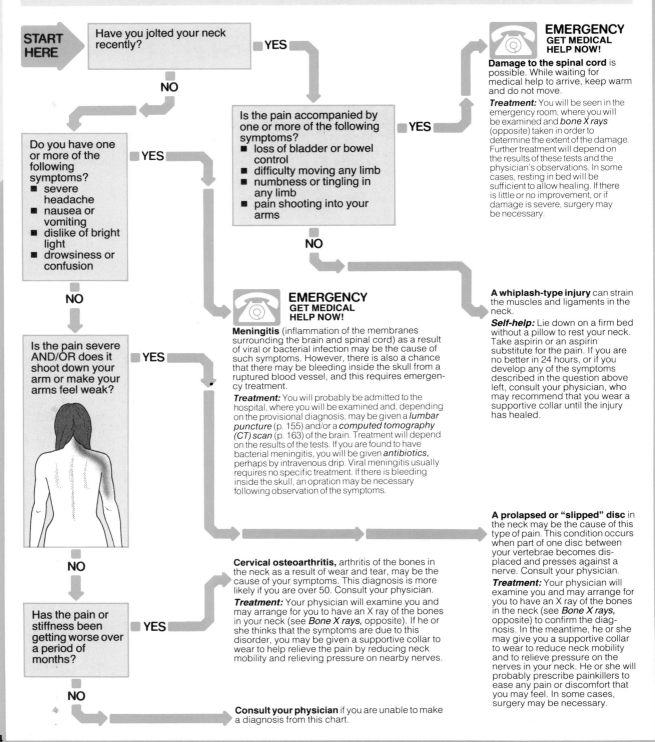

START HERE

Have you jolted your neck recently?

NO

Do you have one or more of the following symptoms?
- severe headache
- nausea or vomiting
- dislike of bright light
- drowsiness or confusion

NO

Is the pain severe AND/OR does it shoot down your arm or make your arms feel weak?

NO

Has the pain or stiffness been getting worse over a period of months?

NO

YES

Is the pain accompanied by one or more of the following symptoms?
- loss of bladder or bowel control
- difficulty moving any limb
- numbness or tingling in any limb
- pain shooting into your arms

NO

YES

EMERGENCY
GET MEDICAL HELP NOW!

Damage to the spinal cord is possible. While waiting for medical help to arrive, keep warm and do not move.

Treatment: You will be seen in the emergency room, where you will be examined and *bone X rays* (opposite) taken in order to determine the extent of the damage. Further treatment will depend on the results of these tests and the physician's observations. In some cases, resting in bed will be sufficient to allow healing. If there is little or no improvement, or if damage is severe, surgery may be necessary.

A whiplash-type injury can strain the muscles and ligaments in the neck.

Self-help: Lie down on a firm bed without a pillow to rest your neck. Take aspirin or an aspirin substitute for the pain. If you are no better in 24 hours, or if you develop any of the symptoms described in the question above left, consult your physician, who may recommend that you wear a supportive collar until the injury has healed.

EMERGENCY
GET MEDICAL HELP NOW!

Meningitis (inflammation of the membranes surrounding the brain and spinal cord) as a result of viral or bacterial infection may be the cause of such symptoms. However, there is also a chance that there may be bleeding inside the skull from a ruptured blood vessel, and this requires emergency treatment.

Treatment: You will probably be admitted to the hospital, where you will be examined and, depending on the provisional diagnosis, may be given a *lumbar puncture* (p. 155) and/or a *computed tomography (CT) scan* (p. 163) of the brain. Treatment will depend on the results of the tests. If you are found to have bacterial meningitis, you will be given *antibiotics*, perhaps by intravenous drip. Viral meningitis usually requires no specific treatment. If there is bleeding inside the skull, an opration may be necessary following observation of the symptoms.

A prolapsed or "slipped" disc in the neck may be the cause of this type of pain. This condition occurs when part of one disc between your vertebrae becomes displaced and presses against a nerve. Consult your physician.

Treatment: Your physician will examine you and may arrange for you to have an X ray of the bones in the neck (see *Bone X rays,* opposite) to confirm the diagnosis. In the meantime, he or she may give you a supportive collar to wear to reduce neck mobility and to relieve pressure on the nerves in your neck. He or she will probably prescribe painkillers to ease any pain or discomfort that you may feel. In some cases, surgery may be necessary.

Cervical osteoarthritis, arthritis of the bones in the neck as a result of wear and tear, may be the cause of your symptoms. This diagnosis is more likely if you are over 50. Consult your physician.

Treatment: Your physician will examine you and may arrange for you to have an X ray of the bones in your neck (see *Bone X rays,* opposite). If he or she thinks that the symptoms are due to this disorder, you may be given a supportive collar to wear to help relieve the pain by reducing neck mobility and relieving pressure on nearby nerves.

Consult your physician if you are unable to make a diagnosis from this chart.

109 Painful arm

Pain in the arm is almost always the result of injury or straining of the muscles and ligaments that hold the various bones and joints in place. Such injuries are particularly likely to occur after any unaccustomed strenuous physical activity, such as participating in a sport for the first time. The pain should disappear if you rest your arm. If any pain in your arm is recurrent or persistent, consult your physician.

START HERE

Did the pain immediately follow an injury, fall or sudden movement?

YES → **Are you unable to move your arm AND/OR is the pain severe, even when resting?**

NO ↓

Is the pain mainly in the upper arm and does it come on only when you move your arm in a certain way?

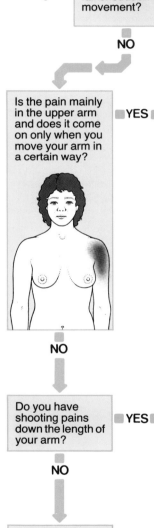

YES →

NO ↓

Do you have shooting pains down the length of your arm?

YES →

NO ↓

Do you have "pins and needles" in your hand, especially at night?

YES →

NO ↓

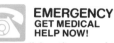

EMERGENCY
GET MEDICAL HELP NOW!

A fracture, dislocation or serious injury to the muscles or ligaments may be causing this pain (see *First aid for suspected broken bones and dislocated joints,* p. 227).

Treatment: The limb will be examined and probably X-rayed (see *Bone X rays,* below) to discover the extent of the damage. Depending on the nature of the injury, you may need to wear a plaster cast or a firm bandage. Sometimes an operation is necessary to reposition the bones.

Injury to the soft tissues (muscles, ligaments and cartilages), such as a sprain or strain or bruising of the arm, is probably causing this pain.

Self-help: Follow the advice on treating such injuries given in the box on p. 231. Consult your physician if the pain is severe or is no better the following day.

Inflammation of the soft tissues or tendons of the shoulder joint (bursitis or tendinitis) as a result of injury or strain is the most likely cause of such pain, although certain forms of arthritis may also cause such symptoms.

Self-help: Take aspirin, an aspirin substitute or an over-the-counter *anti-inflammatory* drug to relieve the pain. Rest the arm while pain persists. Consult your physician if you are no better in 3 days.

CONSULT YOUR PHYSICIAN WITHOUT DELAY
Displacement of a disc between the bones in the neck (see *A prolapsed or "slipped" disc,* opposite) may cause such pain as a result of pressure on a nerve (see *Cervical osteoarthritis,* opposite). There is also likely to be some numbness in the hand.

Treatment: You may be referred for an X ray (see *Bone X rays,* right) of the neck. Your physician will probably prescribe painkillers and may recommend that you wear a supportive collar. In some cases, traction may be necessary.

Carpal tunnel syndrome, a disorder in which a nerve (the median nerve) in the wrist is pinched due to swelling of surrounding tissues, is possible. This condition is particularly common during pregnancy. Consult your physician.

Treatment: The condition often clears up of its own accord. Your physician may refer you for tests to confirm the diagnosis and you may be given injections of *steroids* into the wrist. If the condition is particularly painful and persistent, a simple operation will relieve it.

BONE X RAYS

Because X rays pass through soft tissues such as muscle and fat and clearly show up areas of bone, X-ray pictures are often used to diagnose the extent and nature of damage to any bones from injury or disease. This helps physicians decide on the best form of treatment and, in the case of a broken (fractured) bone, whether or not an operation is necessary to reposition the pieces.

This bone X ray shows a fracture in one of the bones in the lower arm. This type of break is difficult to diagnose without an X ray.

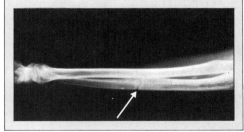

Does the pain mainly affect your joints – for example, your shoulder, elbow or finger joints?

YES →

Go to chart

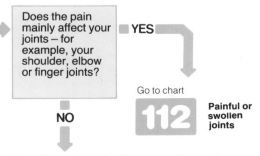
112
Painful or swollen joints

NO ↓

Consult your physician if you are unable to make a diagnosis from this chart and if the pain is severe or persists for more than 24 hours.

110 Painful leg

Pain in the leg is almost always the result of injury or straining of the muscles and ligaments that hold the joints in place. Such injuries are likely if you take part in any unaccustomed activity, such as participating in a sport for the first time. Such pain should disappear if you rest your leg. However, any pain in your leg that is persistent or recurrent may indicate an underlying disorder, so consult your physician.

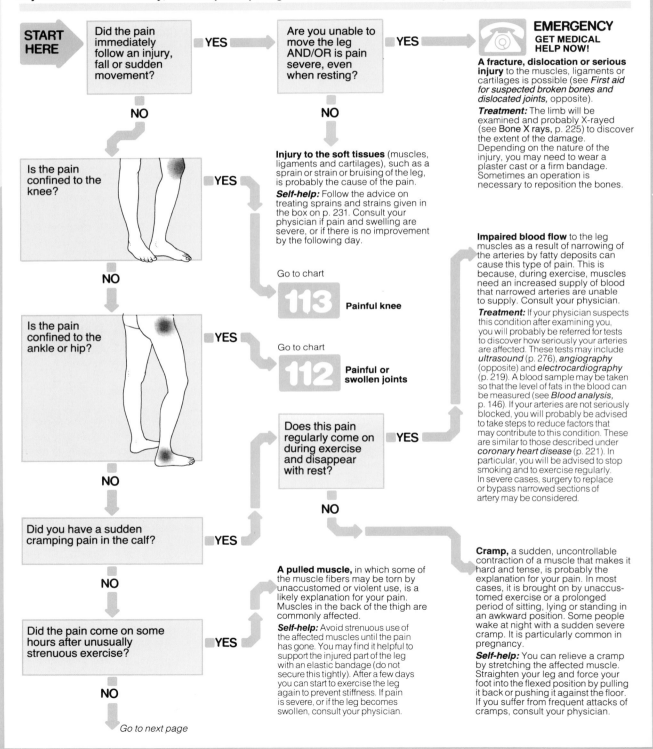

START HERE

Did the pain immediately follow an injury, fall or sudden movement?

YES →

Are you unable to move the leg AND/OR is pain severe, even when resting?

YES →

EMERGENCY
GET MEDICAL HELP NOW!

A fracture, dislocation or serious injury to the muscles, ligaments or cartilages is possible (see *First aid for suspected broken bones and dislocated joints,* opposite).

Treatment: The limb will be examined and probably X-rayed (see **Bone X rays,** p. 225) to discover the extent of the damage. Depending on the nature of the injury, you may need to wear a plaster cast or a firm bandage. Sometimes an operation is necessary to reposition the bones.

NO ↓ (first box)

NO ↓ (second box)

Injury to the soft tissues (muscles, ligaments and cartilages), such as a sprain or strain or bruising of the leg, is probably the cause of the pain.

Self-help: Follow the advice on treating sprains and strains given in the box on p. 231. Consult your physician if pain and swelling are severe, or if there is no improvement by the following day.

Is the pain confined to the knee?

YES →

Go to chart

113 **Painful knee**

NO ↓

Is the pain confined to the ankle or hip?

YES →

Go to chart

112 **Painful or swollen joints**

Impaired blood flow to the leg muscles as a result of narrowing of the arteries by fatty deposits can cause this type of pain. This is because, during exercise, muscles need an increased supply of blood that narrowed arteries are unable to supply. Consult your physician.

Treatment: If your physician suspects this condition after examining you, you will probably be referred for tests to discover how seriously your arteries are affected. These tests may include *ultrasound* (p. 276), *angiography* (opposite) and *electrocardiography* (p. 219). A blood sample may be taken so that the level of fats in the blood can be measured (see *Blood analysis,* p. 146). If your arteries are not seriously blocked, you will probably be advised to take steps to reduce factors that may contribute to this condition. These are similar to those described under *coronary heart disease* (p. 221). In particular, you will be advised to stop smoking and to exercise regularly. In severe cases, surgery to replace or bypass narrowed sections of artery may be considered.

NO ↓

Does this pain regularly come on during exercise and disappear with rest?

YES →

NO ↓

Did you have a sudden cramping pain in the calf?

YES →

NO ↓

A pulled muscle, in which some of the muscle fibers may be torn by unaccustomed or violent use, is a likely explanation for your pain. Muscles in the back of the thigh are commonly affected.

Self-help: Avoid strenuous use of the affected muscles until the pain has gone. You may find it helpful to support the injured part of the leg with an elastic bandage (do not secure this tightly). After a few days you can start to exercise the leg again to prevent stiffness. If pain is severe, or if the leg becomes swollen, consult your physician.

Cramp, a sudden, uncontrollable contraction of a muscle that makes it hard and tense, is probably the explanation for your pain. In most cases, it is brought on by unaccustomed exercise or a prolonged period of sitting, lying or standing in an awkward position. Some people wake at night with a sudden severe cramp. It is particularly common in pregnancy.

Self-help: You can relieve a cramp by stretching the affected muscle. Straighten your leg and force your foot into the flexed position by pulling it back or pushing it against the floor. If you suffer from frequent attacks of cramps, consult your physician.

Did the pain come on some hours after unusually strenuous exercise?

YES →

NO ↓

Go to next page

226

Continued from previous page

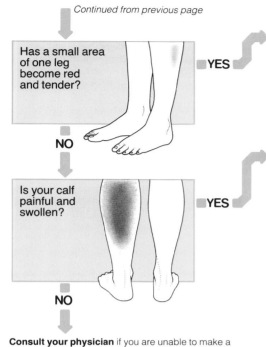

Has a small area of one leg become red and tender?

YES

NO

Is your calf painful and swollen?

YES

NO

Consult your physician if you are unable to make a diagnosis from this chart.

Thrombophlebitis (inflammation of a superficial vein) is the likely cause of such symptoms. Consult your physician.

Treatment: If your physician confirms the diagnosis, he or she will probably prescribe painkillers and, possibly, other medications. A sample of blood may be taken for analysis (see *Blood analysis,* p.146) to find out if there is an underlying reason you have developed this disorder.

CONSULT YOUR PHYSICIAN WITHOUT DELAY!
Deep-vein thrombosis, a condition in which a blood clot blocks a vein in the leg, may be the cause of such symptoms. This disorder is also likely to cause swelling of the ankle. Those taking birth control pills, receiving post menopausal hormone therapy (see *The menopause,* p. 252) or who have been immobilized by injury or illness for a long period are particularly susceptible.

Treatment: Your physician will examine you and, if he or she confirms the possibility of deep-vein thrombosis, will probably arrange for you to be admitted to the hospital for blood-flow tests, and venography (see *Angiography,* below right). Treatment for the condition consists of *anticoagulant* drugs to help dissolve and prevent blood clots. These drugs are usually taken for several months. If you are taking the birth control pill, see chart 136, *Choosing a contraceptive method.*

VARICOSE VEINS

Varicose veins are swollen leg veins causing poor circulation in the legs, usually as a result of damage to the valves in the veins. The veins in the back of the calf and along the inside of the leg are most commonly affected. Varicose veins are likely to cause aching of the leg and swelling of the ankle, especially after long periods of standing. Women often develop varicose veins during pregnancy because of pressure on the pelvic veins from the growing baby.

Self-help measures
If you think that you may be susceptible to varicose veins, especially if you are pregnant, or if you already have swollen veins in the leg, try to keep your weight off your feet as much as possible. Sit with your legs up whenever you can, to help the blood to flow back up your leg. If you have to spend long periods standing up, flex your calf muscles occasionally to help blood circulate in your leg. Wear support stockings or specially prescribed hose. Consult your physician if your varicose veins trouble you, or if the surrounding skin is cracked or sore.

Professional treatment
Your physician may arrange for you to have tests such as venography (see *Angiography,* below). If varicose veins are severe and the self-help measures are not helpful, your physician may recommend surgery to remove the affected veins, or they may be injected with a chemical that seals the vein.

FIRST AID FOR SUSPECTED BROKEN BONES AND DISLOCATED JOINTS

A limb or joint that is very painful or looks misshapen and that will not move following an injury or fall may be broken and/or dislocated. Go to your hospital emergency room. If no help is readily available and/or if you are unable to move, call an ambulance.

General points
- If there is bleeding from the wound, cover it firmly with a clean dressing or cloth.
- Do not try to manipulate the bone or joint back into position yourself; this should only be attempted by a physician.
- While waiting for medical help to arrive, a helper should try to keep the injured person warm and as calm as possible.
- A person with a suspected broken bone or dislocated joint should not eat or drink anything in case a general anesthetic is needed later in order to reset the bone.
- If you have to wait some time for medical attention, immobilize the limb in the most comfortable position, using bandages and splints as described here.

Arm injury
Gently place the injured arm in the most comfortable position across the chest. Some padding, such as a pillow, should be placed between the arm and chest. Support the weight of the arm along its length together with the padding. If the arm cannot be bent, use bandages or tape to secure the arm to the side of the body. A splint (right) may help provide increased support.

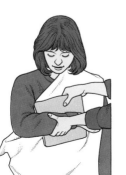

Shoulder, collarbone or elbow injury
Support the weight of the arm in a sling in the most comfortable position.

Leg injury
Secure the injured leg to the undamaged one. If possible, place a well-padded splint (below) between them.

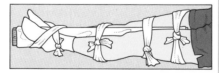

Knee injury
Support the joint in the most comfortable position. If the knee is bent, support it in the bent position. If the knee is unable to bend, support the leg along its length from underneath, using a board or something similar as a splint. Place padding between the knee and the splint and around the heel.

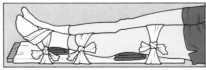

Splints
A splint is a support used to immobilize an injured part of the body (usually an arm or a leg) to reduce pain and the likelihood of further damage. Always secure a splint in at least 2 places not too close to the injury, preferably on either side of it. Use wide lengths of material or tape to do this (not string or rope) and do not secure it too tightly.

ANGIOGRAPHY

Angiography is a procedure that allows physicians to take X-ray pictures of blood vessels that may have become narrowed or blocked. When an artery is under investigation, the procedure is known as arteriography; when it is a vein being examined, it is called venography.

What happens
During angiography, for which you may be sedated, a solution that is visible on X rays is injected into the bloodstream. This is done either by injecting directly into the blood vessel concerned or by means of a fine tube (catheter) inserted through an incision in an accessible blood vessel. The catheter is passed along the blood vessel until it reaches the area where an examination is required. The solution is then released and X rays taken.

111 Foot problems

Problems with feet rarely indicate any serious underlying disorder or disease. Most foot problems are the result of injury or failure to take good care of the feet (see Caring for your feet, below). Consult this chart if you have any pain, irritation or itching of your feet, or if they become deformed in any way.

START HERE

Are you suffering from pain that immediately followed an injury, fall or sudden movement?

YES →

Are you unable to move your foot?

YES →

NO ↓ (from first box)

NO ↓ (from second box)

EMERGENCY
GET MEDICAL HELP NOW!

A fracture, dislocation or serious injury to the ligaments or muscles may be causing this pain. Carry out the first-aid measures for suspected broken bones and dislocated joints as described on p. 227 until medical help arrives.

Treatment: The foot will be examined and probably X-rayed to discover the extent of the damage. Depending on the nature of the injury, you may need to wear a plaster cast or a firm bandage. Sometimes an operation to reposition the bones is necessary.

A soft tissue injury, such as a sprain, strain or bruising, is probably causing this pain.

Self-help: Follow the advice on treating such injuries given in the box on p. 231. Consult your physician if the pain is severe or is no better the following day.

Do both your feet ache all over?

YES →

Have you been walking or standing a long time?

YES →

NO ↓

NO ↓

Did the pain start after you had been walking or running?

YES →

Excessive use of your feet may make them overtired. The pain should stop if you rest your feet. If it recurs, consult your physician, who will examine you to find out if your ligaments have been strained.

NO ↓

A minor fracture of one of the small bones in your foot, often called a stress fracture, is a possibility. Consult your physician.

Treatment: Your physician will examine you and, if he or she suspects this type of injury, you will probably be sent for an X ray to determine the extent and nature of the damage. In most cases, the foot will be firmly bandaged and you will be advised to rest it for a week or so.

Do you have any lumps of hard skin on your toes or on the sides of your feet?

YES →

A corn or callus, caused by pressure from a new or ill-fitting pair of shoes, is probably causing your discomfort. Some people have very little cushioning tissue between the bones and skin of their feet and develop these tender areas easily.

Self-help: To ease the discomfort, soften the hard skin with an over-the-counter corn solvent, and then carefully pare away the top layers of the corn or callus with a corn file. Wear only shoes that fit comfortably. To prevent any direct pressure on the corns, buy some small, spongy, rubber rings from the drugstore to put around them. If these measures do not help, and the corns or calluses persist for several weeks, consult your physician.

NO ↓

Go to next page

CARING FOR YOUR FEET

Ill-fitting shoes can lead to distortion of the toes and may lead to the development of painful conditions such as bunions and corns. When buying shoes, take care to ensure that they fit properly, allowing enough space for the toes to spread. Shoes with pointed toes and high heels should be worn only when you do not expect to be standing or walking for long periods. These shoes are more likely to damage the feet and make you adopt an unnatural posture that may lead to backaches and headaches.

To avoid distorting the toes (right), choose a low-heeled, round-toed shoe (below).

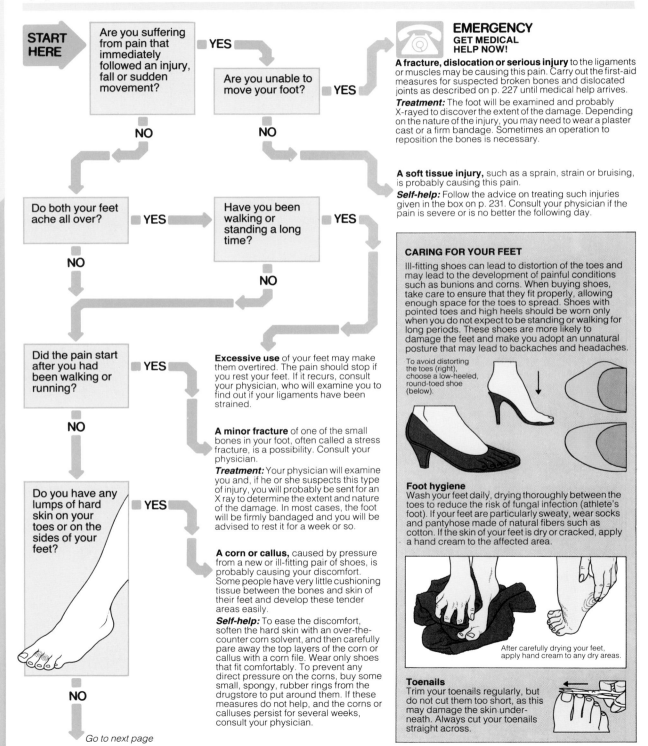

Foot hygiene
Wash your feet daily, drying thoroughly between the toes to reduce the risk of fungal infection (athlete's foot). If your feet are particularly sweaty, wear socks and pantyhose made of natural fibers such as cotton. If the skin of your feet is dry or cracked, apply a hand cream to the affected area.

After carefully drying your feet, apply hand cream to any dry areas.

Toenails
Trim your toenails regularly, but do not cut them too short, as this may damage the skin underneath. Always cut your toenails straight across.

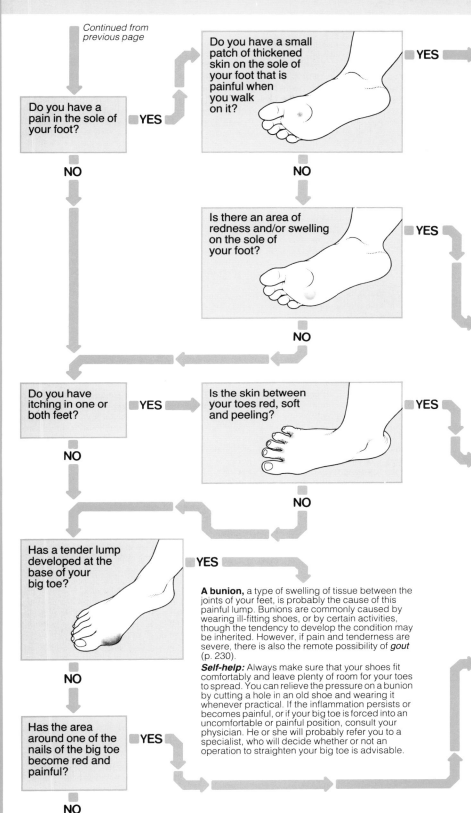

Continued from previous page

Do you have a pain in the sole of your foot?

YES →

Do you have a small patch of thickened skin on the sole of your foot that is painful when you walk on it?

YES →

A plantar wart may have developed as a result of a virus invading the skin cells and causing them to multiply rapidly. They can be spread by touch or by contact with the skin shed from a wart.

Self-help: Most warts disappear naturally in time but, if you find them a nuisance, apply one of the wart remedies available over-the-counter in the form of cream or paint. These preparations should be applied very carefully because they can make the surrounding skin sore – follow the manufacturer's instructions. Afterward, the dead skin should be removed with a pumice stone. If your wart does not respond to this treatment, ask your physician for advice. He or she may refer you to a skin specialist, who may remove the wart by freezing it with liquid nitrogen or carbon dioxide, or burning it off (diathermy).

NO ↓

Is there an area of redness and/or swelling on the sole of your foot?

YES →

An infection, perhaps as a result of a puncture wound, is likely to be the problem. Consult your physician.

Treatment: Your physician will probably arrange for you to have an X ray to see if there is any metal in the wound. If there is, it may need to be removed under local or general anesthetic. You will probably be prescribed *antibiotics* and you may need a tetanus booster shot.

NO

Do you have itching in one or both feet?

YES →

Is the skin between your toes red, soft and peeling?

YES →

Athlete's foot, a fungal infection, is the likeliest cause of these symptoms. In some cases, the nails are also affected and become thickened and discolored.

Self-help: Apply an over-the-counter *antifungal* cream, spray or powder to the affected area and keep your feet as dry as possible. Wear socks made of natural fibers and shoes with porous soles and uppers, or open sandals. If these measures fail to clear up the condition within a week or so, consult your physician, who may prescribe a more vigorous antifungal preparation or a course of antifungal tablets.

NO ↓

Has a tender lump developed at the base of your big toe?

YES →

A bunion, a type of swelling of tissue between the joints of your feet, is probably the cause of this painful lump. Bunions are commonly caused by wearing ill-fitting shoes, or by certain activities, though the tendency to develop the condition may be inherited. However, if pain and tenderness are severe, there is also the remote possibility of *gout* (p. 230).

Self-help: Always make sure that your shoes fit comfortably and leave plenty of room for your toes to spread. You can relieve the pressure on a bunion by cutting a hole in an old shoe and wearing it whenever practical. If the inflammation persists or becomes painful, or if your big toe is forced into an uncomfortable or painful position, consult your physician. He or she will probably refer you to a specialist, who will decide whether or not an operation to straighten your big toe is advisable.

NO ↓

Has the area around one of the nails of the big toe become red and painful?

YES →

An ingrown toenail that has led to infection is likely to be the cause of the problem. This condition may be caused by wearing shoes that are too tight or by cutting the nails incorrectly (see *Caring for your feet,* opposite).

Self-help: Wear shoes that fit comfortably or, if possible, wear open-toed sandals. Cut your toenails straight across without leaving any jagged splinters at the edges and keep the affected area clean and dry. However, if these measures do not help or if your toe becomes very painful, consult your physician. He or she may prescribe an *antibiotic* to clear up any infection. In some cases, minor surgery is necessary.

NO ↓

Consult your physician if you are unable to make a diagnosis from this chart.

112 Painful or swollen joints

Joints occur at the junction of two or more bones and usually allow movement between those bones. The degree and type of movement allowed depends on the structure of the joint. Major joints such as the hips, knees and ankles undergo constant wear and tear, so minor degrees of discomfort or stiffness may occur from time to time. However, severe pain, swelling or limitation of movement may be the result of damage to the bones or soft tissues of the joint from injury, or may indicate an underlying disorder of the joints or skeletal system. Consult this chart if you suffer to any extent from pain, stiffness and/or swelling in or around a joint.

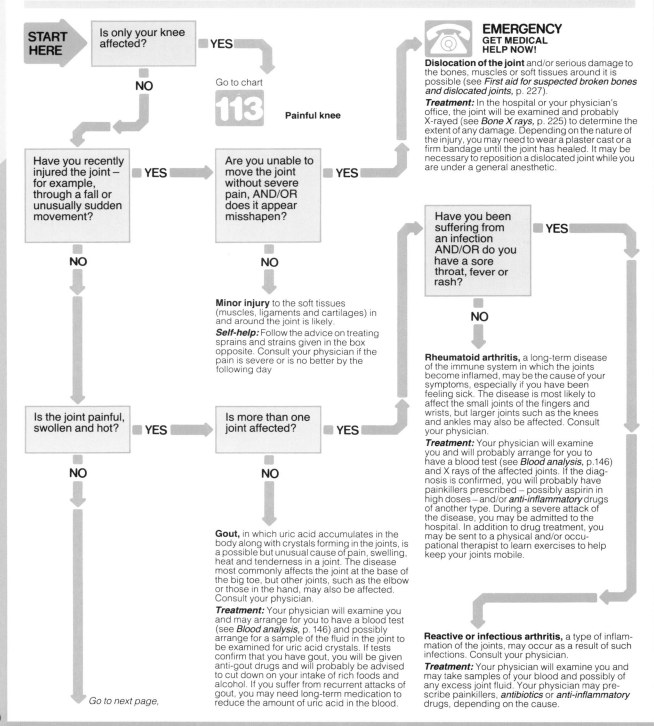

START HERE

Is only your knee affected? → **YES**

Go to chart **113** Painful knee

↓ **NO**

Have you recently injured the joint – for example, through a fall or unusually sudden movement? → **YES**

↓ **NO**

Are you unable to move the joint without severe pain, AND/OR does it appear misshapen? → **YES**

↓ **NO**

EMERGENCY
GET MEDICAL HELP NOW!

Dislocation of the joint and/or serious damage to the bones, muscles or soft tissues around it is possible (see *First aid for suspected broken bones and dislocated joints*, p. 227).

Treatment: In the hospital or your physician's office, the joint will be examined and probably X-rayed (see *Bone X rays*, p. 225) to determine the extent of any damage. Depending on the nature of the injury, you may need to wear a plaster cast or a firm bandage until the joint has healed. It may be necessary to reposition a dislocated joint while you are under a general anesthetic.

Minor injury to the soft tissues (muscles, ligaments and cartilages) in and around the joint is likely.

Self-help: Follow the advice on treating sprains and strains given in the box opposite. Consult your physician if the pain is severe or is no better by the following day

Have you been suffering from an infection AND/OR do you have a sore throat, fever or rash? → **YES**

↓ **NO**

Rheumatoid arthritis, a long-term disease of the immune system in which the joints become inflamed, may be the cause of your symptoms, especially if you have been feeling sick. The disease is most likely to affect the small joints of the fingers and wrists, but larger joints such as the knees and ankles may also be affected. Consult your physician.

Treatment: Your physician will examine you and will probably arrange for you to have a blood test (see *Blood analysis*, p.146) and X rays of the affected joints. If the diagnosis is confirmed, you will probably have painkillers prescribed – possibly aspirin in high doses – and/or *anti-inflammatory* drugs of another type. During a severe attack of the disease, you may be admitted to the hospital. In addition to drug treatment, you may be sent to a physical and/or occupational therapist to learn exercises to help keep your joints mobile.

Is the joint painful, swollen and hot? → **YES** → **Is more than one joint affected?** → **YES**

↓ **NO** (joint painful)   ↓ **NO** (more than one joint)

Gout, in which uric acid accumulates in the body along with crystals forming in the joints, is a possible but unusual cause of pain, swelling, heat and tenderness in a joint. The disease most commonly affects the joint at the base of the big toe, but other joints, such as the elbow or those in the hand, may also be affected. Consult your physician.

Treatment: Your physician will examine you and may arrange for you to have a blood test (see *Blood analysis*, p. 146) and possibly arrange for a sample of the fluid in the joint to be examined for uric acid crystals. If tests confirm that you have gout, you will be given anti-gout drugs and will probably be advised to cut down on your intake of rich foods and alcohol. If you suffer from recurrent attacks of gout, you may need long-term medication to reduce the amount of uric acid in the blood.

Reactive or infectious arthritis, a type of inflammation of the joints, may occur as a result of such infections. Consult your physician.

Treatment: Your physician will examine you and may take samples of your blood and possibly of any excess joint fluid. Your physician may prescribe painkillers, *antibiotics* or *anti-inflammatory* drugs, depending on the cause.

Go to next page,

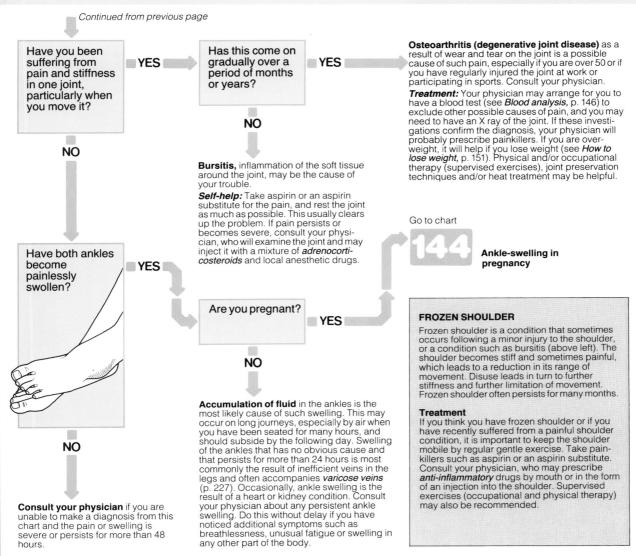

Continued from previous page

Have you been suffering from pain and stiffness in one joint, particularly when you move it? — **YES** → **Has this come on gradually over a period of months or years?** — **YES** →

Osteoarthritis (degenerative joint disease) as a result of wear and tear on the joint is a possible cause of such pain, especially if you are over 50 or if you have regularly injured the joint at work or participating in sports. Consult your physician.
Treatment: Your physician may arrange for you to have a blood test (see *Blood analysis,* p. 146) to exclude other possible causes of pain, and you may need to have an X ray of the joint. If these investigations confirm the diagnosis, your physician will probably prescribe painkillers. If you are overweight, it will help if you lose weight (see *How to lose weight,* p. 151). Physical and/or occupational therapy (supervised exercises), joint preservation techniques and/or heat treatment may be helpful.

NO (from "Has this come on gradually...")

Bursitis, inflammation of the soft tissue around the joint, may be the cause of your trouble.
Self-help: Take aspirin or an aspirin substitute for the pain, and rest the joint as much as possible. This usually clears up the problem. If pain persists or becomes severe, consult your physician, who will examine the joint and may inject it with a mixture of ***adrenocorticosteroids*** and local anesthetic drugs.

NO (from "Have you been suffering...")

Have both ankles become painlessly swollen? — **YES** → **Are you pregnant?** — **YES** →

Go to chart

144

Ankle-swelling in pregnancy

NO (from "Are you pregnant?")

Accumulation of fluid in the ankles is the most likely cause of such swelling. This may occur on long journeys, especially by air when you have been seated for many hours, and should subside by the following day. Swelling of the ankles that has no obvious cause and that persists for more than 24 hours is most commonly the result of inefficient veins in the legs and often accompanies *varicose veins* (p. 227). Occasionally, ankle swelling is the result of a heart or kidney condition. Consult your physician about any persistent ankle swelling. Do this without delay if you have noticed additional symptoms such as breathlessness, unusual fatigue or swelling in any other part of the body.

NO (from "Have both ankles become...")

Consult your physician if you are unable to make a diagnosis from this chart and the pain or swelling is severe or persists for more than 48 hours.

FROZEN SHOULDER

Frozen shoulder is a condition that sometimes occurs following a minor injury to the shoulder, or a condition such as bursitis (above left). The shoulder becomes stiff and sometimes painful, which leads to a reduction in its range of movement. Disuse leads in turn to further stiffness and further limitation of movement. Frozen shoulder often persists for many months.

Treatment
If you think you have frozen shoulder or if you have recently suffered from a painful shoulder condition, it is important to keep the shoulder mobile by regular gentle exercise. Take painkillers such as aspirin or an aspirin substitute. Consult your physician, who may prescribe *anti-inflammatory* drugs by mouth or in the form of an injection into the shoulder. Supervised exercises (occupational and physical therapy) may also be recommended.

FIRST AID FOR SPRAINS AND STRAINS

A joint is said to be sprained when it is wrenched or twisted beyond its normal range of movement – in a fall, for example – thus tearing some or all of the ligaments that support it. Ankles are especially prone to this type of injury. The main symptoms, which may be indistinguishable from those of a minor strain, are pain, swelling and bruising. If you are unable to move the injured part, or if it looks misshapen, a broken bone or dislocated joint is possible and you should carry out first aid as described on p. 227. In other cases, try the following first-aid treatment:

1 For the first 24 hours after the injury, cool the injured part (below).

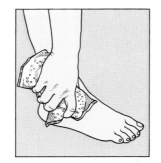

2 Support an injured joint or limb with a firm, but not overtight bandage (below). An arm or wrist may be more comfortable in a sling.

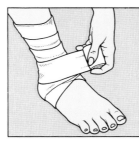

If you have a badly sprained ankle that is still painful the day after the injury, go to your physician, local hospital emergency room or urgent care center to have the joint firmly bandaged to prevent movement while the joint is healing. In this case, you should make sure that you rest the joint for at least a week.

Cooling an injury
Applying cold to any injury causing pain, swelling and/or bruising will help to reduce swelling and relieve pain. This can be done by using an ice bag, a cloth pad soaked in cold water or an unopened packet of frozen vegetables. After the first 24 hours, you should apply warmth to the affected part to reduce inflammation.

3 Rest the injured part for a day or so. A foot, leg or ankle which has been injured should be raised whenever possible.

113 Painful knee

The knee is one of the principal weight-bearing joints in the body and is subject to much wear and tear. If your work involves a great deal of bending or squatting, the risk of damage to the bones, ligaments and cartilages through overuse and/or injury is increased. Consult this chart if you experience pain in one or both knees.

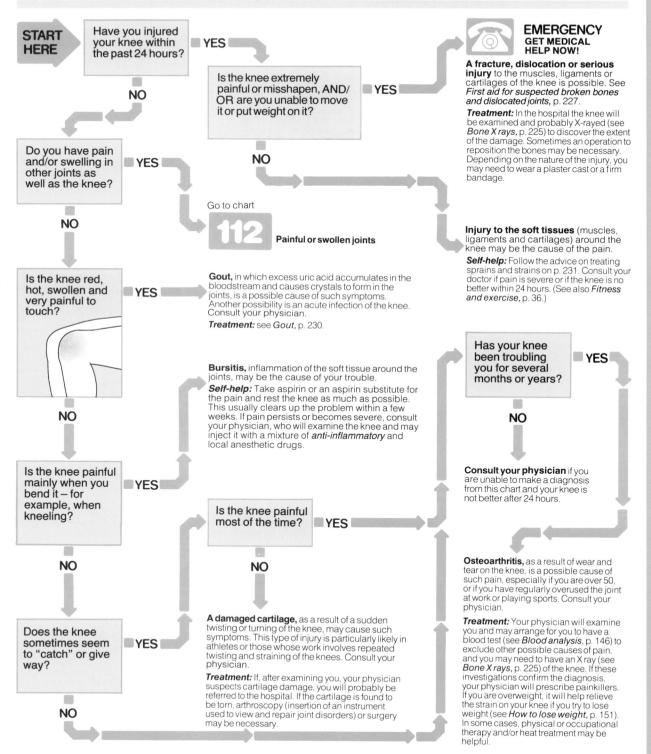

START HERE

Have you injured your knee within the past 24 hours? — YES

Is the knee extremely painful or misshapen, AND/OR are you unable to move it or put weight on it? — YES

NO

NO

Do you have pain and/or swelling in other joints as well as the knee? — YES

NO

Go to chart

112 Painful or swollen joints

EMERGENCY
GET MEDICAL HELP NOW!

A fracture, dislocation or serious injury to the muscles, ligaments or cartilages of the knee is possible. See *First aid for suspected broken bones and dislocated joints,* p. 227.

Treatment: In the hospital the knee will be examined and probably X-rayed (see *Bone X rays,* p. 225) to discover the extent of the damage. Sometimes an operation to reposition the bones may be necessary. Depending on the nature of the injury, you may need to wear a plaster cast or a firm bandage.

Injury to the soft tissues (muscles, ligaments and cartilages) around the knee may be the cause of the pain.

Self-help: Follow the advice on treating sprains and strains on p. 231. Consult your doctor if pain is severe or if the knee is no better within 24 hours. (See also *Fitness and exercise,* p. 36.)

Is the knee red, hot, swollen and very painful to touch? — YES

NO

Gout, in which excess uric acid accumulates in the bloodstream and causes crystals to form in the joints, is a possible cause of such symptoms. Another possibility is an acute infection of the knee. Consult your physician.
Treatment: see *Gout,* p. 230.

Bursitis, inflammation of the soft tissue around the joints, may be the cause of your trouble.
Self-help: Take aspirin or an aspirin substitute for the pain and rest the knee as much as possible. This usually clears up the problem within a few weeks. If pain persists or becomes severe, consult your physician, who will examine the knee and may inject it with a mixture of *anti-inflammatory* and local anesthetic drugs.

Has your knee been troubling you for several months or years? — YES

NO

Consult your physician if you are unable to make a diagnosis from this chart and your knee is not better after 24 hours.

Is the knee painful mainly when you bend it — for example, when kneeling? — YES

NO

Is the knee painful most of the time? — YES

NO

Is the knee painful most of the time? YES

NO

Does the knee sometimes seem to "catch" or give way? — YES

NO

A damaged cartilage, as a result of a sudden twisting or turning of the knee, may cause such symptoms. This type of injury is particularly likely in athletes or those whose work involves repeated twisting and straining of the knees. Consult your physician.

Treatment: If, after examining you, your physician suspects cartilage damage, you will probably be referred to the hospital. If the cartilage is found to be torn, arthroscopy (insertion of an instrument used to view and repair joint disorders) or surgery may be necessary.

Osteoarthritis, as a result of wear and tear on the knee, is a possible cause of such pain, especially if you are over 50, or if you have regularly overused the joint at work or playing sports. Consult your physician.

Treatment: Your physician will examine you and may arrange for you to have a blood test (see *Blood analysis,* p. 146) to exclude other possible causes of pain, and you may need to have an X ray (see *Bone X rays,* p. 225) of the knee. If these investigations confirm the diagnosis, your physician will prescribe painkillers. If you are overweight, it will help relieve the strain on your knee if you try to lose weight (see *How to lose weight,* p. 151). In some cases, physical or occupational therapy and/or heat treatment may be helpful.

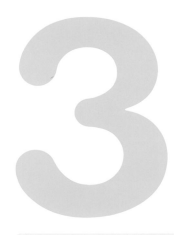

3 Special problems: men

114 Baldness

Male pattern baldness is the term used to describe the type of hair loss that affects many men as they grow older. It is a natural and irreversible part of the aging process. Some men start to lose their hair as early as 20, and the majority have lost their hair to some extent by the age of 60, although some men retain a full head of hair until old age. In most cases hair loss is first noticed when the hairline at the front starts to recede.

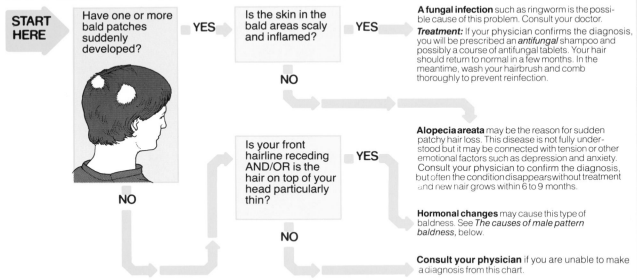

START HERE

Have one or more bald patches suddenly developed? — YES → **Is the skin in the bald areas scaly and inflamed?** — YES →

A fungal infection such as ringworm is the possible cause of this problem. Consult your doctor.

Treatment: If your physician confirms the diagnosis, you will be prescribed an *antifungal* shampoo and possibly a course of antifungal tablets. Your hair should return to normal in a few months. In the meantime, wash your hairbrush and comb thoroughly to prevent reinfection.

NO ↓

Is your front hairline receding AND/OR is the hair on top of your head particularly thin? — YES →

Alopecia areata may be the reason for sudden patchy hair loss. This disease is not fully understood but it may be connected with tension or other emotional factors such as depression and anxiety. Consult your physician to confirm the diagnosis, but often the condition disappears without treatment and new hair grows within 6 to 9 months.

Hormonal changes may cause this type of baldness. See *The causes of male pattern baldness*, below.

NO (from first question) ↓

NO (from hairline question) ↓

Consult your physician if you are unable to make a diagnosis from this chart.

THE CAUSES OF MALE PATTERN BALDNESS

Male pattern baldness occurs when the rate of hair loss in certain areas exceeds the rate of hair replacement. The exact cause of this is not known, although it may be related to an increased production of an androgen, a male sex hormone that is thought to limit hair growth. The tendency to lose hair at a certain age is probably inherited. You may inherit this tendency from one or both sides of your family. If men on both sides of your family have become bald at an early age, you are also likely to lose your hair early. However, if early baldness runs only on one side of the family, your chances of retaining your hair longer are increased.

Concealing hair loss
Because male pattern baldness is irreversible, there is no cure for such hair loss. There is no proof that changes in diet, or that taking large doses of vitamins or minerals, can do anything to reverse or slow down hair loss. Most men simply accept their changing appearance and adopt a new hairstyle to take account of this hair loss.

If you wish to conceal baldness, there are several alternatives with varying degrees of effectiveness. The most straightforward and least risky alternative is a simple hairpiece (toupée). Hair weaving is another possibility. It involves attaching a hairpiece to existing hair on the scalp. The weave requires maintenance throughout its life as your natural hair, which anchors the weave in place, grows. Hair transplantation (below) is an expensive and often difficult alternative.

The development of male pattern baldness

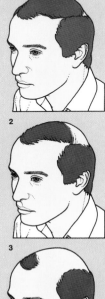

1

2

3

The cycle of hair loss and growth

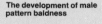

1 When a hair stops growing, the root forms a bulb shape and becomes detached from the base of the follicle.
2 The old hair then moves up the follicle and is shed. A new hair starts to form at the bottom of the follicle.
3 The hair may remain in the growing phase for several years.

Wearing a toupée

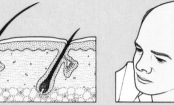
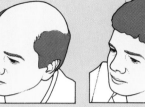
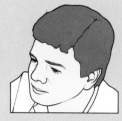

Hair transplantation
In most types of hair transplant, hair from an area of thick growth (donor site) — often the back of the head — is implanted in the bald area (recipient site). This is a lengthy and painful process. Always seek medical advice first.

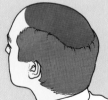
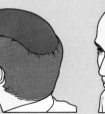

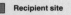 **Recipient site**

Donor site

115 Painful or swollen testicles

Consult this chart if you feel any pain or notice a lump or swelling in one or both of your testicles, or in the whole area within the scrotum (the supportive bag that contains the testicles). It is important to seek your physician's advice because early treatment of an underlying disorder is often necessary to reduce the risk of infertility. Early detection of tumors is also important.

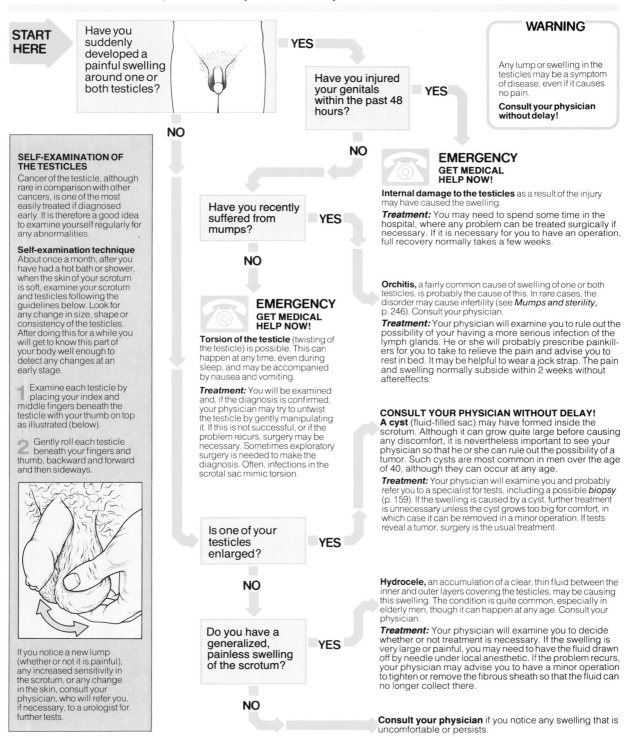

START HERE

Have you suddenly developed a painful swelling around one or both testicles?

YES → Have you injured your genitals within the past 48 hours?

YES →

WARNING

Any lump or swelling in the testicles may be a symptom of disease, even if it causes no pain.

Consult your physician without delay!

NO ↓

NO ↓

EMERGENCY
GET MEDICAL HELP NOW!

Internal damage to the testicles as a result of the injury may have caused the swelling.

Treatment: You may need to spend some time in the hospital, where any problem can be treated surgically if necessary. If it is necessary for you to have an operation, full recovery normally takes a few weeks.

SELF-EXAMINATION OF THE TESTICLES

Cancer of the testicle, although rare in comparison with other cancers, is one of the most easily treated if diagnosed early. It is therefore a good idea to examine yourself regularly for any abnormalities.

Self-examination technique
About once a month, after you have had a hot bath or shower, when the skin of your scrotum is soft, examine your scrotum and testicles following the guidelines below. Look for any change in size, shape or consistency of the testicles. After doing this for a while you will get to know this part of your body well enough to detect any changes at an early stage.

1 Examine each testicle by placing your index and middle fingers beneath the testicle with your thumb on top as illustrated (below).

2 Gently roll each testicle beneath your fingers and thumb, backward and forward and then sideways.

If you notice a new lump (whether or not it is painful), any increased sensitivity in the scrotum, or any change in the skin, consult your physician, who will refer you, if necessary, to a urologist for further tests.

Have you recently suffered from mumps?

YES →

NO ↓

Orchitis, a fairly common cause of swelling of one or both testicles, is probably the cause of this. In rare cases, the disorder may cause infertility (see *Mumps and sterility*, p. 246). Consult your physician.

Treatment: Your physician will examine you to rule out the possibility of your having a more serious infection of the lymph glands. He or she will probably prescribe painkillers for you to take to relieve the pain and advise you to rest in bed. It may be helpful to wear a jock strap. The pain and swelling normally subside within 2 weeks without aftereffects.

EMERGENCY
GET MEDICAL HELP NOW!

Torsion of the testicle (twisting of the testicle) is possible. This can happen at any time, even during sleep, and may be accompanied by nausea and vomiting.

Treatment: You will be examined and, if the diagnosis is confirmed, your physician may try to untwist the testicle by gently manipulating it. If this is not successful, or if the problem recurs, surgery may be necessary. Sometimes exploratory surgery is needed to make the diagnosis. Often, infections in the scrotal sac mimic torsion.

CONSULT YOUR PHYSICIAN WITHOUT DELAY!
A cyst (fluid-filled sac) may have formed inside the scrotum. Although it can grow quite large before causing any discomfort, it is nevertheless important to see your physician so that he or she can rule out the possibility of a tumor. Such cysts are most common in men over the age of 40, although they can occur at any age.

Treatment: Your physician will examine you and probably refer you to a specialist for tests, including a possible *biopsy* (p. 159). If the swelling is caused by a cyst, further treatment is unnecessary unless the cyst grows too big for comfort, in which case it can be removed in a minor operation. If tests reveal a tumor, surgery is the usual treatment.

Is one of your testicles enlarged?

YES →

NO ↓

Hydrocele, an accumulation of a clear, thin fluid between the inner and outer layers covering the testicles, may be causing this swelling. The condition is quite common, especially in elderly men, though it can happen at any age. Consult your physician.

Treatment: Your physician will examine you to decide whether or not treatment is necessary. If the swelling is very large or painful, you may need to have the fluid drawn off by needle under local anesthetic. If the problem recurs, your physician may advise you to have a minor operation to tighten or remove the fibrous sheath so that the fluid can no longer collect there.

Do you have a generalized, painless swelling of the scrotum?

YES →

NO ↓

Consult your physician if you notice any swelling that is uncomfortable or persists.

116 Painful penis

Pain in the penis or soreness of the overlying skin can signal a variety of different disorders of the penis itself or of the urinary tract. Many painful conditions of the penis are the result of minor injuries – perhaps incurred while participating in sports – or from friction with clothing. Nevertheless, it is important that any pain or change in the appearance of your penis not attributable to an injury of this kind be diagnosed by your physician at an early stage so that treatment, if necessary, can be started as soon as possible.

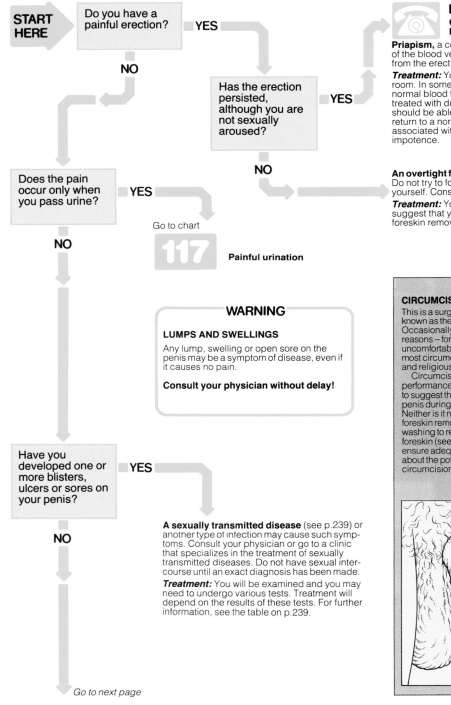

START HERE

Do you have a painful erection? — **YES** →

NO ↓

Has the erection persisted, although you are not sexually aroused? — **YES** →

NO ↓

Does the pain occur only when you pass urine? — **YES** →

NO ↓

Go to chart

117

Painful urination

EMERGENCY
GET MEDICAL HELP NOW!

Priapism, a condition caused by sudden obstruction of the blood vessels so that blood cannot flow away from the erect penis, is possible.

Treatment: You will be examined at the emergency room. In some cases, surgery is necessary to restore normal blood flow. In other cases the condition can be treated with drugs. If priapism is relieved quickly, you should be able to have normal erections again and return to a normal sex life. Prolonged priapism is associated with a high frequency of subsequent impotence.

An overtight foreskin may be the cause of such pain. Do not try to force the foreskin back over the penis yourself. Consult your physician.

Treatment: Your physician will examine you and may suggest that you have a minor operation to have the foreskin removed (see *Circumcision,* below).

WARNING

LUMPS AND SWELLINGS

Any lump, swelling or open sore on the penis may be a symptom of disease, even if it causes no pain.

Consult your physician without delay!

Have you developed one or more blisters, ulcers or sores on your penis? — **YES** →

NO ↓

A sexually transmitted disease (see p.239) or another type of infection may cause such symptoms. Consult your physician or go to a clinic that specializes in the treatment of sexually transmitted diseases. Do not have sexual intercourse until an exact diagnosis has been made.

Treatment: You will be examined and you may need to undergo various tests. Treatment will depend on the results of these tests. For further information, see the table on p.239.

Go to next page

CIRCUMCISION

This is a surgical operation to remove the fold of skin, known as the foreskin, that covers the tip of the penis. Occasionally, the operation is carried out for medical reasons – for example, if the foreskin becomes tight or uncomfortable and is difficult to roll back. However, most circumcisions done in infancy are done for social and religious reasons.

Circumcision has no significant effect on sexual performance – in particular, there is no firm evidence to suggest that it reduces sensitivity at the tip of the penis during intercourse or that it delays orgasm. Neither is it necessarily more hygienic to have the foreskin removed. By paying careful attention when washing to remove all secretions from beneath the foreskin (see *Genital hygiene,* opposite), you will ensure adequate cleanliness. Talk to your physician about the potential risks and possible advantages of circumcision.

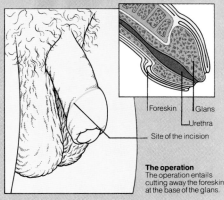

Foreskin | Glans
Urethra
Site of the incision

The operation
The operation entails cutting away the foreskin at the base of the glans.

Continued from previous page

Do you have one or more hard, skin-colored lumps on your penis?

YES → **Anogenital warts,** caused by virus infection, are likely. These often grow quite quickly and can be irritating. They are usually transmitted by sexual contact, but this is not always the case. They may disappear spontaneously, but often recur. Do not attempt to treat this condition yourself with over-the-counter preparations, because the skin of the penis is very sensitive. Consult your physician.

Treatment: Your physician may prescribe a preparation in the form of a cream or paint to apply to the warts. He or she will probably advise you to keep the affected area as clean and dry as possible with regular washing using a mild soap and then gently patting dry. Your physician will also examine you to rule out the possibility of a sexually transmitted disease (p.239) and will also advise you to avoid sexual contact until the warts have disappeared.

NO ↓

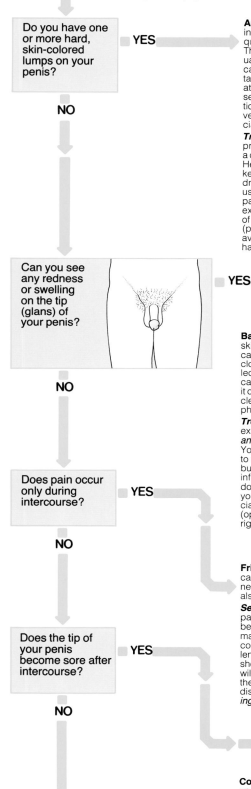

Can you see any redness or swelling on the tip (glans) of your penis?

YES → **Balanitis,** inflammation of the foreskin or glans, is likely. This is usually caused by irritation from infection or clothing or from skin secretions collecting under the foreskin. In some cases, soreness and swelling make it difficult to draw the foreskin back to clean underneath. Consult your physician.

Treatment: Your physician will examine you and may prescribe an *antibiotic* to relieve the inflammation. You will need to pay careful attention to washing underneath the foreskin, but should avoid using soap while inflammation persists. If your foreskin does not draw back easily to allow you to wash thoroughly, your physician may recommend *circumcision* (opposite). See also *Genital hygiene,* right.

NO ↓

Does pain occur only during intercourse?

YES → **Friction during intercourse** may cause pain, especially if your partner's vagina seems dry and if she also complains of discomfort.

Self-help: Try to ensure that your partner is relaxed and aroused before attempting intercourse. You may find it helpful to use an over-the-counter lubricating jelly. If the problem persists, you and your partner should consult your physician, who will examine you both to find out if there is any physical cause for the discomfort. Sometimes *Sex counseling* (p.240) is helpful.

NO ↓

Does the tip of your penis become sore after intercourse?

YES →

NO ↓

Consult your physician if you are unable to make a diagnosis from this chart.

BLOOD IN THE SEMEN

Pinkish, reddish or brownish streaks in your semen may be blood. This uncommon condition is known as hemospermia, and may be barely noticeable. It is caused by the rupture of small veins in the upper part of the urethra during an erection. These heal themselves within a few minutes, although the semen may continue to be slightly discolored for a few days afterward.

What should be done?
There is no need to be concerned if you notice blood in your semen. However, if you notice a blood-stained discharge after ejaculation, or if you notice blood in the urine, consult your physician, who will need to investigate the problem.

GENITAL HYGIENE

Minor irritations of the penis can be avoided by paying attention to genital hygiene, especially if you are sexually active. However, there is no need to be overzealous in your approach to this – the genitals need no more attention than the rest of the body. Washing your penis with warm water and mild soap each time you take a bath or shower is sufficient to maintain hygiene. If you have not been circumcised (see *Circumcision,* opposite), be sure to draw back your foreskin to clean the glans (tip) of your penis.

Cleaning under the foreskin

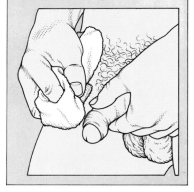

An allergic reaction – for example, to a contraceptive cream or douching solution used by your partner – may be the cause of soreness after intercourse. If you use a condom, there is a possibility that you may be allergic to rubber.

Self-help: Soreness should disappear if you avoid contact with whatever you think may be causing the reaction. It may be necessary for you to choose an alternative form of contraception (see p.248). If you can find no obvious cause for the soreness, or if soreness persists, consult your physician.

117 Painful urination

Consult this chart if you feel pain or discomfort when passing urine. This may be a symptom of infection or inflammation, or may follow injury to the urinary tract, and you should consult your physician without delay.

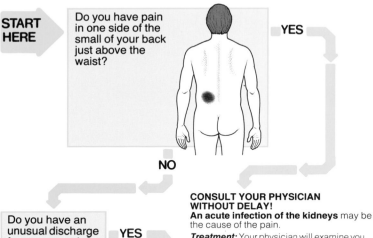

START HERE

Do you have pain in one side of the small of your back just above the waist?

YES →

NO →

Do you have an unusual discharge from your penis?

YES →

NO →

CONSULT YOUR PHYSICIAN WITHOUT DELAY!
An acute infection of the kidneys may be the cause of the pain.

Treatment: Your physician will examine you and take a specimen of your blood and urine and may prescribe *antibiotics*. He or she may also arrange for you to have a special X ray of the kidneys (see *Intravenous pyelography*, right) to try and find an underlying cause of the problem. Further treatment will depend on the results of the tests.

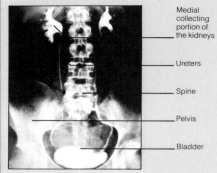

INTRAVENOUS PYELOGRAPHY

Intravenous pyelography provides the physician with a series of X-ray pictures of the urinary tract. A special dye that shows up on X-ray pictures is injected into your bloodstream. It travels through your body until it reaches your kidneys, where it is excreted through the ureters and into the bladder. This process takes an hour or more, and X-ray pictures are taken at regular intervals.

An intravenous pyelogram of a normal urinary tract

- Medial collecting portion of the kidneys
- Ureters
- Spine
- Pelvis
- Bladder

An infection that may have been transmitted sexually may cause pain during urination and also discharge from the penis. See *Sexually transmitted diseases* (opposite) and consult your physician.

ABNORMAL-LOOKING URINE

Color of urine	Possible causes	What action is necessary
Pink, red or smoky	There is a chance that you may have blood in the urine, possibly caused by infection, inflammation or a growth in the urinary tract. However, natural or artificial food colorings can also pass into the urine.	Consult your physician without delay. He or she may need to take samples of urine and blood for analysis (see *Blood analysis*, p.146) in order to make a firm diagnosis. Treatment will depend on the underlying problem.
Dark yellow or orange	If you have not been drinking much fluid, your urine has become concentrated. Loss of fluid caused by diarrhea, vomiting or sweating can also make your urine more concentrated and therefore darker than normal. Certain substances in senna-based laxatives and in rhubarb can also darken your urine temporarily.	This is no cause for concern; as soon as you compensate for any loss of fluid by drinking, your urine will return to its normal color. Substances in laxatives and rhubarb will pass through your system within 24 hours.
Clear and dark brown	Jaundice caused by a disorder of the liver (most commonly hepatitis) or gallbladder is a possibility, especially if your bowel movements are very pale and your skin or the whites of your eyes look yellow.	Consult your physician, who will need to take samples of urine and blood for analysis (see *Blood analysis*, p.146) in order to make a firm diagnosis. Treatment will depend on the underlying problem.
Green or blue	Artificial coloring in food or medicine is almost certainly the cause of this.	This is no cause for concern, as the coloring will pass through your system without harmful effects.

Go to next page

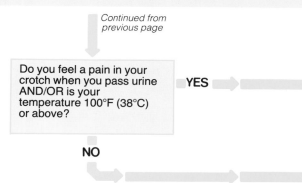

Continued from previous page

Do you feel a pain in your crotch when you pass urine AND/OR is your temperature 100°F (38°C) or above?

YES

NO

Prostatitis (inflammation of the prostate gland, usually caused by an infection) is a possibility. Consult your physician.

Treatment: Your physician will probably feel your prostate gland to find out if it is swollen and tender by inserting a finger into your rectum. You will be asked to provide a urine sample so that it can be analyzed. If the diagnosis is confirmed, your physician will probably advise you to rest and he or she may prescribe *antibiotics* to clear the infection.

A urinary tract infection is the most likely cause of painful urination with no other symptoms. Consult your physician.

Treatment: If your physician suspects infection, he or she may take a sample of urine for analysis. In some cases, further tests such as *intravenous pyelography* (opposite) are necessary. Treatment for infection in the urinary tract is likely to consist of *antibiotics*. You will also be advised to drink plenty of fluids.

SEXUALLY TRANSMITTED DISEASES (STDs)

Infections passed from one person to another during sexual contact (including anal and oral sex) are known as sexually transmitted (venereal) diseases. If you think you have caught a sexually transmitted disease, consult your physician or go to a clinic that specializes in treating such diseases, where you will be treated in the strictest confidence. It is important to seek medical advice promptly because of the risk of passing the infection to someone else. Also, an infection may be less easy to eradicate if there is any delay in starting treatment. If you are found to have a sexually transmitted disease, you will be asked to inform any recent sexual partners so that they too may seek treatment. You should avoid sexual contact until treatment has cleared up your symptoms.

Disease	Incubation period*	Symptoms	Treatment
Gonorrhea	2 to 10 days	Discomfort when passing urine and perhaps a slight discharge of pus from the tip of the penis.	The physician will take a sample of the discharge from the infected urethra for laboratory examination. The usual treatment consists of *antibiotics*.
Nonspecific urethritis	1 to 5 weeks	A slight tingling at the base of the penis – sometimes only felt when urinating first thing in the morning. The tingling may be accompanied by a discharge.	The physician will take a sample of urethral discharge for laboratory examination. The usual treatment is a course of *antibiotics*.
Syphilis	9 to 90 days	In the first stage, a highly infectious, painless sore called a chancre develops on the penis (or in the anus if you have had anal intercourse). This disappears after a few weeks. In the second stage, a rash that does not itch appears all over the body, including the palms and soles. There may also be painless swelling of the lymph glands and infectious wart-like lumps around the anus and maybe the armpits.	The disease is diagnosed by blood tests and samples taken from any sores. The usual treatment is a course of *antibiotic* injections. You will need to have periodic blood tests for 1 to 2 years after treatment to ensure that the disease has not reappeared.
Herpes genitalis	7 days or less	There is usually an itching feeling on the shaft of the penis followed by the appearance of a crop of small, painful blisters. Sometimes these also appear on the thighs and buttocks. The blisters burst after 24 hours, leaving small, red, moist, painful ulcers, which sometimes form a hard crust. The glands in the groin may become enlarged and painful, accompanied by feeling sick and a raised temperature. Outbreaks of blisters are likely to recur.	There is no total cure for this disorder. Your physician may prescribe an *antiviral* drug or ointment to make the ulcers less sore and speed healing. You will be advised to avoid sexual contact while you have an attack so that you do not transmit the infection to your partner. It is not known if someone with herpes is capable of infecting others between attacks, since virus shedding may continue.
Pubic lice (crabs)	0 to 17 days	Many people have no symptoms while others experience itching in the pubic region, particularly at night. You may be able to see the lice; they are brown and about 1/16 in. long.	Your physician will give you a lotion that kills lice and their eggs. At the same time he or she will ensure that you do not have any other sexually transmitted disease.
Acquired immune deficiency syndrome (AIDS)	Varies greatly. May take many months or years to develop	AIDS affects the body's natural defense (immune) system so that it is unable to protect against infections or some cancers. Symptoms include frequent infections, constant feeling of tiredness, weight loss, swollen lymph glands, breathing difficulties, severe diarrhea, skin blotches and rashes.	Reported cases of AIDS have so far been fatal. Research into cures and an effective vaccine is continuing. To date only symptomatic treatment has been available (see p. 37).

*Time between contact with the disease and appearance of symptoms.

118 Erection difficulties

Most men fail to get an erection from time to time, despite feeling sexually aroused in other ways, due to any one of a number of reasons including physical factors, psychological factors or a combination of both. Some men can only get an erection while masturbating or during oral sex, but not when they are trying to have sexual intercourse. Others can get an erection with one woman, but fail to do so with another. Consult this chart if you have noticed problems with getting or maintaining an erection.

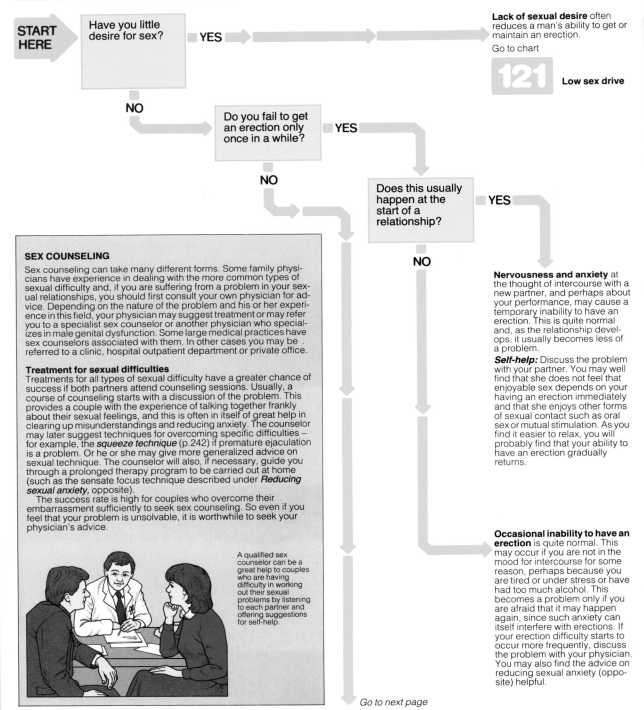

START HERE

Have you little desire for sex?

YES → **Lack of sexual desire** often reduces a man's ability to get or maintain an erection.

Go to chart

121 Low sex drive

NO

Do you fail to get an erection only once in a while?

YES →

NO

Does this usually happen at the start of a relationship?

YES →

NO

Nervousness and anxiety at the thought of intercourse with a new partner, and perhaps about your performance, may cause a temporary inability to have an erection. This is quite normal and, as the relationship develops, it usually becomes less of a problem.

Self-help: Discuss the problem with your partner. You may well find that she does not feel that enjoyable sex depends on your having an erection immediately and that she enjoys other forms of sexual contact such as oral sex or mutual stimulation. As you find it easier to relax, you will probably find that your ability to have an erection gradually returns.

SEX COUNSELING

Sex counseling can take many different forms. Some family physicians have experience in dealing with the more common types of sexual difficulty and, if you are suffering from a problem in your sexual relationships, you should first consult your own physician for advice. Depending on the nature of the problem and his or her experience in this field, your physician may suggest treatment or may refer you to a specialist sex counselor or another physician who specializes in male genital dysfunction. Some large medical practices have sex counselors associated with them. In other cases you may be referred to a clinic, hospital outpatient department or private office.

Treatment for sexual difficulties

Treatments for all types of sexual difficulty have a greater chance of success if both partners attend counseling sessions. Usually, a course of counseling starts with a discussion of the problem. This provides a couple with the experience of talking together frankly about their sexual feelings, and this is often in itself of great help in clearing up misunderstandings and reducing anxiety. The counselor may later suggest techniques for overcoming specific difficulties – for example, the *squeeze technique* (p.242) if premature ejaculation is a problem. Or he or she may give more generalized advice on sexual technique. The counselor will also, if necessary, guide you through a prolonged therapy program to be carried out at home (such as the sensate focus technique described under *Reducing sexual anxiety*, opposite).

The success rate is high for couples who overcome their embarrassment sufficiently to seek sex counseling. So even if you feel that your problem is unsolvable, it is worthwhile to seek your physician's advice.

A qualified sex counselor can be a great help to couples who are having difficulty in working out their sexual problems by listening to each partner and offering suggestions for self-help.

Occasional inability to have an erection is quite normal. This may occur if you are not in the mood for intercourse for some reason, perhaps because you are tired or under stress or have had too much alcohol. This becomes a problem only if you are afraid that it may happen again, since such anxiety can itself interfere with erections. If your erection difficulty starts to occur more frequently, discuss the problem with your physician. You may also find the advice on reducing sexual anxiety (opposite) helpful.

Go to next page

Continued from previous page

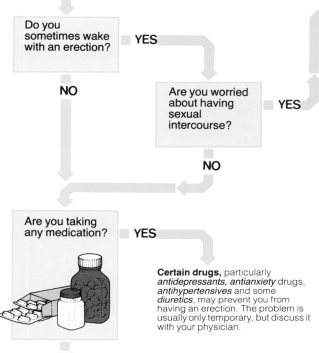

Do you sometimes wake with an erection?

YES → Are you worried about having sexual intercourse?

NO

Are you worried about having sexual intercourse? **YES**

NO

Are you taking any medication? **YES**

Certain drugs, particularly *antidepressants, antianxiety* drugs, *antihypertensives* and some *diuretics,* may prevent you from having an erection. The problem is usually only temporary, but discuss it with your physician.

NO

Consult your physician if you are unable to make a diagnosis from this chart.

If you sometimes wake with an erection, a physical cause for your impotence is highly unlikely. Anxiety is a fairly common cause of erection difficulties. Worry about premature ejaculation, making your partner pregnant or catching a sexually transmitted disease, for example, are all common causes of sexual anxiety. In the majority of cases it is only a temporary difficulty.

Self-help: Discuss your feelings with your partner. You may find that your partner's reassurances are sufficient to help you overcome your difficulty. Meanwhile, try other forms of sexual contact such as mutual stimulation or oral sex. An erection may follow when you begin to feel less anxious. Try also the advice given in *Reducing sexual anxiety* (below). If, after you have tried these measures, the problem persists so that it interferes with you and your partner's sexual enjoyment, consult your physician, who may recommend that you receive counseling (see *Sex counseling,* opposite).

REDUCING SEXUAL ANXIETY

Many sexual difficulties arise out of anxiety in one or both partners, and most forms of *sex counseling* (opposite) involve advice on reducing such anxiety as a basis for improving sexual enjoyment. Sensate focus is often successful in heightening sexual responsiveness without provoking anxiety about performance, and may help you overcome inhibitions and tensions that can mar sexual relationships. The first step is for both partners to agree to abstain from sexual intercourse for, say, 3 weeks.

Sensate focus
Set aside at least 3 evenings (or a period at another time of day) when you can be alone with your partner without fear of interruption for at least 2 hours. Try to create an atmosphere in which you both feel relaxed – playing some favorite music may help. During the time when you are trying this therapy you and your partner must stick to your agreement to refrain from full sexual intercourse.

Stage 1
On the first evening, each partner should take turns gently massaging and caressing the other for a period of about 20 minutes. This is best carried out when you are both naked, and you can use a body lotion or oil if you like. The massage should involve a gentle exploration of all parts of the body except the genital and breast areas. The partner being caressed should concentrate on finding pleasure from being touched, and the partner giving the caresses should concentrate on his or her own pleasure from contact with the partner's body. Once you have gotten over any awkwardness and are finding enjoyment from the sensations you experience during this activity – this may take several sessions – go to stage 2.

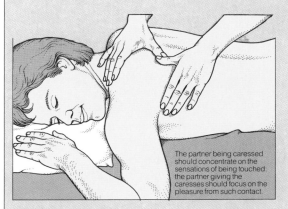

The partner being caressed should concentrate on the sensations of being touched; the partner giving the caresses should focus on the pleasure from such contact.

Stage 2
Stage 2 is similar to stage 1, but this time body massage may include genital and breast areas. Remember, however, to continue to include other parts of the body in your caresses so that direct sexual stimulation can be felt in context with other body sensations.

Stage 3
Most couples find that soon after reaching stage 2 they are ready to resume sexual intercourse, and in most cases they find that they are more relaxed and are more able to enjoy a full range of physical and emotional sexual feelings.

SEX IN LATER LIFE

The majority of men reach their physical sexual peak in their late teens or early twenties. During sexual intercourse they reach orgasm quickly, ejaculate powerfully and are able to have another erection soon after. As a man gets older it may take him longer to get an erection, which may not be as hard as in the past, and more stimulation may be necessary. Ejaculation may be delayed slightly (this can be beneficial for men who have previously suffered from premature ejaculation). The time it takes to develop another erection may be longer. However, there is usually no physical reason why a man should not continue to have an active and happy sex life well into old age.

Possible problems
The changes described above occur only gradually and often go unnoticed. For many men sexual activity becomes more enjoyable with increased experience and confidence. A reduction in the frequency of orgasm is often more than compensated for by the enhanced quality of the sexual experience.

However, some men become anxious about their sexual performance as they approach middle age. This usually occurs when anxiety or depression, possibly connected with other aspects of life – for example, lack of job satisfaction or concern about the future – leads them to compare their current sex life unfavorably with how it was 20 or 30 years before. Some men who have experienced sexual difficulties in the past use their advancing years as an excuse for avoiding sex altogether in later life. This is no cause for concern if both partners are happy not to have sex. But if a reduction in sexual activity causes unhappiness in either partner, it is never too late to seek *sex counseling* (opposite) for this or any other sex problem.

119 Premature ejaculation

There are occasions when men ejaculate before they wish to. This becomes a problem only if you consistently ejaculate so quickly that you and your partner become frustrated by the curtailment of sexual intercourse. The anxiety that often accompanies premature ejaculation tends to make the problem worse and may lead you to avoid sex. This may result in disharmony between you and your partner. However, the tendency to ejaculate prematurely can usually be overcome with time, patience and self-help.

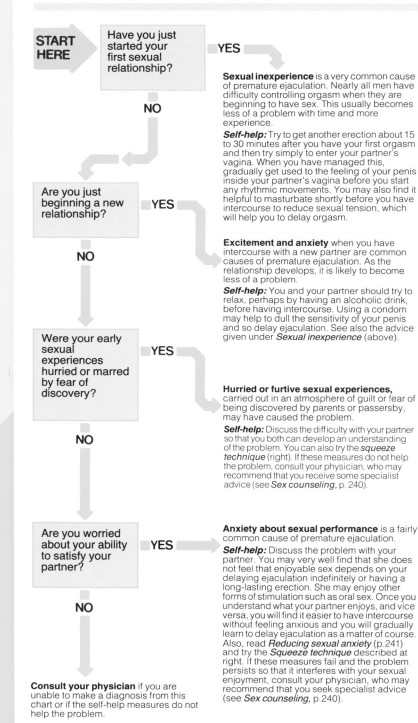

START HERE

Have you just started your first sexual relationship?

YES

Sexual inexperience is a very common cause of premature ejaculation. Nearly all men have difficulty controlling orgasm when they are beginning to have sex. This usually becomes less of a problem with time and more experience.

Self-help: Try to get another erection about 15 to 30 minutes after you have your first orgasm and then try simply to enter your partner's vagina. When you have managed this, gradually get used to the feeling of your penis inside your partner's vagina before you start any rhythmic movements. You may also find it helpful to masturbate shortly before you have intercourse to reduce sexual tension, which will help you to delay orgasm.

NO

Are you just beginning a new relationship?

YES

Excitement and anxiety when you have intercourse with a new partner are common causes of premature ejaculation. As the relationship develops, it is likely to become less of a problem.

Self-help: You and your partner should try to relax, perhaps by having an alcoholic drink, before having intercourse. Using a condom may help to dull the sensitivity of your penis and so delay ejaculation. See also the advice given under *Sexual inexperience* (above).

NO

Were your early sexual experiences hurried or marred by fear of discovery?

YES

Hurried or furtive sexual experiences, carried out in an atmosphere of guilt or fear of being discovered by parents or passersby, may have caused the problem.

Self-help: Discuss the difficulty with your partner so that you both can develop an understanding of the problem. You can also try the *squeeze technique* (right). If these measures do not help the problem, consult your physician, who may recommend that you receive some specialist advice (see *Sex counseling*, p. 240).

NO

Are you worried about your ability to satisfy your partner?

YES

Anxiety about sexual performance is a fairly common cause of premature ejaculation.

Self-help: Discuss the problem with your partner. You may very well find that she does not feel that enjoyable sex depends on your delaying ejaculation indefinitely or having a long-lasting erection. She may enjoy other forms of stimulation such as oral sex. Once you understand what your partner enjoys, and vice versa, you will find it easier to have intercourse without feeling anxious and you will gradually learn to delay ejaculation as a matter of course. Also, read *Reducing sexual anxiety* (p.241) and try the *Squeeze technique* described at right. If these measures fail and the problem persists so that it interferes with your sexual enjoyment, consult your physician, who may recommend that you seek specialist advice (see *Sex counseling*, p.240).

NO

Consult your physician if you are unable to make a diagnosis from this chart or if the self-help measures do not help the problem.

SQUEEZE TECHNIQUE

The squeeze technique is one of the most widely accepted methods for helping a man to delay and control orgasm. It teaches both partners to recognize the sensations that immediately precede ejaculation, so increasing control. Many couples find that it helps to try the technique of sensate focus (see *Reducing sexual anxiety*, p. 241) before undertaking the squeeze technique.

Stage 1
Adopt a position that is comfortable for both you and your partner. Many couples find the best position is one in which the woman sits with her back to the head of the bed, her legs spread out in front. The man lies facing her, with his body between her legs, his legs over hers. Your partner should then caress your penis to full erection and continue until you are close to orgasm. When you feel ready to ejaculate, signal to your partner, who then stops stimulating you and grips the penis firmly with her thumb and index finger just below the glans until your erection subsides. After about half a minute, she can start to stimulate your penis again. Repeat this 2 or 3 times before allowing yourself to ejaculate. With practice, your partner will begin to sense without a signal when you are near to orgasm. After a few sessions, when you both have gained confidence about controlling ejaculation, it is possible to move on to the next stage.

Gripping below the glans delays orgasm

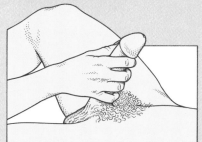

Stage 2
Lie on your back with your partner astride you and your erect penis inside her vagina. Practice holding this position without moving for as long as possible. If you feel you are about to ejaculate, signal to your partner. She then lifts herself away and applies the squeeze grip as before. Repeat this 2 or 3 times. If your erection begins to subside, stimulation of the penis will restore it so that it can be once again be inserted into your partner's vagina.

After a few sessions, when you feel control has improved, normal full intercouse can be attempted so that both partners can reach orgasm. You may find that positions in which your partner is on top allow you to control orgasm most easily. If at any time you feel ready to ejaculate before your partner is ready, she can use the squeeze technique.

120 Delayed ejaculation

Consult this chart if you are able to have a normal erection but are unable to ejaculate as soon as you would like, or if you have lost the ability to ejaculate altogether. There may be physical or emotional reasons for this type of difficulty. Whatever you suspect may be the cause of the problem, frank discussion with your partner is essential so that she can help you to overcome the difficulty.

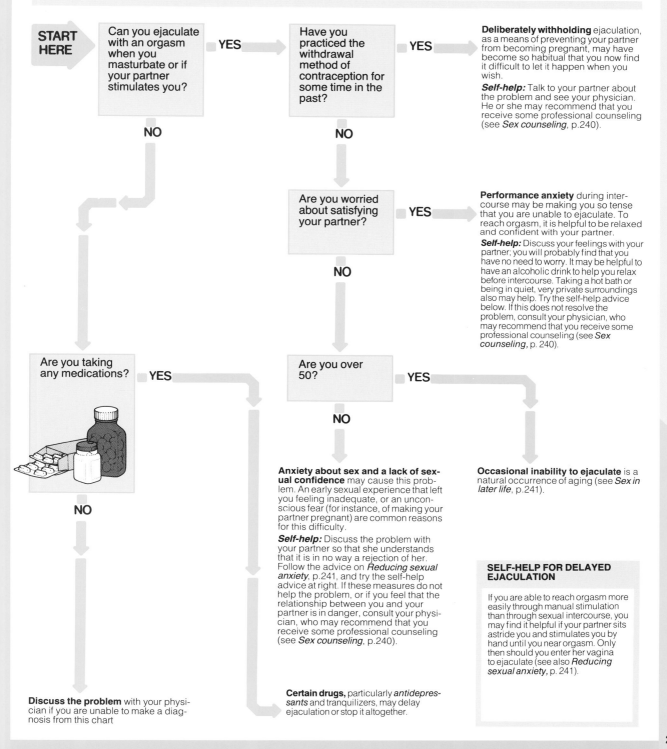

START HERE

Can you ejaculate with an orgasm when you masturbate or if your partner stimulates you? — YES →

Have you practiced the withdrawal method of contraception for some time in the past? — YES →

Deliberately withholding ejaculation, as a means of preventing your partner from becoming pregnant, may have become so habitual that you now find it difficult to let it happen when you wish.
Self-help: Talk to your partner about the problem and see your physician. He or she may recommend that you receive some professional counseling (see *Sex counseling*, p.240).

Are you worried about satisfying your partner? — YES →

Performance anxiety during intercourse may be making you so tense that you are unable to ejaculate. To reach orgasm, it is helpful to be relaxed and confident with your partner.
Self-help: Discuss your feelings with your partner; you will probably find that you have no need to worry. It may be helpful to have an alcoholic drink to help you relax before intercourse. Taking a hot bath or being in quiet, very private surroundings also may help. Try the self-help advice below. If this does not resolve the problem, consult your physician, who may recommend that you receive some professional counseling (see *Sex counseling*, p. 240).

Are you taking any medications? — YES →

Are you over 50? — YES →

Occasional inability to ejaculate is a natural occurrence of aging (see *Sex in later life*, p.241).

Anxiety about sex and a lack of sexual confidence may cause this problem. An early sexual experience that left you feeling inadequate, or an unconscious fear (for instance, of making your partner pregnant) are common reasons for this difficulty.
Self-help: Discuss the problem with your partner so that she understands that it is in no way a rejection of her. Follow the advice on *Reducing sexual anxiety*, p.241, and try the self-help advice at right. If these measures do not help the problem, or if you feel that the relationship between you and your partner is in danger, consult your physician, who may recommend that you receive some professional counseling (see *Sex counseling*, p.240).

SELF-HELP FOR DELAYED EJACULATION

If you are able to reach orgasm more easily through manual stimulation than through sexual intercourse, you may find it helpful if your partner sits astride you and stimulates you by hand until you near orgasm. Only then should you enter her vagina to ejaculate (see also *Reducing sexual anxiety,* p. 241).

Discuss the problem with your physician if you are unable to make a diagnosis from this chart

Certain drugs, particularly *antidepressants* and tranquilizers, may delay ejaculation or stop it altogether.

121 Low sex drive

Male sexual arousal is governed by both psychological factors and by the male sex hormone testosterone. If a man has a very low level of testosterone he is unlikely to have a great interest in sex and may find it difficult to become sexually aroused. However, most cases of reduced sex drive are the result of nonhormonal factors including physical illness, depression, stress, sexual difficulties, boredom, and discontent with a relationship.

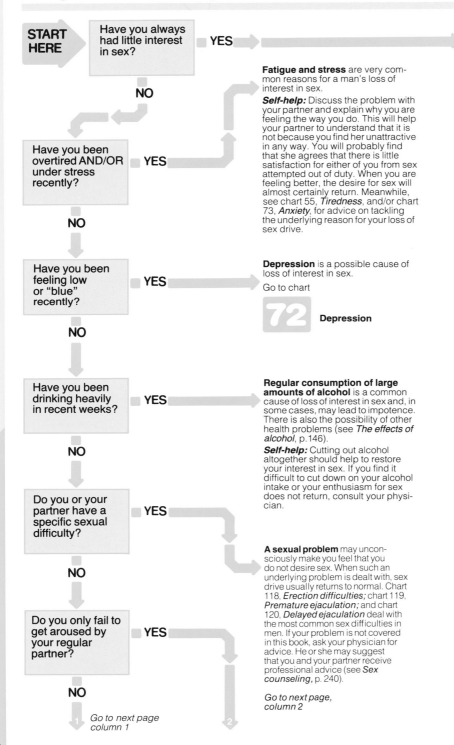

START HERE

Have you always had little interest in sex?

YES →

A naturally low level of interest in sex is a normal part of the personality of some men. This is unlikely to be a cause for concern if you and your partner are happy with your present level of sexual activity. However, if your low sex drive is causing difficulties within your relationship, consult your physician, who may recommend *Sex counseling* (p.240).

NO

Have you been overtired AND/OR under stress recently?

YES →

Fatigue and stress are very common reasons for a man's loss of interest in sex.

Self-help: Discuss the problem with your partner and explain why you are feeling the way you do. This will help your partner to understand that it is not because you find her unattractive in any way. You will probably find that she agrees that there is little satisfaction for either of you from sex attempted out of duty. When you are feeling better, the desire for sex will almost certainly return. Meanwhile, see chart 55, *Tiredness*, and/or chart 73, *Anxiety*, for advice on tackling the underlying reason for your loss of sex drive.

NO

Have you been feeling low or "blue" recently?

YES →

Depression is a possible cause of loss of interest in sex.

Go to chart

72 Depression

NO

Have you been drinking heavily in recent weeks?

YES →

Regular consumption of large amounts of alcohol is a common cause of loss of interest in sex and, in some cases, may lead to impotence. There is also the possibility of other health problems (see *The effects of alcohol*, p.146).

Self-help: Cutting out alcohol altogether should help to restore your interest in sex. If you find it difficult to cut down on your alcohol intake or your enthusiasm for sex does not return, consult your physician.

NO

Do you or your partner have a specific sexual difficulty?

YES →

A sexual problem may unconsciously make you feel that you do not desire sex. When such an underlying problem is dealt with, sex drive usually returns to normal. Chart 118, *Erection difficulties;* chart 119, *Premature ejaculation;* and chart 120, *Delayed ejaculation* deal with the most common sex difficulties in men. If your problem is not covered in this book, ask your physician for advice. He or she may suggest that you and your partner receive professional advice (see *Sex counseling*, p. 240).

NO

Do you only fail to get aroused by your regular partner?

YES →

Go to next page, column 2

NO

Go to next page column 1

SEXUAL ORIENTATION

Sexual orientation – that is, whether you are heterosexual (attracted to people of the opposite sex), homosexual (attracted to people of the same sex) or bisexual (attracted to people of both sexes) is probably determined by a combination of inborn personality traits, upbringing, and family relationships. Some researchers have suggested that there may be hormonal factors that contribute to determining sexual orientation, but these findings have not been generally accepted. Few people are wholly heterosexual or homosexual. In particular, it is common for adolescents to go through a phase of experiencing homosexual feelings before becoming attracted to people of the opposite sex. Some people, however, remain homosexual in their sexual preferences.

Homosexuality

This variation from the mainly heterosexual orientation of the majority is no cause for medical concern among most physicians as long as the individual is happy with his homosexuality. Treatment to change sexual orientation is unlikely to be effective and is seldom recommended unless the individual is determined to make the attempt and has at least some interest in the opposite sex. However, society's attitude toward homosexuality frequently causes homosexuals to feel guilty and abnormal, and therefore leads them to repress their sexual feelings. This can be psychologically damaging. If you think that you are homosexual and are experiencing such problems, consult your physician, who may be able to offer helpful advice and/or refer you for counseling to one of the organizations that specializes in advising homosexuals.

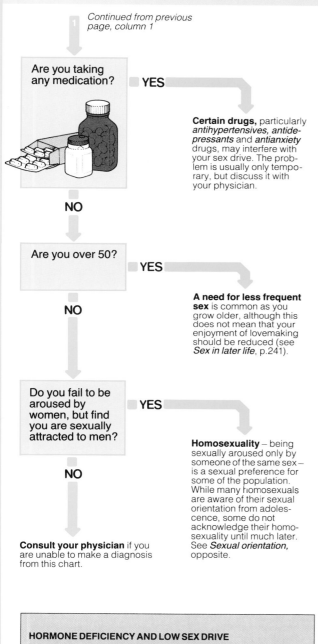

Continued from previous page, column 1

Are you taking any medication? YES

Certain drugs, particularly *antihypertensives, antidepressants* and *antianxiety* drugs, may interfere with your sex drive. The problem is usually only temporary, but discuss it with your physician.

NO

Are you over 50? YES

A need for less frequent sex is common as you grow older, although this does not mean that your enjoyment of lovemaking should be reduced (see *Sex in later life*, p.241).

NO

Do you fail to be aroused by women, but find you are sexually attracted to men? YES

Homosexuality – being sexually aroused only by someone of the same sex – is a sexual preference for some of the population. While many homosexuals are aware of their sexual orientation from adolescence, some do not acknowledge their homosexuality until much later. See *Sexual orientation,* opposite.

NO

Consult your physician if you are unable to make a diagnosis from this chart.

Continued from previous page, column 2

Do you have any other cause for discontent in your relationship? YES

NO

Loss of interest in a sexual relationship once the excitement and novelty have worn off is a common cause of loss of sexual desire.

Self-help: It may help to talk openly with your partner about how you feel so that there is no misunderstanding of the situation. If the relationship is a long-standing one, and sound in every other way, try to inject new life into it (for example, by going away for a weekend together or cooperating in some new venture). You may find trying new approaches to lovemaking helpful. If these measures do not help, consult your physician, who may suggest that you and your partner receive some professional advice (see *Sex counseling*, p.240).

Generalized antagonism or specific disagreements can lead to tension in a relationship that also affects your sexual feelings for each other. There may also be some lack of communication so that you do not fully understand each other's feelings and attitudes toward sex and other matters. This may produce conflict and damage your sexual relationship.

Self-help: Talk to your partner and explain how the problems with your relationship are affecting your feelings. If you find that things do not improve after full and frank discussion, consult your physician, who will examine you to find out if there is an underlying physical problem. If there is no physical disorder, he or she may suggest that you and your partner seek professional guidance about your general difficulties and possibly *sex counseling* (p. 240) for any specific problem you may have.

HORMONE DEFICIENCY AND LOW SEX DRIVE

In rare cases, low sex drive may be a symptom of a deficiency of the male sex hormone testosterone. This type of hormone deficiency often causes additional symptoms such as loss of body hair and unusually small testicles. If your lack of interest in sex is accompanied by such additional symptoms, consult your physician.

Treatment

If tests confirm the diagnosis, hormone treatment will be prescribed and is usually successful in increasing sex drive and reversing such physical changes. Loss of sex drive that is not accompanied by the physical symptoms described here is not likely to be caused by lack of testosterone, and hormone supplements will have no beneficial effect.

MEDICAL PROBLEMS ASSOCIATED WITH HOMOSEXUALITY

While homosexual activity is not in itself a danger to physical or mental health, some diseases seem to be particularly prevalent among male homosexuals. These include hepatitis (liver infection) and all the sexually transmitted diseases, but especially syphilis and AIDS (acquired immune deficiency syndrome). (See also, *Sexually transmitted diseases*, p.239).

These diseases were initially more common among sexually active homosexuals with many different sexual contacts. Homosexual men who have sexual partners outside a long-term monogamous relationship are advised to follow the advice given under *Multiple sex partners*, p.271 and to be especially vigilant for the following symptoms:

- unexplained tiredness
- yellowing of the skin
- unexplained rashes or sores
- abnormally frequent and persistent respiratory and/or digestive-tract infections (diarrhea)
- persistent swelling of the glands

If you notice any of the above symptoms, consult your physician without delay. It is advisable to avoid sexual contact until the cause of the symptoms has been diagnosed and treated.

122 Fertility problems

Consult this chart if you and your partner have had sexual intercourse for more than 12 months without contraception and without your partner having become pregnant. Failure to conceive may be the result of a problem affecting the man or the woman (or both). Male infertility is nearly always the result of insufficient production of sperm or blockage of the passage of sperm during ejaculation. This may be caused by a temporary malfunction of the sperm-producing glands or by a long-term condition.

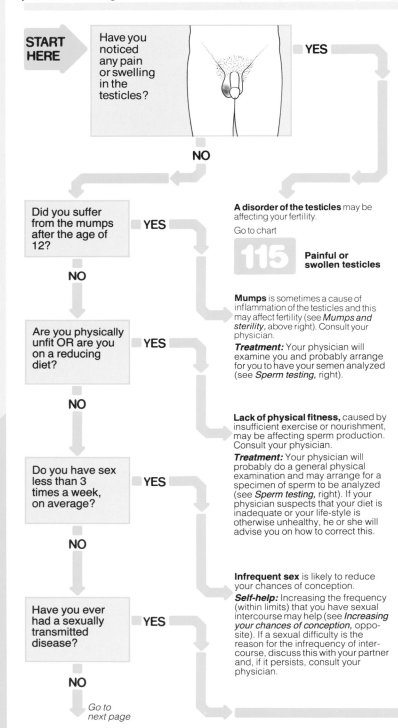

START HERE Have you noticed any pain or swelling in the testicles?

YES → **A disorder of the testicles** may be affecting your fertility.

Go to chart

115 Painful or swollen testicles

NO

Did you suffer from the mumps after the age of 12? — YES

Mumps is sometimes a cause of inflammation of the testicles and this may affect fertility (see *Mumps and sterility,* above right). Consult your physician.

Treatment: Your physician will examine you and probably arrange for you to have your semen analyzed (see *Sperm testing,* right).

NO

Are you physically unfit OR are you on a reducing diet? — YES

Lack of physical fitness, caused by insufficient exercise or nourishment, may be affecting sperm production. Consult your physician.

Treatment: Your physician will probably do a general physical examination and may arrange for a specimen of sperm to be analyzed (see *Sperm testing,* right). If your physician suspects that your diet is inadequate or your life-style is otherwise unhealthy, he or she will advise you on how to correct this.

NO

Do you have sex less than 3 times a week, on average? — YES

Infrequent sex is likely to reduce your chances of conception.

Self-help: Increasing the frequency (within limits) that you have sexual intercourse may help (see *Increasing your chances of conception,* opposite). If a sexual difficulty is the reason for the infrequency of intercourse, discuss this with your partner and, if it persists, consult your physician.

NO

Have you ever had a sexually transmitted disease? — YES

NO

Go to next page

MUMPS AND STERILITY

If you suffered from mumps after the age of 12 and you can remember that you had painful and/or swollen testicles at the time, there is a possibility that the disease has interfered with your ability to produce normal sperm. Your physician will arrange for you to have a sperm count (see *Sperm testing,* below) and will offer you advice.

SPERM TESTING

A sperm count is the standard test for male fertility – that is, whether or not a man has a chance of successfully conceiving. For this test you will be asked to ejaculate into a container. For 2 days prior to the test you will need to refrain from ejaculating so that the number of sperm in the semen is at its highest level. From this sample the number of active, healthy sperm can be assessed.

A count of 100 million sperm per cubic centimeter of semen makes conception likely, providing that your partner is fertile. If a count of 200 million sperm per cubic centimeter is recorded, with 40 percent of them being active and the remainder being of normal shape, then conception is still possible. A "normal" sperm count (with good motility and shape) is considered to begin at about 50 million sperm per cubic centimeter. Because the sperm count varies greatly from day to day, a man found to have a low sperm count may need to have another test to confirm whether or not the result of the low count was a temporary fluctuation in sperm production.

Shape of a sperm

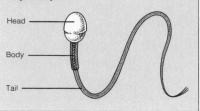

Head
Body
Tail

Sexually transmitted diseases (see p.239) may sometimes cause infertility in both men and women. Consult your physician.

Treatment: If you currently have symptoms, your physician will examine you and take a sample from your blood or urethra. This will be analyzed and, if a sexually transmitted disease is diagnosed, you will probably be given *antibiotics.* If you have had such a disease in the past, tests on sperm (see *Sperm testing,* above) will determine whether or not it has affected your fertility.

Continued from previous page

Are you being treated for any long-term illness?

▶ **YES** ▶ **Certain illnesses** and the drugs used in their treatment may make it difficult for you to father a child. Liver and hormone disorders are particularly likely to have this effect. Discuss the problem with your physician.

NO ▼

Do you wear underpants that are tight-fitting or made of an artificial fiber or do you use saunas or steam baths frequently?

▶ **YES** ▶ **An increased temperature** within the scrotum may be making you less fertile. If the testicles and the sperm they contain are not cooler than normal body temperature, fertility may be reduced (see *Sperm production*, below).

Self-help: Your chances of conception may be improved if you wear loose-fitting underpants made of a natural fiber such as cotton. This material allows air to circulate more freely so that the temperature around your testicles does not get too high. Since there is some evidence that men who use saunas or steam baths often have decreased sperm production due to high temperatures, it might be worthwhile to discontinue use of any saunas or steam baths for a while.

NO ▼

Consult your physician if you are unable to make a diagnosis from this chart.

INCREASING YOUR CHANCES OF CONCEPTION

Although prolonged delay in achieving conception requires professional tests and treatment, you may be able to increase your chances of conception by following the self-help advice given below:

■ Try to ensure that both you and your partner are in good health; eat plenty of fresh, vitamin-rich foods, get plenty of rest, and keep alcohol consumption to a minimum.

■ Have intercourse about 3 times a week; less frequent intercourse may mean that you miss your partner's fertile days, more frequent intercourse may reduce the number of sperm you ejaculate.

■ Try to time intercourse to coincide with your partner's most fertile days (usually midway between menstrual periods).

■ Avoid wearing tight-fitting underpants or those made of artificial fibers, which may damage the sperm by increasing the temperature in the scrotum.

SPERM PRODUCTION

Inside the scrotum (the baggy pouch resting beneath the penis) are the two testicles. Sperm cells are formed in the tiny tubes inside each testicle at the rate of 10 to 30 billion each month. Behind each testicle is a coiled tube called the epididymis. Sperm mature here over a period of 2 to 4 weeks before they are transferred to the seminal vesicles for storage. When you have an orgasm, the sperm pass into the urethra and are then ejaculated in the seminal fluid. Sperm is only a small part of this seminal fluid. On the average, 60 percent of the fluid is produced in the seminal vesicles and 38 percent is produced in the prostate gland. The remaining 2 percent, although nearly all water, contains between 150 and 400 million sperm.

Sperm production is most effective at 6°F (3 to 4°C) below normal body temperature. This is why the testicles are suspended outside the body in the scrotum. A high temperature prevents new sperm from forming and may kill those already in storage. The effect of this is usually only temporary infertility. Very low temperatures also prevent sperm from forming, but this does not damage those already in storage. Under normal conditions, sperm production is continuous, although there may be seasonal variations — sperm concentration seems to be lower in the warm summer months. Severe illness of any kind may temporarily suspend semen production for days or months (for example, in the case of severe infection).

Passage of sperm

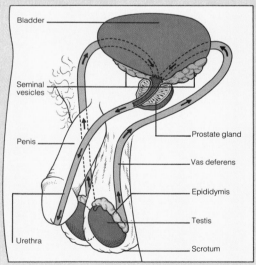

- Bladder
- Seminal vesicles
- Penis
- Urethra
- Prostate gland
- Vas deferens
- Epididymis
- Testis
- Scrotum

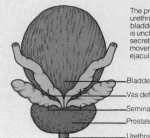

The prostate gland (left) surrounds the urethra at the point where it leaves the bladder. The exact function of the gland is unclear, but it is thought that the secretions it produces stimulate the movement of sperm (right) after ejaculation.

- Bladder
- Vas deferens
- Seminal vesicles
- Prostate gland
- Urethra

Where sperm form and mature

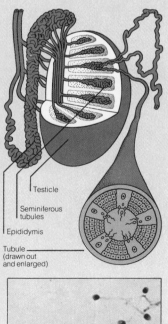

- Testicle
- Seminiferous tubules
- Epididymis
- Tubule (drawn out and enlarged)

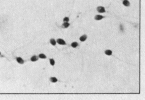

123 Contraception

The complex process by which sperm are produced makes it very difficult for an effective male contraceptive to be developed. It is hard to interfere with the production and development of sperm without affecting male sex drive or reducing the volume of semen ejaculated. Various drugs are being investigated to find a method of reducing sperm count without altering sexual desire or performance, but it will be some time before they can be guaranteed to be safe and effective. Until such a contraceptive has been tried and tested, it is up to you, after reading this chart and discussing contraception with your partner, to decide which is the best method for you or your partner to use (see *Choosing a contraceptive method,* p. 271). The two methods currently available to you if you wish to take sole responsibility are the condom and the vasectomy.

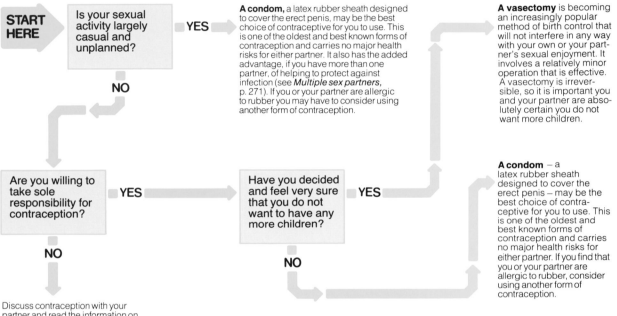

START HERE

Is your sexual activity largely casual and unplanned?

YES → **A condom,** a latex rubber sheath designed to cover the erect penis, may be the best choice of contraceptive for you to use. This is one of the oldest and best known forms of contraception and carries no major health risks for either partner. It also has the added advantage, if you have more than one partner, of helping to protect against infection (see *Multiple sex partners,* p. 271). If you or your partner are allergic to rubber you may have to consider using another form of contraception.

NO

Are you willing to take sole responsibility for contraception?

YES → **Have you decided and feel very sure that you do not want to have any more children?**

YES → **A vasectomy** is becoming an increasingly popular method of birth control that will not interfere in any way with your own or your partner's sexual enjoyment. It involves a relatively minor operation that is effective. A vasectomy is irreversible, so it is important you and your partner are absolutely certain you do not want more children.

NO → **A condom** – a latex rubber sheath designed to cover the erect penis – may be the best choice of contraceptive for you to use. This is one of the oldest and best known forms of contraception and carries no major health risks for either partner. If you find that you or your partner are allergic to rubber, consider using another form of contraception.

NO → Discuss contraception with your partner and read the information on *Choosing a contraceptive method,* p. 271.

VASECTOMY

Who should consider it

It is important to discuss the implications of a vasectomy with your partner. A vasectomy is usually a permanent form of contraception. Therefore, you and your partner need to be absolutely certain that you will not want to have any more children.

Remember that your present circumstances may change in the future. You may divorce and remarry and want to start a family. You may lose the children you already have. Or you may simply decide that you are no longer prepared to live without children. Couples under 30 years of age are usually discouraged from undertaking any form of sterilization. Your physician may suggest that you receive some professional counseling before you make a final decision.

The operation

A vasectomy is a straightforward operation that involves closing off the vas deferens so that sperm are no longer present in the semen. A vasectomy does not interfere with sperm production; sperm continue to be made and still travel along the vas deferens as far as they can but, because they cannot be ejaculated, they eventually dissolve and are absorbed into the system (see *Sperm production,* p. 247). The operation does not affect sex drive or cause impotence. Ejaculation occurs normally because the blockage of the vas deferens does not affect the production of seminal fluid from the prostate gland. The only difference is that after the operation the seminal fluid contains no sperm (this can only be detected by the use of a microscope).

The operation is usually carried out with the help of a local anesthetic. Your pubic hair will be shaved and the surgeon will make two tiny cuts in the scrotum—one on each side, because you have two vas deferens, one for each testicle. Each vas deferens is then tied or clipped in two places and the surgeon snips the length between each knot or clip. You may feel slight discomfort in the groin, but this soon disappears. The whole operation lasts 15 to 25 minutes.

It is a safe procedure, but occasionally there is some bleeding within the scrotum, or a slight infection after the operation. If you notice any swelling in the scrotum in the days following a vasectomy, whether or not it is painful, consult your physician, who may refer you back to the hospital for treatment.

After the operation

A vasectomy does not make you sterile immediately. Sperm produced before the operation remain in the reproductive system beyond the break in the vas deferens until they are expelled by ejaculation over the course of the following months. In the meantime, you and your partner should use some alternative form of contraception until sperm counts (see *Sperm testing,* p. 246) taken during the next three months or so confirm that your seminal fluid is free of sperm.

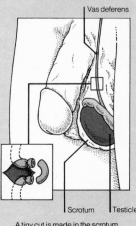

Vas deferens

Scrotum   Testicle

A tiny cut is made in the scrotum, and the vas deferens is tied in two places and snipped in between.

4 Special problems: women

Pregnancy and childbirth,

page 273

124 Breast problems

Each breast consists mainly of fatty tissue in which groups of milk-producing glands are embedded. The size and shape of each breast is determined by the amount of fatty tissue and the condition of the muscles and ligaments that support it. It is common for a woman to have one breast that is slightly larger than the other. Problems affecting the breasts may include pain, tenderness, changes in shape or general appearance (including that of the overlying skin) or the development of one or more lumps in the usually soft breast tissue. Although most breast problems are minor and easily treated, it is essential to watch for any changes (see *Breast self-examination,* below) and to report any change or obvious abnormality to your physician so that the possibility of breast cancer (one of the most common cancers affecting women) can be ruled out.

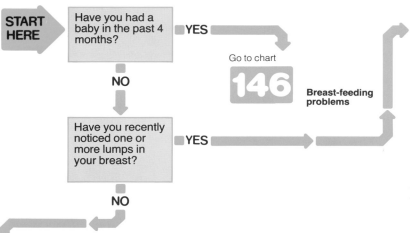

START HERE

Have you had a baby in the past 4 months?

YES → Go to chart **146** Breast-feeding problems

NO ↓

Have you recently noticed one or more lumps in your breast?

YES →

NO ↓

CONSULT YOUR PHYSICIAN WITHOUT DELAY!
Any lump in the breast should be examined by a physician to exclude the possibility of **breast cancer** (opposite), although it is much more likely that there is a less alarming cause for the lump(s), such as a harmless cyst or a thickening of the fibrous breast tissue (fibroadenosis).

Treatment: Your physician will examine you and, if he or she thinks that there is any cause for concern, will refer you for tests, such as those described under *Breast cancer* (opposite). If you are found to have a cyst, it will be examined by drawing off the fluid through a syringe (aspiration). Fibroadenosis often needs no treatment but, if it causes discomfort before periods, you may be offered treatment as described under *Premenstrual breast tenderness* (opposite). Treatments for breast cancer are described in the box opposite.

BREAST SELF-EXAMINATION

Every woman should make breast self-examination a part of her routine. It helps you to become familiar with the shape and feel of your breasts so that any changes will be quickly noticed and any problem dealt with promptly. Follow the routine described here monthly, ideally at the end of each period. Some physicians suggest the 5th day after the onset of the period.

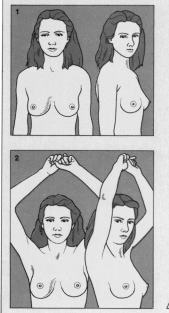

1 Stand in front of a good mirror with your arms by your sides and look at your breasts and nipples from the front and sides for any change in their shape or in the appearance of the skin.

2 Look again with your arms raised.

3 With the left arm still raised, feel all around the left breast using the flat of the fingers of the right hand. Repeat using the left hand to examine the right breast.

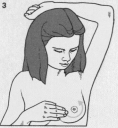

4 Lie down with a pillow under your left shoulder and with your left arm behind your head. Using the right hand as before, feel around the left breast, working from the outside toward the nipple at the center.

5 Check the area between the breast and the armpit and into the armpit itself, first with the left arm raised and then with it by your side.

6 Gently squeeze the nipple to check for any discharge.

Repeat 4, 5 and 6 using the left hand to examine the right breast.

When to consult your physician
If you notice any of the following during the course of your regular breast self-examination – or at any other time – consult your physician without delay:

- a lump in the breast or armpit.
- a change in the outline of the breast.
- discharge from the nipple.
- retraction (indentation) of the nipple.
- any change in the skin of the breast – for example, puckering or dimpling.

Remember, the first few times you examine yourself, you are still becoming familiar with your breasts and many of the lumps you find will be perfectly normal. However, if you are worried that you have found something abnormal, consult your physician.

Go to next page

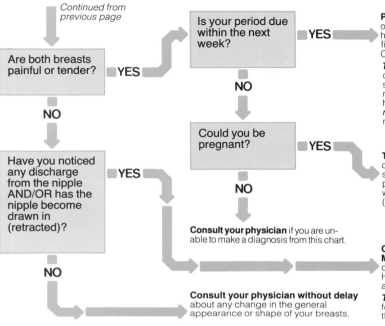

Continued from previous page

Are both breasts painful or tender? ▮ **YES** ▶

NO ↓

Have you noticed any discharge from the nipple AND/OR has the nipple become drawn in (retracted)? ▮ **YES** ▶

NO ↓

Is your period due within the next week? ▮ **YES** ▶

NO ↓

Could you be pregnant? ▮ **YES** ▶

NO ↓

Consult your physician if you are unable to make a diagnosis from this chart.

Consult your physician without delay about any change in the general appearance or shape of your breasts.

Premenstrual breast tenderness is a common occurrence, and is most likely to affect women who have naturally lumpy breasts – a condition known as fibroadenosis (see also *The menstrual cycle*, p.253). Consult your physician.

Treatment: Your physician will examine you. If he or she confirms the diagnosis, depending on the severity of your symptoms and whether you suffer from other unpleasant menstrual symptoms such as irritability or fluid retention, hormone treatment may be suggested (see *Treatment of menstrual problems*, p. 255). Wearing a firm-support bra may also help reduce discomfort.

Tenderness of the breasts and nipples is often one of the earliest signs of pregnancy and may continue for several months while your breasts prepare themselves to produce milk. If discomfort is severe, or you are not sure whether or not you are pregnant, consult your physician (see also *Diagnosis of pregnancy*, p. 252).

CONSULT YOUR PHYSICIAN WITHOUT DELAY!
Most nipple discharges are due to a glandular disorder, a breast infection or a benign growth. However, some may be a sign of *breast cancer* (below) and should be brought to your physician's attention.

Treatment: If your physician thinks there is any cause for concern, he or she will arrange for you to undergo the tests described below.

BREAST CANCER

Breast cancer is the most common cancer affecting women; about 1 woman in 9 develops the disease. It occurs when abnormal (cancerous) cells develop and multiply in the breast, forming a tumor. If untreated, the cancer may spread to other parts of the body. There are several different types of breast cancer; the outlook for anyone affected by the disease depends on the type of cancer present in her case, as well as on how early treatment is started.

Risk factors
Several factors are known to increase the risk of cancer of the breast. The following women may have a higher risk:

- Women who have no children, or who had their first child late in life.
- Women who are overweight.
- Women with close relatives who have had the disease.
- Women who started their periods early.

Screening
Most of the risk factors for developing breast cancer are outside your control, but you can try to ensure that the disease is diagnosed early by regular screening for the disease. The basic form of screening that every adult woman should undertake is monthly breast self-examination (opposite). However, women in high-risk groups may also be advised to undergo regular mammography (below). Even women who are not in high-risk groups are wise to be screened with mammography by age 40. The recommended guidelines are: By 40 years old, at least once; 40 to 50, every 2 years; and over 50 years, once a year.

Symptoms
The most common sign of breast cancer is the appearance of a painless lump in the breast or armpit. However, any of the symptoms listed in the box on *Breast self-examination* (opposite) could indicate cancer.

Confirming the diagnosis
If you notice any change in your breast, you should consult your physician without delay.

Mammography: A low-radiation X ray of the breast.
Aspiration: Used when a cyst is suspected. A fine needle is inserted into the lump to draw off a sample of fluid for examination.
Needle biopsy: A thick needle is inserted into the breast and a sample of tissue is removed for microscopic examination.
Frozen-section biopsy: Carried out under general anesthetic. An incision is made in the breast and all or part of the lump is removed and a section of the lump is frozen and examined under a microscope (see *Breast surgery*, right).

Treatment
Any woman undergoing tests for breast cancer should be aware of all the treatment options for the disease and discuss these fully with her physician. The best treatment will depend on the nature of the cancer and the stage at which it is discovered, but the final choice is a joint decision between the woman and her physician. The main forms of treatment are listed below:

Breast surgery

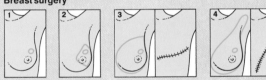

1 Lumpectomy: Removal of the growth alone.
2 Partial mastectomy: Removal of the growth and some of the surrounding breast tissue.
3 Simple mastectomy: Removal of the growth together with the whole breast.
4 Radical mastectomy: Removal of the growth, the breast, the underlying tissue and muscle and the nearby lymph nodes in the armpit.

5 Subcutaneous mastectomy: Occasionally, partial or simple mastectomies may be carried out leaving the overlying skin. Later, reconstructive surgery can be done to restore breast appearance.

Radiotherapy
This may be used on its own or in conjunction with other treatments. The breast and armpit are exposed to radiation to kill cancer cells.

Chemotherapy
Chemotherapy – treatment with anticancer drugs that inhibit multiplication of cancer cells – may be the only treatment used or it may be used with breast surgery and/or radiotherapy. Other drugs, including some that affect hormone activity, may also be given. Some forms of chemotherapy can produce feelings of nausea, reduce the blood count, or cause hair loss as side effects.

After breast surgery
Any woman who loses a breast as a result of breast cancer is naturally upset and worried that it may affect her appearance and femininity. Physicians who treat breast cancer will ensure that as much breast tissue is preserved as possible and may arrange for an implant to preserve breast shape. After a mastectomy you will be advised on the types of artificial breasts that are available. These are undetectable under most types of clothing. Many hospitals have counselors with whom you can discuss your feelings and who will advise about problems before and after breast surgery. Outside support groups also exist for these purposes.

125 Absent periods

Menstrual periods normally start between the ages of 11 and 14. However, for some girls it is normal to start menstruating as early as 10 or as late as 17. Once periods start they may be irregular for the first few years and may not settle down to a regular monthly cycle until the late teens. Once the menstrual cycle is established, it may vary in length from woman to woman from as little as 24 days to about 35 days between periods. Both extremes are normal. Absence of periods (amenorrhea) may occur in healthy women for a variety of reasons, the most common of which is pregnancy. Other factors that may affect your monthly cycle include illness and stress. Strenuous physical activity also may be associated with amenorrhea. Only rarely is absence of periods a sign of an underlying disorder. It is normal for periods to cease permanently as you approach middle age. Consult this chart if you have never had a period or if your period is more than 2 weeks late.

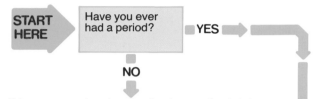

START HERE → Have you ever had a period? ■ **YES** →

NO ↓

Primary amenorrhea describes the absence of periods in a woman or girl who has never started to menstruate. If you are over 16, discuss your absence of periods with your physician.

Treatment: After a physical examination, your physician may arrange for you to undergo tests to uncover the cause. If you want to become pregnant, it is sometimes possible to start menstruation by hormone treatment (see chart 137, *Failure to conceive*).

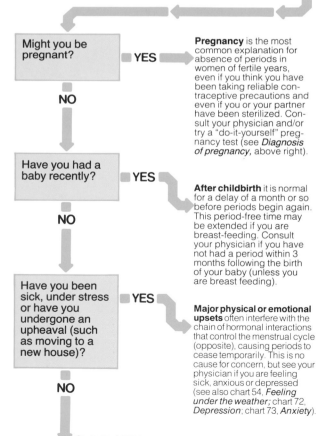

Might you be pregnant? ■ **YES**

Pregnancy is the most common explanation for absence of periods in women of fertile years, even if you think you have been taking reliable contraceptive precautions and even if you or your partner have been sterilized. Consult your physician and/or try a "do-it-yourself" pregnancy test (see *Diagnosis of pregnancy*, above right).

NO ↓

Have you had a baby recently? ■ **YES**

After childbirth it is normal for a delay of a month or so before periods begin again. This period-free time may be extended if you are breast-feeding. Consult your physician if you have not had a period within 3 months following the birth of your baby (unless you are breast feeding).

NO ↓

Have you been sick, under stress or have you undergone an upheaval (such as moving to a new house)? ■ **YES**

Major physical or emotional upsets often interfere with the chain of hormonal interactions that control the menstrual cycle (opposite), causing periods to cease temporarily. This is no cause for concern, but see your physician if you are feeling sick, anxious or depressed (see also chart 54, *Feeling under the weather;* chart 72, *Depression*; chart 73, *Anxiety*).

NO ↓

Go to next page

DIAGNOSIS OF PREGNANCY

For most women, the first indication of pregnancy is missing a menstrual period. However, you may also notice:

- tenderness of the breasts or nipples
- increased frequency of urination
- unusual tiredness
- nausea and/or vomiting

Pregnancy testing

If you think that you may be pregnant, you can either go to your physician (or family planning clinic) for a pregnancy test or try one of the "do-it-yourself" pregnancy testing kits. If you go to your physician, you are likely to be asked for a sample of the first urine you pass in the morning or a blood sample. This will be sent for tests that reveal the presence of certain hormones that occur only during pregnancy. Do-it-yourself pregnancy tests usually work in the same way. Tubal pregnancies can be dangerous and they may not register on a urine pregnancy test.

THE MENOPAUSE

The menopause is signaled by the end of menstrual periods and marks the time when a woman ceases to be fertile. The years surrounding this event are often referred to as the climacteric. The menopause usually occurs around the age of 50 but can happen earlier or later. In general, you can consider that you have reached the menopause if you are over 45 years old and you have not had a period for 6 months. Hormonal fluctuations before and after the menopause often (but not always) give rise to a variety of physical and emotional symptoms. Emotional difficulties may be complicated by social factors that necessitate psychological adjustments as you approach middle age.

Principal symptoms of the menopause

The most common menopausal symptoms are listed below. These normally disappear within a year or so of the cessation of periods.

- irregularity and eventual cessation of periods
- hot flashes (attacks of increased heat and sweating)
- night sweats
- dryness of the vagina as a result of thinning of the vaginal secretions (which may make intercourse uncomfortable)
- emotional upset, including depression and irritability

Treatment for menopausal symptoms

If your symptoms cause you no distress, you probably don't need medical treatment. However, much can be done to alleviate symptoms if they are uncomfortable or embarrassing.

Hormone-replacement therapy

Supplements of estrogen and progesterone may be prescribed for women who are suffering from menopausal symptoms. However, because of the increased risk of blood clots, heart attacks and strokes, such treatment is not suitable for all women. For this reason, your physician may also be unwilling to continue hormone treatment for more than a few years.

Other treatments

Hormone cream or lubricating jelly (for vaginal dryness), *antidepressants* or *antianxiety* drugs (for psychological symptoms) and nonhormonal drugs (to control hot flashes) may also be prescribed in addition to or as an alternative to *hormone*-replacement therapy.

Continued from previous page

Are you underweight according to the chart on p. 303 AND/OR have you recently lost more than 9 lb (4 kg) in weight?

YES →

NO ↓

Have you recently undertaken a rigorous program of exercise?

YES →

Loss of weight or regular strenuous exercise often results in cessation of periods. In these circumstances, absence of periods is not in itself a cause for concern, but it is advisable to discuss the problem with your physician so that he or she can check your general health.

See also chart

56

Loss of weight

NO ↓

Have you recently stopped taking the birth-control pill?

YES →

Re-adjustment of your hormone balance after stopping the birth-control pill may take a month or so. Consult your physician if normal menstruation has not started again after 3 months.

NO ↓

Are you over 40 years old?

YES →

Irregular periods are normal in the years preceding the menopause (opposite). Most women find that periods become increasingly infrequent until they stop altogether. Occasionally, periods continue normally until they suddenly cease. Remember that while you continue to have periods you are probably still fertile. So, if you are sexually active and have missed a period, you should also consider the possibility of pregnancy. You may want to keep a record of your periods to discuss during your medical visits to see if your pattern seems normal for your age.

NO ↓

Consult your physician if you are unable to make a diagnosis from this chart.

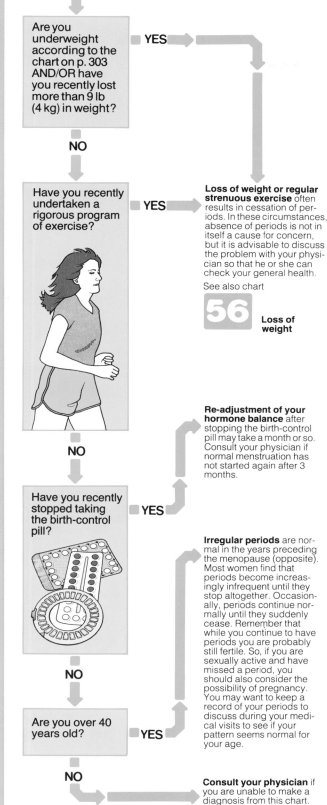

THE MENSTRUAL CYCLE

The menstrual cycle refers to the hormonal interactions that occur approximately every month in women during their childbearing years. This chain of events enables an egg to be released and, if it is fertilized, ensures that the uterus provides a suitable environment for the egg to implant and for the fetus to develop. The most noticeable outward sign of the menstrual cycle is vaginal bleeding – menstruation – during which the lining of the uterus is shed when the previous month's egg is not fertilized. However, many more body changes also take place during the course of the cycle.

A typical cycle
The typical menstrual cycle takes about 28 days, although this varies. The first day of menstrual bleeding is counted as day 1.

Days 1 to 4
Falling levels of the hormone progesterone in the body trigger the start of menstruation – the shedding of the lining of the uterus. During this time, hormones produced in the pituitary gland, prompted by signals from the hypothalamus (part of the brain), stimulate the ripening of an egg in the ovary, which in turn produces increasing levels of another hormone, estrogen.

Days 5 to 14
Menstrual bleeding normally ceases by day 5. For the next few days you may notice a slight vaginal discharge of mucus from the cervix. Between days 9 and 13, estrogen levels reach their peak and the cervical mucus becomes clear and runny. This is the start of the potentially fertile period. On day 13 the levels of the pituitary hormones that stimulate the ripening and release of the egg also reach a peak, temperature rises by about 1°F (½°C), and ovulation takes place on day 14, or approximately 2 weeks before the next menstrual period.

Days 15 to 23
Following ovulation, and if the egg is not fertilized, estrogen levels drop markedly, and the follicle from which the egg has been released forms into a gland called the corpus luteum, which secretes progesterone. On days 15 to 16 you may notice thick, jelly-like cervical mucus, after which there is likely to be little if any mucus for the remainder of the cycle, or the mucus will be pasty rather than jelly-like.

Days 24 to 28
The activity of the corpus luteum begins to decline as the gland degenerates, and progesterone levels begin to fall. Some women may begin to notice premenstrual symptoms such as breast tenderness and mood changes – especially irritability and depression. There may be slight bloating due to fluid retention. The onset of menstruation may be signaled by a drop in temperature of about 1°F (½°C).

Sequence of events

Temperature falls about 1°F

Day of cycle

Temperature rises about 1°F

Vaginal discharge

Hormonal activity

Temperature

General symptoms

Bleeding

Dry or cloudy discharge

Dry days

High progesterone

High estrogen

Clear, thin mucus

Thick mucus

Breast tenderness/lumpiness, mood changes

Ovulation

126 Heavy periods

Heavy periods, a condition sometimes called menorrhagia, are periods in which more than the average amount of blood is lost. Some women naturally lose more blood than others, but for most women bleeding lasts about 5 days, with the heaviest blood loss occurring in the first 3 days. Consult this chart if your periods last longer than this, if normal sanitary napkins or tampons are not sufficient, or if your periods suddenly become heavier than you are used to. Various disorders or devices may cause unusually heavy periods, including disorders of the lining of the uterus and the use of intrauterine contraceptive devices (IUDs). However, whichever reason you suspect for your heavy periods, consult your physician for treatment because there is a risk that regular heavy bleeding may lead to iron-deficiency anemia.

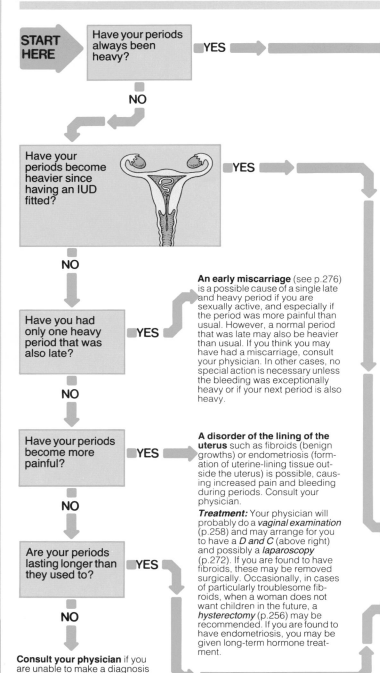

START HERE

Have your periods always been heavy?
— YES →

A thicker-than-usual lining of the uterus may explain why some women have heavier periods than others. This in itself is no cause for concern, but you should discuss the problem with your physician, who may want to rule out the possibility of anemia, and may suggest treatment.

Treatment: If, after examining you, your physician suspects the possibility of anemia, he or she will probably take a blood sample for analysis (see p.146). If you are found to be anemic, your physician will probably prescribe iron tablets and may advise you on a diet. Your physician will also discuss the possibility of treating the heaviness of your periods. In some cases, hormone treatment is suitable. Or you may be advised to have a *D and C* (below).

NO ↓

Have your periods become heavier since having an IUD fitted?
— YES →

NO ↓

Have you had only one heavy period that was also late?
— YES →

An early miscarriage (see p.276) is a possible cause of a single late and heavy period if you are sexually active, and especially if the period was more painful than usual. However, a normal period that was late may also be heavier than usual. If you think you may have had a miscarriage, consult your physician. In other cases, no special action is necessary unless the bleeding was exceptionally heavy or if your next period is also heavy.

NO ↓

Have your periods become more painful?
— YES →

A disorder of the lining of the uterus such as fibroids (benign growths) or endometriosis (formation of uterine-lining tissue outside the uterus) is possible, causing increased pain and bleeding during periods. Consult your physician.

Treatment: Your physician will probably do a *vaginal examination* (p.258) and may arrange for you to have a *D and C* (above right) and possibly a *laparoscopy* (p.272). If you are found to have fibroids, these may be removed surgically. Occasionally, in cases of particularly troublesome fibroids, when a woman does not want children in the future, a *hysterectomy* (p.256) may be recommended. If you are found to have endometriosis, you may be given long-term hormone treatment.

NO ↓

Are your periods lasting longer than they used to?
— YES →

NO ↓

Consult your physician if you are unable to make a diagnosis from this chart.

D AND C

D and C (dilatation and curettage) is a minor operation that is used to discover the cause of heavy periods and may in some cases cure the problem. The technique may also be used for investigation of infertility and for early *elective abortion* (see p. 271). D and C is usually carried out under general anesthetic. The opening of the cervix (neck of the uterus) is dilated (widened) and an instrument called a curette is used to scrape out the lining of the uterus. These scrapings are then taken for laboratory examination. Following the operation, you will have bleeding from the uterus for a few days, and you are likely to experience backache and/or lower abdominal pain. You will probably be advised not to use tampons and to refrain from sexual intercourse for a week or so.

Position of the curette scraping out the uterine lining

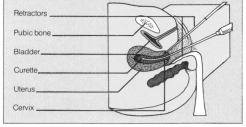

Retractors
Pubic bone
Bladder
Curette
Uterus
Cervix

The IUD (intrauterine contraceptive device) may cause heavier periods as a side effect. This is no cause for concern if the increase in bleeding is slight. If the bleeding is much heavier than usual or if it distresses you, consult your physician, who may suggest that you change to an alternative method of contraception (see chart 136, *Choosing a contraceptive method*).

Fibroids (benign growths inside the uterus) may cause periods to become heavier and longer. This is especially likely if you are over 35 years old. Consult your physician.

Treatment: A physician will usually be able to detect fibroids by a *vaginal examination* (p.258). If the diagnosis is confirmed you may be prescribed hormone treatment to reduce bleeding. If this does not control your symptoms you may need to have a *D and C* (above). Large, troublesome fibroids may need to be removed surgically. Occasionally, a *hysterectomy* (p.256) is advised.

127 Painful periods

Many women experience some degree of pain or discomfort during menstrual periods. The pain – called dysmenorrhea – is usually cramping and is felt in the lower abdomen. In most cases painful periods are not a sign of ill health and do not disrupt everyday activities. However, if you suffer from severe pain or if your periods suddenly start to become much more painful than previously, consult your physician.

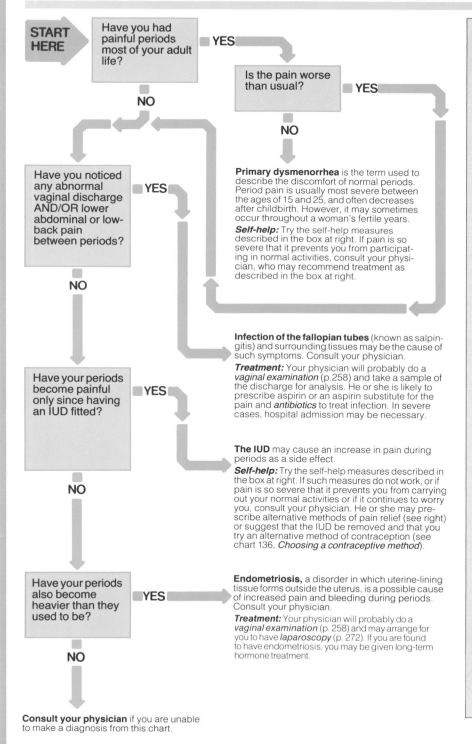

START HERE

Have you had painful periods most of your adult life?

YES →

Is the pain worse than usual? **YES** →

NO ↓

NO ↓

Primary dysmenorrhea is the term used to describe the discomfort of normal periods. Period pain is usually most severe between the ages of 15 and 25, and often decreases after childbirth. However, it may sometimes occur throughout a woman's fertile years.

Self-help: Try the self-help measures described in the box at right. If pain is so severe that it prevents you from participating in normal activities, consult your physician, who may recommend treatment as described in the box at right.

Have you noticed any abnormal vaginal discharge AND/OR lower abdominal or low-back pain between periods? **YES** →

NO ↓

Infection of the fallopian tubes (known as salpingitis) and surrounding tissues may be the cause of such symptoms. Consult your physician.

Treatment: Your physician will probably do a *vaginal examination* (p.258) and take a sample of the discharge for analysis. He or she is likely to prescribe aspirin or an aspirin substitute for the pain and *antibiotics* to treat infection. In severe cases, hospital admission may be necessary.

Have your periods become painful only since having an IUD fitted? **YES** →

NO ↓

The IUD may cause an increase in pain during periods as a side effect.

Self-help: Try the self-help measures described in the box at right. If such measures do not work, or if pain is so severe that it prevents you from carrying out your normal activities or if it continues to worry you, consult your physician. He or she may prescribe alternative methods of pain relief (see right) or suggest that the IUD be removed and that you try an alternative method of contraception (see chart 136, *Choosing a contraceptive method*).

Have your periods also become heavier than they used to be? **YES** →

NO ↓

Endometriosis, a disorder in which uterine-lining tissue forms outside the uterus, is a possible cause of increased pain and bleeding during periods. Consult your physician.

Treatment: Your physician will probably do a *vaginal examination* (p. 258) and may arrange for you to have *laparoscopy* (p. 272). If you are found to have endometriosis, you may be given long-term hormone treatment.

Consult your physician if you are unable to make a diagnosis from this chart.

TREATMENT OF MENSTRUAL PROBLEMS

Unpleasant menstrual symptoms, including premenstrual syndrome (see below), period pain and excessive bleeding, can often be relieved by medical treatment. It is worthwhile to seek your physician's advice if you are distressed by such symptoms.

Premenstrual syndrome
In the week or so before a period, many women experience a variety of symptoms including tension, irritability, depression, a feeling of being bloated – especially in the breasts and abdomen – and headaches. Treatment will depend on your individual symptoms and their severity, but may include one or more of the following:

Counseling may be offered. This may be in the form of sympathetic discussion with your family physician, or through self-help discussion groups.

Progesterone (hormone supplements) may be given in the last part of your *menstrual cycle* (p. 253).

Pyridoxine (vitamin B$_6$) is sometimes given daily to relieve premenstrual symptoms.

Diuretics (see p. 297) **or dietary sodium restriction** may be prescribed in the last half of your menstrual cycle to relieve bloating.

Regular exercise and a diet low in sugar with emphasis on protein and fiber seems to help many women.

Painful periods
If you have painful periods, first try the following self-help suggestions:

■ Take the recommended dose of aspirin or an aspirin substitute.
■ When pain is severe, rest in bed with a well-wrapped hot-water bottle or heating-pad on your abdomen.

If pain continues to trouble you, consult your physician, who may prescribe tablets to inhibit the muscle cramps that lead to period pain. Alternatively, you may be given hormone tablets. If you also require contraception and there is no medical reason that makes it inadvisable, your physician may suggest that you start taking the birth-control pill (see also chart 136, *Choosing a contraceptive method*).

Excessive bleeding
If you suffer from excessive blood loss during periods (menorrhagia), consult your physician, who may advise a *D and C* (opposite) or may prescribe hormone treatment in the form of the birth-control pill (see above) or in another form.

128 Irregular vaginal bleeding

Irregular vaginal bleeding includes irregular menstrual periods and blood loss between normal periods. The latter type of bleeding may consist only of slight "spotting" on one or two days, or it may be heavier. Sometimes, irregular periods may be the result of hormonal fluctuations – for example, in adolescence or as you approach the menopause. However, bleeding between periods, especially if accompanied by pain (or in an older woman), may be a sign of a serious underlying disorder and should be investigated.

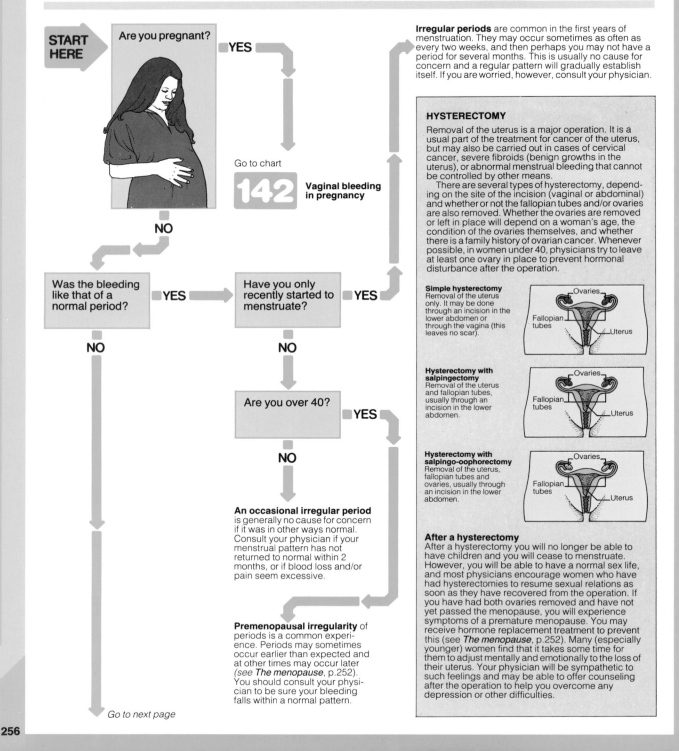

START HERE

Are you pregnant?

YES →

Go to chart

142 **Vaginal bleeding in pregnancy**

NO

Was the bleeding like that of a normal period?

YES → **Have you only recently started to menstruate?** **YES**

NO

NO

Are you over 40? **YES**

NO

An occasional irregular period is generally no cause for concern if it was in other ways normal. Consult your physician if your menstrual pattern has not returned to normal within 2 months, or if blood loss and/or pain seem excessive.

Premenopausal irregularity of periods is a common experience. Periods may sometimes occur earlier than expected and at other times may occur later (see *The menopause*, p.252). You should consult your physician to be sure your bleeding falls within a normal pattern.

Go to next page

Irregular periods are common in the first years of menstruation. They may occur sometimes as often as every two weeks, and then perhaps you may not have a period for several months. This is usually no cause for concern and a regular pattern will gradually establish itself. If you are worried, however, consult your physician.

HYSTERECTOMY

Removal of the uterus is a major operation. It is a usual part of the treatment for cancer of the uterus, but may also be carried out in cases of cervical cancer, severe fibroids (benign growths in the uterus), or abnormal menstrual bleeding that cannot be controlled by other means.

There are several types of hysterectomy, depending on the site of the incision (vaginal or abdominal) and whether or not the fallopian tubes and/or ovaries are also removed. Whether the ovaries are removed or left in place will depend on a woman's age, the condition of the ovaries themselves, and whether there is a family history of ovarian cancer. Whenever possible, in women under 40, physicians try to leave at least one ovary in place to prevent hormonal disturbance after the operation.

Simple hysterectomy
Removal of the uterus only. It may be done through an incision in the lower abdomen or through the vagina (this leaves no scar).

Ovaries
Fallopian tubes
Uterus

Hysterectomy with salpingectomy
Removal of the uterus and fallopian tubes, usually through an incision in the lower abdomen.

Ovaries
Fallopian tubes
Uterus

Hysterectomy with salpingo-oophorectomy
Removal of the uterus, fallopian tubes and ovaries, usually through an incision in the lower abdomen.

Ovaries
Fallopian tubes
Uterus

After a hysterectomy

After a hysterectomy you will no longer be able to have children and you will cease to menstruate. However, you will be able to have a normal sex life, and most physicians encourage women who have had hysterectomies to resume sexual relations as soon as they have recovered from the operation. If you have had both ovaries removed and have not yet passed the menopause, you will experience symptoms of a premature menopause. You may receive hormone replacement treatment to prevent this (see *The menopause*, p.252). Many (especially younger) women find that it takes some time for them to adjust mentally and emotionally to the loss of their uterus. Your physician will be sympathetic to such feelings and may be able to offer counseling after the operation to help you overcome any depression or other difficulties.

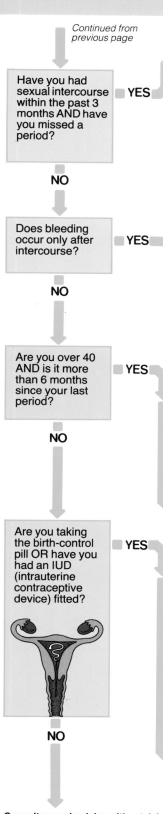

Continued from previous page

Have you had sexual intercourse within the past 3 months AND have you missed a period?

YES →

CALL YOUR PHYSICIAN NOW!
A serious complication of early pregnancy, such as an ectopic pregnancy (pregnancy outside the uterus), is possible, especially if you also have abdominal pain.

Treatment: If your physician suspects an ectopic pregnancy, you will probably be admitted to the hospital. If the diagnosis is confirmed, you will need to have an urgent operation to end the pregnancy.

NO ↓

Does bleeding occur only after intercourse?

YES →

CONSULT YOUR PHYSICIAN WITHOUT DELAY!
Postcoital bleeding may be a sign of a minor abnormality of the cervix (neck of the uterus) but it can also be a sign of other diseases of the cervix.

Treatment: Your physician will do a *vaginal examination* (p.258). If the smear shows the presence of abnormal cells, you may need to have further tests, such as *colposcopy* (below right). Some cervical abnormalities can be treated by laser surgery, freezing, or a minor operation (cone biopsy). However, cancer that seems to have spread may require a *hysterectomy* (opposite) and/or radiotherapy (either in the form of X-ray treatment or by insertion of a radium pellet into the vagina). Treatment of cancer of the cervix is often successful if started early.

NO ↓

Are you over 40 AND is it more than 6 months since your last period?

YES →

CONSULT YOUR PHYSICIAN WITHOUT DELAY!
Postmenopausal bleeding may be caused by a minor vaginal disorder, but it could also be a sign of cancer of the uterus or cervix (neck of the uterus).

Treatment: Your physician will do a *vaginal examination* (p.258) and will probably take a smear of the cervix (see *Cervical screening,* right). He or she may also arrange for you to have a *D and C* (p.254). If cancer is diagnosed, you will probably need to have a *hysterectomy* (opposite). Radiotherapy or the insertion of a radium pellet into the vagina may also be part of your treatment. Hormones may also be given. The earlier treatment is started, the greater the chances of a complete cure.

NO ↓

Are you taking the birth-control pill OR have you had an IUD (intrauterine contraceptive device) fitted?

YES →

Both these contraceptive methods may cause spotting between periods. This is unlikely to be a cause for concern, but you should discuss the symptom with your physician, who may suggest a change of pill, or an alternative form of contraception. (See also chart 136, *Choosing a contraceptive method.*)

NO ↓

Consult your physician without delay if you are unable to make a diagnosis from this chart.

CERVICAL SCREENING

The cells that make up the outer surface of the cervix (neck of the uterus) may sometimes undergo changes for reasons that are not yet fully understood. Such cell abnormalities often present no risk to general health, but in a small proportion of cases the abnormal cells may become cancerous. Cancer of the cervix, although rare compared with other cervical abnormalities, is one of the most common cancers affecting women. It is, however, also one of the most easily treated cancers if diagnosed early. For these reasons it is important for every adult woman to make sure that she has regular screening so that any change in the cells of the cervix can be detected and, when necessary, treated as soon as possible.

Cervical smear (Pap smear)
The standard method of screening is the cervical smear. It is recommended that every woman have this test at least every 3 years unless suspicious cells are found; then it should be done more often. The test can be carried out by your family physician or at a family planning clinic. In the test, the vagina is held open by a speculum, and a spatula is used to scrape away a sample of cells from the surface of the cervix. The sample is then sent for examination.

If the smear shows a mild abnormality, you may simply be asked to return for another smear test in a few months. This is because minor abnormalities often heal without the need for further treatment. If the trouble persists or the smear is suggestive of cancer or precancerous cells, you will probably be referred for a colposcopy.

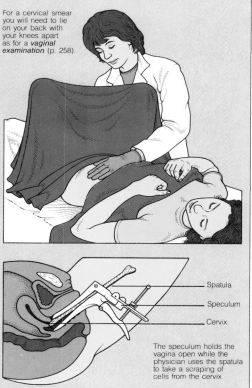

For a cervical smear you will need to lie on your back with your knees apart as for a *vaginal examination* (p. 258).

Spatula
Speculum
Cervix

The speculum holds the vagina open while the physician uses the spatula to take a scraping of cells from the cervix.

Colposcopy
This is a technique that allows the physician to take a close look at the surface of the cervix. An instrument with a magnifying lens and an eyepiece is inserted into the vagina. While the physician is viewing the cervix, he or she will probably also take a *biopsy* (p. 159) of the cervical tissue for further examination. Minor abnormalities can often be treated during colposcopy by laser beam, burning or freezing. More serious abnormalities may require surgery.

129 Abnormal vaginal discharge

The vagina is normally kept moist and clean by secretions from the tissue lining the vagina. Such secretions may be apparent as a thin, whitish discharge from the vagina. This normal discharge may vary in quantity and consistency according to the time of your menstrual cycle, and may increase at times of sexual arousal, during pregnancy and in women using the birth-control pill or intrauterine contraceptive device (IUD). A discharge that looks abnormal, especially if it is accompanied by itching or burning around the vagina, may be a sign of infection and needs medical diagnosis and treatment. Consult this chart if you notice any increase in vaginal discharge or change in its color or consistency.

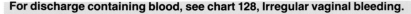

For discharge containing blood, see chart 128, Irregular vaginal bleeding.

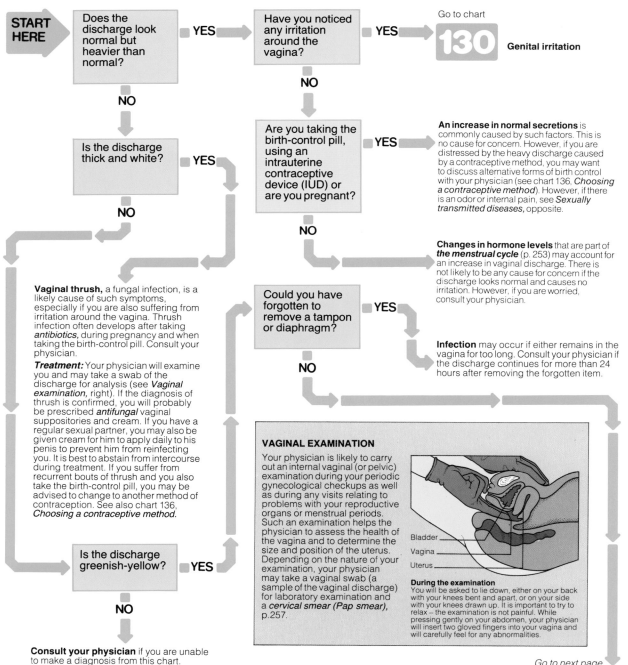

START HERE

Does the discharge look normal but heavier than normal?

YES → **Have you noticed any irritation around the vagina?**

YES → Go to chart **130** Genital irritation

NO ↓

Is the discharge thick and white? — YES

NO ↓

Are you taking the birth-control pill, using an intrauterine contraceptive device (IUD) or are you pregnant? — YES

An increase in normal secretions is commonly caused by such factors. This is no cause for concern. However, if you are distressed by the heavy discharge caused by a contraceptive method, you may want to discuss alternative forms of birth control with your physician (see chart 136, *Choosing a contraceptive method*). However, if there is an odor or internal pain, see *Sexually transmitted diseases*, opposite.

NO ↓

Could you have forgotten to remove a tampon or diaphragm? — YES

Changes in hormone levels that are part of *the menstrual cycle* (p. 253) may account for an increase in vaginal discharge. There is not likely to be any cause for concern if the discharge looks normal and causes no irritation. However, if you are worried, consult your physician.

Infection may occur if either remains in the vagina for too long. Consult your physician if the discharge continues for more than 24 hours after removing the forgotten item.

NO ↓

Vaginal thrush, a fungal infection, is a likely cause of such symptoms, especially if you are also suffering from irritation around the vagina. Thrush infection often develops after taking *antibiotics*, during pregnancy and when taking the birth-control pill. Consult your physician.

Treatment: Your physician will examine you and may take a swab of the discharge for analysis (see *Vaginal examination*, right). If the diagnosis of thrush is confirmed, you will probably be prescribed *antifungal* vaginal suppositories and cream. If you have a regular sexual partner, you may also be given cream for him to apply daily to his penis to prevent him from reinfecting you. It is best to abstain from intercourse during treatment. If you suffer from recurrent bouts of thrush and you also take the birth-control pill, you may be advised to change to another method of contraception. See also chart 136, *Choosing a contraceptive method.*

VAGINAL EXAMINATION

Your physician is likely to carry out an internal vaginal (or pelvic) examination during your periodic gynecological checkups as well as during any visits relating to problems with your reproductive organs or menstrual periods. Such an examination helps the physician to assess the health of the vagina and to determine the size and position of the uterus. Depending on the nature of your examination, your physician may take a vaginal swab (a sample of the vaginal discharge) for laboratory examination and a *cervical smear (Pap smear)*, p.257.

Bladder
Vagina
Uterus

During the examination
You will be asked to lie down, either on your back with your knees bent and apart, or on your side with your knees drawn up. It is important to try to relax – the examination is not painful. While pressing gently on your abdomen, your physician will insert two gloved fingers into your vagina and will carefully feel for any abnormalities.

Is the discharge greenish-yellow? — YES

NO ↓

Consult your physician if you are unable to make a diagnosis from this chart.

Go to next page

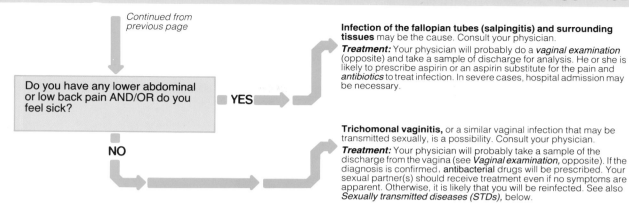

Continued from previous page

Do you have any lower abdominal or low back pain AND/OR do you feel sick?

YES →

Infection of the fallopian tubes (salpingitis) and surrounding tissues may be the cause. Consult your physician.
Treatment: Your physician will probably do a *vaginal examination* (opposite) and take a sample of discharge for analysis. He or she is likely to prescribe aspirin or an aspirin substitute for the pain and *antibiotics* to treat infection. In severe cases, hospital admission may be necessary.

NO →

Trichomonal vaginitis, or a similar vaginal infection that may be transmitted sexually, is a possibility. Consult your physician.
Treatment: Your physician will probably take a sample of the discharge from the vagina (see *Vaginal examination,* opposite). If the diagnosis is confirmed, **antibacterial** drugs will be prescribed. Your sexual partner(s) should receive treatment even if no symptoms are apparent. Otherwise, it is likely that you will be reinfected. See also *Sexually transmitted diseases (STDs),* below.

SEXUALLY TRANSMITTED DISEASES (STDs)

Infections passed from one person to another during sexual contact (including sexual intercourse, and anal or oral sex) are known as sexually transmitted (or venereal) diseases. If you think you have caught a sexually transmitted disease and/or if your sexual partner has, consult your physician or go to a clinic that specializes in such diseases (STD clinic), where you will be treated in the strictest confidence. It is important to seek medical advice promptly because of the risk of serious damage to your reproductive organs from many such diseases even when symptoms are not severe. (Some like AIDS may be life-threatening, see chart 117.) Also, you may unknowingly pass on the infection to someone else. You should avoid sex until your physician confirms that treatment has cleared your symptoms and inform any partners so they can seek treatment if necessary.

Disease	Incubation period*	Symptoms	Treatment
Nonspecific genital infection (*Chlamydia*)	14 to 21 days	Often causes few or no symptoms. There may be a slightly abnormal vaginal discharge. If untreated, *Chlamydia* infection may lead to infertility. Suspect the disease if you have a sexual partner who has nonspecific urethritis (a disease usually caused by the *Chlamydia* microbe).	Your physician may take a swab from your vagina for culture (see *Vaginal examination,* opposite). Treatment is usually with *antibiotics*.
Trichomonal vaginitis	Variable	An infected-looking (greenish-yellow) vaginal discharge, usually causing irritation around the vagina. Pain on intercourse.	The diagnosis is confirmed by analysis of a sample of discharge taken from the vagina (see *Vaginal examination,* opposite). The usual treatment is a course of *antibiotics*.
Gonorrhea	2 to 10 days	May be symptomless in women. It may sometimes cause abnormal vaginal or urethral discharge and/or painful urination. Persistent untreated infection may spread to the uterus and fallopian tubes, causing lower abdominal pain.	The disease is diagnosed by a urethral/vaginal swab (see *Vaginal examination,* opposite). Treatment consists of a course of *antibiotics*.
Herpes genitalis	7 days or less	There is usually an itching feeling in the genital area followed by the appearance of a crop of small, painful blisters. Sometimes these also appear on the thighs and buttocks. The blisters burst after 24 hours, leaving small, red, moist, painful ulcers that sometimes crust over. The glands in the groin may become enlarged and painful. This may be accompanied by a feeling of being sick and a raised temperature. Outbreaks of blisters are likely to recur.	There is no complete cure for this disorder. Your physician may prescribe an *antiviral* drug or ointment to make the ulcers less sore and to speed healing. You will be advised to avoid close sexual contact while you have blisters or sores so you do not transmit the infection to your partner.
Syphilis	9 to 90 days	In the first stage, a highly infectious, painless sore called a chancre develops, usually in the genital area (or in some cases in the anus). This disappears after a few weeks. In the second stage a rash that does not itch appears all over the body, including the palms and soles. There may also be painless swelling of the lymph glands and infectious wartlike lumps around the anus and/or mouth.	The disease is diagnosed by blood tests and samples taken from any sores. The usual treatment is a course of *antibiotic* injections. You will need to have periodic blood tests for 1 to 2 years after treatment to check that the disease has not reappeared.
Pubic lice	0 to 17 days	Usually there is intense itching in the pubic region, particularly at night. You may be able to see the lice; they are brown and 1/16 in. (1 to 2 mm) long.	Your physician will give you a lotion or ointment that kills lice and their eggs. He or she will also check that you do not have any other sexually transmitted disease. Often, other family members may be treated. Bedding and clothing should be thoroughly laundered at the time of treatment.

*Time between contact with the disease and the appearance of symptoms.

130 Genital irritation

Consult this chart if you have been suffering from itching and/or soreness in the vagina or around the vulva (external genital area). Such irritation may also cause stinging during urination and discomfort during intercourse. This symptom is known medically as pruritus vulvae. It may be brought on by infection in the vagina or urinary tract, by local irritation from soaps or deodorants, or by various skin conditions.

Consult this diagnostic chart only after reading chart 61, Itching.

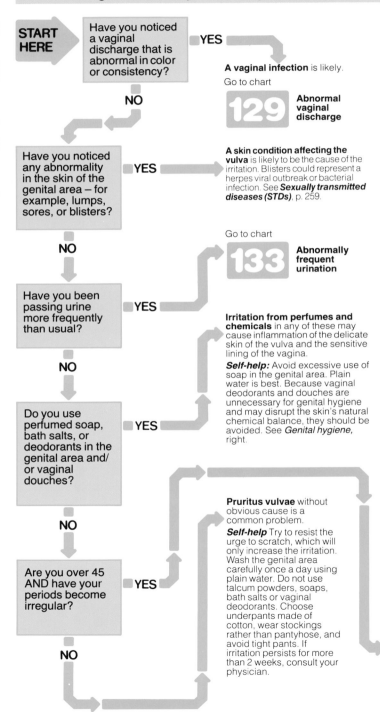

START HERE

Have you noticed a vaginal discharge that is abnormal in color or consistency?

YES → **A vaginal infection** is likely.

Go to chart **129** **Abnormal vaginal discharge**

NO

Have you noticed any abnormality in the skin of the genital area – for example, lumps, sores, or blisters?

YES → **A skin condition affecting the vulva** is likely to be the cause of the irritation. Blisters could represent a herpes viral outbreak or bacterial infection. See *Sexually transmitted diseases (STDs)*, p. 259.

NO

Have you been passing urine more frequently than usual?

YES → Go to chart **133** **Abnormally frequent urination**

NO

Do you use perfumed soap, bath salts, or deodorants in the genital area and/or vaginal douches?

YES → **Irritation from perfumes and chemicals** in any of these may cause inflammation of the delicate skin of the vulva and the sensitive lining of the vagina.

Self-help: Avoid excessive use of soap in the genital area. Plain water is best. Because vaginal deodorants and douches are unnecessary for genital hygiene and may disrupt the skin's natural chemical balance, they should be avoided. See *Genital hygiene,* right.

NO

Are you over 45 AND have your periods become irregular?

YES → **Pruritus vulvae** without obvious cause is a common problem.

Self-help Try to resist the urge to scratch, which will only increase the irritation. Wash the genital area carefully once a day using plain water. Do not use talcum powders, soaps, bath salts or vaginal deodorants. Choose underpants made of cotton, wear stockings rather than pantyhose, and avoid tight pants. If irritation persists for more than 2 weeks, consult your physician.

NO

GENITAL HYGIENE

Everyday care
Cleansing the genital area should be part of your normal daily washing routine. However, the skin in this area is delicate and needs to be treated gently so that it does not become inflamed and irritated. Use only plain water; bath salts and soaps, even mild ones, may be irritating. It should only be necessary to wash the external skin of the vulva. The internal lining of the vagina is kept clean by its natural secretions, which also help to protect against infection. Vaginal douches and deodorants are unnecessary for hygiene and health and may cause irritation. They may also disrupt the chemical balance inside the vagina.

Menstrual hygiene
Your choice of method of sanitary protection during menstrual periods is largely a matter of personal preference. In normal circumstances there is no medical reason for preferring external sanitary pads to internal tampons or vice versa. Sanitary pads may be more suitable for women who have heavy periods because they usually provide greater absorbency. Pads should also be used to absorb blood loss in the weeks following childbirth to minimize the chances of infection. Young girls may also find pads easier to use in the first years of menstruation. Tampons have the advantage of being unnoticeable even under close-fitting clothes, and do not interfere with participation in sports such as swimming. Whichever method you choose, you will need to change your pad or tampon every 3 to 6 hours depending on the heaviness of the menstrual flow.

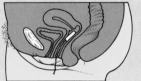

Choose the method that feels best for you – the easy-to-insert tampon or the absorbent press-on pad.

Toxic shock syndrome
Some women were discouraged from using tampons by reports of serious illness as a result of their use. This occurred when women experienced abnormal bacterial growth in the vagina while using certain high-absorbency tampons. Toxins (poisons) produced by the bacteria were absorbed into the bloodstream leading to life-threatening blood poisoning (toxic shock). The chance of toxic shock syndrome occurring is very slim with presently available tampons. A forgotten tampon of normal absorbency may cause an offensive discharge, but is unlikely to be a serious risk to health. Symptoms of toxic shock syndrome include fatigue, fever and skin rash. Your physician should be consulted immediately if you have these symptoms.

Falling levels of estrogen (a female hormone) as you approach *the menopause,* (p. 252) may lead to genital irritation. Consult your physician.

Treatment: If your physician finds that your irritation is due to hormonal changes he or she may prescribe a hormone cream to apply to the vagina and vulva. Alternatively, the physician may recommend hormone replacement therapy. If the irritation causes discomfort during sexual intercourse, a lubricating jelly may help.

131 Poor bladder control

Difficulty controlling your bladder or involuntary passing of urine may be a sign of infection in the urinary tract or it may be due to weak muscle control. Always seek your physician's advice about this symptom.

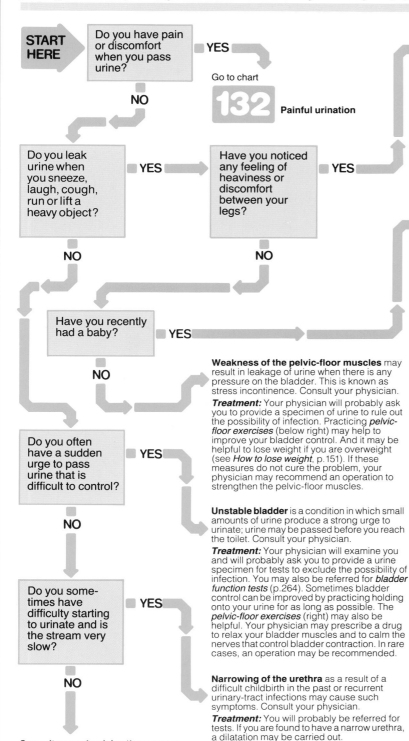

START HERE

Do you have pain or discomfort when you pass urine?

YES — Go to chart **132** Painful urination

NO

Do you leak urine when you sneeze, laugh, cough, run or lift a heavy object?

YES — **Have you noticed any feeling of heaviness or discomfort between your legs?**

NO

NO

Have you recently had a baby?

YES

NO

Do you often have a sudden urge to pass urine that is difficult to control?

YES

NO

Do you sometimes have difficulty starting to urinate and is the stream very slow?

YES

NO

Consult your physician if you are unable to make a diagnosis from this chart.

Prolapse of the uterus or vagina may be causing these symptoms. This occurs when the muscles and ligaments supporting the uterus become weak and slack. This is particularly likely if you are over 50. Consult your physician.

Treatment: Your physician will examine you and may ask you to provide a specimen of urine for analysis to rule out the possibility of infection. If you are suffering from prolapse, your physician will probably recommend that you try *pelvic-floor exercises* (below). If you are overweight, you will also be advised to lose weight (see *How to lose weight*, p. 151). In some cases, a specially designed vaginal device will also be fitted. If these measures do not improve your condition, you may need to have an operation.

Childbirth may have temporarily weakened your pelvic-floor muscles. This is a common occurrence and nearly always improves within a few months without special treatment. Consult your physician.

Treatment: Your physician will examine you and may ask you to provide a urine sample for tests to rule out the possibility of infection. In most cases, no treatment is necessary. However, *pelvic-floor exercises* (below) may help your muscle tone return to normal more quickly. Your condition will also improve if you lose any excess weight you may have gained during pregnancy (see *How to lose weight*, p.151).

Weakness of the pelvic-floor muscles may result in leakage of urine when there is any pressure on the bladder. This is known as stress incontinence. Consult your physician.

Treatment: Your physician will probably ask you to provide a specimen of urine to rule out the possibility of infection. Practicing *pelvic-floor exercises* (below right) may help to improve your bladder control. And it may be helpful to lose weight if you are overweight (see *How to lose weight*, p.151). If these measures do not cure the problem, your physician may recommend an operation to strengthen the pelvic-floor muscles.

Unstable bladder is a condition in which small amounts of urine produce a strong urge to urinate; urine may be passed before you reach the toilet. Consult your physician.

Treatment: Your physician will examine you and will probably ask you to provide a urine specimen for tests to exclude the possibility of infection. You may also be referred for *bladder function tests* (p.264). Sometimes bladder control can be improved by practicing holding onto your urine for as long as possible. The *pelvic-floor exercises* (right) may also be helpful. Your physician may prescribe a drug to relax your bladder muscles and to calm the nerves that control bladder contraction. In rare cases, an operation may be recommended.

Narrowing of the urethra as a result of a difficult childbirth in the past or recurrent urinary-tract infections may cause such symptoms. Consult your physician.

Treatment: You will probably be referred for tests. If you are found to have a narrow urethra, a dilatation may be carried out.

WARNING

INABILITY TO PASS URINE

If you find that you are unable to urinate even though you feel the urge to urinate, you need urgent medical attention. Try taking a warm bath, which may enable you to pass some urine.

SUDDEN LOSS OF BLADDER CONTROL

Sudden inability to control urination may be a sign of damage to the spinal cord or nervous system, especially if you have recently had a back injury or have experienced weakness in your legs.

Seek medical help at once!

PELVIC-FLOOR EXERCISES

These exercises are useful for toning up the pelvic floor muscles that support the bladder and reproductive organs. While the exercises are particularly useful during pregnancy, after childbirth or if you are suffering from weak bladder control, they are worth practicing at any time. When you go to the toilet to pass urine, follow this procedure at least twice a day:

1 Contract the muscles around the vagina upward and inward so that you can stop the flow of urine.
2 Hold this position for a count of 6.
3 Now let the flow of urine continue for another count of 6.
4 Finally, interrupt the flow of urine again for the count of 6, before totally emptying your bladder of urine.

132 Painful urination

A burning or stinging pain or discomfort when you pass urine is usually the result of infection in the lower urinary tract or inflammation around the urethral opening. Such disorders are more common in women and in most cases are easily cured by a combination of home and professional treatments.

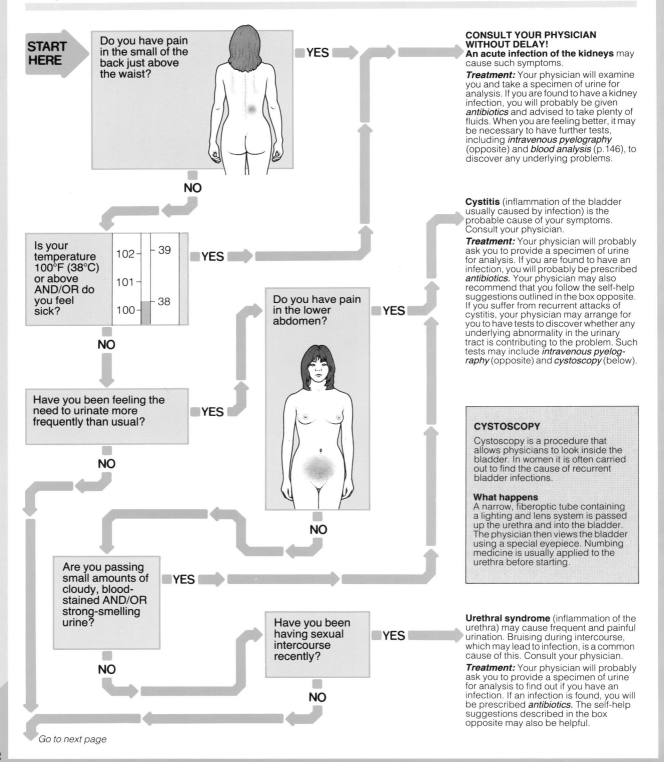

START HERE

Do you have pain in the small of the back just above the waist?

YES →

CONSULT YOUR PHYSICIAN WITHOUT DELAY!
An acute infection of the kidneys may cause such symptoms.

Treatment: Your physician will examine you and take a specimen of urine for analysis. If you are found to have a kidney infection, you will probably be given *antibiotics* and advised to take plenty of fluids. When you are feeling better, it may be necessary to have further tests, including *intravenous pyelography* (opposite) and *blood analysis* (p.146), to discover any underlying problems.

NO ↓

Is your temperature 100°F (38°C) or above AND/OR do you feel sick?

102 — 39
101
100 — 38

YES →

NO ↓

Have you been feeling the need to urinate more frequently than usual?

YES →

Do you have pain in the lower abdomen?

YES →

Cystitis (inflammation of the bladder usually caused by infection) is the probable cause of your symptoms. Consult your physician.

Treatment: Your physician will probably ask you to provide a specimen of urine for analysis. If you are found to have an infection, you will probably be prescribed *antibiotics.* Your physician may also recommend that you follow the self-help suggestions outlined in the box opposite. If you suffer from recurrent attacks of cystitis, your physician may arrange for you to have tests to discover whether any underlying abnormality in the urinary tract is contributing to the problem. Such tests may include *intravenous pyelography* (opposite) and *cystoscopy* (below).

NO ↓

NO ↓

CYSTOSCOPY

Cystoscopy is a procedure that allows physicians to look inside the bladder. In women it is often carried out to find the cause of recurrent bladder infections.

What happens
A narrow, fiberoptic tube containing a lighting and lens system is passed up the urethra and into the bladder. The physician then views the bladder using a special eyepiece. Numbing medicine is usually applied to the urethra before starting.

Are you passing small amounts of cloudy, blood-stained AND/OR strong-smelling urine?

YES →

NO ↓

Have you been having sexual intercourse recently?

YES →

Urethral syndrome (inflammation of the urethra) may cause frequent and painful urination. Bruising during intercourse, which may lead to infection, is a common cause of this. Consult your physician.

Treatment: Your physician will probably ask you to provide a specimen of urine for analysis to find out if you have an infection. If an infection is found, you will be prescribed *antibiotics.* The self-help suggestions described in the box opposite may also be helpful.

NO ↓

Go to next page

Continued from previous page

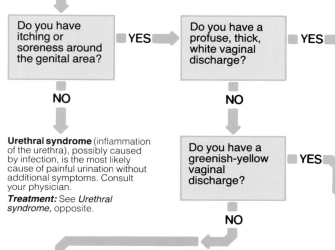

Do you have itching or soreness around the genital area?

YES → **Do you have a profuse, thick, white vaginal discharge?**

YES →

NO ↓   **NO** ↓

Urethral syndrome (inflammation of the urethra), possibly caused by infection, is the most likely cause of painful urination without additional symptoms. Consult your physician.

Treatment: See *Urethral syndrome,* opposite.

Do you have a greenish-yellow vaginal discharge?

YES →

NO ↓

Vaginal thrush, a fungal (yeast) infection, is a likely cause of such symptoms. Consult your physician.

Treatment: Your physician will examine you and may take a swab of the discharge from the inside of the vagina for analysis (see *Vaginal examination,* p. 258). If the diagnosis of thrush is confirmed, you will probably be prescribed *antifungal* vaginal suppositories. If you have a regular sexual partner, you will also be given cream for him to apply daily to his penis to prevent him from reinfecting you. If you suffer from recurrent bouts of thrush and you also take the birth control pill, you may be advised to change to another method of contraception. This is because the pill sometimes causes an increase in vaginal secretions, which makes fungal infection more likely. See also chart 136, *Choosing a contraceptive method.*

Trichomonal vaginitis, a vaginal infection that may be transmitted sexually, is a possibility. Consult your physician.

Treatment: Your physician will examine you and will probably take a sample of the discharge from the vagina for analysis (see *Vaginal examination,* p.258). If trichomonal vaginitis is confirmed, you will be prescribed a course of *antibiotics.* It is important that your sexual partner(s) also receive treatment, even if no symptoms are apparent. Otherwise, it is possible that you will be reinfected. See also *Sexually transmitted diseases,* p.259.

Pruritis vulvae (irritation of the vulva) may cause urination to become painful. There is often no obvious cause for this condition, but, in women who are past the menopause, it may be linked to a drop in hormone levels, causing the vagina to become dry. In younger women, an allergic reaction – to soap, for example – or irritation may be responsible.

Self-help: Try not to scratch the irritated area; this will only aggravate the condition. Wash the genital area gently once a day and apply a soothing cream. Do not use soap, talcum powder, vaginal deodorants or douches because these may increase irritation. Wear cotton underwear and avoid nylon pantyhose and close-fitting pants that restrict ventilation. If your vagina feels dry during intercourse, use a lubricating jelly. If the problem persists for more than a few days, consult your physician.

SELF-HELP FOR INFECTIONS OF THE BLADDER AND URETHRA

If you are suffering from cystitis or the urethral syndrome, the following self-help suggestions, in addition to whatever treatment your physician may prescribe, will help to relieve your symptoms, hasten recovery, and prevent the trouble from recurring.

- To relieve abdominal pain and fever, take aspirin or an aspirin substitute. A hot-water bottle wrapped in a towel or a heating pad on the abdomen is often comforting. Sitz baths two or three times daily are beneficial.
- Make sure that you drink plenty of fluids and urinate frequently.
- Cranberry juice or vitamin C will acidify the urine, thereby inhibiting the growth of many of the cystitis-causing bacteria.

- If you use a diaphragm, ask your physician or clinic to check that it fits properly; ill-fitting diaphragms may bruise the urethra, leading to infection.

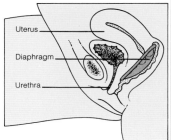

Uterus
Diaphragm
Urethra

- Keep the genital area clean and dry, but do not use vaginal douches or deodorants, or heavily scented soaps.
- When you go to the toilet, always wipe from front to back to keep germs from the bowel away from the urethral opening.
- Avoid wearing nylon pantyhose or underpants. Cotton underpants are preferable. No undergarment should be too tight-fitting or snug.

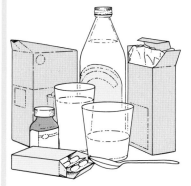

- Try to empty your bladder completely each time you pass urine to prevent a residue from remaining in the bladder, which could encourage infection.
- If sexual intercourse is sometimes painful, use a vaginal lubricant and experiment with different positions.
- Always empty your bladder after sexual intercourse.

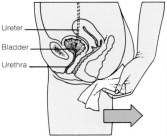

Ureter
Bladder
Urethra

INTRAVENOUS PYELOGRAPHY

Intravenous pyelography (excretory urography) is a procedure that provides physicians with a series of X-ray pictures of the urinary tract. A dye that shows up on X rays is injected into the bloodstream. It travels around the body until it is absorbed by the kidneys. This process may take an hour or so. X-ray pictures are taken as the chemical works its way through the kidneys, down the ureters, and into the bladder.

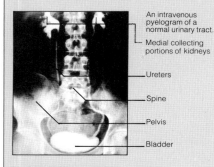

An intravenous pyelogram of a normal urinary tract.

Medial collecting portions of kidneys

Ureters

Spine

Pelvis

Bladder

Micturating cystogram or voiding cystourethrogram
This is a series of X rays that show the action of the bladder during urination. This is often done following an intravenous pyelogram when dye is already in the bladder. However, sometimes the dye is passed directly into the bladder through a fine tube (catheter) inserted into the urethra.

133 Abnormally frequent urination

The number of times you need to pass urine each day depends on a number of factors, including habit, the amount of fluid consumed and the strength of your bladder muscles. Most women need to pass urine between 2 and 6 times a day. You will know what is normal for you. Consult this chart if you find that you are having to pass urine more frequently than you are used to. This is rarely a symptom of serious disease, but simple treatment can often clear up this disruptive and sometimes embarrassing symptom.

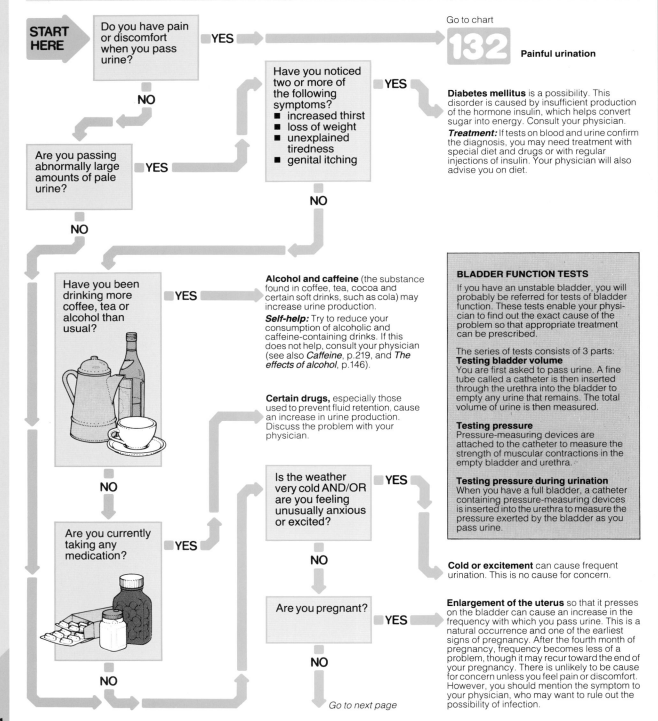

START HERE → Do you have pain or discomfort when you pass urine?

YES → Go to chart **132** Painful urination

NO ↓

Are you passing abnormally large amounts of pale urine?

YES → Have you noticed two or more of the following symptoms?
- increased thirst
- loss of weight
- unexplained tiredness
- genital itching

YES → **Diabetes mellitus** is a possibility. This disorder is caused by insufficient production of the hormone insulin, which helps convert sugar into energy. Consult your physician.

Treatment: If tests on blood and urine confirm the diagnosis, you may need treatment with special diet and drugs or with regular injections of insulin. Your physician will also advise you on diet.

NO (from symptoms box) ↓

NO (from pale urine box) ↓

Have you been drinking more coffee, tea or alcohol than usual?

YES → **Alcohol and caffeine** (the substance found in coffee, tea, cocoa and certain soft drinks, such as cola) may increase urine production.

Self-help: Try to reduce your consumption of alcoholic and caffeine-containing drinks. If this does not help, consult your physician (see also *Caffeine*, p.219, and *The effects of alcohol*, p.146).

NO ↓

Are you currently taking any medication?

YES → **Certain drugs,** especially those used to prevent fluid retention, cause an increase in urine production. Discuss the problem with your physician.

Is the weather very cold AND/OR are you feeling unusually anxious or excited?

YES → **Cold or excitement** can cause frequent urination. This is no cause for concern.

NO ↓

Are you pregnant?

YES → **Enlargement of the uterus** so that it presses on the bladder can cause an increase in the frequency with which you pass urine. This is a natural occurrence and one of the earliest signs of pregnancy. After the fourth month of pregnancy, frequency becomes less of a problem, though it may recur toward the end of your pregnancy. There is unlikely to be cause for concern unless you feel pain or discomfort. However, you should mention the symptom to your physician, who may want to rule out the possibility of infection.

NO ↓

NO ↓

Go to next page

BLADDER FUNCTION TESTS

If you have an unstable bladder, you will probably be referred for tests of bladder function. These tests enable your physician to find out the exact cause of the problem so that appropriate treatment can be prescribed.

The series of tests consists of 3 parts:

Testing bladder volume
You are first asked to pass urine. A fine tube called a catheter is then inserted through the urethra into the bladder to empty any urine that remains. The total volume of urine is then measured.

Testing pressure
Pressure-measuring devices are attached to the catheter to measure the strength of muscular contractions in the empty bladder and urethra.

Testing pressure during urination
When you have a full bladder, a catheter containing pressure-measuring devices is inserted into the urethra to measure the pressure exerted by the bladder as you pass urine.

Continued from previous page

Do you often have a sudden, strong urge to pass urine, but pass only a small amount?

YES → **Unstable bladder** is a condition in which even small amounts of urine in the bladder produce a strong urge to urinate, and urine may be passed before you can reach the toilet. Consult your physician.

Treatment: Your physician will examine you and will probably ask you to provide a urine specimen for tests to exclude the possibility of infection. You may also be referred for *bladder function tests* (opposite). Sometimes bladder control can be improved by practicing holding your urine for as long as possible. The *pelvic-floor exercises* on p.261 may also be helpful. Your physician may prescribe a drug to relax your bladder muscles and to calm the nerves that control bladder contraction. In rare cases, an operation may be recommended.

NO ↓

Do you sometimes have difficulty controlling your bladder?

YES → Go to chart **131** **Poor bladder control**

NO ↓

Consult your physician if you are unable to make a diagnosis from this chart and the frequency of urination is such that it wakes you at night or continues for more than a week.

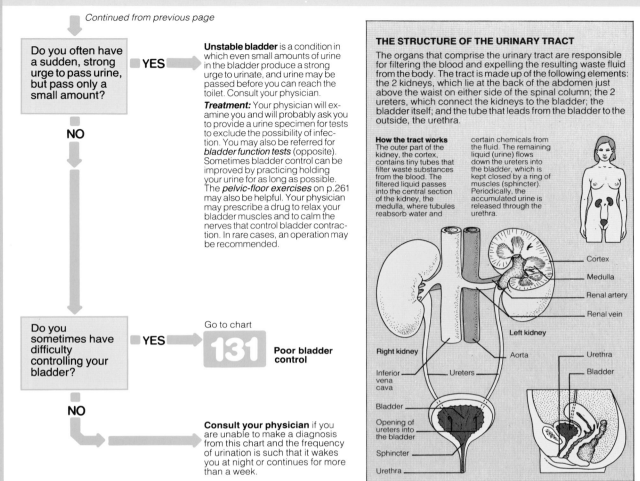

THE STRUCTURE OF THE URINARY TRACT

The organs that comprise the urinary tract are responsible for filtering the blood and expelling the resulting waste fluid from the body. The tract is made up of the following elements: the 2 kidneys, which lie at the back of the abdomen just above the waist on either side of the spinal column; the 2 ureters, which connect the kidneys to the bladder; the bladder itself; and the tube that leads from the bladder to the outside, the urethra.

How the tract works
The outer part of the kidney, the cortex, contains tiny tubes that filter waste substances from the blood. The filtered liquid passes into the central section of the kidney, the medulla, where tubules reabsorb water and certain chemicals from the fluid. The remaining liquid (urine) flows down the ureters into the bladder, which is kept closed by a ring of muscles (sphincter). Periodically, the accumulated urine is released through the urethra.

Labels: Cortex, Medulla, Renal artery, Renal vein, Left kidney, Right kidney, Aorta, Urethra, Bladder, Inferior vena cava, Ureters, Bladder, Opening of ureters into the bladder, Sphincter, Urethra

ABNORMAL-LOOKING URINE

Color of urine	Possible causes	What action is necessary
Pink, red or smoky	There is a chance that you may have blood in the urine, possibly caused by infection, inflammation or a growth in the urinary tract. However, natural or artificial red food colorings can also pass into the urine.	Consult your physician without delay. He or she may need to take samples of urine and blood for analysis (see *Blood analysis*, p.146) in order to make a firm diagnosis. Treatment will depend on the underlying problem.
Dark yellow or orange	If you have not been drinking much fluid, your urine has become concentrated. Loss of fluid caused by diarrhea, vomiting or sweating can make your urine more concentrated and therefore darker than usual. Certain substances in senna-based laxatives and in rhubarb can also darken your urine.	This is no cause for concern. As soon as you compensate for any loss of fluid by drinking, your urine will return to its normal color. Substances in laxatives and rhubarb will pass through your system within 24 hours.
Clear and dark brown	Jaundice caused by a disorder of the liver (most commonly hepatitis) or gallbladder is a possibility, especially if your bowel movements are very pale and your skin or eyes look yellow.	Consult your physician. He or she will need to take samples of urine and blood for analysis (see *Blood analysis*, p.146) in order to make a firm diagnosis. Treatment will depend on the underlying problem.
Green or blue	Artificial coloring in food or medicines is almost certainly the cause of this.	This is no cause for concern; the coloring will pass through without harmful effects.

134 Painful intercourse

A woman may feel pain or discomfort in or around the vagina at the time of penetration, or during or following sexual intercourse. This symptom is known medically as dyspareunia. It is a relatively common problem among women of all ages, and may occur for a variety of physical (muscle spasms or problems with the vaginal lining) or emotional reasons. Whatever cause you suspect, it is worthwhile seeking medical help if this symptom persists because, if intercourse is repeatedly painful for you, there is a risk that it will affect your desire for sex and so damage your relationship with your partner.

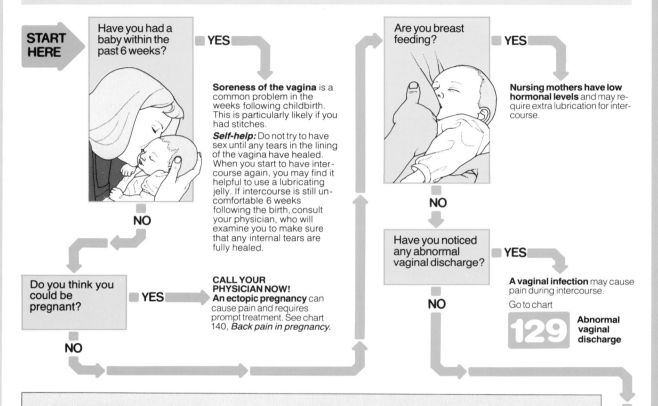

START HERE

Have you had a baby within the past 6 weeks?

YES

Soreness of the vagina is a common problem in the weeks following childbirth. This is particularly likely if you had stitches.

Self-help: Do not try to have sex until any tears in the lining of the vagina have healed. When you start to have intercourse again, you may find it helpful to use a lubricating jelly. If intercourse is still uncomfortable 6 weeks following the birth, consult your physician, who will examine you to make sure that any internal tears are fully healed.

NO

Do you think you could be pregnant?

YES

CALL YOUR PHYSICIAN NOW!
An ectopic pregnancy can cause pain and requires prompt treatment. See chart 140, *Back pain in pregnancy.*

NO

Are you breast feeding?

YES

Nursing mothers have low hormonal levels and may require extra lubrication for intercourse.

NO

Have you noticed any abnormal vaginal discharge?

YES

A vaginal infection may cause pain during intercourse.

Go to chart

129 Abnormal vaginal discharge

NO

REDUCING SEXUAL ANXIETY

Many sexual difficulties arise out of anxiety in one or both partners, and most forms of sex counseling involve advice on reducing such anxiety as a basis for improving sexual enjoyment. The following technique, called sensate focus, is often successful in heightening sexual responsiveness without provoking anxiety about performance, and may help you to overcome inhibitions and tensions that can mar sexual relationships. Usually the first step in reducing anxiety is for both partners to agree to abstain from sexual intercourse for, say, 3 weeks.

Sensate focus

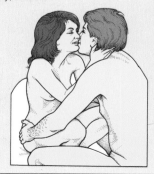

Set aside at least 3 evenings (or a period at another time of day) when you can be alone with your partner without fear of interruption for at least 2 hours. Try to create an atmosphere in which you both feel relaxed — playing some favorite music may help. During the time when you are trying this therapy you and your partner must stick to your agreement to refrain from full sexual intercourse.

Stage 1

On the first evening, each partner should take turns gently massaging and caressing the other for a period of about 20 minutes. This is best carried out when you are both naked, and you can use a body lotion or oil if you like. The massage should involve gentle exploration of all parts of the body except the genital and breast areas. The partner being caressed should concentrate on finding pleasure from being touched, and the partner giving the caresses should concentrate on his or her own pleasure from contact with the partner's body. Once you have got over any awkwardness and are finding enjoyment from the sensations you experience during this activity — this may take several sessions — go on to stage 2.

Stage 2

Stage 2 is similar to stage 1, but this time body massage may include genital and breast areas. Remember, however, to continue to include other parts of the body in your caresses, so that direct sexual stimulation can be felt in context with other body sensations.

Stage 3

Most couples find that soon after reaching stage 2 they are ready to resume sexual intercourse, and in most cases find that they are more relaxed and are more able to enjoy a full range of physical and emotional sexual feelings. Couples who still are experiencing difficulties may want to consult a marital counselor or sex therapist.

Go to next page

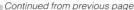

Continued from previous page

Does your vagina feel dry and tight so that penetration is difficult and painful?

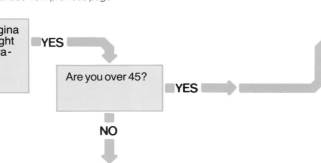

YES → **Are you over 45?** — **YES** →

NO ↓

NO ↓

Hormonal changes around the time of the *menopause* (p.252) can cause the lining of the vagina to become thinner and less well lubricated, and this often makes intercourse uncomfortable. Consult your physician.

Treatment: Your physician will examine you and, depending on whether you are suffering from additional menopausal symptoms and on the state of your general health, may prescribe hormone replacement therapy (see *The menopause,* p. 252) and/or recommend that you use a lubricating jelly. He or she may also advise you and your partner on sexual techniques to assist arousal and prevent discomfort. See also *Sex in later life,* below.

Sexual anxiety and/or lack of arousal can lead to tension during lovemaking that prevents normal lubrication of the vagina and relaxation of the surrounding muscles and tissues. Anxiety can arise out of a specific difficulty experienced by you or your partner, or may be the result of generalized stress within the relationship.

Self-help: Discuss the problem with your partner. You may find that talking openly about the difficulty is in itself enough to reduce tension and help overcome the problem. Use of a lubricating jelly during intercourse may be helpful. You could also try the advice given opposite on reducing sexual anxiety. If the problem persists, consult your physician. He or she will examine you to rule out the possibility of a physical cause for your difficulty and may, if necessary, arrange for you and your partner to receive *sex counseling* (p.268). See also chart 135, *Loss of interest in sex.*

Do you feel pain during intercourse only occasionally or only in certain positions?

YES →

NO ↓

Endometriosis, a disorder in which uterine lining tissue forms outside the uterus, is a possible, although rare, cause of increased pain during periods and pain during intercourse. Consult your physician.

Treatment: Your physician will probably do a *vaginal examination* (p.258) and may arrange for you to have a *laparoscopy* (p.272). If you are found to have endometriosis, you may be given long-term hormone treatment.

A cyst (fluid-filled sac) of an ovary can sometimes cause pain if touched during intercourse. Such cysts may also cause abdominal swelling. Alternatively, such pain may be due to inflammation (erosion) of the cervix. Consult your physician.

Treatment: Your physician will examine your abdomen and probably do a *vaginal examination* (p.258). He or she may do a cervical smear (Pap) test (see *Cervical screening,* p.257) and may arrange for you to have tests such as an *ultrasound scan* (p.276) and possibly a *laparoscopy* (p.272). If you are found to have an ovarian cyst, you may need to have an operation to remove it. This can sometimes be done without damaging the ovary, but in other cases it is necessary to remove the ovary and perhaps the fallopian tube as well. However, if the remaining ovary is healthy, you will still be able to have children. If you have a cervical erosion, it may be treated by laser, freezing or a minor operation.

Pressure on an ovary or on another tender spot during deep penetration may be the cause of such pain. If you have always noticed such pain when you have intercourse in a certain position, this is unlikely to be a cause for concern and simply trying alternative positions may overcome the problem. However, it is wise to mention the symptom to your physician, who may examine you to rule out the possibility of an underlying disorder.

Have you just started your first or a new sexual relationship?

YES →

NO ↓

Bruising and soreness of the genital area commonly follows unaccustomed or unusually enthusiastic sex. This is no cause for concern and the discomfort will soon pass. If soreness is severe, abstaining from sex for a day or so may help.

Consult your physician if you are unable to make a diagnosis from this chart.

SEX IN LATER LIFE

Most women who have enjoyed an active and happy sex life in the first part of their lives continue to do so during middle and old age. Provided your relationship with your partner is sound, there is no physical reason why your capacity for enjoying the full range of physical and emotional sexual feelings should be diminished. In a loving relationship there is no reason why the physical changes associated with aging should reduce the attraction you and your partner feel for each other. Many women find their sex lives improve with greater experience and more leisure to enjoy their partner's company, and without the fear of pregnancy.

Possible problems
Although many women have no sex difficulties as they grow older, problems may arise. A common complaint of women past the menopause is discomfort during intercourse as a result of reduced vaginal lubrication. In the short term, this can sometimes be helped by hormone replacement therapy (see *The menopause,* p. 252). In the longer term, use of a lubricating jelly and adapting new and different lovemaking techniques are usually the best solutions.

Obviously, if either partner has a disabling disease, this can inhibit sexual relations. In such cases experimenting with different positions and a variety of forms of sexual contact – for example, mutual caresses and oral sex – can be helpful. You should not be embarrassed to seek your physician's advice.

Some women who have experienced sexual difficulties in the past use their advancing years as an excuse for avoiding sex altogether in later life. (Men commonly find it may take longer to achieve an erection and to ejaculate. This is normal and need not be cause for alarm.) This is no cause for concern if both partners are happy not to have sex, but if a reduction in sexual activity causes unhappiness in either partner, it is never too late to seek *sex counseling* (p. 268) for this or any other sex problem.

135 Loss of interest in sex

The frequency with which a woman feels the need for sex is determined by a range of inborn psychological and physiological factors, as well as being affected by experiences in early life. Some women feel the need for sex every day, others only once or twice a week or less. Both ends of the spectrum are normal. Once a normal pattern exists, changes may be questioned. A sudden falling off in the frequency of your normal level of sexual desire may be a sign of a number of problems. There may be a physical cause – for example, sickness or an infection that makes intercourse painful. Or the cause may be emotional – for example, overwork, depression, anxiety about a specific sexual difficulty or discord within the relationship. Consult this chart if you are aware of a reduction in the frequency with which you want sex and/or if you notice that you are not as easily aroused as you used to be, leading to discomfort during intercourse.

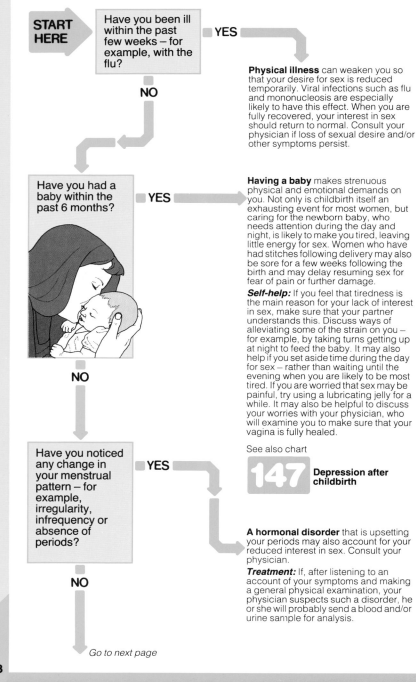

START HERE

Have you been ill within the past few weeks – for example, with the flu?

YES →

NO

Physical illness can weaken you so that your desire for sex is reduced temporarily. Viral infections such as flu and mononucleosis are especially likely to have this effect. When you are fully recovered, your interest in sex should return to normal. Consult your physician if loss of sexual desire and/or other symptoms persist.

Have you had a baby within the past 6 months?

YES →

NO

Having a baby makes strenuous physical and emotional demands on you. Not only is childbirth itself an exhausting event for most women, but caring for the newborn baby, who needs attention during the day and night, is likely to make you tired, leaving little energy for sex. Women who have had stitches following delivery may also be sore for a few weeks following the birth and may delay resuming sex for fear of pain or further damage.

Self-help: If you feel that tiredness is the main reason for your lack of interest in sex, make sure that your partner understands this. Discuss ways of alleviating some of the strain on you – for example, by taking turns getting up at night to feed the baby. It may also help if you set aside time during the day for sex – rather than waiting until the evening when you are likely to be most tired. If you are worried that sex may be painful, try using a lubricating jelly for a while. It may also be helpful to discuss your worries with your physician, who will examine you to make sure that your vagina is fully healed.

See also chart

147 **Depression after childbirth**

Have you noticed any change in your menstrual pattern – for example, irregularity, infrequency or absence of periods?

YES →

NO

A hormonal disorder that is upsetting your periods may also account for your reduced interest in sex. Consult your physician.

Treatment: If, after listening to an account of your symptoms and making a general physical examination, your physician suspects such a disorder, he or she will probably send a blood and/or urine sample for analysis.

Go to next page

SEX COUNSELING

Sex counseling can take many different forms. Some family physicians have experience in dealing with the more common types of sexual difficulty and, if you are suffering from a problem in your sexual relationships, you should first consult your own physician for advice. Depending on the nature of the problem and his or her experience in this field, your physician may suggest treatment or may refer you to a specialist sex counselor or another physician who specializes in this field. Some large medical practices have sex counselors associated with them. In other cases you may be referred to a clinic, hospital outpatient department or private office.

Treatments for sexual difficulties
Treatments for all types of sexual difficulty have a greater chance of success if both partners attend counseling sessions. Usually, a course of counseling starts with a discussion with the counselor about the nature of the problem. In many cases this provides a couple with their first experience of talking together frankly about their sexual feelings, and this is often in itself of great help in clearing up misunderstandings and reducing anxiety. The counselor may later suggest techniques for overcoming specific difficulties or he or she may give more generalized advice on sexual technique. The counselor will also, if necessary, guide you through a prolonged therapy program to be carried out at home, such as the sensate focus technique described under *Reducing sexual anxiety* (p.266).
The success rate is high for couples who overcome their embarrassment sufficiently to seek sex counseling. So, even if you feel that your problem is unsolvable, it is worthwhile to seek your physician's advice.

Partners take part in sex counseling together.

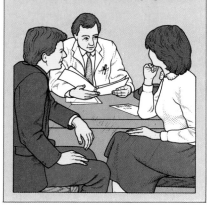

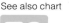

Continued from previous page

Have you any reason to feel under stress – for example, are you having problems at work or upheavals at home?

■ **YES**

Generalized stress (see *What is stress?* p.175) can easily affect your desire for sex. Once the cause of worry has been dealt with, you should find that your interest in sex revives. Meanwhile, make sure that your partner understands your feelings. If your difficulties cannot easily be resolved, or if your interest in sex does not return to normal, consult your physician.

See also chart

 Anxiety

NO

Have you been feeling low or "blue" lately?

■ **YES**

Depression is a possible cause of loss of interest in sex.

Go to chart

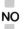 **Depression**

NO

Are you worried that you may become pregnant?

■ **YES**

Fear of pregnancy can cause some women to reject sex. Consult your physician.

Treatment: Your physician will discuss your fears with you and recommend the most reliable method of contraception in your case. There are several forms of contraception that provide excellent protection against pregnancy if used properly (see *Choosing a contraceptive method,* p. 271). If your physician is unable to allay your fears, or if reliable contraception is unsuitable or unacceptable in your case, he or she may refer you for specialized counseling.

NO

Do you or your partner have a specific sexual difficulty?

■ **YES**

Sexual difficulties – for example, failure to achieve orgasm in a woman, or premature ejaculation in a man – can often cause one or both partners to lose interest in sex. Consult your physician.

Treatment: Your physician will want to discuss the problem with both you and your partner. Depending on the nature of the underlying difficulty, he or she may offer advice and treatment, and/or refer you for specialized *sex counseling* (opposite).

NO

Do you have any other cause for discontent in your relationship?

YES ▷

NO

Do you fail to become aroused only by your regular partner?

■ **YES**

NO

Loss of interest in a sexual relationship, once the excitement and novelty have worn off, is a common cause of loss of sexual desire.

Self-help: It may help to talk openly with your partner about how you feel so that there is no misunderstanding. If the relationship is a long-standing one and sound in every other way, try to inject new life into it – for example, by going away on a vacation together or cooperating in some new venture. You may find adopting new approaches to lovemaking may be helpful. If these suggestions do not improve matters, consult your physician, who may recommend *sex counseling* (opposite).

Do you fail to be aroused by men, but find you are sexually attracted to other women?

■ **YES**

Homosexuality – being sexually attracted only to those of the same sex – is a sexual preference for some of the population. While many homosexual women (lesbians) are aware of their orientation from adolescence, others do not recognize their homosexuality until much later. See *Sexual orientation,* right.

NO

Consult your physician if you are unable to make a diagnosis from this chart.

Generalized antagonism or specific disagreements can lead to tension in a relationship that also affects your sexual feelings for each other.

Self-help: Talk to each other and explain how the problems with your relationship are affecting your feelings. If you find that things do not improve after a full and frank discussion, consult your physician. He or she will probably examine you to rule out any underlying physical problem, and may suggest that you and your partner seek counseling about your general difficulties, and possibly *sex counseling* (opposite) for any specific sex problems you may have.

SEXUAL ORIENTATION

Sexual orientation – that is, whether you are heterosexual (attracted to people of the opposite sex), homosexual (attracted to people of the same sex) or bi-sexual (attracted to people of both sexes) – is probably determined by a combination of in-born personality traits, upbringing and family relationships. Some researchers have suggested that there may be hormonal factors that contribute to homosexuality, but these findings have not been generally accepted. Few people are wholly heterosexual or homosexual. In particular, it is common for adolescents to go through a phase of experiencing homosexual feelings before becoming attracted to people of the opposite sex. Some, however, remain homosexual in their sexual preferences. This variation from the mainly heterosexual orientation of the majority is no cause for medical concern among most physicians as long as the individual woman is happy with her homosexuality. Treatment to change sexual orientation is unlikely to be effective and is seldom recommended. However, society's attitude toward homosexuality frequently causes homosexuals to feel guilty and abnormal, and therefore leads them to repress their sexual feelings. This can be psychologically damaging. If you think that you are homosexual and are experiencing such problems, consult your physician, who may be able to offer helpful advice and/or refer you for counseling or to one of the organizations that specializes in advising homosexuals.

136 Choosing a contraceptive method

Although no method of preventing pregnancy is problem-free, most couples can find a method that suits them. In most relationships it is the woman who takes responsibility for contraception. This is probably because a woman who wants to be sure of avoiding pregnancy is likely to be more confident with a method that she controls herself, and because there are more contraceptive choices available to women. However, some methods of contraception carry slight risks, so a couple in a stable relationship may wish to consider the

male options that are available. In evaluating the risks of birth control, it is important to realize that pregnancy itself has substantial medical risks. This self-diagnosis chart is intended as a broad guide to help you decide which methods may be most suitable in your case, but the right contraceptive decision can only be reached through careful discussion with your physician and your partner, taking into account the possible side effects and risks of each method and your attitude toward an unplanned pregnancy.

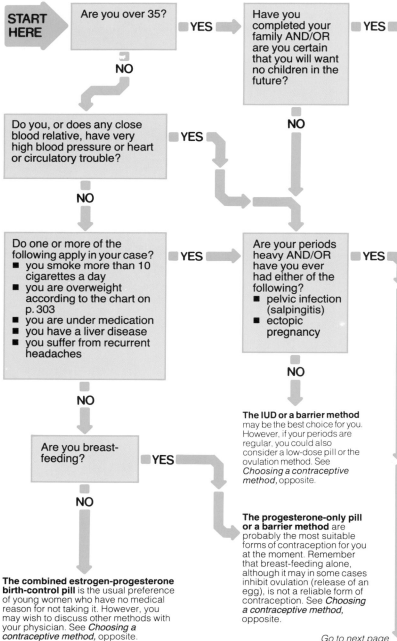

START HERE

Are you over 35?

YES →

Have you completed your family AND/OR are you certain that you will want no children in the future?

YES →

Sterilization, either for you or your partner, may be worth considering (see *Sterilization,* below). If this option is not acceptable to you, answer "No" to the previous question and follow the pathway.

NO ↓

NO ↓

Do you, or does any close blood relative, have very high blood pressure or heart or circulatory trouble?

YES →

NO ↓

Do one or more of the following apply in your case?
- you smoke more than 10 cigarettes a day
- you are overweight according to the chart on p. 303
- you are under medication
- you have a liver disease
- you suffer from recurrent headaches

YES →

Are your periods heavy AND/OR have you ever had either of the following?
- pelvic infection (salpingitis)
- ectopic pregnancy

YES →

NO ↓

NO ↓

Are you breast-feeding?

YES →

The IUD or a barrier method may be the best choice for you. However, if your periods are regular, you could also consider a low-dose pill or the ovulation method. See *Choosing a contraceptive method,* opposite.

NO ↓

The progesterone-only pill or a barrier method are probably the most suitable forms of contraception for you at the moment. Remember that breast-feeding alone, although it may in some cases inhibit ovulation (release of an egg), is not a reliable form of contraception. See *Choosing a contraceptive method,* opposite.

The combined estrogen-progesterone birth-control pill is the usual preference of young women who have no medical reason for not taking it. However, you may wish to discuss other methods with your physician. See *Choosing a contraceptive method,* opposite.

Go to next page

STERILIZATION

Sterilization is almost always a permanent form of contraception. For this reason it is not a contraceptive option that should be chosen without careful consideration. Usually, couples thinking about sterilization are offered counseling before reaching a final decision. You will need to consider not only your present situation, but also the possibility that your life-style might change (for example, through divorce or death of a partner). Those under 35 are generally discouraged from undertaking such a final step. Sterilization may, however, be a good solution for an older couple who have completed their family or for a couple for whom pregnancy presents a serious risk.

Female sterilization
The usual method of sterilization for women is tubal ligation. This procedure is usually done under general anesthesia and is carried out using a laparoscope (see *Laparoscopy,* p. 272). Each fallopian tube is clipped, tied and sealed off, preventing eggs from traveling down the tubes. Recovery usually takes only a few days and there are no lasting side effects. Sterilization has no documented effect on the production of female sex hormones, sexual desire or performance, or menstrual periods, although some women have claimed it has changed their menstrual cycle. You may find that it may take a little while to adjust psychologically to your loss of fertility.

Male sterilization
Male sterilization is achieved through a vasectomy. It is a simpler operation than that required for female sterilization and, because it does not require an abdominal incision, carries fewer risks. Usually, 2 small incisions are made in the scrotum and each vas deferens is cut and sealed so that sperm produced in the testicles can no longer pass out of the body. Because sperm may remain in the male reproductive system for several months, you will need to take additional contraceptive precautions until test results confirm that the seminal fluid is free of sperm. A vasectomy has no effect on sexual performance or ejaculation.

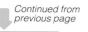

Continued from previous page

Are your periods regular?

YES

NO

A barrier method could be the best method for you. See *Choosing a contraceptive method*, below.

A barrier method or the ovulation method may be suitable options in your case. If you are a nonsmoker and are free of other medical problems, a low-dose pill also may be suitable. See *Choosing a contraceptive method*, below.

MULTIPLE SEX PARTNERS

There are certain medical risks associated with having sex with a number of partners. The chief risk is that of contracting a sexually transmitted disease (STD, p.259). There is also evidence that women who have many sex partners have a greater-than-average risk of developing cancer of the cervix, especially if they started having sex in their teens. This is because the viruses that are now thought to cause cervical cancer may be sexually transmitted. There are precautions you can take to reduce the risk of infection and cervical abnormalities.

- Encourage your partner to wear a condom, whether or not you are using other precautions. This may help to prevent the transmission of infection and may protect the cervix. Use of a diaphragm may reduce the likelihood of cervical abnormalities.
- Make sure you have regular Pap smears (p.257.)
- Report any suspicious symptoms to your physician at once. If one of your partners mentions that he has had an infection, consult your physician.
- Avoid IUDs, as they seem to increase the risk of pelvic infection. Birth-control pills and barrier methods may offer some protection against some STDs (p.259.)

ELECTIVE ABORTION

If you discover that you are pregnant and you do not want to be, you should discuss this with your physician immediately. Planned Parenthood or a local family planning clinic may be able to offer advice also.

Methods of elective abortion
Elective abortion is best carried out before the 14th week of pregnancy when the usual procedure is similar to a *D and C* (p.254). After 14 weeks you may undergo a similar procedure or be given prostaglandin by vaginal suppository, which stimulates the uterus to contract (as if in labor) and expel the fetus. Other riskier methods exist for more advanced pregnancies.

CHOOSING A CONTRACEPTIVE METHOD

Combined estrogen-progesterone pills

How do they act?
There are many different types of combined pills containing various dosages of estrogen and progesterone. They all act primarily by increasing the level of estrogen and progesterone in the body, which prevents the release of an egg (ovulation).

For whom are they recommended?
The combined pills are usually recommended for young women. They are particularly useful for those who suffer from painful or heavy periods. They are not usually advised for women over 35, who smoke, are overweight, who suffer from migraines, or who have a history of circulatory disorders (e.g., phlebitis), high blood pressure, or heart or liver disease.

Medical supervision
The combined pills are available only on prescription from your physician or family planning clinic. You will need to have regular medical checkups (usually every 6 months).

Possible side effects and risks
Possible side effects include headaches, an increase in blood pressure, depression, loss of sex drive, weight gain, breast fullness, stroke, gallstones and benign liver tumors. The combined pills may cause "spotting" between periods (breakthrough bleeding). If this is a nuisance, you may need to change your prescription. Occasionally it may take several months for ovulation to restart after stopping these pills. The main medical risk associated with prolonged use of these pills is that of circulatory problems. In particular, there seems to be an increase in the frequency of blood clots (thromboembolisms) in regular pill-takers.

Progesterone-only pill

How does it act?
The progesterone-only pill is used infrequently. It increases the level of progesterone in the body, and this may prevent eggs from ripening and being released. Its important contraceptive effect is that it causes thickening of the mucus at the entrance to the cervix, thus preventing penetration by sperm.

For whom is it recommended?
The progesterone-only pill is usually recommended for women who want to use an oral contraceptive but for whom an estrogen-containing pill is unsuitable for any reason. In particular, it is useful for breast-feeding mothers because it does not reduce milk production. Because this type of pill needs to be taken at precisely the same time each day to be effective, it may not be suitable for those who have an irregular life-style or who tend to be forgetful.

Medical supervision
Same as for the combined estrogen-progesterone birth-control pills.

Possible side effects and risks
There is a likelihood of irregular periods and "spotting" between periods (breakthrough bleeding).

Postcoital ("morning-after") pill

How does it act?
The postcoital pill contains estrogen or combined estrogen-progestin which, taken (usually in 2 separate doses) following intercourse without contraception, provokes a shedding of the uterine lining. This expels the egg and so prevents a pregnancy from developing. This should not be used as a major form of contraception.

For whom is it recommended?
The postcoital pill is usually used only in unusual circumstances (for rape victims or when couples have a single, unprotected episode, e.g., a damaged condom). Since the hormones are potentially hazardous and will fail to interrupt a preexisting pregnancy, "morning-after" contraception is an emergency measure and should not be used as your regular method of contraception.

Medical supervision
The postcoital pill needs to be prescribed by a physician.

Possible side effects and risks
Some women experience nausea for a day or so after taking this type of pill.

Intrauterine contraceptive device (IUD)

How does it act?
The IUD (usually made of plastic and sometimes covered with copper wire) is inserted in the uterus. It prevents a fertilized egg from becoming implanted in the uterus.

For whom is it recommended?
The IUD is usually recommended for women in stable relationships who need effective and convenient contraception, but cannot or do not wish to use the combined pill or a barrier device. It may not be suitable for the very young, those who have had an ectopic pregnancy or those who have had pelvic infections. Many physicians feel that women who have never had children should not use the IUD.

Medical supervision
An IUD is prescribed and fitted by a physician. It can be inserted during a normal visit. You will be taught to see that it remains in position and will need to have yearly checkups. Depending on type, an IUD needs to be replaced every 2 to 10 years. The new copper IUDs should be replaced every 3 years.

Possible side effects and risks
Many women notice a slight increase in bleeding and sometimes pain during periods. There is also a slightly increased risk of pelvic infections and of ectopic pregnancy. Occasionally, an IUD may be displaced or expelled from the uterus.

Barrier methods

A barrier method is any device that prevents sperm from entering the uterus and so fertilizing an egg. Barrier methods used by women include the sponge, diaphragm and cervical cap. Both these devices are placed over the entrance to the cervix. Used with spermicidal foam, cream or jelly, they provide an effective barrier to sperm. The condom used by men is also a barrier method. The sponge is a disc-shaped disposable, spermicide-containing barrier that a women places in her vagina. Foam and contraceptive suppositories used alone offer some protection against pregnancy, but are less effective than the diaphragm, sponge or condom.

For whom are they recommended?
Barrier methods are suitable for almost all women, and may be the best methods for women who cannot or do not want to use the pill or IUD. Because a diaphragm, sponge or cap needs to be inserted each time you have intercourse, such methods may not be the best for the very young or those for whom sex is usually unplanned.

Medical supervision
A diaphragm or cap needs to be fitted by a physician or nurse, who will also teach you how to use it properly with spermicides. Yearly checkups are needed. You will also need to have your size checked again if you gain or lose a significant amount of weight or if you have a baby. Condoms, sponges, contraceptive foam and suppositories can be bought over-the-counter.

Possible side effects
There are few adverse side effects, although some women find them inconvenient. A few women are allergic to rubber or to chemicals in spermicides and may need to switch brands. Beneficial side effects of using a barrier method include the possible protection they may provide to the cervix. Barriers, particularly condoms, may offer some protection against sexually transmitted diseases.

Ovulation (rhythm) methods

How do they work?
There are various ovulation methods of birth control, all of which are based on the principle of a woman predicting when ovulation (release of an egg) will occur, allowing her to abstain from sex on fertile days. Ovulation can be predicted by monitoring changes in body temperature and observation of the appearance and consistency of the mucus produced by the cervix (see *The menstrual cycle*, p. 253).

For whom are they recommended?
Women who are reluctant to use internal or barrier methods for personal or religious reasons may find these methods attractive. However, ovulation methods may be unreliable for women whose periods are irregular, and they may be unacceptable to couples who do not wish to abstain from sex for at least 7 days each month.

Medical supervision
Women using ovulation methods of birth control need to be carefully taught (by a physician or other specialist trained in these methods) how to monitor and record the changes that indicate ovulation.

Possible side effects and risks
There are no physical side effects, but ovulation methods can lead to frustration for both partners during the fertile period.

137 Failure to conceive

Consult this chart if you and your partner have been having regular sexual intercourse for more than 12 months without contraception and without your having become pregnant. Failure to conceive may be the result of a problem affecting the woman or man (or both); this chart deals only with possible problems affecting the woman. Female infertility is usually the result of a failure to produce eggs or of a blockage in the fallopian tubes. More rarely, an allergy to your partner's semen may be a factor. Failure to conceive usually requires extensive tests on both partners, usually by a specialist, to find the underlying reason for the problem.

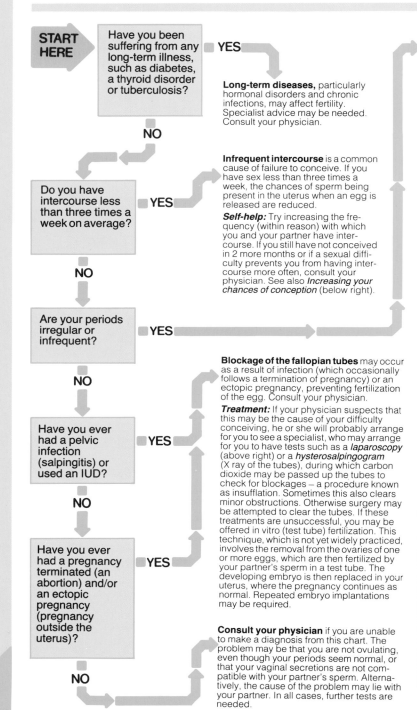

START HERE

Have you been suffering from any long-term illness, such as diabetes, a thyroid disorder or tuberculosis?

YES → **Long-term diseases,** particularly hormonal disorders and chronic infections, may affect fertility. Specialist advice may be needed. Consult your physician.

NO ↓

Do you have intercourse less than three times a week on average?

YES → **Infrequent intercourse** is a common cause of failure to conceive. If you have sex less than three times a week, the chances of sperm being present in the uterus when an egg is released are reduced.
Self-help: Try increasing the frequency (within reason) with which you and your partner have intercourse. If you still have not conceived in 2 more months or if a sexual difficulty prevents you from having intercourse more often, consult your physician. See also *Increasing your chances of conception* (below right).

NO ↓

Are your periods irregular or infrequent?

YES →

NO ↓

Have you ever had a pelvic infection (salpingitis) or used an IUD?

YES → **Blockage of the fallopian tubes** may occur as a result of infection (which occasionally follows a termination of pregnancy) or an ectopic pregnancy, preventing fertilization of the egg. Consult your physician.
Treatment: If your physician suspects that this may be the cause of your difficulty conceiving, he or she will probably arrange for you to see a specialist, who may arrange for you to have tests such as a *laparoscopy* (above right) or a *hysterosalpingogram* (X ray of the tubes), during which carbon dioxide may be passed up the tubes to check for blockages – a procedure known as insufflation. Sometimes this also clears minor obstructions. Otherwise surgery may be attempted to clear the tubes. If these treatments are unsuccessful, you may be offered in vitro (test tube) fertilization. This technique, which is not yet widely practiced, involves the removal from the ovaries of one or more eggs, which are then fertilized by your partner's sperm in a test tube. The developing embryo is then replaced in your uterus, where the pregnancy continues as normal. Repeated embryo implantations may be required.

NO ↓

Have you ever had a pregnancy terminated (an abortion) and/or an ectopic pregnancy (pregnancy outside the uterus)?

YES →

NO ↓

Consult your physician if you are unable to make a diagnosis from this chart. The problem may be that you are not ovulating, even though your periods seem normal, or that your vaginal secretions are not compatible with your partner's sperm. Alternatively, the cause of the problem may lie with your partner. In all cases, further tests are needed.

A hormone imbalance that either prevents ovulation (release of an egg) or reduces the frequency with which you ovulate may explain your failure to conceive. Consult your physician.
Treatment: Your physician may refer you to a specialist for tests and treatment. If the tests, which may include *blood analysis* (p.146), urine analysis, a *D and C* (p.254) and *laparoscopy* (below), show a hormone imbalance, you may be prescribed hormone supplements (fertility drugs).

LAPAROSCOPY

Laparoscopy is an endoscopic technique (see *Endoscopy*, p. 201) for investigating abdominal disorders. In women it is commonly used to discover the cause of gynecological problems such as infertility or to assist in surgical procedures such as *sterilization* (p. 270). Laparoscopy may also be used when other tests such as *barium X rays* (p. 207) and *ultrasound scan* (p. 276) fail to show the cause of symptoms such as recurrent abdominal pain.

The procedure is usually carried out under general anesthetic. Two small slits are made in the abdomen, and carbon dioxide is passed through a hollow needle inserted into one slit to distend the abdomen. An endoscope is inserted into the second slit, enabling the surgeon to see inside and find the cause of the trouble.

PREVIOUS PREGNANCY

If you have been pregnant before by the same or by a different partner, the chances of your present failure to conceive being a result of a problem affecting you are reduced. It is nevertheless possible for any one of the disorders discussed in this chart to develop after a previous pregnancy and therefore complete testing of both partners is still required.

INCREASING YOUR CHANCES OF CONCEPTION

Although prolonged delay in achieving conception requires professional tests and treatment, you may be able to increase your chances of becoming pregnant by following the self-help advice given below:

- Have intercourse about 3 times a week; less frequent intercourse may mean that you miss your fertile days, more frequent intercourse may reduce your partner's sperm count.
- Time intercourse to coincide with your most fertile days (see *The menstrual cycle*, p. 253).
- Discourage your partner from wearing tight-fitting or nylon briefs or undershorts, which may in some cases damage the sperm by increasing the temperature within the scrotum.

Pregnancy and childbirth

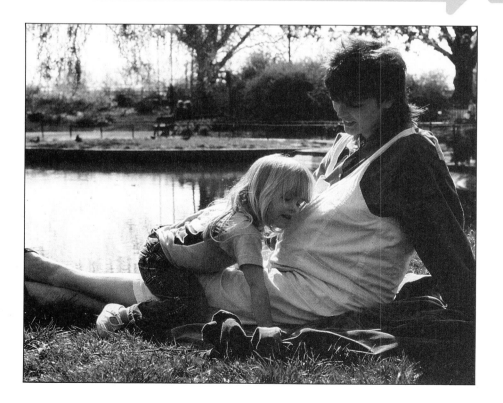

138 Nausea and vomiting in pregnancy

Most women experience some nausea during the first three months of pregnancy and may actually vomit. Usually these symptoms fade after the 12th week, but they may persist. "Morning sickness" is probably the result of the dramatic increase in hormones (estrogen, progesterone and human chorionic gonadotropin [HCG]) during the early part of pregnancy. Although it commonly occurs in the morning, sickness can come at any time of day, especially when you are tired or hungry. Most women learn to control their nausea, but a few need medical treatment.

Consult this diagnostic chart only after reading chart 94, Vomiting.

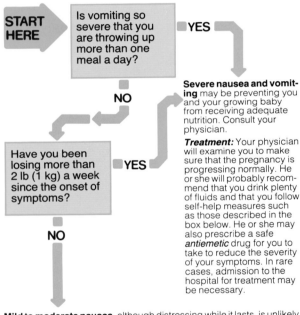

START HERE Is vomiting so severe that you are throwing up more than one meal a day?

YES

NO

Have you been losing more than 2 lb (1 kg) a week since the onset of symptoms?

YES

NO

Severe nausea and vomiting may be preventing you and your growing baby from receiving adequate nutrition. Consult your physician.

Treatment: Your physician will examine you to make sure that the pregnancy is progressing normally. He or she will probably recommend that you drink plenty of fluids and that you follow self-help measures such as those described in the box below. He or she may also prescribe a safe *antiemetic* drug for you to take to reduce the severity of your symptoms. In rare cases, admission to the hospital for treatment may be necessary.

Mild to moderate nausea, although distressing while it lasts, is unlikely to present a risk to your general health or to that of your baby.
Self-help: Try the self-help measures suggested in the box below. If these do not help, and especially if you find that nausea is preventing you from eating so that you are losing weight, consult your physician.

COPING WITH NAUSEA AND VOMITING

The following self-help suggestions may help to reduce the severity of nausea and vomiting during pregnancy:

- Have a light snack – for example, crackers or toast – before you get out of bed in the morning.
- Eat small, frequent meals of foods that seem to agree with you.
- Try to avoid sweet or fatty foods.
- Give up smoking and drinking alcohol.
- Get as much rest as possible.
- Take regular, light exercise in the fresh air.
- Do not take any drugs or over-the-counter medicines without first consulting your physician.

Consult your physician if nausea and vomiting are so severe that you are unable to eat a proper diet or if you are losing weight.

139 Skin changes in pregnancy

The hormonal changes of pregnancy may have a variety of effects on your skin, including changes in color. Some women find that their skin becomes more oily, others find that it becomes drier. Skin conditions (such as eczema) you have suffered from before pregnancy may either improve or get worse. The way in which your skin is affected depends on the balance of hormones and on your basic skin type.

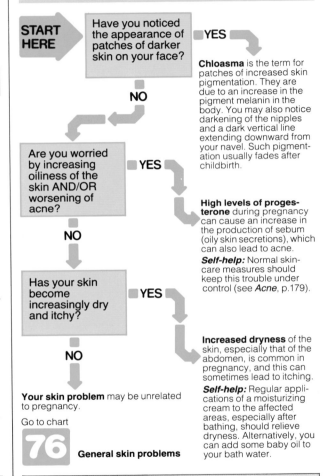

START HERE Have you noticed the appearance of patches of darker skin on your face?

YES

NO

Are you worried by increasing oiliness of the skin AND/OR worsening of acne?

YES

NO

Has your skin become increasingly dry and itchy?

YES

NO

Your skin problem may be unrelated to pregnancy.

Go to chart

76 General skin problems

Chloasma is the term for patches of increased skin pigmentation. They are due to an increase in the pigment melanin in the body. You may also notice darkening of the nipples and a dark vertical line extending downward from your navel. Such pigmentation usually fades after childbirth.

High levels of progesterone during pregnancy can cause an increase in the production of sebum (oily skin secretions), which can also lead to acne.
Self-help: Normal skin-care measures should keep this trouble under control (see *Acne*, p.179).

Increased dryness of the skin, especially that of the abdomen, is common in pregnancy, and this can sometimes lead to itching.
Self-help: Regular applications of a moisturizing cream to the affected areas, especially after bathing, should relieve dryness. Alternatively, you can add some baby oil to your bath water.

STRETCH MARKS

Stretch marks are red marks on the skin that later fade, leaving silvery, scarlike lines. They occur when the skin is stretched beyond its normal range of elasticity when weight is gained rapidly. In pregnancy, stretch marks commonly occur on the breasts and on the abdomen. If too much weight is gained, they may also appear on the thighs, buttocks and upper arms.

Avoiding stretch marks
The best way to reduce your chances of developing stretch marks is to avoid putting on too much weight. However, even those who manage to limit their weight gain to a healthy 20 to 28 lb (9 to 13 kg) may develop some marks. The regular application of any type of cream or oil does not prevent or heal stretch marks, although it may alleviate dryness of the skin.

140 Back pain in pregnancy

Backache is one of the most common symptoms of pregnancy. It usually occurs as a dull pain and stiffness in the middle and lower back and may make it difficult to get up from a sitting or lying position. It is likely to become more troublesome as pregnancy progresses. Most such backaches do not signify any troublesome condition. Occasionally, however, the sudden onset of pain in the back, especially if accompanied by additional symptoms such as vaginal bleeding, may be a sign of an impending miscarriage. Toward the end of a pregnancy, back pain may herald the onset of labor. If you are concerned about a backache, consult your physician.

Consult this diagnostic chart only after reading chart 107, Back pain.

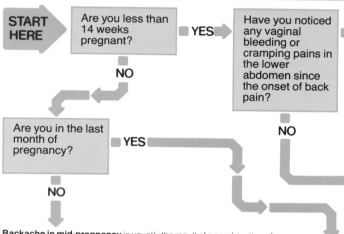

START HERE

Are you less than 14 weeks pregnant? → **YES** → Have you noticed any vaginal bleeding or cramping pains in the lower abdomen since the onset of back pain? → **YES**

NO

Are you in the last month of pregnancy? → **YES**

NO

NO

CALL YOUR PHYSICIAN NOW!
A serious complication, such as an impending miscarriage or ectopic pregnancy (pregnancy outside the uterus), is a possibility.

Treatment: If your physician suspects either of these possibilities, you will probably be admitted to the hospital for rest and tests. If you have an ectopic pregnancy, an operation to end the pregnancy will be carried out. See also *Miscarriage,* p.276.

Relaxation of the ligaments supporting the spine, as a result of hormonal changes, can lead to backache even in early pregnancy. Pressure on the back from the enlarging uterus can also cause pain.
Self-help: Pay attention to the advice given under *Preventing backache* (p.223). You may also find it helpful to try some gentle yoga-style exercises. Consult your physician if pain becomes severe enough to restrict your day-to-day activities.

The start of labor is sometimes marked by the onset of persistent back pain, especially if the pain is different from any backache you have experienced before.
Go to chart

145 Am I in labor?

Backache in mid-pregnancy is usually the result of a combination of relaxation of ligaments supporting the spine (see above right) and changes in posture to accommodate the increasing weight of the baby. Sometimes the enlarging uterus puts pressure on a nerve and you may experience a pain that shoots down the back of a leg (sciatica).
Self-help: Read the suggestions for *preventing backache* on p. 223. Be careful how you lift heavy objects, such as young children. At this stage in your pregnancy, good posture is especially important. You may find prenatal and gentle yoga-style exercises helpful. Consult your physician if pain becomes severe enough to restrict your day-to-day activities.

141 Heartburn in pregnancy

Heartburn, a burning pain in the center of the chest or upper abdomen, is usually caused by the slight backflow of acid juices from the stomach into the esophagus. It is common throughout pregnancy, but may be more severe in the later months when the growing baby and expanding uterus take up more space. Although heartburn may be uncomfortable, it is not a danger to the general health of you or your baby.

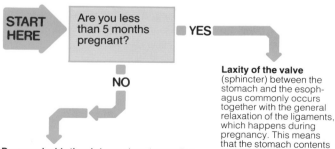

START HERE

Are you less than 5 months pregnant? → **YES**

NO

Laxity of the valve (sphincter) between the stomach and the esophagus commonly occurs together with the general relaxation of the ligaments, which happens during pregnancy. This means that the stomach contents can more easily flow back up into the esophagus, which becomes inflamed, leading to pain (heartburn).
Self-help: See *Self-help for heartburn,* right.

Pressure inside the abdomen from the growing baby during the later stages of pregnancy can cause leakage of the stomach contents back into the esophagus. Laxity of the sphincter between the stomach and esophagus (right) also contributes to this problem, and there may be some degree of *hiatal hernia* (see p. 213).
Self-help: See *Self-help for heartburn,* right.

SELF-HELP FOR HEARTBURN

If you are suffering from heartburn, whatever the stage of your pregnancy, the following self-help measures should help to prevent and relieve the discomfort:

- Avoid eating large meals, especially of fried or highly spiced foods.
- Give up smoking and alcohol.
- Do not wear tight maternity girdles.
- If heartburn is troublesome at night, drink a glass of milk before going to bed and sleep propped up with pillows.
- Do not lie down after meals.

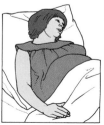

If such self-help measures do not help to alleviate the problem, consult your physician, who may prescribe a safe antacid medicine for you to take.

142 Vaginal bleeding in pregnancy

Consult this chart if you notice any vaginal bleeding while you are pregnant, whether it consists of only slight spotting or more profuse blood loss. This is a serious symptom that should always be reported to your physician promptly, although in a large proportion of cases there is no danger to the pregnancy. If you notice vaginal bleeding, go to bed and rest until you have received medical attention.

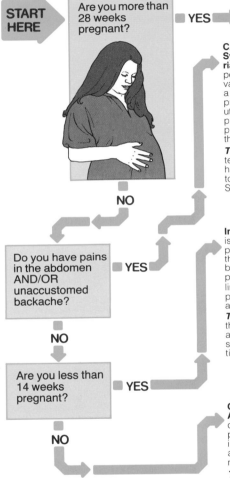

START HERE → **Are you more than 28 weeks pregnant?** — **YES** →

NO ↓

Do you have pains in the abdomen AND/OR unaccustomed backache? — **YES** →

NO ↓

Are you less than 14 weeks pregnant? — **YES** →

NO ↓

CALL YOUR PHYSICIAN NOW!
Symptoms of an impending miscarriage are cramping abdominal pains or persistent backache with accompanying vaginal bleeding. There is, however, also a possibility that you may have an ectopic pregnancy (pregnancy outside the uterus) if you are less than 12 weeks pregnant, particularly if the onset of pain preceded blood loss and is sharp rather than cramping.
Treatment: You will probably be admitted to the hospital for rest and tests. If you have an ectopic pregnancy, an operation to end the pregnancy will be carried out. See also *Miscarriage,* below right.

In early pregnancy, spotting of blood is common and often occurs when a period would have been due and when the level of certain hormones produced by the placenta is not high enough to prevent slight shedding of the uterine lining. Usually there is no risk to the pregnancy, but you should go to bed and consult your physician.
Treatment: If your physician confirms the diagnosis, he or she will probably advise you to rest until the bleeding stops. Hormone supplements are sometimes given.

CALL YOUR PHYSICIAN NOW!
A threatened miscarriage is the usual diagnosis when bleeding occurs without pain in mid pregnancy. However, bleeding may also occur as a result of an abnormality involving the cervix or inflammation of the vagina.
Treatment: See *Miscarriage,* right.

CALL YOUR PHYSICIAN NOW!
Antepartum hemorrhage is the term used to describe any vaginal bleeding in the later stages of pregnancy. It may be due to partial separation of the placenta from the wall of the uterus, especially if the placenta is low-lying, to bleeding from a vein in the vagina or to abnormalities of the cervix. Sometimes the discharge of a blood-stained plug of mucus is the first sign of impending labor (see chart 145, *Am I in labor?*). Spotting in late pregnancy can be due to simple stretching of the cervix and may not be serious. However, your physician should be consulted.
Treatment: Your physician is likely to recommend a careful examination and tests, which may include an ultrasound scan (below left). Often no treatment other than bed rest is needed but, if bleeding is severe or continues, you may need to be delivered early by induction of labor (p. 278) or cesarean section.

MISCARRIAGE

Miscarriage (spontaneous abortion) is the expulsion of the embryo or fetus from the uterus before the 28th week of pregnancy. It occurs in a high proportion of pregnancies, often before a woman knows that she is pregnant.

Causes
The cause of a miscarriage is not always easy to discover. It may sometimes be due to an abnormality of the fetus, or to a hormonal imbalance. Occasionally, miscarriages in mid pregnancy are due to failure of the cervix to hold the fetus inside the uterus (incompetent cervix).

Symptoms
The first sign of a threatened miscarriage is usually vaginal bleeding. Often this bleeding stops and the pregnancy continues as normal. However, bleeding may sometimes be followed by cramping pains in the abdomen or, in some cases, backache.

Treatment
A threatened miscarriage is usually treated by complete bed rest. If there is reason to suspect a hormone deficiency, you may be given hormone supplements. Sometimes hospital admission is advised. If bleeding stops, you may need to have an ultrasound scan (left) to confirm that the pregnancy is continuing normally. If your physician thinks that a miscarriage is inevitable or if you have already lost the baby but some matter remains in the uterus, you will probably be admitted to the hospital, where the contents of the uterus may be removed (see also *D and C*, p.254). Most women who have had a miscarriage are able to conceive again without difficulty and subsequently go through a normal pregnancy.

ULTRASOUND SCAN

Ultrasound provides a safe, painless way of examining internal organs and is often used during pregnancy to examine the uterus, placenta and fetus. The technique involves sending a beam of very high-pitched sound (ultrasound) through the tissues of the body. These sound waves are deflected off the internal organs and converted by computer into a picture that can be seen on a screen or printed on paper. Ultrasound may reveal cysts, tumors or other swellings, and in pregnancy helps to determine the position of the placenta, the size of the fetus and the stage of the pregnancy. Ultrasound scanning can reveal the presence of twins.

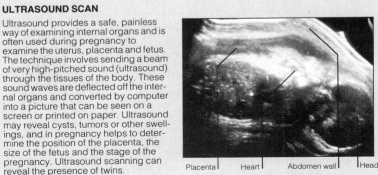

Placenta | Heart | Abdomen wall | Head

Ultrasound picture of fetus at 35 weeks.

143 Shortness of breath in pregnancy

Shortness of breath on exertion is noticed by many women after the 28th week of pregnancy. It is usually caused by restriction of the normal movement of the diaphragm and by restriction of the lungs as a result of the enlarged uterus pushing the abdominal organs up into the chest cavity. Breathlessness is often eased in the last month of pregnancy when the baby's head descends into the pelvis.

Consult this diagnostic chart only after reading chart 90, Difficulty breathing.

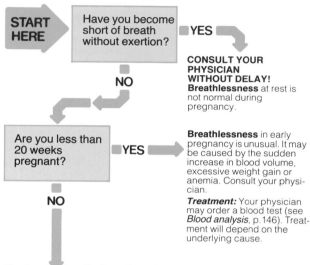

START HERE → **Have you become short of breath without exertion?** → **YES**

CONSULT YOUR PHYSICIAN WITHOUT DELAY! Breathlessness at rest is not normal during pregnancy.

NO ↓

Are you less than 20 weeks pregnant? → **YES**

Breathlessness in early pregnancy is unusual. It may be caused by the sudden increase in blood volume, excessive weight gain or anemia. Consult your physician.

Treatment: Your physician may order a blood test (see *Blood analysis*, p.146). Treatment will depend on the underlying cause.

NO ↓

Shortness of breath after only moderate exertion is normal after the 28th week of pregnancy, and may occasionally occur earlier, especially if you are physically unfit, if you have gained too much weight or if you smoke.

Self-help: You can take steps to minimize breathlessness in late pregnancy. Try to control wieght gain, give up smoking and avoid tight clothes and girdles that constrict the abdomen. Consult your physician if breathlessness is severe enough to restrict your daily activities or if you are also feeling unusually tired or sick.

PRENATAL CHECKUPS

If you are pregnant, go to your physician for regular checkups, where progress will be carefully monitored. In addition to a physical examination to assess the size of the uterus and the position of the fetus, the following tests are carried out:

- **Weight gain** Regular weighing enables you and your physician to ensure that you are putting on enough, but not too much, weight. Most women can expect to gain 20 to 28 lb (9 to 13 kg) during pregnancy. Usually, during the first weeks of pregnancy, little weight is gained and some may be lost (see *Weight loss in pregnancy*, p. 148). After the 12th week, weight is usually gained at the rate of about 1 lb (0.5 kg) a week.
- **Urine** Urine is tested regularly for the presence of protein, which may be a sign of preeclampsia (below) and for the presence of sugar, which may indicate diabetes.
- **Blood pressure** This is tested at every prenatal visit. A sudden rise may be a sign of preeclampsia.
- **Blood tests** At the beginning of pregnancy your blood may be tested to determine whether you have syphilis, are diabetic or have had German measles and whether you may be susceptible to anemia. Black couples may be screened for sickle cell trait. Couples of Jewish extraction may be screened for Tay-Sachs disease. At 16 to 18 weeks, a blood test for malformation of the spinal column in the baby may also be carried out.
- **Ultrasound** Many women will undergo ultrasound screening (see *Ultrasound scan*, opposite).
- **Amniocentesis** In this test a sample of the amniotic fluid surrounding the baby is drawn off by syringe. Analysis of the fluid reveals if the baby is affected by certain abnormalities. This test is normally carried out only when there is a higher-than-average risk of disorders (e.g., if there is a family history of genetic disorder or if the mother is over 35 years old), because it may provoke a miscarriage.

144 Ankle-swelling in pregnancy

During pregnancy the body tends to retain more water than usual. Ankle-swelling is likely to become more marked toward the end of pregnancy. Slight ankle-swelling at the end of the day is usually no cause for concern, but it may occasionally be a sign of excessive fluid retention and high blood pressure.

Consult this chart only after consulting chart 112, Painful or swollen joints.

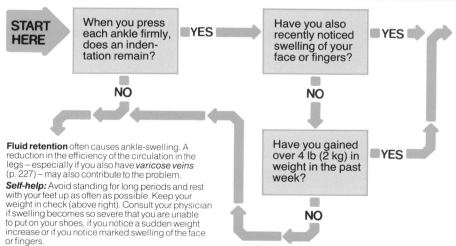

START HERE → **When you press each ankle firmly, does an indentation remain?** → **YES** → **Have you also recently noticed swelling of your face or fingers?** → **YES**

NO ↓ ... **NO** ↓

Have you gained over 4 lb (2 kg) in weight in the past week? → **YES**

NO ↓

CONSULT YOUR PHYSICIAN WITHOUT DELAY! Preeclampsia is a condition in which blood pressure rises, excessive fluid is retained and protein leaks into the urine. It may cause ankle-swelling, especially if accompanied by swelling elsewhere or sudden weight gain. Preeclampsia needs prompt treatment because it may develop into eclampsia (toxemia), in which blood pressure reaches such high levels that the health of mother and baby is threatened.

Treatment: Your physician will take your blood pressure and also a urine sample. If your physician diagnoses preeclampsia, you may be advised to rest and may be given diuretics and/or medication to reduce blood pressure. You also may be advised to limit your salt intake. If your symptoms are severe, hospital admission may be necessary and your baby may need to be delivered early by *induction of labor* (p. 278) or cesarean section.

Fluid retention often causes ankle-swelling. A reduction in the efficiency of the circulation in the legs – especially if you also have *varicose veins* (p. 227) – may also contribute to the problem.

Self-help: Avoid standing for long periods and rest with your feet up as often as possible. Keep your weight in check (above right). Consult your physician if swelling becomes so severe that you are unable to put on your shoes, if you notice a sudden weight increase or if you notice marked swelling of the face or fingers.

145 Am I in labor?

The average duration of pregnancy is 40 weeks, but it is quite normal for a baby to be born as early as 36 weeks or as late as 42 weeks. The onset of labor – the series of events leading to the expulsion of the baby from the uterus – is heralded by a number of different signs, including abdominal or back pains, rupture of the amniotic sac (the "bag of waters") and the passage of a plug of thick,

perhaps blood-stained, mucus. The symptoms of labor experienced by each woman and the order in which they appear may vary. The diagnostic chart is designed to help you decide whether or not the symptoms you are experiencing indicate that labor has started and how urgently you should notify your physician or hospital.

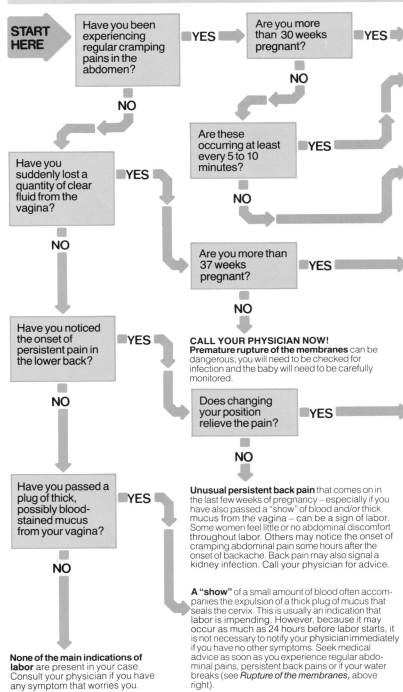

START HERE

Have you been experiencing regular cramping pains in the abdomen?

YES → Are you more than 30 weeks pregnant? **YES** →

CALL YOUR PHYSICIAN NOW!
Premature labor can often be stopped if you seek immediate medical attention.

NO ↓ (from "Are you more than 30 weeks pregnant?")

CALL YOUR PHYSICIAN NOW!
Regular contractions of the muscles of the uterus are the principal indication that labor is established. Rupture of the membranes (below) and the passage of the mucus plug from the cervix may occur before contractions start or, sometimes, after. Your physician or hospital will advise you on what further action to take.

NO ↓ (from "Have you been experiencing regular cramping pains in the abdomen?")

Have you suddenly lost a quantity of clear fluid from the vagina?

Are these occurring at least every 5 to 10 minutes? **YES** →

Early labor may be signaled by intermittent cramping pains in the abdomen caused by contraction of the uterine muscles. Contractions will become stronger and more frequent. Ask your physician what to do when contractions are regular. First labors are often very slow; subsequent births can be rapid. Call your physician if your membranes have ruptured, releasing clear fluid from the vagina.

NO ↓ (from "Are these occurring at least every 5 to 10 minutes?")

YES → (from "Have you suddenly lost a quantity of clear fluid from the vagina?")

NO ↓

Are you more than 37 weeks pregnant? **YES** →

Rupture of the membranes ("breaking of the waters") – bursting of the fluid-filled amniotic sac, which encloses the baby – usually occurs early in labor but may sometimes happen several hours before the uterus starts to contract. Contact your physician when this happens. You may be admitted to the hospital or be instructed to wait for labor to begin. When rupture of the membranes occurs and the uterus does not start to contract spontaneously, *induction of labor* (below) is usually recommended. Rupture of the membranes before the start of labor does not have any effect on the level of pain you will experience.

NO ↓ (from "Are you more than 37 weeks pregnant?")

Have you noticed the onset of persistent pain in the lower back?

YES →

CALL YOUR PHYSICIAN NOW!
Premature rupture of the membranes can be dangerous; you will need to be checked for infection and the baby will need to be carefully monitored.

NO ↓ (from "Have you noticed the onset of persistent pain in the lower back?")

Does changing your position relieve the pain? **YES** →

Low back pain that is relieved by changing your position is unlikely on its own to be an indication that labor has started. However, if you are more than 36 weeks pregnant and you have suffered from continuous backache for more than an hour, or if you have also passed a "show" of blood and/or thick mucus from the vagina, call your physician or hospital for advice. See also chart 140, *Back pain in pregnancy.*

NO ↓ (from "Does changing your position relieve the pain?")

Have you passed a plug of thick, possibly blood-stained mucus from your vagina?

YES →

Unusual persistent back pain that comes on in the last few weeks of pregnancy – especially if you have also passed a "show" of blood and/or thick mucus from the vagina – can be a sign of labor. Some women feel little or no abdominal discomfort throughout labor. Others may notice the onset of cramping abdominal pain some hours after the onset of backache. Back pain may also signal a kidney infection. Call your physician for advice.

NO ↓ (from "Have you passed a plug of thick, possibly blood-stained mucus from your vagina?")

A "show" of a small amount of blood often accompanies the expulsion of a thick plug of mucus that seals the cervix. This is usually an indication that labor is impending. However, because it may occur as much as 24 hours before labor starts, it is not necessary to notify your physician immediately if you have no other symptoms. Seek medical advice as soon as you experience regular abdominal pains, persistent back pains or if your water breaks (see *Rupture of the membranes,* above right).

None of the main indications of labor are present in your case. Consult your physician if you have any symptom that worries you.

INDUCTION OF LABOR

If labor does not start spontaneously by the 42nd week of pregnancy, or if your physician considers it dangerous for you or your baby for the pregnancy to continue, you may be advised to have the delivery of the baby induced.

What happens
Labor may be induced by a hormone called oxytocin given intravenously. Alternatively, a vaginal gel or suppository containing prostaglandins may be given to soften and dilate the cervix, or the amniotic sac may be broken (artificial rupture of the membranes). Occasionally, if these procedures fail to bring about delivery or if your or the baby's medical condition requires very rapid delivery, a cesarean section will be performed.

146 Breast-feeding problems

Medical authorities agree that breast milk is the best form of nutrition for newborn babies. It contains all the essential nutrients in their ideal proportions and in the most easily assimilated form for your baby. Breast-fed babies develop fewer allergies than babies fed on formula and are less subject to gastroenteritis. Antibodies (substances that fight infection) are present in breast milk and provide some natural protection for your baby against germs in the newborn period. It is rare for a mother to be medically unable to breast-feed, and any problems can be overcome with perseverance on your part and support and encouragement from your physician and family. Consult this chart if you have had a baby in the past few months and have any problems related to breast-feeding such as pain, engorged breasts, or inadequate milk supply.

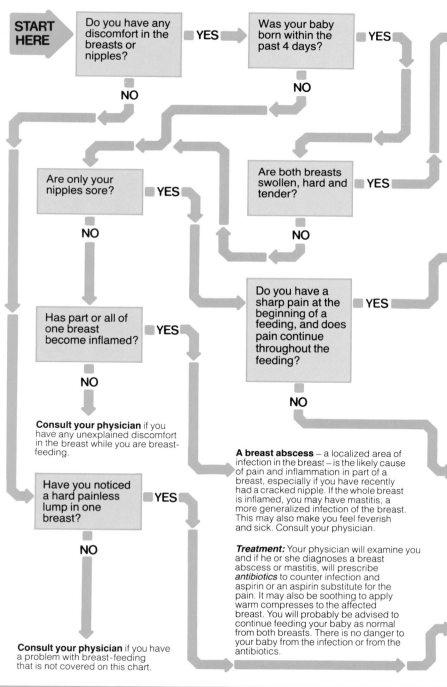

START HERE

Do you have any discomfort in the breasts or nipples? — YES → Was your baby born within the past 4 days? — YES →

NO ↓

Are only your nipples sore? — YES →

NO ↓

Has part or all of one breast become inflamed? — YES →

NO ↓

Consult your physician if you have any unexplained discomfort in the breast while you are breast-feeding.

Have you noticed a hard painless lump in one breast? — YES →

NO ↓

Consult your physician if you have a problem with breast-feeding that is not covered on this chart.

Was your baby born within the past 4 days? — NO ↓

Are both breasts swollen, hard and tender? — YES →

NO ↓

Do you have a sharp pain at the beginning of a feeding, and does pain continue throughout the feeding? — YES →

NO ↓

A breast abscess – a localized area of infection in the breast – is the likely cause of pain and inflammation in part of a breast, especially if you have recently had a cracked nipple. If the whole breast is inflamed, you may have mastitis, a more generalized infection of the breast. This may also make you feel feverish and sick. Consult your physician.

Treatment: Your physician will examine you and if he or she diagnoses a breast abscess or mastitis, will prescribe *antibiotics* to counter infection and aspirin or an aspirin substitute for the pain. It may also be soothing to apply warm compresses to the affected breast. You will probably be advised to continue feeding your baby as normal from both breasts. There is no danger to your baby from the infection or from the antibiotics.

Engorgement is the term used to describe excessive fullness of the breasts. It is common when the milk starts to come in around the third day after the birth. This can make it difficult for your baby to take the whole nipple into his or her mouth, and this can lead to soreness of the nipple.

Self-help: Continue to feed as often as your baby seems to want. You can make it easier for your baby to take the nipple by expressing a little milk at the start of each feeding. But you should be careful not to express too much as this will only stimulate the breast to produce more milk. Warm baths or warm compresses on the breasts may help to relieve the discomfort of breast fullness. In most cases, engorgement usually ceases within a week. Consult your physician if engorgement continues for more than 2 weeks.

A crack around the base of the nipple is possible. This is usually caused by the baby failing to take the whole of the colored area of the nipple into the mouth when he or she is feeding. This may also cause bleeding.

Self-help: Do not allow the baby to feed from the affected breast for at least 24 hours because of the danger of infection entering the breast through the crack. Instead, express milk from the affected breast and feed it to your baby by bottle. It may help if you apply a lanolin ointment to the nipple. Once the crack has healed you can return to normal feeding, but try to prevent the problem from recurring by ensuring that your baby is latching on to the whole of the nipple when he or she sucks. Consult your physician if you notice pain or redness in the breast itself, or if the crack has not healed within 3 days.

Soreness of the nipples is common, especially in the first 2 weeks following the birth. Discomfort is often felt at the start of a feeding as the baby latches on, and it wears off as the feeding continues.

Self-help: At first do not allow your baby to feed for more than 10 minutes on each breast at each feeding. Keep your breasts as dry as possible between feedings by using breast pads inside your bra and changing them frequently. Expose your breasts to the air as often as possible. Regular applications of lanolin ointment may be helpful. Consult your physician if soreness persists.

A blocked milk duct is the most likely explanation for such a lump. This should clear itself within a few days without special treatment and you should continue feeding. Consult your physician if the lump becomes painful or inflamed, or if it persists for more than a week.

147 Depression after childbirth

Childbirth is a traumatic event for a woman, both physically and emotionally. Not only is labor an exhausting physical experience, but it initiates a dramatic alteration in the body's hormone balance as you begin to readjust to no longer being pregnant. Your emotions are also likely to be in turmoil following this event as you start to come to terms with the reality of motherhood and the demands that a new baby will make on you and your family. It is therefore natural that

childbirth should be followed by a period of emotional instability. In the first day or so following the birth the most common feeling is that of elation, but in the subsequent days and sometimes weeks some women become sad, withdrawn, and apathetic, and they may also suffer from guilt that they cannot respond with more enthusiasm to the arrival of their baby. Consult this chart if you suffer from such feelings of depression.

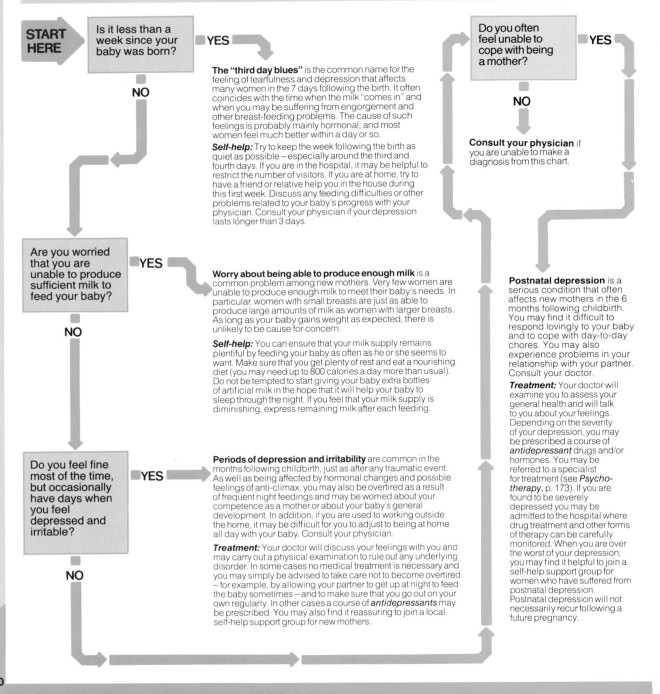

START HERE

Is it less than a week since your baby was born?

YES

The **"third day blues"** is the common name for the feeling of tearfulness and depression that affects many women in the 7 days following the birth. It often coincides with the time when the milk "comes in" and when you may be suffering from engorgement and other breast-feeding problems. The cause of such feelings is probably mainly hormonal, and most women feel much better within a day or so.

Self-help: Try to keep the week following the birth as quiet as possible – especially around the third and fourth days. If you are in the hospital, it may be helpful to restrict the number of visitors. If you are at home, try to have a friend or relative help you in the house during this first week. Discuss any feeding difficulties or other problems related to your baby's progress with your physician. Consult your physician if your depression lasts longer than 3 days.

NO

Are you worried that you are unable to produce sufficient milk to feed your baby?

YES

Worry about being able to produce enough milk is a common problem among new mothers. Very few women are unable to produce enough milk to meet their baby's needs. In particular, women with small breasts are just as able to produce large amounts of milk as women with larger breasts. As long as your baby gains weight as expected, there is unlikely to be cause for concern.

Self-help: You can ensure that your milk supply remains plentiful by feeding your baby as often as he or she seems to want. Make sure that you get plenty of rest and eat a nourishing diet (you may need up to 800 calories a day more than usual). Do not be tempted to start giving your baby extra bottles of artificial milk in the hope that it will help your baby to sleep through the night. If you feel that your milk supply is diminishing, express remaining milk after each feeding.

NO

Do you feel fine most of the time, but occasionally have days when you feel depressed and irritable?

YES

Periods of depression and irritability are common in the months following childbirth, just as after any traumatic event. As well as being affected by hormonal changes and possible feelings of anti-climax, you may also be overtired as a result of frequent night feedings and may be worried about your competence as a mother or about your baby's general development. In addition, if you are used to working outside the home, it may be difficult for you to adjust to being at home all day with your baby. Consult your physician.

Treatment: Your doctor will discuss your feelings with you and may carry out a physical examination to rule out any underlying disorder. In some cases no medical treatment is necessary and you may simply be advised to take care not to become overtired – for example, by allowing your partner to get up at night to feed the baby sometimes – and to make sure that you go out on your own regularly. In other cases a course of **antidepressants** may be prescribed. You may also find it reassuring to join a local self-help support group for new mothers.

NO

Do you often feel unable to cope with being a mother?

YES

NO

Consult your physician if you are unable to make a diagnosis from this chart.

Postnatal depression is a serious condition that often affects new mothers in the 6 months following childbirth. You may find it difficult to respond lovingly to your baby and to cope with day-to-day chores. You may also experience problems in your relationship with your partner. Consult your doctor.

Treatment: Your doctor will examine you to assess your general health and will talk to you about your feelings. Depending on the severity of your depression, you may be prescribed a course of **antidepressant** drugs and/or hormones. You may be referred to a specialist for treatment (see **Psychotherapy**, p. 173). If you are found to be severely depressed you may be admitted to the hospital where drug treatment and other forms of therapy can be carefully monitored. When you are over the worst of your depression, you may find it helpful to join a self-help support group for women who have suffered from postnatal depression. Postnatal depression will not necessarily recur following a future pregnancy.

Useful information

Essential first aid

Caring for a sick child

When you are ill

Health checkups

Medication guide

Children's growth charts

Adult weight tables

Children's medical records

Children's development records

Adult medical records

Useful addresses

Useful telephone numbers

Essential first aid

Many accidental injuries are minor and easily treated with simple first-aid techniques. However, every person should be prepared for the possibility of a more serious accident that may require immediate lifesaving first-aid treatment—perhaps even resuscitation of someone whose breathing has stopped. Accurate and rapid assessment of what must be done is crucial and requires good judgment and common sense. For example, rushing to help a victim of electric shock before eliminating the power source would be dangerous. It is equally important to know what must be done first (see **Emergency checklist,** below right). In any situation, the goals of first aid are to preserve life, to prevent an injury or condition from becoming worse, and to promote recovery. The task of the person administering first aid is to find out what happened without endangering himself or herself, to reassure and protect the affected person from any further danger, to deal with the injury or condition as required, and to arrange for transport home or to the hospital. An ambulance will be needed for anyone who has difficulty breathing, heart failure, or serious burns, or is bleeding severely, unconscious, or in shock, or has been poisoned.

The more knowledge you have, the more useful you can be in an emergency. On the following pages you will find instructions for the major lifesaving techniques. This information cannot substitute for the practical experience you gain if you attend classes in first aid. However, if you become familiar with the techniques described here, you will be able to act more swiftly and efficiently in an emergency situation.

Getting emergency help
Usually, the quickest way to obtain emergency medical treatment is to take the person by car to the emergency department of your local hospital. DO NOT transport an injured person in the following circumstances:

- If the person has a suspected neck or back injury and/or any other injury (such as a broken leg) that makes moving him or her without a stretcher inadvisable.
- If you are alone, and the person needs supervision because he or she is very distressed or unconscious.

In such cases, or if you have no means of transportation, call for an ambulance immediately. If you are in any doubt or live far away from a hospital, call a doctor or a hospital emergency department for advice.

Emergency checklist

If a person is seriously injured, give emergency first-aid treatment according to the priorities listed below before seeking emergency help. If possible, send someone else for help while you perform first aid.
1 Check the person's airway and breathing. If the airway is not obstructed and the person is not breathing, perform artificial ventilation or complete *cardiopulmonary resuscitation* (*CPR,* page 283) as necessary.
2 Attempt to control any severe bleeding (page 284).
3 If the person is unconscious and does not have a neck or back injury, place him or her in the recovery position (page 283).
4 Treat any severe burns (page 286).
5 Look for signs of shock (page 285) and treat if necessary.

First-aid index

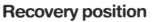

Cardiopulmonary resuscitation (CPR)

Our brief description of the emergency procedures cannot substitute for training from the American Heart Association or the American Red Cross. If an adult or child stops breathing, whether conscious or unconscious, call for emergency help. If the person is struggling to breathe, get emergency help. If the person is unconscious, check the mouth and throat for obstruction, and begin artificial ventilation (steps 1-4 below). You can also begin CPR (steps 1-6) if you are sure the person does not have a pulse.

1 Gently position the person on his or her back. Open airway by pushing head back. Place your hand on person's forehead and your fingers under chin. (For a child, tilt chin and push head slightly back.)

2 Look, listen, and feel for breathing (see *Choking*, p. 285).

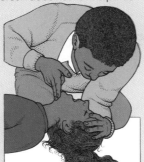

3 If the person still is not breathing, seal your mouth around person's mouth (and nose, if small child). Give 2 slow breaths, each lasting 1 to 1½ seconds.

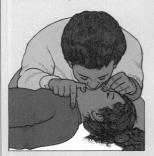

4 Feel for a pulse. If pulse is present in neck of an adult or child, breathe for the adult with 1 breath every 5 seconds and for the child with 1 breath every 4 seconds. If victim is an infant, check pulse on the inside of the upper arm between elbow and shoulder. If pulse is present, breathe for baby, giving 1 breath every 3 seconds. If there is no pulse, start chest compressions.

5 CPR for adult: Put heel of one hand two thirds of the way down breastbone and your other hand on top. Compress chest 1 to 2 inches. Continue compressing 3 times every 2 seconds (80 to 100 per minute). After 15 chest compressions, give 2 breaths. Repeat until a pulse returns or medical help arrives.

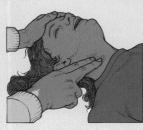

6 CPR for child: Put heel of hand on chest and compress 1 to 1½ inches at point of lowest ribs. On an infant, compress 1 to 1½ inches between nipples. After every 5 compressions, give 2 breaths. Repeat until trained help arrives.

Recovery position

If a person is unconscious, the recovery position allows him or her to breathe freely and prevents choking and inhalation of vomit. The limbs support the body in a stable and comfortable position. Place the victim in the recovery position after you have ensured that he or she is breathing normally and you have dealt with any obvious injury. DO NOT use the recovery position if you have any reason to suspect a neck or back injury.

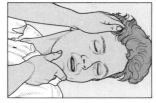
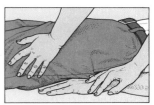

1 Check the mouth of the unconscious person to make sure there are no foreign objects or loose dentures inside.

2 Place the near arm of the person close to his or her body, tucking the hand under the near leg.

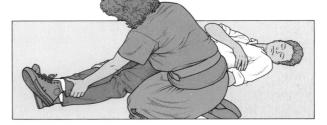

3 Cross the far arm over the chest toward you and cross the far leg over the near leg at the knee.

4 Protect and support the head with one hand. With the other hand, grasp the clothing at the hip farthest from you and pull the person quickly toward you, keeping him or her supported against you.

5 Readjust the head to make certain the airway is still open.

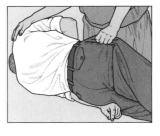

6 Bend the person's uppermost arm into a position to support the upper body. Bend his or her uppermost leg at the knee, bringing the thigh forward to support the lower body. Carefully pull the other arm out from under the person, working from the shoulder down. Leave it lying parallel to the body to prevent the person from rolling back.

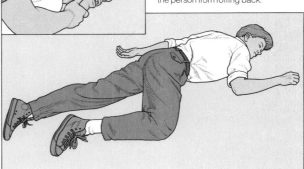

Drowning

In a drowning accident, check the person's breathing as soon as you reach him or her. If the person is not breathing, start artificial ventilation immediately (see *CPR*, page 283). Do not wait to get the person out of the water and do not try to remove water from the lungs. Once you have restored breathing and are out of the water, place the victim in the *recovery position* (see page 283) and keep him or her warm by covering with blankets or clothes. Seek medical help.

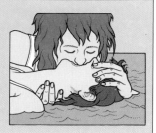

1 Quickly remove any obstructions, such as seaweed, from the person's mouth and begin mouth-to-mouth resuscitation immediately.

2 If the person is still in the water and you can stand comfortably, use one arm to support the person's body and the other hand to support his or her head and seal the nose.

Bleeding

Bleeding, whether from a cut or more serious wound, should be dealt with promptly and calmly. Treat bleeding as severe:

- If blood spurts forcefully from the wound.
- If you estimate that more than 1/2 pint of blood has been lost.
- If bleeding continues for more than 5 minutes.

Severe bleeding

In a severe wound, blood may be flowing so freely that it cannot clot before spurting from the body. Your goal is to reduce blood flow to encourage the clotting of blood in the wound to seal the damaged blood vessels. You can do this by applying pressure to the wound itself, as described below. As a rule, you should try to keep the injured part raised above the level of the heart. Do not try to clean a wound that is bleeding profusely with water or antiseptic. As soon as you have performed first aid, seek emergency medical help.

How to stop severe bleeding

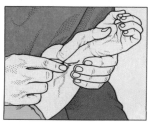

1 Lay the person down and raise the injured part.

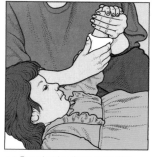

2 Remove any obvious foreign objects such as pieces of glass from the wound, but do not probe for anything that is deeply embedded.

3 Press hard on the wound with a cloth pad, holding any gaping edges together. If anything is still embedded in the wound, avoid exerting direct pressure on it.

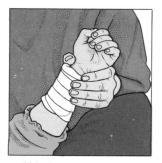

4 Maintain pressure on the wound by binding the pad firmly over the wound, using a bandage or strips of material.

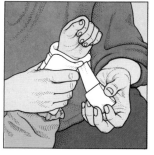

5 If the pad becomes soaked with blood, do not remove it. Instead, apply more padding over the wound and hold it in place firmly with another bandage.

Nosebleeds

Nosebleeds are a common occurrence and may be brought on by a minor injury to the nose.

If you have a nosebleed, sit down, leaning slightly forward. Make sure that you breathe through the mouth. Place your thumb and index finger as high on the softer part of your nose as you can and pinch both nostrils firmly closed for about 10 minutes. This pressure allows a blood clot to form and seal the damaged blood vessels. Do not blow your nose for several hours after the bleeding has stopped because you may dislodge the blood clot.

Seek medical help if bleeding continues for longer than 20 minutes or if you suspect that the nose may be broken—for example, if bleeding followed a severe blow to the nose. Get emergency medical attention if bleeding from the nose follows a blow to another part of the head; this may indicate a fractured skull.

Minor cuts and scrapes

Bleeding from a minor cut or scrape helps clean the wound and usually stops on its own after a few minutes. Press a clean pad over the wound for a few minutes to help stop bleeding. When bleeding has stopped, clean around the cut, wiping from the edges outward with a clean gauze or cotton pad. There is no need to clean inside the wound itself. Small cuts and even large grazes heal more rapidly if left uncovered. You can hold gaping edges closed with strips of surgical tape, but any cut more than about 1/2 inch long may need stitches to minimize scarring. Consult your doctor or local hospital emergency department if you think that the wound might need stitching, if it is very dirty, if it is a deep puncture wound (for example, from a nail), or if you have not been vaccinated against tetanus within 5 years.

Treating minor cuts

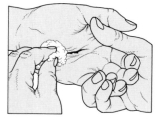

Wipe from the edges of the wound outward, using a clean swab of cotton for each stroke. Put any antiseptics on the cleansing pad, not directly on the cut.

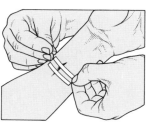

Small cuts heal best if left uncovered. However, if the edges of the cut gape, draw them together and put one or two strips of surgical tape across the wound.

Puncture wounds

A deep wound caused by something dirty—such as a rusty nail or an animal's tooth—has a high risk of infection, because dirt is pressed deep into the tissues and the wound bleeds very little to carry it back out. If numbness, tingling, or weakness in a limb follows a deep cut or puncture wound, underlying nerves or tendons may have been damaged. Antibiotics and a tetanus shot (if you have not been vaccinated in 5 years) are recommended for all deep wounds.

Choking

If your child chokes on a piece of food or any object, take immediate action to remove the obstruction. Always call for medical help. If the child stops breathing you may need to start chest compressions (see below) to dislodge the object from the airway. The technique used on an adult choking victim is shown on page 199.

Infant

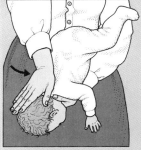

1 Place the baby face down on your arm with the head low. Support the head with your hand on the jaw. Give 4 blows between the shoulder blades with heel of your hand.

2 Turn the baby over. Alternate 4 chest compressions with 4 back blows until trained help arrives or the object is dislodged. If the baby becomes unconscious, begin artificial ventilation (see *CPR,* page 283).

Unconscious child

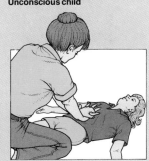

1 Place the child on his or her back. Put heel of one hand above navel and below ribs. Put other hand on top; straighten your elbows. Give 4 quick, downward and forward thrusts.

2 Only if the object is visible, try to remove the obstruction by sweeping your index finger across the back of the throat.

3 Repeat these steps until the object is dislodged or medical help arrives.

Conscious child

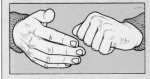

1 Stand behind the child; put your arms around his or her waist. Place your fist, thumb inward, against the child's stomach above the navel and below the ribs.

2 Give 4 quick, upward and inward thrusts. Repeat this movement 6 to 10 times until the child coughs up the object or becomes unconscious.

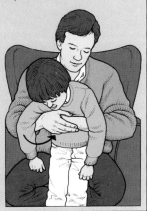

Shock

Shock is a life-threatening condition that may occur with severe injury or illness. In a person in shock, the flow of blood to vital organs and tissues is inadequate. The person's blood pressure drops sharply. Suspect that an injured or ill person is in shock if he or she becomes pale and sweaty, and drowsy or confused. Call for emergency medical help immediately. Do not give food or fluids.

Treating shock
Lay the person down on his or her back with legs raised. Loosen any tight clothing and cover the person to keep him or her warm. Offer reassurance while you wait for help to arrive.

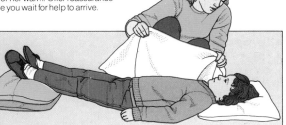

Electric shock

A severe electric shock is likely to knock a person unconscious and breathing may stop. Deep burns at the point where the current entered and exited the body and internal damage may result. Always seek medical advice after an electric shock even if the person seems to have only minor burns.

What to do
First turn off the current or break the contact between the person and the appliance. Do not try to pull the person away or you may receive a shock yourself. Instead, use a dry, nonmetal object such as a wooden broom handle to push away the source of the current. Check the person's airway and breathing. If breathing has stopped, start artificial ventilation (see *CPR,* page 283) at once and feel for a pulse. You may need to continue for half an hour or more. Once the person is breathing, place him or her in the *recovery position* (see page 283), treat any *burns* (see page 286), and get medical help.

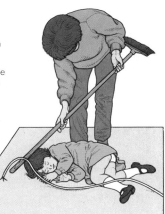

Unconsciousness

Unconsciousness refers not only to unrousable coma, but also to a state in which someone is drowsy and confused and does not respond to your presence. Unconsciousness may result from such conditions as brain damage, loss of blood, lack of oxygen, chemical changes in the blood, or an overdose of drugs. The main danger with unconsciousness is obstruction of the airway, either because the tongue has become limp and has fallen backward (blocking the airway) or because the person can no longer cough adequately to clear vomit or other matter from the back of the throat.

First check to see whether the unconscious person is breathing. If not, begin artificial ventilation (see *CPR,* page 283). If the person is breathing but respiration sounds noisy or gurgling, check deep inside the mouth to make certain there is no obstruction. Loosen any tight clothing around the neck and chest as soon as normal breathing resumes. Place the person in the *recovery position* (see page 283). If possible, place a coat or blanket under the person and cover with another to minimize heat loss. Try not to leave the person unattended until medical help arrives.
Note: If the person lost consciousness after a fall or collision and a spinal injury is possible, do not place the person in the recovery position unless he or she is vomiting. In such cases, try not to flex the person's neck or back.

Burns

Burns may be caused by dry heat (fire), moist heat (steam or hot liquids), electricity, or corrosive chemicals. For treatment of *electric shock,* see page 285.

To treat a burn, first remove the cause. For example, extinguish flames. The affected area should then be cooled as rapidly as possible by holding it under cold running water or by immersing the area in cold water. DO NOT ever apply butter or any type of ointment or cream to the burn or burst any blisters that may form on the skin.

After doing first aid, get emergency medical help if the burn affects an extensive area; if the skin is broken, severely blistered, or charred; or if the person is in severe pain. Even small burns on the face or hands may cause scarring, so you should always seek medical advice promptly. Burns are prone to tetanus, so a tetanus shot may be required.

Minor burns and scalds
A burn or scald can be treated safely at home—even if it causes reddening and blistering—if it damages only the superficial layer of skin over a fairly small area. Sunburn is usually considered a minor burn.

Superficial burns are very painful, so first aid is performed mainly by cooling the area to relieve pain. Hold the burned area under cold, running water; immerse it in cold water; or place cool, wet towels on the area for at least 10 minutes or until the pain stops. If blisters form over a burn, do not break them. If they are on a part of the skin that can be rubbed by clothing, cover them with a padded dressing. Do not apply any cream, grease, or ointment. The exception is mild sunburn, which can often be soothed with calamine lotion or an anesthetic lotion or spray.

Treating burns

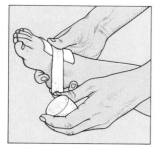

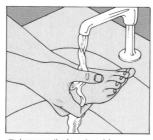

1 Clothing that has been soaked by boiling water or chemical agents should be removed from the burned area unless it is firmly stuck to the skin. Dry, burned clothing should be left on.

2 Immerse the burn in cold, preferably running, water for at least 10 minutes. If the area affected is large, cover it with a clean towel or sheet soaked in cold water.

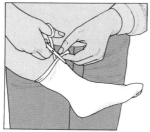

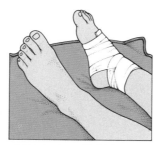

3 After you have cooled the burn, cover it with a clean, dry gauze or cloth dressing. Do not use cotton balls or other fluffy materials. If you are taking the person to the hospital, do not cover the burn; any dressing will have to be removed, possibly causing him or her more pain.

4 Elevate a burned limb to keep swelling to a minimum.

Poisoning

Accidental poisoning is one of the most common reasons that children, especially those under 5, need emergency treatment in the hospital. In adults, poisoning is more likely to be due to a drug overdose, either deliberate or accidental. Children can be poisoned by swallowing alcohol, medicines, household cleaning fluids or chemicals, or poisonous plants or berries. A person may not tell you that he or she has taken something poisonous; always suspect that your child, or an older person, has swallowed poison if he or she starts to vomit suddenly and inexplicably, becomes drowsy or confused, loses consciousness, or starts to breathe abnormally.

If you think that someone may have taken any type of poison, even if he or she seems well at the moment, seek expert advise at once. Call your local poison control center or hospital emergency department. You should try to give them the following information:

- What has been swallowed.
- How much has been swallowed. In the case of medicines, try to find out how many tablets were taken.
- When it was swallowed.
- If you take the person to the hospital or to a doctor, take with you any containers you think may have held the poison. If you are unable to obtain expert advice and cannot easily get to a hospital, follow the steps below.

Household poisons
(including household cleaning fluids, kerosene, gasoline, polishes, and paint). Read the product label for specific first-aid instructions.

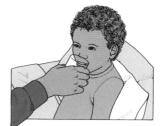

1 If the person is conscious, give a glass of milk or water to drink at once.

2 DO NOT try to induce vomiting but, if the person vomits spontaneously, put him or her face down (hold over your lap, if a child) to prevent inhalation of chemicals in the vomit.

3 If the person loses consciousness, place him or her in the *recovery position* (p. 283). If breathing stops, perform artificial ventilation and feel for a pulse to evaluate the need for *CPR* (p. 283).

4 Get medical help immediately.

Medicines, alcohol, poisonous plants and berries

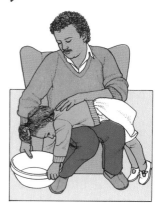

1 If the person is conscious, try to induce vomiting (see below).

2 If the person is unconscious, do not give anything by mouth. Lay the person down in the *recovery position* (p. 283) and, if breathing stops, perform artificial ventilation and evaluate the need for *CPR* (p. 283).

3 Seek medical help immediately.

How to induce vomiting
Never try to induce vomiting in a person who is unconscious or who has swallowed chemical products such as cleaning fluids, kerosene, or gasoline. Do not try to induce vomiting by giving salt water or by sticking a finger down the person's throat.

In other cases, give syrup of ipecac (2 teaspoons for infants, 3 teaspoons for children, and 6 teaspoons for older children and adults) followed by 2 glasses of water or another liquid. If this does not lead to vomiting within 20 minutes, repeat the dose only once. When the person vomits, keep his or her face down, with head lowered, to prevent choking or inhalation of vomit.

Hypothermia

Body temperature is normally constant at about 98°F. During prolonged exposure to cold, more body heat may be lost than can be replaced, so the body temperature drops. This condition is known as hypothermia. Babies and the elderly are especially vulnerable to chilling. They may lose a dangerous amount of body heat in conditions that may not seem particularly cold to a younger adult. In healthy people, hypothermia occurs after prolonged exposure to cold, windy conditions. The drop in body temperature causes a gradual physical and mental slowing. The person will become increasingly clumsy, unreasonable, irritable, confused, and drowsy; speech will become slurred. Eventually, unconsciousness results, with slow, weak breathing and a barely discernible heartbeat. Hypothermia requires immediate medical attention but, before professional help arrives, you can assist the person by following the steps below. If the person is unconscious and breathing regularly, he or she should be placed in the *recovery position* (see page 283).

Treatment for chilling

1 If the person is unconscious, check the airway and breathing and begin artificial ventilation (see *CPR*, p. 283) if needed. Check the pulse and evaluate the need for *CPR* (see p. 283).

2 Once breathing is regular, shelter the person from the cold, insulating him or her from the ground if you are outside. If you are indoors, remove any wet clothes and exchange them for warm, dry ones or wrap the person in warm blankets.

3 If the person is conscious, give sips of warm, sweet liquids but do not give any alcohol. Do not put the person in a hot bath or use hot water bottles or electric blankets.

Heat exhaustion

If someone who is not accustomed to heat neglects to consume plenty of salt and extra fluids, heat exhaustion can result from excessive sweating. The person will become exhausted, with pale, clammy skin and may feel sick, dizzy, and faint. His or her pulse rate and breathing will become rapid and headache or muscle cramps may develop. Untreated heat exhaustion may develop into heat stroke, a more serious condition that always requires medical attention.

Treatment for heat exhaustion

1 Lay the person down in a cool, quiet place with his or her feet raised a little.

2 Loosen any tight clothing. If the person is conscious, give him or her clear liquids to drink. If the person is unconscious or lethargic, get medical help promptly.

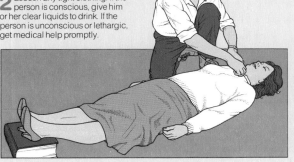

Frostbite

This serious condition requires immediate medical attention. Frostbitten skin is hard, pale, cold, and painless; when thawed out, it becomes red and painful. Get the person inside as soon as possible and summon medical help. Meanwhile, shelter the person from wind and give him or her warm drinks. Cover the frozen part with clothing or blankets, or warm it against your body. Cover the face with your dry, gloved hands; the person's hands should be tucked inside his or her armpits; frostbitten feet should be raised. Do not use direct heat and do not rub the affected area. Encourage the person to exercise warmed, frostbitten parts. Do not start the warming process if there is a possibility that refreezing could occur.

Bites and stings

Most animal bites and insect bites or stings are minor and are no threat to your general health. When traveling, know how to identify animals and insects that have poisonous bites or stings. Occasionally, a person may develop a severe allergic reaction to an apparently minor bite or sting. This situation requires emergency treatment (see *Anaphylactic shock,* below).

Animal bites: If you are bitten by a wild or domestic animal, seek medical advice immediately. Most bite wounds will become infected if not quickly treated. You may need an antitetanus injection and/or stitches; antirabies injections may also be needed.

Snake bites: If you are bitten by a snake, wash the wound, take aspirin (or give a child an aspirin substitute) to relieve any pain, and rest. Call a doctor. If you think the snake may have been poisonous, immobilize the affected part and keep it below the level of the heart, to reduce the circulation of the poison.

Insect bites or stings: Bites or stings from most common insects—such as bees and mosquitoes—cause itching, redness, and swelling. Apply calamine lotion to relieve discomfort. If stung by a bee or hornet, first try to remove the stinger from the wound by gently scraping it out with a clean fingernail or knife blade. Use ice packs and antihistamines to minimize pain and swelling. Watch for signs of anaphylactic shock (below).

Jellyfish stings: Though seldom dangerous, a jellyfish sting may cause painful burning and swelling. Calamine lotion or an antihistamine cream are best for relief of burning and swelling. The Portuguese man-of-war may cause a more serious reaction. The person may experience shortness of breath and may faint. Wrap your hand in cloth and scrape off the tentacles. Place the person in the *recovery position* (page 283) and keep him or her warm while you call for medical help.

Anaphylactic shock

In rare cases, a person may become hypersensitive to a particular type of bite or sting—usually after having been bitten or stung previously. Subsequent bites or stings cause a severe allergic reaction known as anaphylactic shock. Symptoms may include difficulty breathing and/or any of the signs of *shock* (page 285). Other symptoms may include tightening of the throat, difficulty swallowing, or a rash. If a person shows such symptoms after being bitten or stung, treat as you would for shock and get emergency medical help immediately.

Caring for a sick child

A child who is ill is often anxious and in need of comfort, even if the disease or disorder is not painful or serious. Reassurance is an important part of caring for your child, whether he or she is at home or in a hospital (see *Children in the hospital* and *Treating the most common symptoms and disorders at home,* opposite). Advice on dealing with specific disorders is given in the symptom charts (see *How to use the charts,* page 38). On these pages you will find general advice on caring for a sick child at home.

How to tell when your child is sick

Most parents know immediately when their child is sick. Apart from obvious signs such as a rash, vomiting, or pain, other less specific indicators of illness include loss of appetite (particularly in young babies), irritability and crying, or unusual lethargy. If you suspect that your baby or child is sick, consult the appropriate chart in this book (see *How to find the correct chart,* pages 40 to 48) to discover the possible cause and to find out whether you need to call your doctor. If your child's symptoms are vague, start with chart 9, *Feeling sick.*

Bed rest

For most illnesses, it is not essential that your child stay in bed all day. If he or she feels well enough to get up and play in the house, it is usually safe. However, if your child does not feel like getting out of bed or if your doctor has advised rest, try to prevent boredom by providing special attention. A sick child may not be able to concentrate for long and will not want to play games that are too demanding. Your child will probably need extra reassurance from you and you may have to spend more time with him or her than usual. Often, a child is happier resting in a bed made up on the sofa, where he or she can feel closely involved with other members of the family, rather than in an out-of-the-way bedroom. This arrangement will also allow you to watch your child more closely.

Keeping a sick child occupied
Keeping your child amused will help raise his or her spirits. If your child needs or wants to stay in bed, a variety of activities such as drawing or putting pictures in a scrapbook may pass the time. Your child may be happier in a bed made up on a sofa in a room with other people.

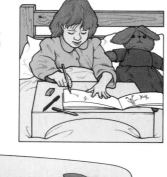

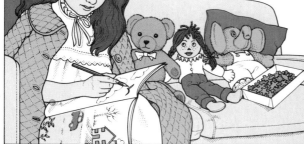

Lowering your child's temperature

You can safely try to reduce your child's temperature in the following way:

- Remove as much clothing as possible.
- Keep the room temperature at a comfortable level.
- Sponge your child repeatedly with lukewarm water, or give him or her a lukewarm bath if his or her temperature is 102°F or more.
- Give the recommended dose of an aspirin substitute.
- Have your child drink plenty of fluids daily.

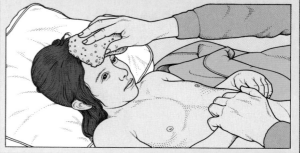

Food and fluid intake

A sick child usually has a smaller appetite than usual, which in the short term is not a cause for concern. No special diet is necessary for most illnesses but, if you are worried that your child is not eating enough, you may be able to coax him or her to eat by fixing a favorite meal (even if the meal is not particularly nourishing). If loss of appetite continues through a long illness, ask your doctor for advice. In most cases, it is important that your child drink plenty of fluids, especially if he or she is feverish, has been vomiting, or has diarrhea. Although water or fruit juices are preferable, offer whatever fluids your child seems to enjoy, including carbonated drinks.

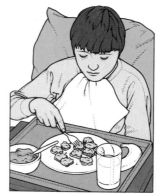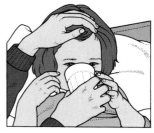

Giving your child food and fluids
Your child will probably not feel like eating, though you may successfully encourage him or her to eat a favorite food. Make sure he or she drinks plenty of fluids.

Fresh air

The room your child is resting in should be at a moderate temperature—68 to 70°F—and have plenty of ventilation. If your child is well enough to play in the house, he or she may be allowed to play outside, providing the weather is not too cold and he or she does not have a fever. However, your child should not play near others if he or she has an infectious disease (see opposite).

Infectious diseases

If your child has an infectious illness, such as a cold, measles, or whooping cough, he or she can pass it on to others. In the early stages of an infectious illness, keep him or her away from children and any adults who may be vulnerable to infection. In the case of rubella (German measles), keep your child out of public places and especially away from pregnant women, who are at risk of contracting the disease. The table on page 97 gives the infectious period of the common childhood infectious diseases. Your doctor will advise you on any disease not covered there. If your child is lonely, you may want to invite children who have already had the disease to play at your house. The danger of their developing the disease again is remote.

When to call your doctor

The charts in this book give advice on when to call your doctor about particular symptoms. However, as a general rule, you should seek medical advice about your child's condition in the following cases:

- If you are unsure about the cause of the symptoms
- If home treatment does not help or the symptoms worsen
- If you are worried because your child is still an infant
- If your child refuses to drink or is very drowsy
- If your child has abdominal pain

Remember that diseases tend to develop more quickly in a child than in an adult, so a delay in seeking medical help that may be acceptable for an adult may not be safe for a young child. It is better to call your doctor than to risk serious complications.

Medicines

Medicines for children are usually prescribed in flavored, liquid form or chewable tablets to encourage the child to take the medicine more readily. You can give a baby accurately measured amounts of medicine in a calibrated dropper. For an older child, use a measuring spoon. Try to put the medicine on the back of the tongue (the taste buds are at the front). Never give aspirin to children or teenagers. Acetaminophen is the preferred painkiller for them.

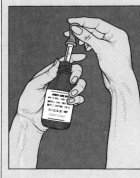

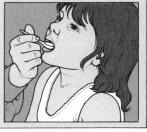

Giving your child medicine
To give your baby medicine, fill a calibrated dropper with the exact dosage and empty it down the back of the throat. An older child should be given the medicine in a measuring spoon while sitting up. Make sure that the dosage is accurate and that your child completes the whole course.

Treating the most common symptoms and disorders at home

The following boxes give advice on treatment to combat childhood infection and when to consult your doctor.
Feverish convulsions (babies), p. 54
Feverish convulsions (children), p. 76
Treating gastroenteritis (babies), p. 63
Relieving your child's headache, p. 83
Treating your child's cold, p. 106
Treatment of a sore throat, p. 107
What to do when your child vomits, p. 115
Treating your child's gastroenteritis, p. 121
How to relieve your child's toothache, p. 113

Children in the hospital

Admission to the hospital—even for a short time—is a difficult experience for a young child. It may be the first time he or she has been away from home overnight, and the surroundings are likely to be strange and frightening. The fact that your child feels sick will increase any distress. It is extremely important for parents to spend as much time as possible at the hospital with their child. Most pediatric facilities allow unlimited visiting for parents and often provide overnight accommodations as well. You will usually be able to participate in the day-to-day care (such as feeding or bathing) of your child. This care will provide valuable reassurance for him or her and may help speed recovery. If your child needs to have an operation, you should arrange to be present if possible when he or she is given general anesthesia and when he or she awakens afterward.

Preparing for a hospital stay
You can prepare your child for a planned stay in the hospital by talking about what is going to happen, visiting the hospital beforehand, and reassuring him or her that you will be there. Spending time with your child in the hospital, bringing familiar toys, and providing him or her with plenty of favorite activities will help your child during the stay.

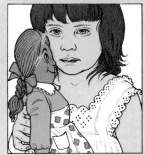

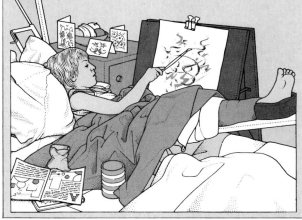

When you are ill

You will recover from most illnesses more quickly if you stop work, stay at home, and take it easy. While you are ill, do not smoke and do not drink alcohol. Drink plenty of fluids, especially if you have a fever or diarrhea. Unless your doctor has advised a particular kind of diet, eat whatever you choose but eat small, frequent meals. There is no need to stay in bed if you are not seriously ill, as long as you stay in a comfortable, well-ventilated environment. If you have a fever, you may sweat profusely and feel hot, sticky, and uncomfortable. This is because the sweat glands in the skin are more active than usual during illness. You will feel better if you bathe often.

Bed rest
If it is necessary to stay in bed while you are ill, make sure that the room is comfortable and free of drafts. Try to have everything you may need within easy reach. Have your telephone and your doctor's phone number close by so that you can call to ask questions or report any abrupt changes in your symptoms. Never smoke in bed.

Food and fluid intake
Small helpings of simple, nutritious foods may be all that you will feel like eating and it is wise to drink as much fluid (such as water, fresh juices, or tea) as possible. It is particularly important when you are ill to ensure that your diet is well balanced and includes all of the essential vitamins and nutrients (see *Safeguarding your health,* diet, page 35).

Fresh air
When you are ill it may help you to feel more comfortable if a window is left slightly open. This will ensure that the room is properly ventilated and will clear the air of unpleasant odors. As long as the room is reasonably warm (especially if the patient is elderly) and free of drafts, a daily dose of fresh air can sometimes do wonders.

Your temperature

Normal body temperature is about 98.6°F but may vary by up to 1 to 2°F throughout the day, dropping to its lowest point in the early hours of the morning. A rise in temperature (a fever) is not dangerous unless it exceeds 104°F.

The clinical thermometer
The best way to take your temperature is by mouth with a clinical thermometer. The thermometer is a small glass tube marked by a scale and with a mercury-filled bulb at one end. As the mercury is heated by your body, it expands and rises up the tube to a point on the scale that has an arrow indicating normal body temperature. A small kink in the tube prevents the mercury from sinking back into the bulb when the thermometer is removed from the warmth of your body. Before you buy a clinical thermometer, examine it carefully, warming the bulb in your hand and checking to see that the mercury column and the markings are clearly visible. Never take your temperature immediately after a bath, meal, hot drink, or cigarette, because you will probably get a false reading.

Taking your child's temperature
A thermometer in the mouth gives a fairly accurate reading of body temperature, but it is easier to take the temperature of a young child by placing the thermometer bulb in the armpit.

This reading will be about 1°F lower than that given when the thermometer is in the mouth.

However, the most accurate reading for a young child comes from taking the temperature in the rectum. (See *How to take a baby's temperature,* page 55 and *Taking your child's temperature,* page 77.)

Temperature indicator strips can be purchased at your drug store but, because they do not give as precise a reading as a thermometer, they should be used only to get an approximate idea of body temperature. The indicator strip is heat sensitive but tends to underestimate a fever, so add at least 1°F to any reading.

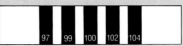

Using a temperature indicator strip
Place the strip firmly against the person's forehead for at least 1 minute until the heat-sensitive panels have settled on one color. Read the temperature printed at the very bottom of the colored panel, and remember to add 1°F to the reading.

How to take your temperature

1 Shake the thermometer in the direction of the bulb with several downward flicks of the wrist until the mercury level is well below the normal mark.

2 Place the thermometer under your tongue and close your mouth. Do not bite down on the thermometer.

3 Remove the thermometer after 3 minutes and hold it up to the light. The top of the mercury column marks the temperature against the scale.

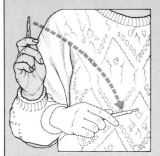

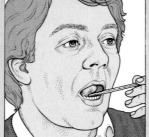

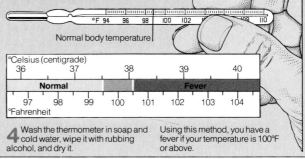

Normal body temperature

°Celsius (centigrade)				
36	37	38	39	40
Normal			**Fever**	
97 98	99	100 101	102	103 104
°Fahrenheit				

4 Wash the thermometer in soap and cold water, wipe it with rubbing alcohol, and dry it.

Using this method, you have a fever if your temperature is 100°F or above.

A raised temperature

It is important to know when you have a fever and what to do to keep it under control. In addition to taking your temperature with a thermometer, there are obvious signs of fever to look for. If you have a fever you will probably feel very hot, flushed, and sweaty. Your eyes will appear bright and may feel hot. You will probably experience dryness in the mouth, thirst, and possibly a headache. Because of increased fluid loss through sweating, you may pass smaller quantities of urine than usual and it may be darker than usual. If your headache is severe, a cold cloth and an aspirin or an aspirin substitute may be soothing.

How to reduce fever

It is important to keep a raised temperature under control to speed recovery. The following self-help measures should help to reduce your fever, whatever its cause.

- Take the recommended dose of aspirin or an aspirin substitute.
- Drink plenty of cool, nonalcoholic fluids.
- For a high fever, sponge your body with lukewarm water and/or use a fan.

Consult your doctor if your temperature continues to rise in spite of these measures.

Applying a cold compress

Fold a washcloth into a strip and soak it in a bowl containing water and ice cubes.

Wring the cloth out and apply to the forehead, leaving a second cloth to soak. Replace as necessary.

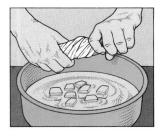

Infectious diseases

Infectious diseases are caused by bacteria, viruses, or fungi that invade and multiply in the body. Many of these organisms are contagious—that is, they are spread between people in close contact or by sneezing or coughing into the air. In the early stages of an infection, it is best to avoid other adults and children.

When to call your doctor

The self-diagnosis charts contained in this book give advice on when to call your doctor about particular symptoms. However, as a general rule, you should seek medical advice about your condition in the following cases:

- If you do not start to feel better after 48 hours despite your self-help efforts
- If your temperature exceeds 104°F
- If, after taking medicine, symptoms develop that seem unrelated to your illness
- If you have young children at home and are worried that you may infect them

Your doctor can more easily diagnose your illness if you record your temperature and the time it was taken. Also write down exactly when various symptoms started.

Treating the most common symptoms and disorders at home

The following boxes appear alongside the charts in this book and provide self-help measures that deal with common symptoms and disorders at home. Listed in alphabetical order, they include recommendations for:

In the hospital

Your doctor may admit you into a hospital for treatment if necessary. In general, you consent to overall medical treatment when you are admitted to the hospital. Any special procedures will require your informed consent, which means that you must sign a document stating that you fully understand the benefits and risks of treatment.

When you go into the hospital you will be given information explaining regular hospital routine and available services. If information is sent to you prior to your admission, it may include a list of what you should take to the hospital with you (see illustration below). You might want to bring something to read, although many hospitals have a lending library for patient use.

Things to take to the hospital

Shaving kit or cosmetics case
Nightgown or pajamas
Robe
Towel
Washcloth or sponge

Soap
Toothpaste
Toothbrush
Brush or comb
Slippers
Deodorant
Sanitary napkins
Money

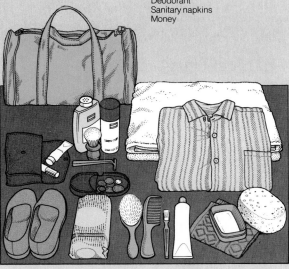

Health checkups

These recommendations are not absolute. Your age and previous medical problems will determine the frequency with which you need specific tests.

 Men  Women

EYE EXAMINATION
 To detect any visual defects or eye muscle disorders and to look for any signs of disease.
At high risk Anyone diagnosed as having diabetes or high blood pressure or who has a family history of glaucoma.

DENTAL CHECKUP
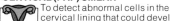 To check on the health of the teeth, gums, tongue, and mouth and to look for oral cancer.
At high risk Tobacco smokers or chewers.

CERVICAL (PAP) SMEAR
To detect abnormal cells in the cervical lining that could develop into cancer.
At high risk Women already diagnosed and treated for precancerous changes or for herpes or genital warts.

MEASUREMENT OF BLOOD PRESSURE
To detect high blood pressure at an early stage, before complications develop.
At high risk Anyone with a family history of hypertension, heart or kidney disease, or stroke or diabetes, or who is overweight or taking oral contraceptives.

BLOOD CHOLESTEROL TEST
To detect people at high risk of coronary heart disease.
At high risk Anyone with a family history of early-onset coronary heart disease.

MAMMOGRAPHY (BREAST X-RAY)
To detect breast cancer early, before it can be detected by physical examination.
At high risk Anyone with a close relative who has had cancer of the breast or colon.

EXAMINATION OF THE RECTUM AND COLON
To detect cancer of the rectum and colon. There are three separate tests—
a) digital rectal examination,
b) tests for hidden blood in the stool,
and c) sigmoidoscopy.
At high risk Anyone with an immediate family member who has had cancer of the colon or rectum; polyps of the colon; or long-standing, extensive ulcerative colitis.

COMPLETE PHYSICAL EXAMINATION
To determine your health status and develop your relationship with your doctor.

TEST	FREQUENCY	
	NOT AT HIGH RISK	**AT HIGH RISK**
TEENAGERS TO AGE 30		
♂♀	Every 2 years if you have problems with your vision.	At least once a year.
♂♀	Every 6 months until age 21, then at least once a year.	As your dentist recommends.
♀	Annually for women over 18 and all sexually active women, or as your doctor recommends.	Annually.
♂♀	Begin at age 20; after 20, at 3- to 5-year intervals.	Annually.
♂♀	At the time of your first physical examination.	If abnormal, follow your doctor's advice.
♂♀	Usually not necessary.	a) Annually after age 20.
♂♀	Twice in your 20s.	
ADULTS 30 TO 50		
♂♀	Every 2 years. If you have good vision, start at 40.	About once a year.
♂♀	At least once a year.	As your dentist recommends.
♀	Every 1 to 3 years.	Annually.
♂♀	Every 3 to 5 years.	Annually.
♂♀	Depends on results of last test. If normal, repeat in 3 to 5 years.	If abnormal, follow your doctor's advice.
♀	Once between 35 and 40; every 1 to 2 years between 40 and 50.	Every 1 to 2 years, beginning at age 35.
♂♀	a) Annually after 40.	a) Annually. b) Annually. c) Every 3 to 5 years.
♂♀	Every 1 to 2 years, as your doctor recommends.	
ADULTS 50 AND OVER		
♂♀	Every 2 years.	At least once a year.
♂♀	Every 1 to 2 years.	As your dentist recommends.
♀	Every 3 to 5 years.	Annually.
♂♀	Annually.	As your doctor recommends.
♂♀	Depends on results of last test. If normal, repeat in 3 to 5 years.	If abnormal, follow your doctor's advice.
♀	Annually.	Same as for those not at high risk.
♂♀	a) Annually. b) Annually. c) Every 3 to 5 years.	Same as for those not at high risk.
♂♀	Every 1 to 2 years to age 65; after 65, every year.	

Specialized tests

You may be given some tests, such as blood and urine tests, as part of a routine physical checkup. Other tests, such as X-rays or bronchoscopy, will only be given to confirm or rule out a particular disorder that your doctor is investigating. Recently, some tests that carried a risk or caused discomfort—for example, X-rays during pregnancy—have been replaced by new tests that are low-risk and painless, such as ultrasound. The introduction of fiberoptics (the transmission of images through lighted, flexible threads) has also been a major advance, allowing examination of body cavities without major surgery. Many of the tests listed below, as well as those described elsewhere in the book, use fiberoptic techniques.

Index of tests

CHOLECYSTOGRAPHY

This procedure is used to diagnose disorders of the gallbladder and bile duct.

What happens

The patient takes a substance, visible on X-rays, by mouth, and it is photographed as it passes through the gallbladder and bile duct. The X-ray below shows a gallbladder with gallstones.

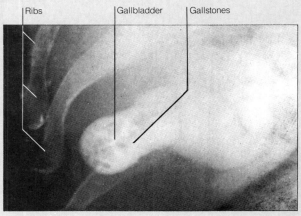

Ribs | Gallbladder | Gallstones

CYSTOSCOPY

Cystoscopy is a procedure for diagnosing the cause of recurrent infections and other disorders of the bladder.

What happens

Local anesthetic is usually applied to the urethra before insertion of a narrow, fiberoptic tube that enables the doctor to view the bladder and to treat some conditions, as well.

LAPAROSCOPY

Laparoscopy is a technique that uses a viewing tube (see *Endoscopy,* page 201) for investigating abdominal disorders. It is often used in women to discover the cause of gynecological problems, such as infertility, or to assist in sterilization procedures. It is also used, in some patients, for other abdominal operations (for example, removal of the gallbladder).

What happens

The procedure is usually done while the patient is under general anesthesia. Two small incisions are made in the abdomen, and carbon dioxide is passed through a hollow needle into one incision to distend the abdomen, while an endoscope is inserted into the second incision, enabling the surgeon to view the interior.

LAPAROTOMY

Laparotomy is an exploratory operation that gives the doctor an inside view of the abdomen. It is usually done when there are signs of a severe abdominal disorder that cannot be firmly diagnosed.

What happens

An incision is made through the abdominal wall (the exact site depends on the suspected problem). Treatment—such as removing an inflamed appendix—can usually be done at the same time.

MYELOGRAPHY

Myelography is a procedure that is used to diagnose disorders of the spine and spinal cord, such as a prolapsed (slipped) disc. It can take up to an hour and requires sedation because it may be uncomfortable.

What happens

A solution that is visible on X-rays is injected into the fluid-filled space that surrounds the spinal cord. The patient is then tilted into different positions so that the movement of the solution inside the spinal column can be recorded by X-ray.

ULTRASOUND

Ultrasound provides a safe, painless way of examining internal organs, especially abdominal and pelvic organs such as the liver and kidneys. It is often used during pregnancy to examine the uterus, placenta, and fetus.

What happens

A wave of very high-pitched sound—ultrasound—is sent through the tissues of the body. These sound waves are deflected off the internal organs and converted into an image that can be shown on a screen or printed on paper. Ultrasound can reveal cysts, tumors, or other swellings (see *Ultrasound scan,* special problems, women, page 276). The ultrasound scan below shows a healthy liver.

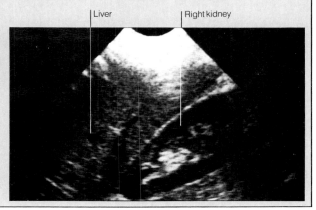

Liver | Right kidney

Medication guide

New drugs are constantly being discovered. Many drugs in common use 20 years ago have been replaced by newer, safer compounds with broader applications. This medication guide is an index of major groups of drugs; it gives their uses and possible side effects and, in many cases, children's dose information and warnings about when medicines should not be taken. This list is selective; it does not include trade names. Check with your doctor before you or a member of your family uses any drug.

When taking any medicine, a few precautionary measures can ensure the drug's effectiveness and your safety. Never exceed the recommended dosage. Always check with your doctor or pharmacist if you are unsure when or how frequently to take the medicine (for example, some drugs work best when taken with a meal). Avoid drinking alcohol when taking any medicine, because some drugs enhance the effects of alcohol, and alcohol can affect the actions of some drugs, causing side effects or adverse reactions. Also, even if your symptoms disappear, complete the prescribed course of medicine. Failure to do so may prevent complete recovery. Make sure your pharmacist puts all prescription drugs in childproof containers, and keep all drugs in a locked medicine cabinet (see opposite).

In general, the fewer drugs you take, the better. Except for minor symptoms (such as an occasional cough or headache), let your doctor prescribe all the medicines you need. He or she will balance the potential benefits of the medicine against its side effects.

Drugs during pregnancy

During pregnancy it is important to avoid any substances that could endanger the development of the fetus. Most drugs pass from the woman's circulation to the fetus. While some are known to be harmless, others can, in certain instances and at certain times during pregnancy, threaten the health of the fetus. If you are pregnant or are contemplating pregnancy, ask your doctor for advice before taking any drugs, including aspirin, acetaminophen, or any other over-the-counter preparation. If you have a chronic condition for which you are receiving medication, your doctor will advise you on the best treatment while you are pregnant. Both alcohol and smoking are known to have harmful effects on the developing fetus.

Drugs and breast-feeding

While breast-feeding, do not take any over-the-counter drugs without your doctor's approval. Your doctor will try to avoid prescribing drugs at this time unless they are absolutely necessary. However, many drugs either pass into the breast milk in insignificant quantities or are known to be safe. When there is a risk of harm to the baby, you can switch to bottle-feeding while you take the drug. If you want to resume breast-feeding later, you will need to express and discard your milk while you are bottle-feeding in order to maintain the milk supply.

Drugs for children

If your child becomes ill, part of the treatment may include prescription or over-the-counter drugs. Special care should be taken when giving drugs to babies and children because their livers, which process chemicals from the bloodstream, are immature. Potentially dangerous levels of a drug may build up more quickly in a child than in an adult, so it is important to accurately measure medicines and to give only the exact dose prescribed. Never dilute your child's medicines or add them to your baby's bottle.

Never give a child any drug that has been prescribed for an adult or for another child. If you are giving over-the-counter medicines, make sure that you read the instructions carefully and ask your doctor or pharmacist for advice. Do not give a child aspirin unless prescribed by a doctor; aspirin can cause a severe reaction in children. Never give over-the-counter medicines for prolonged periods without seeking medical advice. Never give your child a drug to which he or she has exhibited previous sensitivity with symptoms such as nausea, vomiting, diarrhea, rash, or swollen joints. Replace over-the-counter drugs after 1 year.

Tips for giving medicines

Babies and toddlers

- Place a little of the medicine in the baby's mouth at one time.
- If the baby spits out the medicine, put the medicine into one cheek and then, gently but firmly, close the mouth.

Older children

- Crush tablets between two spoons and mix the powder with honey, peanut butter, or ice cream, and make sure your child takes it all.
- Try to put liquid medicine on the back of the tongue.
- Have your child's favorite drink ready to wash the taste of the medicine away.

Prescription drugs

When your doctor prescribes a drug, make sure that you ask the following:

- How much should be taken in each dose.
- How often a dose should be taken.
- How and when the drug should be taken in relation to meals and whether or not sleep should be interrupted to take the medication.
- If there are any side effects.
- If there are any unusual or dangerous reactions to the drug.
- How soon you should expect to see an improvement.
- How long the drug should be taken before consulting your doctor again.

Over-the-counter medicines

Many medications are available over-the-counter. They may come in the form of tablets, capsules, liquids, drops, sprays, creams, ointments, or inhalers. These drugs seldom have any direct effect on the cause of a condition, but they may relieve painful or uncomfortable symptoms. For instance, some of the remedies for coughs and colds are soothing, and mild analgesics such as aspirin and acetaminophen relieve pain.

In most cases, the speed of your recovery depends more on your age and general health than on any such treatment. However, if such products make you feel better, they are unlikely to be harmful if you follow the instructions on the package. In some cases your doctor may recommend a particular over-the-counter preparation. If you are unsure about any aspect of an over-the-counter medication, ask your pharmacist or doctor.

Home medical supplies

The two lists below tell you what items to keep at home to deal with common problems such as indigestion and muscle strain, and to be prepared for accidents and emergencies.

Home medicine cabinet
The best place to keep presciption medications and over-the-counter remedies is in a medicine cabinet that can be locked. The items will stay dry and will be out of the reach of children. Many over-the-counter preparations have a shelf life of 1 year and should be replaced regularly. You are likely to need:

Thermometer
Antiseptic cream (cuts and scrapes)
Insect-sting treatment
Antacid liquid or tablets (indigestion)
Antidiarrheal medication
Motion-sickness tablets
Sunscreen
Lotion (itching rashes)
Petroleum jelly (chafing)
Elastic bandage
Aspirin or acetaminophen

Home first-aid kit
In an emergency, a home first-aid kit provides additional supplies. These should be stored in a well-sealed metal or plastic box that is clearly labeled and easy for you to open. It should be kept in a dry place, out of reach of children, and should include:

1 Packet of sterile cotton
2 Sterile prepared bandages (2 large, 2 medium, 2 small)
3 Sterile gauze in several sizes
4 Sterile triangular bandages (2)
5 Gauze bandages (2) and at least 1 elastic bandage
6 Tubular gauze with applicator
7 Antiseptic
8 Waterproof adhesive bandages in assorted sizes
9 Wide and narrow adhesive tape
10 Safety pins
11 Tweezers
12 Scissors

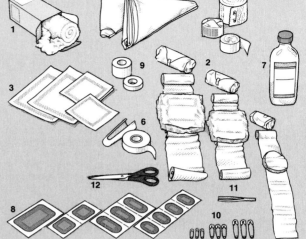

Safety note: It is important to keep all medicines out of the reach of children. A locked wall cabinet is usually the safest place.

Medications

ANALGESICS
Drugs that relieve pain. Many also reduce inflammation (see ANTI-INFLAMMATORIES) and fever (see ANTIPYRETICS). There are 3 main types: simple analgesics—usually containing aspirin or acetaminophen—for mild pain; anti-inflammatories, often given for muscle aches and pains and arthritis; and narcotic analgesics—usually chemically related to morphine—for severe pain.
Possible side effects: Nausea, stomach irritation, constipation, dizziness, drug dependence, and development of tolerance to the drug (narcotic analgesics only). For side effects of other types, see ANTI-INFLAMMATORIES and ANTIPYRETICS.
Children's doses: Acetaminophen is the safest over-the-counter analgesic to use for pain and feverish symptoms in children. Aspirin, another analgesic often used by adults, is no longer considered safe for children because it may be linked with Reye's syndrome, a rare and dangerous condition affecting the brain and liver. For more severe pain—such as after an operation—a narcotic analgesic (such as codeine) may be prescribed. Some analgesics can make a child sleepy and cause constipation, nausea, and dizziness.

ANTACIDS
Drugs that neutralize stomach acid (relieving heartburn and similar conditions). They contain simple chemicals such as sodium bicarbonate, calcium carbonate, aluminum hydroxide, and/or magnesium trisilicate.
Possible side effects: Belching (sodium bicarbonate preparations), constipation (aluminum or calcium preparations), and diarrhea (magnesium preparations).

Warning: If you are taking any other medication, consult your doctor before taking antacids; antacids can reduce the effects of some other drugs.

ANTI-ANXIETY DRUGS
Drugs that reduce feelings of anxiety and relax muscles. Sometimes called anxiolytics, sedatives, or minor tranquilizers. May be used to help you sleep and to relieve premenstrual tension.
Possible side effects: Drowsiness, dizziness, confusion, unsteadiness, and lack of coordination.
Children's doses: These drugs are rarely used to treat children. As an emergency treatment for seizures, diazepam is used intravenously. The newer anti-anxiety drugs may occasionally be used to treat older children suffering from psychological stress. Side effects include drowsiness and confusion; these drugs may be habit-forming.
Warning: Not to be taken if you intend to drive or operate potentially dangerous machinery. Anti-anxiety drugs may increase the effects of alcohol. They can be habit-forming and should not be used for more than a few weeks. After prolonged use, withdrawal symptoms may occur if treatment is halted abruptly.

ANTIBIOTICS
Substances (often derived from living organisms such as molds or bacteria) that kill or inhibit the growth of bacteria in the body. Some of the newer antibiotics are synthetic versions of naturally occurring substances. Any single antibiotic is effective only against certain strains of bacteria, although some broad-spectrum antibiotics combat a wide range of bacterial infections. Sometimes a strain of bacteria becomes resistant to a

particular antibiotic and an alternative is prescribed. No antibiotic is effective against viruses.
Possible side effects: Nausea, vomiting, and diarrhea. Some people may be allergic to certain antibiotics and may experience symptoms such as rashes, fever, joint pain, swelling, and wheezing. Following treatment with broad-spectrum antibiotics, fungal infection of the vagina sometimes occurs.
Children's doses: The following are the antibiotics most commonly used to treat children: ampicillin, amoxicillin, erythromycin, and penicillin. Antibiotics may cause side effects, and some children may be particularly sensitive to penicillin and similar antibiotics. Side effects may include rashes, nausea, vomiting, diarrhea, and wheezing. Always consult your doctor about any reaction to an antibiotic.
Warning: Always take all of the antibiotics that your doctor prescribes. Failure to do so, even when symptoms have cleared, may lead to a recurrence of infection that is more difficult to treat (due to resistance of the bacteria to the antibiotic).

ANTICOAGULANTS
Drugs that prevent and/or disperse blood clots; used to treat conditions that make dangerous clots likely.
Possible side effects: Increased tendency to bleed from the nose or gums or under the skin (bruising). Blood may also appear in the urine or stools.
Warning: Anticoagulants may react more intensely in the presence of other drugs, including aspirin. Consult your doctor before taking any medicines, so that the effectiveness of the anticoagulant is not altered. If you are taking anticoagulants, you will be

advised to carry a warning card or identification tag.

ANTICONVULSANTS
Drugs used to prevent and treat epileptic seizures. These usually are given at least twice a day. Careful calculation of the best dose for the individual is necessary to minimize side effects. Blood or saliva tests are usually given to monitor drug concentrations. Usually, the drug is given over a prolonged period until the person has gone 2 to 4 years without a seizure.
Possible side effects: Drowsiness, rashes, dizziness, headache, nausea, and thickening of the gums.
Children's doses: The drugs most commonly used to treat children who have grand mal seizures are phenytoin, valproate sodium, and carbamazepine. Their side effects may include drowsiness, gastrointestinal disturbances, rashes, an increase in body hair, overgrowth of the gums, enlargement of the lymph glands, blood abnormalities, and liver damage. Phenobarbital is less often prescribed for children because it may cause behavior disturbances. Petit mal seizures (periods in which the child stares off into space and does not seem to hear or see) may be treated with valproate sodium or ethosuximide.
Warning: Alcohol may increase the likelihood and severity of side effects and is best avoided, as are ANTIHISTAMINES. Consult your doctor before driving and/or operating potentially dangerous machinery.

ANTIDEPRESSANTS
Drugs that treat depression and are also effective for other problems such as anxiety disorders, chronic pain, some types of headache, and chronic fatigue syndrome. These drugs fall into

two main groups: tricyclics and their derivatives, and monoamine oxidase (MAO) inhibitors. Because their side effects are likely to be more serious, MAO inhibitors are usually only prescribed for those types of severe depression that are less likely to respond to treatment with tricyclics. A newer type of antidepressant (fluoxetine) is now available to treat some forms of depression. It generally has fewer side effects than other products.

Possible side effects: Drowsiness, dry mouth, blurred vision, constipation, difficulty urinating, faintness, sweating, trembling, rashes, palpitations, and headaches.

Children's doses: Antidepressants may occasionally be prescribed for older children suffering from depression. In addition, some doctors may prescribe antidepressants such as amitriptyline for bed-wetting in children over the age of 12 when other forms of treatment have failed. This use of antidepressants is controversial, however. Side effects may include behavioral disturbances and abnormal heart rate and rhythm.

Warning: MAO inhibitors react adversely with a number of foods and drugs, possibly leading to a serious rise in blood pressure. Your doctor will advise you and may recommend that you carry a warning card or identification tag. During both types of antidepressant treatment, alcohol intake should be limited. Ask your doctor whether it is advisable to drive or operate machinery.

ANTIDIARRHEALS

Drugs used to control and treat diarrhea. There are two main types: those that absorb excess water and toxins in the bowel (for example, those containing kaolin, bismuth compounds, chalk, or charcoal) and those that reduce the contractions of the bowel, thus decreasing the frequency with which stools are passed (including codeine, morphine, and opium mixtures).

Possible side effects: Constipation.

Warning: Antidiarrheals relieve symptoms but do not treat the underlying cause of diarrhea and may prolong the course of toxic or infectious diarrhea. They should not be taken for more than a day or so before seeking medical advice. When treating diarrhea, always drink plenty of fluids. See also REHYDRATION TREATMENTS.

ANTIEMETICS

Drugs used to suppress nausea and vomiting. Most also suppress dizziness. The main groups of drugs in this category include certain ANTIHISTAMINES (especially for nausea caused by motion sickness or ear disorders), ANTISPASMODICS, and certain tranquilizers. Because antiemetic treatment may hinder diagnosis, such drugs are not usually prescribed when the cause of vomiting is unknown or when vomiting is unlikely to persist for longer than a day or so, as in cases of gastroenteritis.

Possible side effects: These vary according to the drug group prescribed. Prolonged treatment with certain tranquilizers may cause involuntary movement of the facial muscles. These drugs should never be taken for more than a few days at a time.

Warning: Because most antiemetics

may cause drowsiness, do not drink alcohol and seek your doctor's advice before driving or operating potentially dangerous machinery.

ANTIFUNGALS

Drugs to treat fungal conditions such as ringworm, athletes' foot, vaginal infection, and some diaper rash. They may be applied directly to the skin or taken by mouth over a prolonged period.

Possible side effects: Oral antifungals may cause nausea, vomiting, diarrhea, and/or headaches; locally applied (topical) preparations may cause irritation.

Warning: Always finish a course of antifungal treatment as prescribed; otherwise the infection may recur. Some infections, especially of the nails, may require treatment with oral antifungals for many months.

ANTIHISTAMINES

Drugs to counteract allergic symptoms produced by the release of a substance called histamine in the body. Such symptoms may include runny nose and watery eyes (allergic rhinitis), itching, and urticaria (hives). Antihistamines may be given orally or applied to skin rashes in the form of creams or sprays. Antihistamine drugs also act on the organs of balance in the middle ear and therefore are often used to prevent motion sickness. Their sedative effect may also be used to treat sleeplessness (on your doctor's advice). They are also given as a medication before operations to ensure that a person is in a relaxed, drowsy state. Another class of antihistamine interferes with gastric acid secretion and is used to treat peptic ulcers.

Possible side effects: Drowsiness, dry mouth, and blurred vision.

Children's doses: Antihistamines most commonly given to children are chlorpheniramine and promethazine hydrochloride. The main side effect is drowsiness, but some children may become unusually excited instead.

Warning: Driving or drinking alcohol should be avoided after taking an antihistamine.

ANTIHYPERTENSIVES

Drugs that lower blood pressure. BETA BLOCKERS and DIURETICS and, more recently, angiotensin-converting enzyme (ACE) inhibitors (which reduce the formation of a substance produced in the kidney and liver that can raise blood pressure) and calcium channel blockers (which decrease the calcium in the heart muscle and increase the oxygen supply to the heart) are some examples.

Possible side effects: Dizziness, rashes, impotence, nightmares, and lethargy.

ANTI-INFLAMMATORIES

Drugs used to reduce inflammation, which is the redness, heat, swelling, pain, and increased blood flow that is found in infections and in many chronic noninfective diseases such as rheumatoid arthritis and gout. Three main types of drugs are used as anti-inflammatories: ANALGESICS such as aspirin, CORTICOSTEROIDS, and nonsteroidal anti-inflammatory drugs such as indomethacin, which is used especially in the treatment of arthritis and muscle disorders. CORTICOSTEROIDS may be applied locally as cream or eyedrops for inflammation of the skin or eyes, but

they are not generally prescribed for chronic rheumatic conditions except in unusual circumstances.

Possible side effects: Rashes, stomach irritation, (occasionally) bleeding, disturbances in hearing, and wheezing.

Children's doses: There are two main categories of anti-inflammatory drugs used to treat children: CORTICO-STEROIDS and nonsteroidal anti-inflammatories. Commonly prescribed drugs of the latter type include aspirin (not used for the treatment of children—see ANALGESICS), ibuprofen, and mefenamic acid. These drugs may cause constipation, minor digestive disturbances, and possible bleeding in the stomach and intestines.

ANTIPYRETICS

Drugs that reduce fever. The most commonly used are aspirin and acetaminophen, which are both also ANALGESICS. This double action makes them particularly effective for relieving the symptoms of an illness such as flu. Take with food.

Possible side effects: Rashes, stomach irritation, (occasionally) bleeding, disturbances in hearing, and wheezing.

ANTISPASMODICS

Drugs for reducing spasm of the bowel to relieve the pain of conditions such as irritable colon or diverticular disease.

Possible side effects: Dry mouth, palpitations, difficulty urinating, constipation, and blurred vision.

ANTIVIRALS

Drugs that combat viral infections. Effective drug treatment is not yet available for the majority of viral infections, such as colds and flu. However, severe cold sores caused by the herpes simplex virus can be treated by the application of idoxuridine ointment as soon as symptoms appear. Idoxuridine is also used to treat shingles. Another antiviral drug, acyclovir, may be given orally or by injection or applied directly to the skin in the form of a cream to treat most severe types of herpes infection. Since the outbreak of acquired immune deficiency syndrome (AIDS), new antiviral drugs have been developed, including zidovudine (AZT), which slows the progression of the virus that causes AIDS.

Possible side effects: Antivirals used to treat cold sores, genital herpes, and shingles may cause a stinging sensation, rashes, and (occasionally) loss of sensation in the skin.

BETA BLOCKERS

Beta-adrenergic blocking agents (beta blockers for short) reduce oxygen needs of the heart by reducing heartbeat rate. They are used as ANTIHYPERTENSIVES and antiarrhythmics, for treating angina due to exertion, and for easing symptoms such as palpitations and tremors in some people. Beta blockers may be taken as tablets or given by injection.

Possible side effects: Nausea, insomnia, fatigue, and diarrhea.

Warning: Overdose can cause dizziness and fainting spells. Discontinuation of treatment should be gradual, not abrupt. Beta blockers are not prescribed for people with asthma or heart failure.

BRONCHODILATORS

Drugs that open up bronchial tubes

narrowed by muscle spasm. Bronchodilators, which ease breathing in diseases such as asthma, are most often taken as aerosol sprays, but they are also available in tablet, liquid, or suppository form. In emergencies—such as a severe attack of asthma—they may be given by injection. Effects usually last for 3 to 5 hours.

Possible side effects: Rapid heartbeat, palpitations, tremor, headache, and dizziness.

Children's doses: In children, narrowing of the bronchial tubes usually occurs as a result of asthma or respiratory infections (such as bronchitis or bronchiolitis). Two primary groups of drugs are used to treat asthma. First are those that treat an acute attack (bronchodilators), including terbutaline and the theophyllines. These may also be routinely given orally or by injection. Second are those that act to prevent an attack (cromolyn sodium). These are not effective in an acute attack. CORTICOSTEROIDS (see ANTI-INFLAMMATORIES), either taken by mouth, inhaled, or injected, can be used to treat asthma that is resistant to the above-mentioned drugs. Children over 3 can be taught to use inhalers very effectively. Side effects of the anti-asthmatics include increased heart rate, tremor, and irritability.

Warning: Because of possible effects on the heart, prescribed doses should never be exceeded; when asthma does not respond to the prescribed doses, emergency medical treatment is needed.

COLD REMEDIES

Although there is no drug that can cure a cold, symptoms can be effectively relieved by aspirin or acetaminophen, taken with plenty of fluid. For drying up nasal secretions and unblocking nasal passages, many preparations contain ANTIHISTAMINES and DECONGES-TANTS. However, these drugs are unlikely to be effective when taken by mouth, unless swallowed in doses high enough to produce side effects that outweigh any benefits.

Possible side effects: Drowsiness, dizziness, headache, nausea, vomiting, sweating, thirst, palpitations, difficulty passing urine, weakness, trembling, anxiety, and insomnia.

Warning: Cold remedies should be avoided by people who have angina, high blood pressure, diabetes, or thyroid disorders, and by anyone taking monoamine oxidase inhibitors. It is inadvisable to drive or use potentially dangerous machinery after taking a remedy containing an antihistamine.

CORTICOSTEROIDS

A group of anti-inflammatory drugs (see ANTI-INFLAMMATORIES) that is chemically similar to certain naturally produced hormones from the adrenal glands that help the body respond to stress. They may be given orally, injected, applied to the skin as a cream, or inhaled into the lungs. Corticosteroid inhalations such as beclomethasone may be prescribed when other anti-asthmatic drugs have failed. There are few side effects to such treatment when used for limited periods of time. Corticosteroids such as hydrocortisone or prednisolone given orally or by injection are used for acute conditions (e.g., shock, severe allergic reactions, or severe asthma). They are used in the long-term

treatment of a wide variety of inflammatory conditions. They are not curative but do reduce inflammation, which sometimes enables the body to repair itself. Corticosteroids may be useful for treating certain types of cancer or in compensating for a deficiency of natural hormones.
Possible side effects: Weight gain, fluid retention, stomach irritation, mental disturbances and development of diabetes with long-term use.
Children's doses: The conditions of children who are prescribed these drugs should be carefully monitored because of the side effects. These include fluid retention with excessive weight gain, a moon-shaped face, and growth retardation.

COUGH SUPPRESSANTS
Medicines that relieve coughing— usually as a result of a cold. There are many over-the-counter products, including lozenges and syrups, that contain soothing substances (such as honey and glycerin to act on the surface of the throat), pleasant-tasting flavorings, and minute doses of antiseptic chemicals. They may give temporary relief to a ticklish throat and the taste may be comforting. Many cough suppressants contain alcohol; non-alcoholic products are available.

CYTOTOXICS
Drugs that kill or damage multiplying cells. Cytotoxics are used in treatment of cancer and as IMMUNOSUPPRESSIVES. They are taken as tablets or given by injection or by intravenous drip. Several cytotoxics, with different types of action, may be used in combination.
Possible side effects: Nausea, vomiting, and loss of hair.
Children's doses: Cytotoxics are used in the treatment of some types of cancer in children, notably leukemia. These powerful drugs are given under close supervision. The most effective dosage is calculated to cause minimal side effects.
Warning: Because cytotoxic action can affect healthy as well as cancerous cells, these drugs may also have dangerous side effects. For example, they can damage bone marrow and affect the production of blood cells, causing anemia, increased susceptibility to infection, and hemorrhage. Frequent blood counts are advisable for anyone taking cytotoxics.

DECONGESTANTS
Drugs that act on the mucous membranes lining the nose to reduce mucus production and so relieve a runny or stuffy nose resulting from the common cold or an allergy. These drugs can be applied directly in the form of nose drops or spray or may be taken by mouth. Decongestants taken by mouth can raise blood pressure. People with high blood pressure should consult their doctors.
Children's doses: Decongestants are usually recommended only for occasional use on your doctor's advice—for example, when a stuffy nose prevents a young baby from sucking. If used excessively or for prolonged periods, nose drops may cause increased congestion.

DIURETICS
Drugs that increase the quantity of urine produced by the kidneys and passed out of the body, thus ridding the body of excess fluid. Diuretics reduce excess fluid that has collected in the tissues as a result of any disorder of the heart, kidneys, and liver. They are useful for treating mildly raised blood pressure.
Possible side effects: Rashes, dizziness, weakness, numbness, tingling in the hands and feet, and excessive loss of potassium.

HORMONES
Chemicals produced naturally by the endocrine (pituitary, thyroid, adrenal, ovary/testicle, pancreas, or parathyroid) glands. When they are not produced naturally (because of some disorder), they can be replaced by natural or synthetic hormones. See SEX HORMONES.
Possible side effects: There may be an exaggeration of the secondary sexual characteristics. Estrogens given to a man may increase the size of his breasts and androgens given to a woman may cause increased body hair and deepening of the voice. Estrogens also affect blood clotting and so may cause heart attack, stroke, or blood clots in the legs.
Children's doses: Hormones may occasionally be given to children when a glandular disorder prevents sufficient quantities of that hormone from being produced by the body. The most common deficiencies are in thyroid-stimulating hormone, growth hormone, and insulin (diabetes). If your child needs to take supplements of any of these hormones, regular blood tests will be taken so that the dosage can be accurately controlled.

HYPOGLYCEMICS
Drugs that lower the level of glucose in the blood. Oral hypoglycemic drugs are used in the treatment of diabetes mellitus that cannot be controlled by diet alone yet does not require treatment with injections of insulin.
Possible side effects: Loss of appetite, nausea, indigestion, numbness or tingling in the skin, fever, and rashes.
Warning: If the glucose level falls too low, weakness, dizziness, pallor, sweating, increased saliva flow, palpitations, irritability, and trembling may result. If such symptoms occur several hours after eating, the dose may be too high. Report symptoms to your doctor.

IMMUNOSUPPRESSIVES
Drugs that prevent or reduce the body's normal reaction to invasion by disease organisms or by foreign proteins such as those in a transplanted organ. Immunosuppressives are used to treat autoimmune diseases (in which the body's defenses work abnormally and attack the body's own tissues) and to help prevent rejection of organ transplants.
Possible side effects: Susceptibility to infection (especially chest infections, fungal infections of the mouth and skin, and virus infections) is increased. Some immunosuppressives may damage the bone marrow, causing anemia, and may cause nausea and vomiting.

LAXATIVES
Drugs that increase the frequency and ease of bowel movements. They work by stimulating the bowel wall, by increasing the bulk of bowel contents, or by increasing the fluid content of the stool.

Children's doses: Laxatives should never be given to children except on the advice of a doctor.
Warning: Laxatives are not to be taken regularly; the bowel may become unable to work properly without them.

REHYDRATION TREATMENTS
These specially formulated powders and solutions contain glucose and essential mineral salts in measured quantities that, when added to boiled water, can be used to prevent and treat dehydration resulting from diarrhea or vomiting. These powders and solutions are useful for home treatment of stomach and intestinal infections in babies and children. Similar solutions may be given intravenously in the hospital.

SEX HORMONES (FEMALE)
The hormones responsible for the development of secondary sexual characteristics and regulation of the menstrual cycle. There are two main types of hormone drugs: estrogens and progestogens. Estrogens may be used for treating breast or prostate cancer; progestogens may be used for treating endometriosis. Postmenopausal estrogen replacement can help slow or prevent development of coronary artery disease and osteoporosis in some women. Sex hormones may be applied as skin patches, taken as tablets, given by injection, or implanted in muscle tissue.
Possible side effects: Nausea, weight gain, headache, depression, breast enlargement and tenderness, rashes and skin pigmentation changes, alterations in sex drive, and abnormal blood-clotting that can cause heart disorders.
Warning: Estrogens are not prescribed for anyone with circulatory or liver trouble, and estrogen treatment must be carefully controlled for people who have had jaundice, diabetes, epilepsy, or kidney or heart disease. Progestogen treatment is not prescribed for people with liver trouble and must be carefully controlled for anyone who has asthma, epilepsy, or heart or kidney disease.

SEX HORMONES (MALE)
The hormones (of which the most powerful is testosterone) responsible for the development of male secondary sexual characteristics. Small quantities are also produced in females. As drugs, male sex hormones are given to compensate for hormonal deficiency in hypopituitarism or testicular disorders. They may be used for treating breast cancer in women, but synthetic derivatives—the anabolic steroids, which have less marked side effects— and specific antiestrogens are often preferable. Anabolic steroids also have a body-building effect that has led to their usually illicit use, by both men and women, in competitive sports. Such use can cause heart, liver, or kidney disease, sterility, and violent behavior. Male sex hormones can be taken by mouth or by injection, or implanted in muscle tissue.
Possible side effects: Edema, weight gain, weakness, loss of appetite, drowsiness, and nausea. High doses in women may cause cessation of menstruation, deepening of the voice, shrinking of the breasts, hairiness, and male-pattern baldness.
Warning: Treatment is inadvisable for people with kidney or liver trouble and

must be carefully controlled for anyone who has epilepsy or migraine.

SKIN CREAMS
A wide variety of skin creams, ointments, and lotions are available to treat and/or prevent skin disorders (for example, to combat infection or relieve irritation). They usually consist of a base to which various active ingredients are added. Creams commonly used include: antiseptics containing a drug such as cetrimonium bromide to prevent infection of minor wounds; soothing barriers such as zinc oxide, vitamin-based products, or petroleum jelly to prevent and treat diaper rash; ANTIBIOTICS to treat skin infections such as impetigo; CORTICOSTEROIDS; ANTIFUNGALS; acne preparations; and local anesthetic and antipruritic (itch-relieving) creams containing calamine, ANTIHISTAMINES, or a local anesthetic such as benzocaine.
Children's doses: When selecting a cream to treat a child's skin condition, always ask your doctor for advice.

SLEEPING DRUGS
Two main groups of drugs are used to induce sleep: ANTI-ANXIETY DRUGS and barbiturates. All such drugs have a sedative effect in low doses and are effective sleeping preparations in higher doses. Anti-anxiety drugs are used more widely than barbiturates because they are safer, and have fewer side effects, and there is less risk of eventual physical and psychological dependence.
Possible side effects: "Hangover," dizziness, dry mouth, and, especially in the elderly, clumsiness and confusion.
Children's doses: Adult sleeping drugs are not used to treat sleeplessness in children. A young child who persistently wakes at night may be given ANTIHISTAMINES, which cause drowsiness. In rare cases, an older child may be prescribed an ANTI-ANXIETY DRUG to promote sleep during a period of psychological distress.
Warning: Sleeping drugs are habit-forming, should be taken for short periods only, and should be discontinued gradually. Broken, restless sleep and vivid dreams may follow withdrawal and may persist for weeks. It is inadvisable to drive, handle dangerous machinery, or drink alcohol until the effects of a sleeping drug have completely worn off.

VASODILATORS
Drugs that dilate blood vessels. Most widely used to prevent and treat angina, but also to treat heart failure and circulatory disorders.
Possible side effects: Headache, palpitations, flushing, faintness, nausea, vomiting, diarrhea, and stuffy nose.

VITAMINS
Vitamins are complex chemicals needed by the body in minute quantities. They are often prescribed for babies and young children, but are usually unnecessary for healthy children and adults eating an adequate diet. Vitamins do not make a person feel more energetic. Small doses of vitamin supplements are harmless, but exceeding the recommended daily dose can have adverse effects and interfere with the action of other drugs.

Children's growth charts

These growth charts and those on pages 300 and 301 are based on the standard growth charts used by doctors in the U.S. You can use these charts to keep a record of your child's growth as measured by your pediatrician.

The growth charts on this and the facing page are for recording the progress of babies of both sexes up to the age of 36 months. The charts on pages 300 and 301 are for boys and girls from 3 to 18 years.

Standard growth curves

On each chart you will find seven solid lines already drawn. These lines are the standard growth curves for small to large children. The standard curves enable you to compare your child's progress with the expected growth of children of similar size at birth. Remember that there is wide variation among children. If you have any concerns about your child's growth, discuss them with your pediatrician.

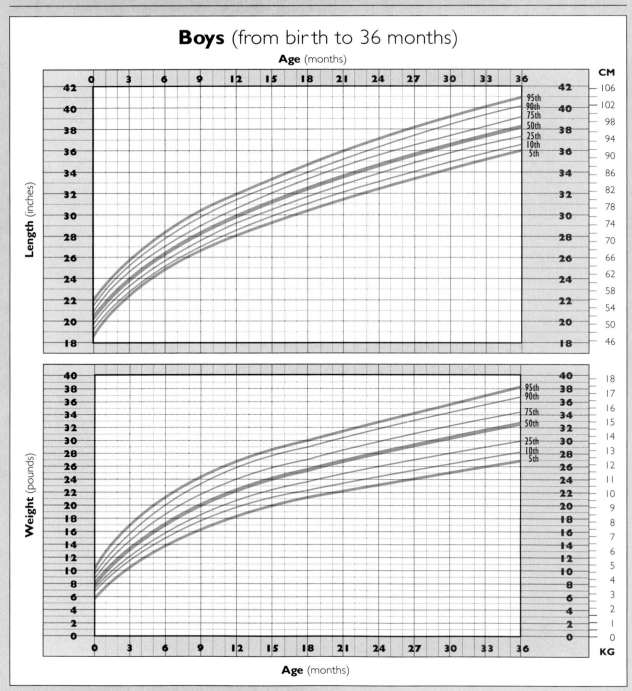

Boys (from birth to 36 months)

Recording your child's growth

When your pediatrician weighs and measures your child during his or her visits, mark the results on the appropriate chart. You may even want to take the charts, along with his or her immunization record, to the office with you. Use a ruler to help you read horizontally across from the scales on the left and right of the chart to the point where it meets the vertical line up from your child's age at the top or bottom of the chart.

Mark the point where the two lines cross. By linking this mark with the previous result, you will soon build a curve showing your child's growth.

Also consult symptom chart 1, *Slow weight gain;* chart 10, *Slow growth;* chart 11, *Excessive weight gain;* or chart 53, *Adolescent weight problems.*

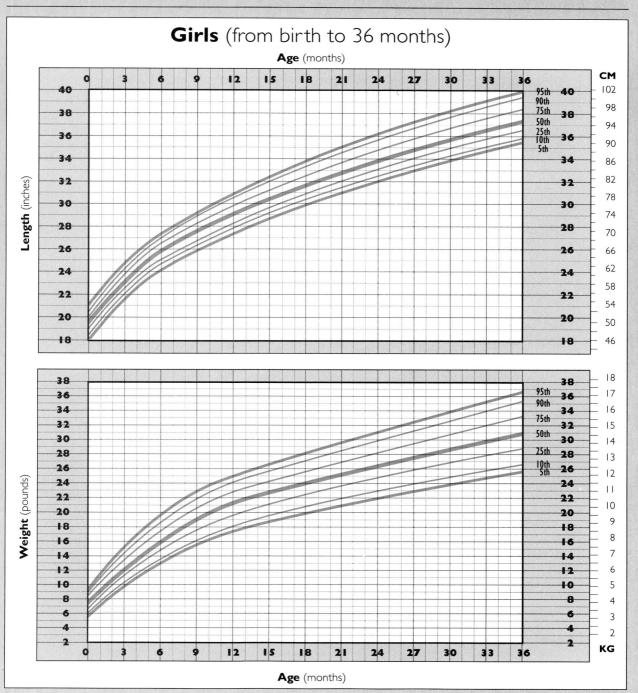

Girls (from birth to 36 months)

Growth charts

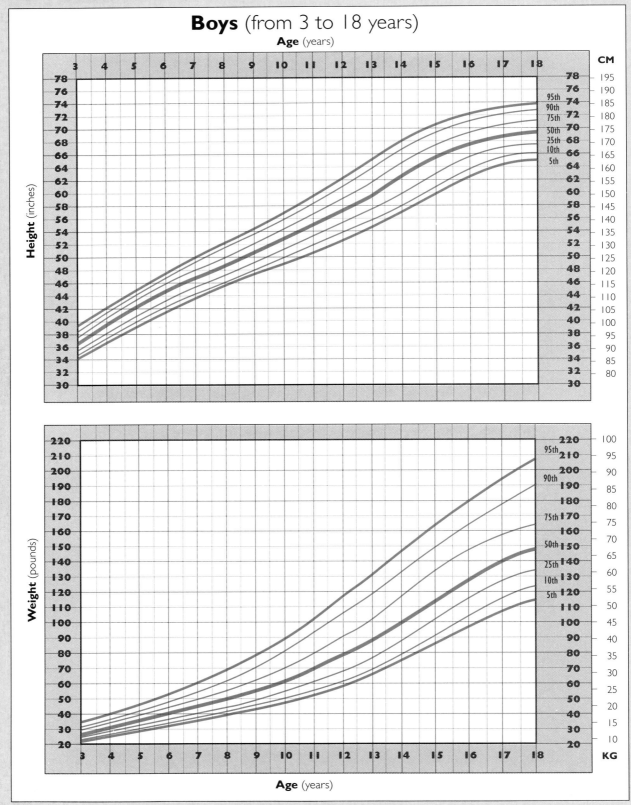

Boys (from 3 to 18 years)

Girls (from 3 to 18 years)

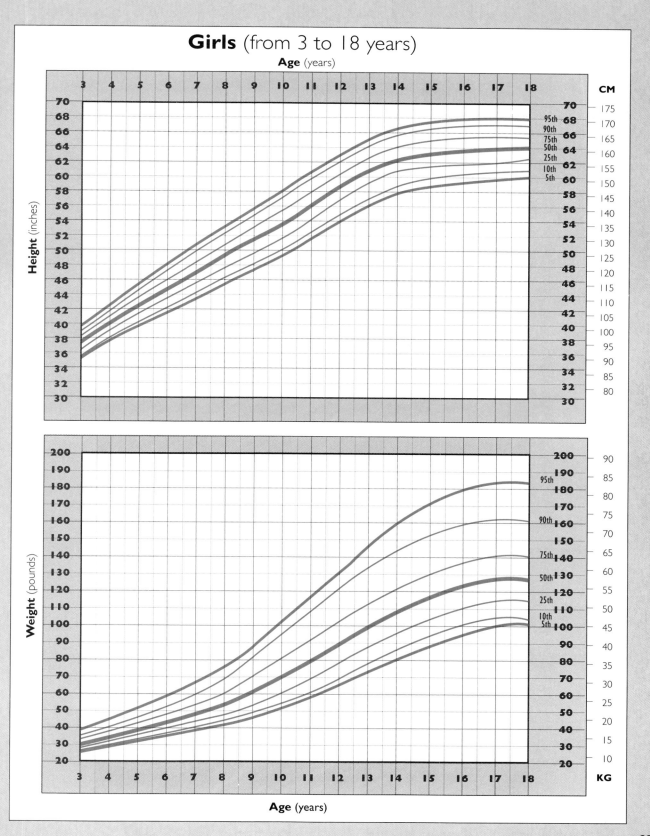

Adult weight tables

Fat usually accounts for about 10 to 20 percent of the weight of an adult male, and 25 percent of the weight of an adult female. Much more fat than this is both unnecessary and unhealthy. The weight chart below shows an approximate healthy weight range for different heights. Your weight should remain roughly constant after the age of 25, although most people gradually gain weight as they grow older, and are heaviest around the age of 50. Weight gain is more likely if you exercise less at this time in life, when your body is beginning to take longer to burn calories. Matching food intake with energy output is the best way to maintain your weight over the years (see *Age and increasing weight,* page 150). If you fall into the overweight range on the weight chart, see *How to lose weight* (page 151) and learn how to lose the extra pounds sensibly. If you are not convinced that you need to lose weight, try the fat-fold thickness test described on the opposite page. It is important to take a pinch of skin on the abdomen above the navel or on the side just over the lower ribs because both sexes have an equal amount of fat there. In other areas, such as the upper arm and thigh, women have more fat than men. To check your actual weight against a healthy weight for someone of your height, first find your height to the left of the weight table. Then draw a line across from your height and a line up from your weight on the bottom of the chart. If the point where your height and weight lines meet is in the colored central band, your weight is healthy for someone of your height. If you are overweight, you are more susceptible than trimmer people to coronary artery disease, high blood pressure, diabetes, and other disorders. For further information, consult the relevant symptom chart (see *Overweight,* page 150) and discuss the matter with your doctor. If you are seriously underweight, this too may be cause for concern (see *Loss of weight,* page 148); you should discuss the matter with your doctor.

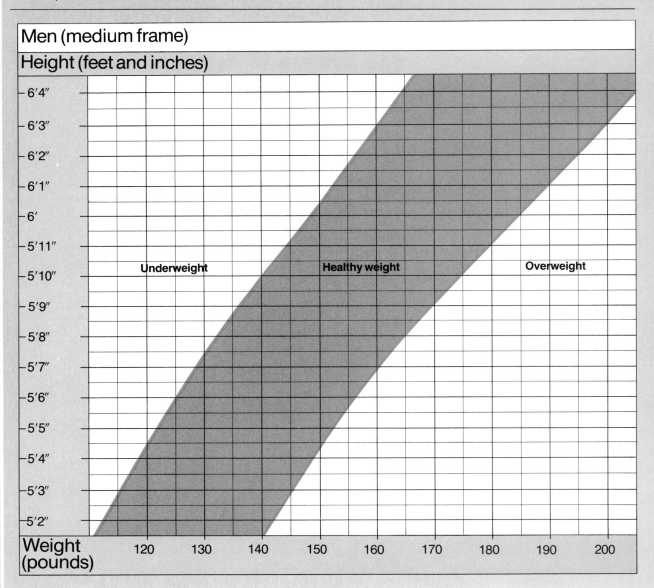

Men (medium frame)

Height (feet and inches)

Underweight   Healthy weight   Overweight

Weight (pounds): 120 130 140 150 160 170 180 190 200

FAT DISTRIBUTION

Fat is deposited in a layer underneath the skin and within the tissues in some parts of the body, including the buttocks, breasts, and inside the chest and abdominal cavities. Fat comprises more of a woman's weight than a man's weight. It is distributed in such a way as to give male and female bodies their characteristic contours. Fat is stored when food intake is greater than is needed to fuel the body's energy requirements. It is burned when food intake fails to equal the body's energy output. Fat also serves as insulation against the cold.

Both too much and too little fat can be unhealthy. Being too fat can lead to heart and circulation problems. Being too thin is less of a health risk, but may be a sign of undernourishment and can reduce your resistance to a variety of diseases. Fluctuations in the level of fat deposits are almost always the result of an imbalance between food intake and energy expenditure.

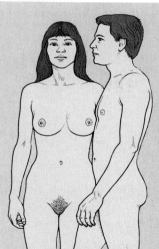

The best place to measure the thickness of a fold of fat for both men and women is just above the navel. Or you can take a deep pinch of skin on your side just over the lower ribs. Most men and women have roughly the same amounts of fat there. If the distance between thumb and index finger is greater than 1 inch thick, you are probably overweight and should adjust your diet and exercise regularly.

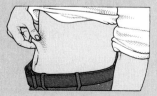

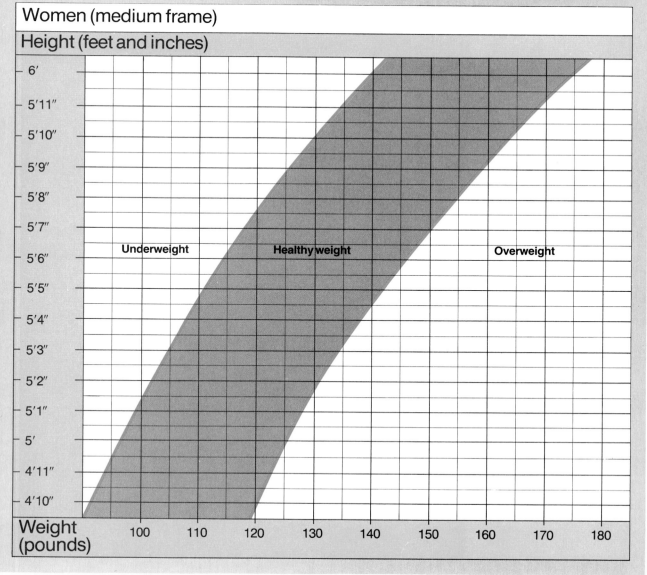

Women (medium frame)

Height (feet and inches)

Underweight   Healthy weight   Overweight

Weight (pounds)

Children's medical records

Birth record

Name _____ Weight _____
Time of birth _____ Blood type _____
Date of birth _____ Type of feeding _____
Height _____   Breast _____ Bottle _____

Details of pregnancy

Mother's health during pregnancy:
Illness _____
Medication _____
Problems _____
Delivery:
Type _____ Drugs _____
Monitoring _____ Pediatrician _____
Problems _____ Hospital _____
_____ Length of stay _____

Illness and injury record

Illnesses	Date/age	Duration of treatment
Injuries		

Immunization record

Disease	Date/age	Booster dates
Diphtheria, tetanus, pertussis (DTP)		
Poliomyelitis		
Measles, mumps, rubella		
Haemophilus influenzae type b (Hib)		

Birth record

Name ————————————————   Weight ————————————————
Time of birth ——————————————   Blood type ——————————————
Date of birth ——————————————   Type of feeding ——————————
Height ————————————————   Breast ————— Bottle ————

Details of pregnancy

Mother's health during pregnancy:
Illness ————————————————
Medication ———————————————
Problems ————————————————
Delivery:
Type ————————————————   Drugs ————————————————
Monitoring ——————————————   Pediatrician ——————————————
Problems ——————————————   Hospital ——————————————
————————————————   Length of stay ——————————————

Illness and injury record

Illnesses	Date/age	Duration of treatment
Injuries		

Immunization record

Disease	Date/age	Booster dates
Diphtheria, tetanus, pertussis (DTP)		
Poliomyelitis		
Measles, mumps, rubella		
Haemophilus influenzae type b (Hib)		

Children's development records

Name _____

Developmental milestones	Date/age
Smiles _____	_____
Rolls over _____	_____
Raises head and shoulders from a facedown position _____	_____
Sits unsupported _____	_____
Passes objects from one hand to the other _____	_____
Crawls _____	_____
First tooth _____	_____
Starts solid foods _____	_____
Is weaned _____	_____
Stands unsupported _____	_____
Sleeps through the night _____	_____
Walks unaided _____	_____
First words _____	_____
Talks in simple sentences _____	_____
First visit to the dentist _____	_____
Gets dressed and undressed (with a little help) _____	_____
Draws a recognizable figure _____	_____
Starts playschool/nursery school _____	_____

Name

Developmental milestones	Date/age
Smiles	
Rolls over	
Raises head and shoulders from a facedown position	
Sits unsupported	
Passes objects from one hand to the other	
Crawls	
First tooth	
Starts solid foods	
Is weaned	
Stands unsupported	
Sleeps through the night	
Walks unaided	
First words	
Talks in simple sentences	
First visit to the dentist	
Gets dressed and undressed (with a little help)	
Draws a recognizable figure	
Starts playschool/nursery school	

Adult medical records

Female

Name

Examinations	Date/result	Date/result	Date/result
Cervical (pap) smear			
Vaginal examination			
Mammogram			
Eye test			
Dental checkup			
Complete physical			
Blood pressure			
Stool test for hidden blood			
Serum cholesterol			
Triglycerides			

Medications	Dose	Side effects

Contraceptives

Allergies	Treatment

Injuries and/or illnesses	Date

Operations and/or procedures	Date

Name

Examinations	Date/result	Date/result	Date/result
Eye test			
Dental checkup			
Complete physical			
Blood pressure			
Stool test for hidden blood			
Serum cholesterol			
Triglycerides			

Medications	Dose	Side effects

Allergies	Treatment

Injuries and/or illnesses	Date

Operations and/or procedures	Date

Immunization records

Name _____

Disease	Date of immunization/ illness	Date of booster
Hepatitis*		
Measles*		
Mumps*		
Rubella*		
Whooping cough (pertussis)*		
Diphtheria*		
Poliomyelitis*		
Tetanus†		
Influenza‡		
Pneumococcal pneumonia§		
Other		

Name _____

Hepatitis*		
Measles*		
Mumps*		
Rubella*		
Whooping cough (pertussis)*		
Diphtheria*		
Poliomyelitis*		
Tetanus†		
Influenza‡		
Pneumococcal pneumonia§		
Other		

* All of these immunizations should be completed by age 16 or by young adulthood. Women considering pregnancy should be certain that they have been immunized against rubella before they become pregnant.

† Adults should be reimmunized against tetanus every 10 years (for example, first immunization at age 15, then at 25, 35, and so on) or if they have a dirty wound.

‡ Immunization against influenza (a "flu" shot) every fall is advisable for people over 65; people with lung disease, heart disease, diabetes, or another chronic illness; and people who work in a health care or other institution where people may be ill.

§ People over 65 or with chronic illness, especially lung disease, should be immunized against pneumococcal pneumonia. One vaccination lasts for at least 5 years.

Useful addresses

Adolescence

THE NATIONAL CLEARINGHOUSE
FOR ALCOHOL AND DRUG
INFORMATION
P.O. Box 2345
Rockville, MD 20847
(800) 729-6686

PLANNED PARENTHOOD
FEDERATION OF AMERICA
810 Seventh Avenue
New York, NY 10019
(212) 541-7800

Aging

NATIONAL ASSOCIATION FOR
HOME CARE
519 C Street NE
Washington, DC 20002
(202) 547-7424

THE NATIONAL COUNCIL ON THE
AGING, INC.
409 Third Street SW
Washington, DC 20024
(202) 479-1200

NATIONAL INSTITUTE ON AGING
Public Information Office
Federal Building, Room 6C12
Bethesda, MD 20892
(301) 496-4000

AIDS

THE NATIONAL AIDS HOTLINE
(800) 342-2437

Alcohol abuse

ALCOHOLICS ANONYMOUS
468 Park Avenue South
New York, NY 10016
(212) 686-1100

AL-ANON FAMILY GROUP
HEADQUARTERS
P.O. Box 862 Midtown Station
New York, NY 10018
(800) 356-9996

NATIONAL COUNCIL ON
ALCOHOLISM AND DRUG
DEPENDENCE, INC.
12 West 21st Street
New York, NY 10010
(800) NCA-CALL; (212) 206-6770 in NY

Alzheimer's disease

ALZHEIMER'S ASSOCIATION
919 N. Michigan Avenue, Suite 1000
Chicago, IL 60611
(800) 272-3900; (312) 335-8700 in IL

Arthritis

ARTHRITIS FOUNDATION
1314 Spring Street NW
Atlanta, GA 30309
(404) 872-7100

Birth control and abortion

PLANNED PARENTHOOD
FEDERATION OF AMERICA
810 Seventh Avenue
New York, NY 10019
(212) 541-7800

Blindness and visual impairment

AMERICAN FOUNDATION FOR THE
BLIND, INC.
15 West 16th Street
New York, NY 10011
(212) 620-2000

ASSOCIATION FOR EDUCATION
AND REHABILITATION OF THE
BLIND AND VISUALLY IMPAIRED
206 North Washington Street, Suite 320
Alexandria, VA 22314
(703) 548-1884

NATIONAL SOCIETY TO PREVENT
BLINDNESS
500 East Remington Road
Schaumburg, IL 60173
(708) 843-2020

Cancer

AMERICAN CANCER SOCIETY
1599 Clifton Road NE
Atlanta, GA 30329
(800) ACS-2345; (404) 320-3333 in
Atlanta

CANCER INFORMATION SERVICE
Building 31, Room 10A24
9000 Rockville Pike
Bethesda, MD 20892
(800) 4-CANCER

CANDLELIGHTERS CHILDHOOD
CANCER FOUNDATION
1312 18th Street NW, Suite 200
Washington, DC 20036
(202) 659-5136

NATIONAL COALITION FOR
CANCER SURVIVORSHIP
1010 Wayne Avenue, 5th floor
Silver Spring, MD 20910
(301) 585-2616

Child health

NATIONAL INSTITUTE OF CHILD
HEALTH AND HUMAN
DEVELOPMENT
9000 Rockville Pike
Bethesda, MD 20892
(301) 496-4000

MATERNAL AND CHILD HEALTH
BUREAU
5600 Fishers Lane, Room 948
Parklawn Building
Rockville, MD 20857
(301) 443-2370

Chronic fatigue syndrome

NATIONAL CHRONIC FATIGUE
SYNDROME ASSOCIATION, INC.
3521 Broadway, Suite 222
Kansas City, MO 64111
(816) 931-4777

Deafness and hearing impairment

NATIONAL ASSOCIATION OF
THE DEAF
814 Thayer Avenue
Silver Spring, MD 20910
(301) 587-1788

SELF-HELP FOR HARD OF
HEARING PEOPLE, INC.
7800 Wisconsin Avenue
Bethesda, MD 20814
(301) 657-2248

Dental health

AMERICAN DENTAL ASSOCIATION
Dept. of Public Information and
Education
211 East Chicago Avenue
Chicago, IL 60611
(312) 440-2593

Depression

NATIONAL DEPRESSIVE AND
MANIC DEPRESSIVE ASSOCIATION
730 N. Franklin Street, Suite 501
Chicago, IL 60610
(312) 642-0049; (800) 826-3632 in IL

Diabetes

AMERICAN DIABETES
ASSOCIATION
1660 Duke Street
Alexandria, VA 22314
(800) 232-3472

NATIONAL DIABETES
INFORMATION CLEARINGHOUSE
Box NDIC
9000 Rockville Pike
Bethesda, MD 20892
(301) 468-2162

Heart disease

AMERICAN HEART ASSOCIATION
7320 Greenville Avenue
Dallas, TX 75231
(214) 706-1220 or your local chapter

Lyme disease

LYME BORRELIOSIS FOUNDATION
P.O. Box 462
Tolland, CT 06084
(203) 871-2900

Mental health

NATIONAL ALLIANCE FOR THE
MENTALLY ILL
2101 Wilson Boulevard, Suite 302
Arlington, VA 22201
(703) 524-7600; (800) 950-6264

NATIONAL INSTITUTE OF MENTAL
HEALTH
Public Inquiries
5600 Fishers Lane, Room 15C-05
Rockville, MD 20857
(301) 443-4513

NATIONAL MENTAL HEALTH
ASSOCIATION
1021 Prince Street
Alexandria, VA 22314
(703) 684-7722; (800) 969-6642

Pregnancy

MARCH OF DIMES BIRTH DEFECTS
FOUNDATION
1275 Mamaroneck Avenue
White Plains, NY 10605
(914) 428-7100

Public health

AMERICAN PUBLIC HEALTH
ASSOCIATION
1015 15th Street NW
Washington, DC 20005
(202) 789-5600

AMERICAN RED CROSS
430 17th Street NW
Washington, DC 20006
(202) 737-8300 or your local chapter

CENTERS FOR DISEASE CONTROL
1600 Clifton Road NE, Mailstop A23
Atlanta, GA 30333
(404) 639-3286

Substance abuse

THE AMERICAN COUNCIL FOR
DRUG EDUCATION
204 Monroe Street, Suite 110
Rockville, MD 20850
(301) 294-0600; (800) 488-DRUG

NAR-ANON FAMILY GROUPS, INC.
P.O. Box 2562
Palos Verdes, CA 90274
(213) 547-5800

Suicide

AMERICAN ASSOCIATION OF
SUICIDOLOGY
2459 South Ash Street
Denver, CO 80222
(303) 692-0985

Violence and abuse

CHILDHELP USA
P.O. Box 630
Hollywood, CA 90028
(800) 422-4453

NATIONAL DOMESTIC VIOLENCE
HOTLINE
P.O. Box 463100
Mount Clemens, MI 48046
(800) 333-SAFE

PARENTS ANONYMOUS
520 S. Lafayette Park Place, Suite 316
Los Angeles, CA 90057
(800) 421-0353

Worksite health

WASHINGTON BUSINESS GROUP
ON HEALTH
777 N. Capitol Street NE, Suite 800
Washington, DC 20020
(202) 408-9320

WELLNESS COUNCILS OF
AMERICA
Historic Library Plaza
1823 Harney Street, Suite 201
Omaha, NE 68102
(402) 444-1711

Other self-help resources

You may wish to use these health-care
resources to find information about
conditions or disabilities not listed
above.

AMERICAN SELF-HELP
CLEARINGHOUSE
St. Clares-Riverside Medical Center
Pocono Road
Denville, NJ 07834
(201) 625-9565; (800) 367-6274

COMBINED HEALTH INFORMATION
DATABASE
National Institutes of Health
Box CHID
9000 Rockville Pike
Bethesda, MD 20892
(301) 468-6555

NATIONAL HEALTH INFORMATION
CENTER
P.O. Box 1133
Washington, DC 20013
(800) 336-4797; (301) 565-4167 in MD

NATIONAL SELF-HELP
CLEARINGHOUSE
(includes Women's Self-Help
Clearinghouse)
City University of New York Graduate
Center
33 West 42nd Street
New York, NY 10036
(212) 840-1259

Useful telephone numbers

911 or emergency number in your community

	Telephone	Name	Address	Hours
Doctor or health center				
Local hospital				
Hospital emergency department				
Poison control center				
Fire station				
Police station				
Pharmacist				
Mother's work				
Father's work				
Child-care center or babysitter				
Family friend or neighbor				

INDEX

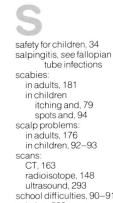